PRIMARY IMMUNODEFICIENCY DISEASES

RECENT TITLES PUBLISHED BY ALAN R. LISS, INC.
FOR MARCH OF DIMES BIRTH DEFECTS FOUNDATION

Birth Defects Compendium, Second Edition, Daniel Bergsma, *Editor*

BIRTH DEFECTS: ORIGINAL ARTICLE SERIES

1982 — Volume 18

- No. 1 **Craniofacial Anomalies: New Perspectives,** Carlos F. Salinas, *Editor*
- No. 3A **Annual Review of Birth Defects, 1981, Prenatal Diagnosis and Mechanisms of Teratogenesis,** William L. Nyhan and Kenneth Lyons Jones, *Editors*
- No. 3B **Annual Review of Birth Defects, 1981, Dysmorphology,** William L. Nyhan and Kenneth Lyons Jones, *Editors*
- No. 4 **Children With Sex Chromosome Aneuploidy: Follow-Up Studies,** Donald A. Stewart, *Editor*
- No. 5 **Cumulative Index: Birth Defects: Original Article Series Volumes I (1965)–XVI (1980),** Natalie W. Paul, *Editor*
- No. 6 **Genetic Eye Diseases: Retinitis Pigmentosa and Other Inherited Eye Disorders,** Edward Cotlier, Irene H. Maumenee, and Elaine R. Berman, *Editors*
- No. 7 **Thalassemia: Recent Advances in Detection and Treatment,** Antonio Cao, Ugo Carcassi, and Peter T. Rowley, *Editors*

1983 — Volume 19

- No. 1 **Dentition: Genetic Effects,** Ronald J. Jorgenson, *Editor*
- No. 3 **Primary Immunodeficiency Diseases,** Ralph J. Wedgwood, Fred S. Rosen, and Natalie W. Paul, *Editors*
- No. 4 **Nervous System Regeneration,** Bernard Haber, J. Regino Perez-Polo, George A. Hashim, and Anna Maria Giuffrida Stella, *Editors*
- No. 5 **Annual Review of Birth Defects, 1982, Birth Defects: Clinical and Ethical Considerations,** Sara C. Finley, Wayne H. Finley, and Charles E. Flowers, Jr., *Editors*

See pages following the index for previous titles in this series published by Alan R. Liss, Inc.

March of Dimes Birth Defects Foundation
Birth Defects: Original Article Series, Volume 19, Number 3, 1983

PRIMARY IMMUNODEFICIENCY DISEASES

International Workshop held September 12 – 15, 1982,
at Rosario Resort, Orcas Island, Washington, U.S.A.
Sponsored by the March of Dimes Birth Defects Foundation

Editors: **Ralph J. Wedgwood, MD**
University of Washington
Seattle, Washington

Fred S. Rosen, MD
Children's Hospital Medical Center
Boston, Massachusetts

Natalie W. Paul
March of Dimes Birth Defects Foundation
White Plains, New York

Assistant Editors: **Florence Dickman**
Elizabeth O'Brien Eakin
Sue Conde Greene
March of Dimes Birth Defects Foundation

ALAN R. LISS, INC., NEW YORK

To enhance medical communication in the birth defects field, the March of Dimes Birth Defects Foundation publishes the *Birth Defects Compendium (Second Edition)*, an *Original Article Series*, *Syndrome Identification*, a *Reprint Series*, and provides a series of films and related brochures.

Further information can be obtained from:

Professional Education Department
March of Dimes Birth Defects Foundation
1275 Mamaroneck Avenue
White Plains, New York 10605

Published by:
Alan R. Liss, Inc.
150 Fifth Avenue
New York, New York 10011

Copyright © 1983 by March of Dimes Birth Defects Foundation

All rights reserved. No part of this publication may be reproduced or transmitted in any form or by any means, electronic or mechanical, including photocopying and recording, or by any information storage and retrieval system, without permission in writing from the copyright holder.

Views expressed in articles published are the authors', and are not to be attributed to the March of Dimes Birth Defects Foundation or its editors unless expressly so stated.

Library of Congress Cataloging in Publication Data

Main entry under title:

Primary immunodeficiency diseases.

   (Birth defects original article series; v. 19, no. 3)
   Sponsored by March of Dimes Birth Defects Foundation.
   Includes index.
   1. Immunological deficiency syndromes—Congresses.
2. Immunological deficiency syndromes in children—Congresses. I. Wedgwood, Ralph J. II. Rosen, Fred S.
III. Paul, Natalie W. IV. March of Dimes Birth Defects
Foundation. V. Series. [DNLM: 1. Immunologic
deficiency syndromes—Congresses. WI BI966 v.19 no.3
WD 308 P952 1982]
RG626.B63 vol. 19, no. 3   616'.043s [616.9]   83-13563
[RC606]
ISBN 0-8451-1054-3

Printed in the United States of America.

The **March of Dimes Birth Defects Foundation** is dedicated to the goals of preventing birth defects and ameliorating their consequences for patients, families, and society.

As part of our efforts to achieve these goals, we sponsor, or participate in, a variety of scientific meetings where all questions relating to birth defects are freely discussed. Through our professional education program we speed the dissemination of information by publishing the proceedings of these and other meetings. From time to time, we also reprint pertinent journal articles to help achieve our goals. Now and then, in the course of these articles or discussions, individual viewpoints may be expressed which go beyond the purely scientific and into controversial matters. It should be noted, therefore, that personal viewpoints about such matters will not be censored but this does not constitute an endorsement of them by the **March of Dimes Birth Defects Foundation.**

Contents

Contributors xi
Introduction
   Ralph J. Wedgwood xv
List of Abbreviations xvii

SECTION 1: CLINICAL IMMUNOBIOLOGY

The Role of Macrophages in the Immune Process
Ralph van Furth 3

The Identification and Function of T Cells, T-Cell Subsets, and Their Factors
Raif S. Geha 9

Suppressor T-Cell Circuit in Man
Cobi J. Heijnen and Rudy E. Ballieux 15

A Formula to Assess Lymphocyte Responsiveness In Vitro
Clifford S. Hosking and Anne Balloch 21

B-Cell Differentiation
Max D. Cooper 25

The Regulation of the Human Humoral Immune Response and Functional Assays for Its Assessment
Thomas A. Waldmann 31

Human T-Cell Hybridomas Secreting Factors for B-Cell Differentiation and Proliferation
Shu Man Fu, Lloyd Mayer, and Henry G. Kunkel 37

Specific In Vitro Anti-Mannan Antibody Production by Human Blood Lymphocytes
Anne Durandy, Alain Fischer, and Claude Griscelli 41

Appearance of Antibody-Producing Cells in the Peripheral Blood in Response to Immunization With a Specific Antigen
Hans D. Ochs, John Bohnsack, Samuel R. Heller, and Ralph J. Wedgwood 47

The Regulatory Role of Human Neonatal Monocytes in the In Vitro Antigen-Specific Plaque-Forming Cell Response
M.J.D. van Tol, J. Zijlstra, B.J.M. Zegers, and R.E. Ballieux 51

Immune Regulation in the Hyper-IgE/Job Syndrome
Hans D. Ochs, Michael J. Kraemer, Catherine G. Lindgren, Clifton T. Furukawa, and Ralph J. Wedgwood 57

SECTION 2: SEVERE COMBINED IMMUNODEFICIENCIES (SCID)

Diagnosis and Classification of Severe Combined Immunodeficiency Disease
Erwin W. Gelfand and Hans-Michael Dosch 65

Genetic Deficiencies of Adenosine Deaminase and Purine Nucleoside Phosphorylase: Overview, Genetic Heterogeneity and Therapy
Rochelle Hirschhorn 73

The Bare Lymphocyte Syndrome: Immunodeficiency Resulting From the Lack of Expression of HLA Antigens
Jean-Louis Touraine and Hervé Bétuel 83

Combined Immunodeficiency With Defective Expression of HLA: Modulation of an Abnormal HLA Synthesis and Functional Studies
Barbara Lisowska-Grospierre, Anne Durandy, Jean-Louis Virelizier, Alain Fischer, and Claude Griscelli 87

Defective Expression of Mononuclear Cell Membrane HLA Antigens Associated With Combined Immunodeficiency: Impaired Cellular Interactions
B.J.M. Zegers, C.J. Heijnen, J.J. Roord, W. Kuis, R.K.B. Schuurman, J.W. Stoop, and R.E. Ballieux 93

GPL-115 Deficiency: A New Class of Immunodeficiencies
Robertson Parkman, Eileen Remold-O'Donnell, Dianne M. Kenney, and Fred S. Rosen 97

Severe Combined Immunodeficiency (SCID) With Natural Killer (NK) Cell Predominance
Rebecca H. Buckley, Sherrie Gard, Barton F. Haynes, Lawrence J. Sindel, Kathryn Davis, Hugh A. Sampson, Michael E. Ruff, and Hillel S. Koren 101

Selective Deficiency of OKT4+ Lymphocytes in a Child With Combined Immunodeficiency
Marzia Duse, Rita Maccario, Luigi Nespoli, Alessandro Plebani, and Alberto G. Ugazio 105

T-Cell Subsets and Natural Killer Cells in DiGeorge and SCID Patients
M.C. Sirianni, L. Businco, L. Fiore, R. Seminara, and F. Aiuti 107

Does an Interferonopathy Underlie a Severe Combined Immunodeficiency Disease (SCID) Syndrome?
James F. Jones, Linda M. Minnich, David O. Lucas, Marlyn P. Langford, and G. John Stanton 109

Impaired Production of Interleukins in Patients With Cellular Immunodeficiency (Abstract)
R.J. Levinsky, R. Paganelli, F. Aiuti, and P.C.L. Beverley 115

Dipyridamole and Intravenous Deoxycytidine Therapy in a Patient With Adenosine Deaminase Deficiency
Arthur J. Ammann, Morton J. Cowan, David W. Martin, and Diane W. Wara 117

Prenatal Diagnosis for Severe Combined Immunodeficiency
D.C. Linch, C.H. Rodeck, H.A. Simmonds, and R.J. Levinsky ... 121

Prenatal Diagnosis of Severe Combined Immunodeficiency and X-Linked Agammaglobulinemia
Anne Durandy and Claude Griscelli ... 125

Transplantation of Hematopoietic Cells for Lethal Congenital Immunodeficiencies
Richard J. O'Reilly, Neena Kapoor, Dahlia Kirkpatrick, Neal Flomenberg, Marilyn S. Pollack, Bo Dupont, Robert A. Good, and Yair Reisner ... 129

European Experience With Fetal Tissue Transplantation in Severe Combined Immunodeficiency (SCID)
Jean-Louis Touraine ... 139

Chimerism Following Fetal Liver Transplantation: Cell Cooperation Despite HLA Mismatch
Jean-Louis Touraine, Claude Griscelli, Hervé Bétuel, Anne Durandy, Bruno Bétend, and Gérard Souillet ... 143

Problems of Mismatched Bone Marrow Transplantation for Severe Combined Immunodeficiency After Soybean Lectin Fractionation
Roland J. Levinsky, E.G. Davies, M. Butler, A. Abai, D.C. Linch, and A.H. Goldstone ... 147

SECTION 3: DISORDERS AFFECTING B LYMPHOCYTES

Diagnosis Criteria and Classification of Human Primary Defects of Humoral Immunity
Maxime Seligmann and Jean-Jacques Ballet ... 153

A National Registry for Primary Immunodeficiency Syndromes in Italy: A Report for the Period 1972–1982
G. Luzi, L. Businco, and F. Aiuti ... 161

Failure of Isotype Progression in Hypogammaglobulinemia and During Normal B-Cell Ontogeny
R. Scott Pereira, Susan R. Wilkins, A. David Webster, Geoffrey L. Asherson, and Thomas A.E. Platts-Mills ... 165

Recurrent Infections in Children With "Selective" IgA Deficiency: Association With IgG2 and IgG4 Deficiency
Alberto G. Ugazio, Theo A. Out, Alessandro Plebani, Marzia Duse, Virginia Monafo, Luigi Nespoli, and G. Roberto Burgio ... 169

IgG$_2$ and IgG$_3$ Subclass Deficiencies in Selective IgA Deficiency in the United States
Charlotte Cunningham-Rundles, Vivi-Anne Oxelius, and Robert A. Good ... 173

Pre-B Cells in X-Linked Agammaglobulinemia
Jerrold Schwaber ... 177

Lymphoid Cell-Derived Lectin-Like Receptor Molecules as Immunoregulatory Signals in Immunodeficiency
R. Michael Blaese, Andrew V. Muchmore, and Giovanna Tosato ... 183

T Cells and T-Cell Subsets in a Large Population of Patients With Primary Immunodeficiency
Rebecca H. Buckley, Sherrie Gard, Richard I. Schiff, and Hugh A. Sampson ... 187

Treatment of Defects of Humoral Immunity
Martha Eibl ... 193

Use of Intravenous pH 4.0 Treated Gamma Globulin in Humoral Immunodeficiency Disease
Charlotte Cunningham-Rundles, Elizabeth M. Smithwick, Frederick P. Siegal, Noorbibi K. Day, Alise Lion, Joseph O'Malley, Silvio Barandun, and Robert A. Good ... 201

Intramuscular and Intravenous Administration of Immunoglobulin to Patients With Hypogammaglobulinemia
L.Å. Hanson, J. Björkander, and C. Wadsworth ... 205

Individualization of Gamma Globulin Dosage in Patients With Humoral Immunodeficiency
Richard I. Schiff, Christine Rudd, Ruby Johnson, and Rebecca H. Buckley ... 209

Subcutaneous Infusion of Gamma Globulins in the Management of Agammaglobulinemic Patients
Alberto G. Ugazio, Marzia Duse, Alessandro Plebani, Luigi D. Notarangelo, and G. Roberto Burgio ... 213

Treatment of Antibody Deficiency Syndromes With Subcutaneous Infusion of Gamma Globulin
John J. Roord, Jos W.M. van der Meer, Wietse Kuis, and Ralph van Furth ... 217

Epidemiology and Treatment of Hypogammaglobulinemia
C.S. Hosking and D.M. Roberton ... 223

Oral Administration of Secretory Immunoglobulin A and Its Clinical Significance
Shuzo Matsumoto, Tohru Watanabe, Shunzo Chiba, Wataru Abo, and Tooru Nakao ... 229

Dietary Protein Antigenemia in Hypogammaglobulinemia: Relationship to Splenomegaly
Charlotte Cunningham-Rundles, Ronald I. Carr, and Robert A. Good ... 239

SECTION 4: THE ROLE OF THE THYMUS

The Thymus in Immunodeficiency Diseases: New Therapeutic Approaches
Jean-François Bach ... 245

Demonstration of Abnormalities in Expression of Thymic Epithelial Surface Antigens in Severe Cellular Immunodeficiency Diseases
Barton F. Haynes, Robert W. Warren, Rebecca H. Buckley, John E. McClure, Allan L. Goldstein, Frederick W. Henderson, Lucinda L. Hensley, and George S. Eisenbarth ... 255

Thymus Transplantation
Richard Hong ... 259

Therapy With Thymopoietin Pentapeptide (TP-5) in 26 Patients With Primary Immunodeficiencies
Fernando Aiuti, Luisa Businco, M. Fiorilli, E. Galli, I. Quinti, S. Le Moli, R. Seminara, and G. Goldstein ... 267

Effect of Synthetic Thymic Hormone (TP5) in Children With T-Cell Immunodeficiencies
Roland J. Levinsky, E. Graham Davies, and Gideon Goldstein ... 273

Delayed Marrow Aplasia Following Treatment for Thymic Hypoplasia: Correction by Marrow Transplant Without Immunosuppression
Anthony R. Hayward, John Githens, Shirley Murphy, Bennie McWilliams, Peter Lane, and Daniel R. Ambruso 277

Immunologic Reconstitution With Bone Marrow Transplantation and Thymic Hormones in Two Patients With Severe Pure T-Cell Defect
Luisa Businco, P. Rossi, R. Paganelli, R. Seminara, and F. Aiuti 281

SECTION 5: OTHER STATES ASSOCIATED WITH PRIMARY IMMUNODEFICIENCY

The Human Fetus and Newborn: Development of the Immune Response
Anthony R. Hayward 289

Deficient DR Antigen Expression on Human Neonatal Monocytes: Reversal With Lymphokines
E. Richard Stiehm, Dean Mann, Carolyn Newland, Marcelo B. Sztein, Patricia S. Steeg, Joost J. Oppenheim, and R. Michael Blaese 295

T-Cell Cytotoxicity and Chemiluminescence Abnormalities in Newborns and Chronic Granulomatous Disease
Allen G. Peerless and E. Richard Stiehm 299

Protean Appearances of Immunodeficiencies: Syndromes and Inborn Errors Involving Other Systems Which Express Associated Primary Immunodeficiency
Walter H. Hitzig 307

Hereditary Orotic Aciduria: A Defect of Pyrimidine Metabolism With Cellular Immunodeficiency
Robert Girot, Anne Durandy, Jean-Louis Perignon, and Claude Griscelli 313

Heterogeneity of Immunologic and Enzymatic Deficiencies in the Familial Reticuloendotheliosis Syndrome
Alain Fischer, Françoise Ledeist, Anne Durandy, Michèle Hamet, Frank Arnaud-Battandier, and Claude Griscelli 317

X-Linked Lymphoproliferative Syndrome: Abnormal Antibody Responses to Bacteriophage ϕX 174
Hans D. Ochs, John L. Sullivan, Ralph J. Wedgwood, Janet K. Seeley, Kiyoshi Sakamoto, and David T. Purtilo 321

Down Syndrome: A Model of Immunodeficiency
G. Roberto Burgio, Alberto Ugazio, Luigi Nespoli, and Rita Maccario 325

Hypogammaglobulinemia and Malakoplakia—Effect of Bethanechol
John F. Soothill, B.A.M. Harvey, M. Webb, W.C. Marshall, L. Spitz, and J.R. Pincott 329

Basophil and Eosinophil Deficiency in a Patient With Hypogammaglobulinemia Associated With Thymoma
E. Bruce Mitchell, Thomas A.E. Platts-Mills, R. Scott Pereira, Vera Malkovska, and A. David Webster 331

Bone Marrow Transplantation in a Patient With Chédiak-Higashi Syndrome
Claude Griscelli and Jean-Louis Virelizier 333

Humoral Immune Deficiency and Recurrent Otitis Media
C.S. Hosking, M.J. Shelton, J. Ward, and D.M. Roberton 335

Immunization Reactions and Immunodeficiency
John F. Soothill and J.A. Dudgeon 339

SECTION 6: SUMMARY

Primary Immunodeficiency Diseases 345

Index 361

Contributors

A. Abai, BSc, Institute of Child Health, London WC1N 1EH, England **[147]**

Wataru Abo, MD, Department of Pediatrics, Sapporo Medical College, Sapporo, Japan **[229]**

Fernando Aiuti, MD, Department of Clinical Immunology, Institute of Internal Medicine III, University of Rome, 00185 Rome, Italy **[107,115,161,267,281]**

Daniel R. Ambruso, MD, Department of Pediatrics, University of Colorado School of Medicine, Denver, CO 80262 **[277]**

Arthur J. Ammann, MD, Departments of Pediatrics, Biochemistry and Medicine, University of California, San Francisco, San Francisco, CA 94143 **[117]**

Frank Arnaud-Battandier, MD, Unité de Gastro-Enterologie et Nutrition, Département de Pédiatrie, Hôpital Necker-Enfants Malades, 75730 Paris Cedex 15, France **[317]**

Geoffrey L. Asherson, FRCP, FRCPath, Division of Immunological Medicine, Clinical Research Centre, Harrow HA1 3UJ, England **[165]**

Jean-François Bach, MD, Hôpital Necker, 75015 Paris Cedex 15, France **[245]**

Jean-Jacques Ballet, MD, Laboratory of Immunochemistry and Immunopathology, Research Institute on Blood Diseases of University Paris VII, and Laboratory of Oncology and Immunohematology of CNRS, Hôpital Saint-Louis, 75475 Paris Cedex 10, France **[153]**

Rudy E. Ballieux, PhD, Department of Clinical Immunology, University Hospital, 3500 CG Utrecht, The Netherlands **[15,51,93]**

Anne Balloch, Department of Immunology, Royal Children's Hospital, Parkville, Victoria 3052, Australia **[21]**

Silvio Barandun, MD, University of Berne, Berne, Switzerland **[201]**

Bruno Bétend, MD, Service de Pédiatrie, Hôpital Edouard Herriot, 69374 Lyon Cedex 2, France **[143]**

Hervé Bétuel, MD, Centre de Transfusion Sanguine, Transplantation and Immunobiology Unit, Hôpital Edouard Herriot, 69374 Lyon Cedex 2, France **[83,143]**

P.C.L. Beverley, BSc, MB, BS, University College Hospital, London WC1, England **[115]**

J. Björkander, MD, Division of Allergy, Department of Medicine I, University of Göteborg, Göteborg, Sweden **[205]**

R. Michael Blaese, MD, Cellular Immunology Section, National Cancer Institute, National Institutes of Health, Bethesda, MD 20205 **[183,295]**

John Bohnsack, MD, Department of Pediatrics, University of Washington, Seattle, WA 98195 **[47]**

Rebecca H. Buckley, MD, Departments of Pediatrics, Microbiology and Immunology, Duke University Medical Center, Durham, NC 27710 **[101,187,209,255]**

G. Roberto Burgio, MD, Department of Pediatrics, University of Pavia, 27100 Pavia, Italy **[169,213,325]**

Luisa Businco, MD, Institute of Pediatrics, University of Rome, 00185 Rome, Italy **[107,161,267,281]**

M. Butler, FIMLS, Institute of Child Health, London WC1N 1EH, England **[147]**

Ronald I. Carr, MD, PhD, National Jewish Hospital, Denver, CO 80206 **[239]**

Shunzo Chiba, MD, Department of Pediatrics, Sapporo Medical College, Sapporo, Japan **[229]**

Max D. Cooper, MD, Departments of Pediatrics and Microbiology, and The Comprehensive Cancer Center, University of Alabama in Birmingham, Birmingham, AL 35294 **[25]**

Morton J. Cowan, MD, Departments of Pediatrics, Biochemistry and Medicine, University of California, San Francisco, San Francisco, CA 94143 **[117]**

Charlotte Cunningham-Rundles, MD, PhD, Memorial Sloan-Kettering Cancer Institute, New York, NY 10021 **[173,201,239]**

E. Graham Davies, MRCP, Department of Immunology, Institute of Child Health, University of London, London WC1N 1EH, England **[147,273]**

Kathryn Davis, BS, Department of Pediatrics, Duke University School of Medicine, Durham, NC 27710 **[101]**

Noorbibi K. Day, PhD, Oklahoma Medical Research Foundation, Oklahoma City, OK 73104 **[201]**

Hans-Michael Dosch, MD, Division of Immunology, The Hospital for Sick Children, Toronto, Ontario, Canada M5G 1X8 **[65]**

J.A. Dudgeon, MD, Department of Microbiology, The Hospital for Sick Children, London WC1, England **[339]**

Bo Dupont, MD, Memorial Sloan-Kettering Cancer Institute, New York, NY 10021 **[129]**

Anne Durandy, MD, Unité d'Immunologie et d'Hématologie Pédiatriques, Département de Pédiatrie, Hôpital des Enfants Malades, 75730 Paris Cedex 15, France **[41,87,125,143,313,317]**

Marzia Duse, MD, Clinica Pediatrica, Università di Pavia, Policlinico S. Matteo, 27100 Pavia, Italy **[105,169,213]**

Martha Eibl, MD, Institute of Immunology, University of Vienna, Vienna, Austria **[193]**

George S. Eisenbarth, MD, PhD, Joslin Diabetes Center, Research Department, Boston, MA 02215 **[255]**

L. Fiore, MD, Institute of Pediatrics, University of Rome, 00185 Rome, Italy **[107]**

M. Fiorilli, MD, Department of Clinical Immunology, University of Rome, 00185 Rome, Italy **[267]**

The boldface number in brackets indicates the opening page number of that contributor's article.

Alain Fischer, MD, Unité d'Immunologie et d'Hématologie Pédiatriques, Département de Pédiatrie, Hôpital des Enfants Malades, 75730 Paris Cedex 15, France [41,87,317]

Neal Flomenberg, MD, Memorial Sloan-Kettering Cancer Institute, New York, NY 10021 [129]

Shu Man Fu, MD, PhD, Oklahoma Medical Research Foundation, Oklahoma City, OK 73104 [37]

Clifton T. Furukawa, MD, Department of Pediatrics, University of Washington, Seattle, WA 98195 [57]

E. Galli, MD, Department of Pediatrics I, University of Rome, 00185 Rome, Italy [267]

Sherrie Gard, BS, Department of Pediatrics, Duke University Medical Center, Durham, NC 27710 [101,187]

Raif S. Geha, MD, Division of Allergy and Immunology, Children's Hospital Medical Center, Department of Pediatrics, Harvard Medical School, Boston, MA 02115 [9]

Erwin W. Gelfand, MD, FRCP(C), Division of Immunology, The Hospital for Sick Children, Toronto, Ontario, Canada M5G 1X8 [65]

Robert Girot, MD, Laboratoire Central d'Hématologie et d'Immunologie Necker, Paris, France [313]

John Githens, MD, Department of Pediatrics, University of Colorado School of Medicine, Denver, CO 80262 [277]

Allan L. Goldstein, PhD, Department of Biochemistry, George Washington University, Washington, DC 20037 [255]

Gideon Goldstein, MD, Ortho Pharmaceutical Corp., Raritan, NJ 08869 [267,273]

A.H. Goldstone, MRCP, University College Hospital, London, England [147]

Robert A. Good, MD, PhD, Oklahoma Medical Research Foundation, Oklahoma City, OK 73104 [129,173,201,239]

Claude Griscelli, MD, Unité d'Immunologie et d'Hématologie Pédiatriques, Département de Pédiatrie, Hôpital des Enfants Malades, 75730 Paris Cedex 15, France [41,87,125,143,313,317,333]

Michèle Hamet, PhD, Unité d'Immunologie et d'Hématologie Pédiatriques, Département de Pédiatrie, Hôpital Necker-Enfants Malades, 75730 Paris Cedex 15, France [317]

L.Å. Hanson, MD, Department of Clinical Immunology, Institute of Medical Microbiology, University of Göteborg, Göteborg, Sweden [205]

B.A.M. Harvey, FIMLT, Department of Immunology, Institute of Child Health, London WC1N 1EH, England [329]

Barton F. Haynes, MD, Department of Medicine, Duke University School of Medicine, Durham, NC 27710 [101,255]

Anthony R. Hayward, MD, PhD, MRCP, Department of Pediatrics, University of Colorado School of Medicine, Denver, CO 80262 [277,289]

Cobi J. Heijnen, PhD, Department of Immunology, University Children's Hospital, "Het Wilhelmina Kinderziekenhuis," 3512 LK Utrecht, The Netherlands [15,93]

Samuel R. Heller, MS, Department of Pediatrics, University of Washington, Seattle, WA 98195 [47]

Frederick W. Henderson, MD, Pediatric Infectious Diseases, North Carolina Memorial Hospital, Chapel Hill, NC 27514 [255]

Lucinda L. Hensley, MT, 5011 Timmons Dr., Durham, NC 27713 [255]

Rochelle Hirschhorn, MD, Department of Medicine, New York University School of Medicine, New York, NY 10016 [73]

Walter H. Hitzig, MD, Department of Pediatrics, University of Zurich, 8032 Zurich, Switzerland [307]

Richard Hong, MD, Departments of Pediatrics and Medical Microbiology, University of Wisconsin Center for Health Sciences, Madison, WI 53792 [259]

Clifford S. Hosking, MD, FRACP, FRCPA, Department of Immunology, Royal Children's Hospital, Parkville, Victoria 3052, Australia [21,223,335]

Ruby Johnson, Department of Pediatrics, Duke University School of Medicine, Durham, NC 27710 [209]

James F. Jones, MD, Department of Pediatrics, University of Arizona School of Medicine, Tucson, AZ 85724 [109]

Neena Kapoor, MD, Oklahoma Medical Research Foundation, Oklahoma City, OK 73104 [129]

Dianne M. Kenney, PhD, Center for Blood Research, Boston, MA 02115 [97]

Dahlia Kirkpatrick, MD, Memorial Sloan-Kettering Cancer Institute, New York, NY 10021 [129]

Hillel S. Koren, PhD, Department of Microbiology and Immunology, Duke University School of Medicine, Durham, NC 27710 [101]

Michael J. Kraemer, MD, Department of Pediatrics, University of Washington, Seattle, WA 98195 [57]

Wietse Kuis, MD, Department of Immunology, University Children's Hospital, "Het Wilhelmina Kinderziekenhuis," 3512 LK Utrecht, The Netherlands [93,217]

Henry G. Kunkel, MD, Rockefeller University, New York, NY 10021 [37]

Peter Lane, MD, Department of Pediatrics, University of Colorado School of Medicine, Denver, CO 80262 [277]

Marlyn P. Langford, PhD, Department of Microbiology, University of Texas Medical Branch, Galveston, TX 77550 [109]

Françoise Ledeist, MD, Unité d'Immunologie et d'Hématologie Pédiatriques, Département de Pédiatrie, Hôpital Necker-Enfants Malades, 75730 Paris Cedex 15, France [317]

S. Le Moli, PhD, Department of Clinical Immunology, University of Rome, 00185 Rome, Italy [267]

Roland J. Levinsky, MD, FRCP, Department of Immunology, Institute of Child Health, University of London, London WC1N 1EH, England [115,121,147,273]

D.C. Linch, MRCP, Department of Hematology, University College Hospital, London WC1, England [121,147]

Catherine G. Lindgren, BS, Department of Pediatrics, University of Washington, Seattle, WA 98195 [57]

Alise Lion, RN, Memorial Sloan-Kettering Cancer Institute, New York, NY 10021 [201]

Barbara Lisowska-Grospierre, MD, Unité d'Immunologie et d'Hématologie Pédiatriques, Département de Pédiatrie, Hôpital des Enfants Malades, 75730 Paris Cedex 15, France [87]

David O. Lucas, PhD, Department of Molecular and Medical Microbiology, University of Arizona School of Medicine, Tucson, AZ 85724 [109]

G. Luzi, MD, Department of Clinical Immunology, University of Rome, 00185 Rome, Italy [161]

Rita Maccario, PhD, Department of Pediatrics, University of Pavia, 27100 Pavia, Italy [105,325]

Vera Malkovska, Division of Pathology, Clinical Research Centre, Harrow HA1 3UJ, England [331]

Dean Mann, MD, National Cancer Institute and the Uniformed Services University for the Health Sciences, Bethesda, MD 20205 [295]

W.C. Marshall, MD, Hospital for Sick Children, London WC1, England [329]

David W. Martin, MD, Departments of Pediatrics, Biochemistry and Medicine, University of California, San Francisco, San Francisco, CA 94143 [117]

Shuzo Matsumoto, MD, Department of Pediatrics, Hokkaido University School of Medicine, Sapporo, Japan [229]

Lloyd Mayer, MD, Rockefeller University, New York, NY 10021 [37]

John E. McClure, PhD, Department of Biochemistry, George Washington University, Washington, DC 20037 [255]

Bennie McWilliams, MD, Department of Pediatrics, University of New Mexico School of Medicine, Albuquerque, NM 87131 [277]

Linda M. Minnich, MS, Department of Pathology, University of Arizona School of Medicine, Tucson, AZ 85724 [109]

E. Bruce Mitchell, MD, FRCP(C), Division of Immunological Medicine, Clinical Research Centre, Harrow HA1 3UJ, England [331]

Virginia Monafo, MD, Department of Pediatrics, University of Pavia, 27100 Pavia, Italy [169]

Andrew V. Muchmore, MD, Cellular Immunology Section, Metabolism Branch, National Institutes of Health, Bethesda, MD 20205 [183]

Shirley Murphy, MD, Department of Pediatrics, University of New Mexico School of Medicine, Albuquerque, NM 87131 [277]

Tooru Nakao, MD, Department of Pediatrics, Sapporo Medical College, Sapporo, Japan [229]

Luigi Nespoli, MD, Department of Pediatrics, University of Pavia, 27100 Pavia, Italy [105,169,325]

Carolyn Newland, PhD, Uniformed Services University for the Health Sciences, Bethesda, MD 20205 [295]

Luigi D. Notarangelo, MD, Department of Pediatrics, University of Pavia, 27100 Pavia, Italy [213]

Hans D. Ochs, MD, Department of Pediatrics, University of Washington, Seattle, WA 98195 [47,57,321]

Joseph O'Malley, MD, The American Red Cross, Washington, DC [201]

Joost J. Oppenheim, MD, National Institute of Dental Research, National Institutes of Health, Bethesda, MD 20205 [295]

Richard J. O'Reilly, MD, Memorial Sloan-Kettering Cancer Institute, New York, NY 10021 [129]

Theo A. Out, PhD, Central Laboratory of the Netherlands Red Cross Blood Transfusion Service, and Laboratory for Experimental and Clinical Immunology, University of Amsterdam, Amsterdam, The Netherlands [169]

Vivi-Anne Oxelius, MD, PhD, Institute of Medical Microbiology, University of Lund, Lund, Sweden [173]

R. Paganelli, MD, Department of Clinical Immunology, University of Rome, 00185 Rome, Italy [115,281]

Robertson Parkman, MD, Divisions of Immunology and Hematology-Oncology, Children's Hospital Medical Center, and Division of Pediatric Oncology, Sidney Farber Cancer Institute, Boston, MA 02115 [97]

Allen G. Peerless, MD, Department of Pediatrics and the Center for Interdisciplinary Research in Immunologic Diseases, UCLA School of Medicine, Los Angeles, CA 90024 [299]

R. Scott Pereira, MRCPath, Division of Rheumatology, Clinical Research Centre, Harrow HA1 3UJ, England [165,331]

Jean-Louis Perignon, MD, Laboratoire de Biochemie, Faculté de Médecine Necker, Paris, France [313]

J.R. Pincott, MRCPath, Department of Histopathology, Hospital for Sick Children, London WC1, England [329]

Thomas A.E. Platts-Mills, FRCP, Division of Allergy and Clinical Immunology, Department of Medicine, University of Virginia, Charlottesville, VA 22908 [165,331]

Alessandro Plebani, PhD, Department of Pediatrics, University of Pavia, 27100 Pavia, Italy [105,169,213]

Marilyn S. Pollack, PhD, Memorial Sloan-Kettering Cancer Institute, New York, NY 10021 [129]

David T. Purtilo, MD, Department of Pathology and Laboratory Medicine, University of Nebraska Medical Center, Omaha, NE 68105 [321]

I. Quinti, MD, Department of Clinical Immunology, University of Rome, 00185 Rome, Italy [267]

Yair Reisner, PhD, Weizmann Institute of Science, Rehovot, Israel [129]

Eileen Remold-O'Donnell, PhD, Center for Blood Research, Boston, MA 02115 [97]

D.M. Roberton, MD, FRACP, Department of Immunology, Royal Children's Hospital, Parkville, Victoria 3052, Australia [223,335]

C.H. Rodeck, MRCOG, Department of Obstetrics, Kings College Hospital, London SE5, England [121]

John J. Roord, MD, Department of Immunology, University Children's Hospital, "Het Wilhelmina Kinderziekenhuis," 3512 LK Utrecht, The Netherlands [93,217]

Fred S. Rosen, MD, Division of Immunology, Children's Hospital Medical Center, Boston, MA 02115 [97]

P. Rossi, MD, Department of Clinical Immunology, University of Rome, 00185 Rome, Italy [281]

Christine Rudd, DPhar, Department of Pharmacy, Duke University, Durham, NC 27710 [209]

Michael E. Ruff, MD, Department of Pediatrics, Duke University School of Medicine, Durham, NC 27710 [101]

Kiyoshi Sakamoto, MD, Department of Pathology and Laboratory Medicine, University of Nebraska Medical Center, Omaha, NE 68105 [321]

Hugh A. Sampson, MD, Department of Pediatrics, Duke University School of Medicine, Durham, NC 27710 [101,187]

Richard I. Schiff, MD, PhD, Department of Pediatrics, Duke University School of Medicine, Durham, NC 27710 [187,209]

R.K.B. Schuurman, MD, Department of Immunology, University Children's Hospital, "Het Wilhelmina Kinderziekenhuis," 3512 Utrecht, The Netherlands [93]

Jerrold Schwaber, PhD, Children's Hospital Medical Center, Harvard Medical School, Boston, MA 02115 [177]

Janet K. Seeley, PhD, Department of Pediatrics, Health Center, The University of Connecticut, Farmington, CT 06032 [321]

Maxime Seligmann, MD, Laboratory of Immunochemistry and Immunopathology, Research Institute on Blood Diseases of University Paris VII, and Laboratory of Oncology and Immunohematology of CNRS, Hôpital Saint-Louis, 75475 Paris Cedex 10, France [153]

R. Seminara, MD, Department of Clinical Immunology, Institute of Internal Medicine III, University of Rome, 00185 Rome, Italy [107,267,281]

M.J. Shelton, MSc, Department of Immunology, Royal Children's Hospital, Parkville, Victoria 3052, Australia [335]

Frederick P. Siegal, MD, Mt. Sinai Hospital, New York, NY 10029 [201]

H.A. Simmonds, PhD, Guy's Hospital, London SW1 1EH, England **[121]**

Lawrence J. Sindel, MD, Department of Pediatrics, Duke University School of Medicine, Durham, NC 27710 **[101]**

M. C. Sirianni, MD, Department of Clinical Immunology, Institute of Internal Medicine III, 00185 Rome, Italy **[107]**

Elizabeth M. Smithwick, MD, Memorial Sloan-Kettering Cancer Institute, New York, NY 10021 **[201]**

John F. Soothill, FRCP, Department of Immunology, Institute of Child Health, London WC1N 1EH, England **[329,339]**

Gérard Souillet, MD, Service de Pédiatrie, Hôpital de Brousse, 69005 Lyon Cedex 2, France **[143]**

L. Spitz, FRCS, Department of Surgery, Institute of Child Health, London WC1N 1EH, England **[329]**

G. John Stanton, PhD, Department of Microbiology, University of Texas Medical Branch, Galveston, TX 77550 **[109]**

Patricia S. Steeg, PhD, National Institute of Dental Research, National Institutes of Health, Bethesda, MD 20205 **[295]**

E. Richard Stiehm, MD, Department of Pediatrics and the Center for Interdisciplinary Research in Immunologic Diseases, UCLA School of Medicine, Los Angeles, CA 90024 **[295,299]**

J.W. Stoop, MD, Department of Immunology, University Children's Hospital, "Het Wilhelmina Kinderziekenhuis," 3512 LK Utrecht, The Netherlands **[93]**

John L. Sullivan, MD, University of Massachusetts Medical Center, Worcester, MA 01605 **[321]**

Marcelo B. Sztein, MD, National Institute of Dental Research, National Institutes of Health, Bethesda, MD 20205 **[295]**

Giovanna Tosato, MD, Cellular Immunology Section, Metabolism Branch, National Institutes of Health, Bethesda, MD 20205 **[183]**

Jean-Louis Touraine, MD, Transplantation and Immunobiology Unit, Hôpital Edouard Herriot, 69374 Lyon Cedex 2, France **[83,139,143]**

Alberto G. Ugazio, MD, Department of Pediatrics, University of Pavia, 27100 Pavia, Italy **[105,169,213,325]**

Jos W.M. van der Meer, MD, Department of Infectious Diseases, University Hospital, Leiden, The Netherlands **[217]**

Ralph van Furth, MD, PhD, Department of Infectious Diseases, University Hospital, Leiden, The Netherlands **[3,217]**

M.J.D. van Tol, PhD, Department of Immunology, University Children's Hospital, "Het Wilhelmina Kinderziekenhuis," 3512 LK Utrecht, The Netherlands **[51]**

Jean-Louis Virelizier, MD, Unité d'Immunologie et d'Hématologie Pédiatriques, Département de Pédiatrie, Hôpital des Enfants Malades, 75730 Paris Cedex 15, France **[87,333]**

C. Wadsworth, PhD, Department of Clinical Immunology, Institute of Medical Microbiology, University of Göteborg, Göteborg, Sweden **[205]**

Thomas A. Waldmann, MD, Metabolism Branch, NCI, National Institutes of Health, Bethesda, MD 20205 **[31]**

Diane W. Wara, MD, Departments of Pediatrics, Biochemistry and Medicine, University of California, San Francisco, San Francisco, CA 94143 **[117]**

J. Ward, MD, Department of Immunology, Royal Children's Hospital, Parkville, Victoria 3052, Australia **[335]**

Robert W. Warren, MD, PhD, Duke University Medical Center, Durham, NC 27710 **[255]**

Tohru Watanabe, MD, Department of Pediatrics, Hokkaido University School of Medicine, Sapporo, Japan **[229]**

M. Webb, MB, Hospital for Sick Children, London WC1, England **[329]**

A. David Webster, FRCP, Division of Immunological Medicine, Clinical Research Centre, Harrow HA1 3UJ, England **[165,331]**

Ralph J. Wedgwood, MD, Department of Pediatrics, School of Medicine, University of Washington, Seattle, WA 98195 **[xv,47,57,321]**

Susan R. Wilkins, BSc, Division of Immunological Medicine, Clinical Research Centre, Harrow HA1 3UJ, England **[165]**

B.J.M. Zegers, PhD, Department of Immunology, University Children's Hospital, "Het Wilhelmina Kinderziekenhuis," 3512 LK Utrecht, The Netherlands **[51,93]**

J. Zijlstra, Department of Immunology, University Children's Hospital, "Het Wilhelmina Kinderziekenhuis," 3512 LK Utrecht, The Netherlands **[51]**

Introduction

It is now 30 years since Bruton described his famous patient with agammaglobulinemia and initiated the study of patients with primary defects of immunity—the primary immunodeficiency syndromes. The finding, coming on the wave of biomedical research after World War II, carried with it enormous impetus. The observation and the tools to study the observation were fortunately juxtaposed; plasma cells had been identified as the source of antibodies and immunoglobulins; the structure and function of immunoglobulins were emerging; the distinction between cellular and humoral immunity had been demonstrated; the term "experiments of nature" as an exemplar for clinical research was in common currency. Publications on lymphocytes entered into a logarithmic growth phase.

In 1967, the First International Workshop—supported by the then National Foundation, now the March of Dimes Birth Defects Foundation—was held on Sanibel Island, Florida, bringing together many of the investigators involved in the rapidly growing field. The results of the workshop delineated clearly, from clinical and experimental study, the two-component concept of immunity [1]. Stimulated in part by concerns of the World Health Organization and its Expert Committee on Immunodeficiency, a Second International Workshop, again under the sponsorship of the March of Dimes, was held in St. Petersburg, Florida in 1973. At this meeting the sophistication of the field became apparent; T- and B-cell markers and the ontogeny of these cell lines led to emphasis on classification and differentiation defects [2]. By 1980, the types of cells involved in the immune responses and the importance of immunoregulation resulted in a Third International Workshop – this time aptly termed a Symposium – held at the Abbey de Royaumont near Paris [3]. And now, a short two years later, the rapid advances in immunobiology bring together a group who have worked in the field since the onset with the new generation of clinical immunologists and immunobiologists. All have in common the view that these fascinating patients hold answers to basic biologic questions – and conversely, that through these patients recent findings from the bench can be given new relevance.

Is then the term "experiments of nature" as valid in 1982 as it was in 1952? The concept is much older than that. William Harvey [4], in the last year of his life (1657), wrote:

"Nature is nowhere accustomed more openly to display her secret mysteries than in cases where she shows tracings of her workings apart from the beaten paths; nor is there any better way to advance the proper practice of medicine than to give our minds to the discovery of the usual law of nature, by careful investigation of cases of rarer forms of disease."

Ten generations later – as I believe this workshop will again show – the concept continues as the hallmark for excellence in biomedical research.

ACKNOWLEDGMENTS

We appreciate the assistance of the National Institute of Allergy and Infectious Disease at NIH and of the World Health Organization who, in addition to the March of Dimes Birth Defects Foundation, assisted in defraying the costs of the meeting. Thanks are also due to Joan Palmer, Anne Junker, and Brian Hamilton for their extraordinary help in setting up and running the meeting, and to Joan Palmer and Anne Junker for their labors in the preparation of the final summary.

REFERENCES

1. Bergsma D, Good RA, Finstad J, Miescher PA, Smith RT, Nusser JL, (eds): "Immunologic Deficiency Diseases in Man." The National Foundation – March of Dimes: Birth Defects Original Article Series, Vol IV, No. 1, 1968.
2. Bergsma D, Good RA, Finstad J, Paul NW, (eds): "Immunodeficiency in Man and Animals," Vol. XI, No. 1. Birth Defects: Original Article Series. Sunderland, Mass.: Sinauer Associates, Inc, 1975.
3. Seligmann M, Hitzig WH (eds): "Primary Immunodeficiencies." New York: Elsevier/North-Holland Biomedical Press, 1980.
4. I wish that I could claim to have found this reference in the original – and that I had the time and wit to trace the origin of the phrase through the labyrinth of time like R.K. Merton in his splendid book, "On the Shoulders of Giants" (Harcourt Brace and World, Inc, 1965). I cannot. I found the quotation quite by accident in Maurice B. Strauss' "Familiar Medical Quotations" (Little Brown and Company, 1968). The book has a number of other, equally good quotations – which I have resisted.

Ralph J. Wedgwood

List of Abbreviations

AC–adherent cell(s)
ACC–antibody containing cell(s)
ADA–adenosine deaminase
ADCC–antibody-dependent cell-mediated cytotoxicity
ADNIg–antibody deficiency and normal immunoglobulin
AET–aminoethylisothiouronium
ALG–antilymphocyte globulin
ALL–acute lymphatic leukemia
ALS–antilymphocyte serum
ANA–antinuclear antibody
AT–ataxia telangiectasia
ATCS–antihuman T-cell serum
ATP–adenosine 5′-triphosphate

BCG–bacillus Calmette-Guérin
BFUe–erythroid burst forming activity unit
BGG–bovine gamma globulin
BMT–bone marrow transplant(ation)(s)
BSA–bovine serum albumin
bw–body weight
$\beta_2 m$–β_2 microglobulin

CBMC–cord blood mononuclear cell(s)
CDF–cytotoxic differentiation factor
CFU_{GM}–granulocyte/monocyte colony forming units
CGD–chronic granulomatous disease
CHD(S)–Chédiak-Higashi disease (syndrome)
CID–combined immunodeficiency
CMCC–chronic mucocutaneous candidiasis
CMCM–chronic mucocutaneous moniliasis
CMI–cell-mediated immunity
CML–cell-mediated lymphocytolysis
Con A–concanavalin A
CRM–cross-reacting material
CTL–cytolytic T-cell line
CVH–common variable hypogammaglobulinemia
CVID–common variable immunodeficiency

DHR–delayed hypersensitivity reaction
DiG–DiGeorge syndrome

EBV–Epstein-Barr virus
ELISA–enzyme-linked immunoassay
E-RFC–erythrocyte rosette-forming cell

FACS–fluorescent activated cell sorter
FCS–fetal calf serum
FLT–fetal liver transplant(ation)
FTT–fetal thymus transplant(ation)

GALT–gut-associated lymphoid system
GVH(D)–graft-vs-host (disease)

HLA–human lymphocyte antigens
HSG–human standard globulin
HypE–hyper IgE syndrome
HypM–hyper IgM

ID–immunodeficiency
IFN–interferon
Ig–immunoglobulin
IL–interleukin

KLH–keyhole limpet hemocyanin

LGL–large granular lymphocyte(s)

MBLA–mouse specific B-lymphocyte antigen
MHC–major histocompatibility complex
MLC–mixed lymphocyte/leukocyte culture
MLR–mixed leukocyte reaction
MNC–mononuclear cell(s)

NEZ–Nezelof syndrome
NK–natural killer
NP–nucleoside phosphorylase

OA–ovalbumin
ODC–orotidine 5′-phosphate decarboxylase
OPRT–orotate phosphoribosyltransferase

PBL–peripheral blood lymphocyte(s)
PBMC–peripheral blood mononuclear cell(s)
PEG/HES–polyethylene glycol/hydroxy ethyl starch
PFC–plaque-forming cell
PGE-2–prostaglandin E2
PHA–phytohemagglutinin
PMA–phorbol myristate acetate
PMN–polymorphonuclear neutrophil leukocytes
PMNL–polymorphonuclear leukocytes
PNA–peanut agglutinin
PNP–purine nucleoside phosphorylase
PPD–purified protein derivative
PRPP–5′-phosphoribosyl 1-pyrophosphate
PWM–pokeweed mitogen

RFC–rosette-forming cells

SBA–soybean agglutinin
SCID–severe combined immunodeficiency
SE–sheep erythrocytes
SI–stimulation index
SIg–surface membrane immunoglobulins
SLA–X-linked agammaglobulinemia
SRBC–sheep red blood cells

TF–transfer factor
Th–T helper
TH–thymic hormone
ThF–T helper factor
Ts–T suppressor
TT–tetanus toxoid

URI–upper respiratory infection

WAS–Wiskott-Aldrich syndrome

SECTION 1
CLINICAL IMMUNOBIOLOGY

The Role of Macrophages in the Immune Process

Ralph van Furth, MD, PhD

Department of Infectious Diseases, University Hospital, Leiden, The Netherlands

In vivo, the immune response to microbial antigens is not elicited by the microorganisms themselves but by antigen molecules liberated after degradation of the microorganisms. Macrophages play an important role in the initiation of the immune processes, because these cells cannot only ingest and kill, but also can degrade ingested microorganisms. Then, antigen molecules or fragments are available to stimulate lymphocytes either directly, when present at the surface of the macrophages, or indirectly, when transferred to other antigen-presenting cells.

The sequence of events occurring between the contamination of a subject with microorganisms and a humoral or cell-mediated immune response includes several phases (Table 1). Phases 4 and 5 are important for limitation of the infection; phases 6 and 7 are concerned with the specific immune responses; and phase 8 provides persistent immunity.

This report will cover the origin and kinetics of macrophages, the humoral regulation of monocytopoiesis during inflammation, some aspects of the intracellular killing of microorganisms by monocytes and macrophages, and the role of macrophages in antigen presentation.

ORIGIN AND KINETICS OF MONOCYTES AND MACROPHAGES

Mononuclear phagocytes form a cell line that starts with a pluripotent stem cell in the bone marrow. The most immature cell of this line is the monoblast (Fig. 1). In the mouse, the duration of the cell cycle of the monoblast is about 12 hr, and by division one cell gives rise to 2 promonocytes. The promonocyte divides only once (cell-cycle time about 16 hr) and gives rise to 2 monocytes. Monocytes leave the bone marrow randomly within 24 hr after they are formed; these cells remain in the circulation for a relatively long time (half-time about 17 hr) compared with granulocytes (half-time about 7 hr), and leave this compartment randomly [1].

The bone-marrow origin of the macrophages in the various tissues and serous cavities has been proven by a large number of chimera studies [2]. In addition, in vitro and in vivo labeling studies with the DNA precursor, ^{3}H-thymidine, showed a labeling index of $< 5\%$ for macro-

TABLE 1.

Phase 1:	Contamination of body surface with (pathogenic) microorganisms
Phase 2:	Penetration of the body via skin or mucous membranes by microorganisms
Phase 3:	Multiplication of microorganisms in tissues or circulation
Phase 4:	Inflammatory response in the tissue
	a. Exudation of plasma proteins: Igs and complement components
	b. Accumulation of leukocytes: granulocytes, monocytes, and lymphocytes
Phase 5:	Interaction between microorganisms and humoral and cellular defense mechanisms
	a. Killing of microorganisms by humoral microbicidal factors (antibodies and complement)
	b. Complement activation
	c. Opsonization of microorganisms by antibodies and/or complement
	d. Phagocytosis and intracellular killing of microorganisms by granulocytes and (exudate) macrophages
	e. Digestion of killed microorganisms by macrophages
	f. Transport of antigens to cell surface of macrophages
Phase 6:	Antigen presentation by macrophages or dendritic cells and specific immune responses
	a. Proliferation of, and antibody production by, B lymphocytes
	b. Proliferation of T-helper and T-suppressor lymphocytes and secretion of soluble products
	c. Proliferation (sensitization) of T lymphocytes involved in CMI
	d. Production of humoral factors by macrophages Lymphocyte-activating factor (ie interleukin-1), prostaglandins (PGE), interferon, endogenous pyrogen and other factors
Phase 7:	CMI response
	a. Antigen presentation to sensitized T lymphocytes
	b. Production of lymphokines (γ-interferon and other molecules) by sensitized T lymphocytes
	c. Activation of macrophages
	d. Increased phagocytosis, intracellular killing, and digestion by macrophages
Phase 8:	Persistence of antigen in macrophages
	a. Continuation B-lymphocyte response and antibody formation (humoral immunity)
	b. Continuation T-lymphocyte response and macrophage activation (CMI)

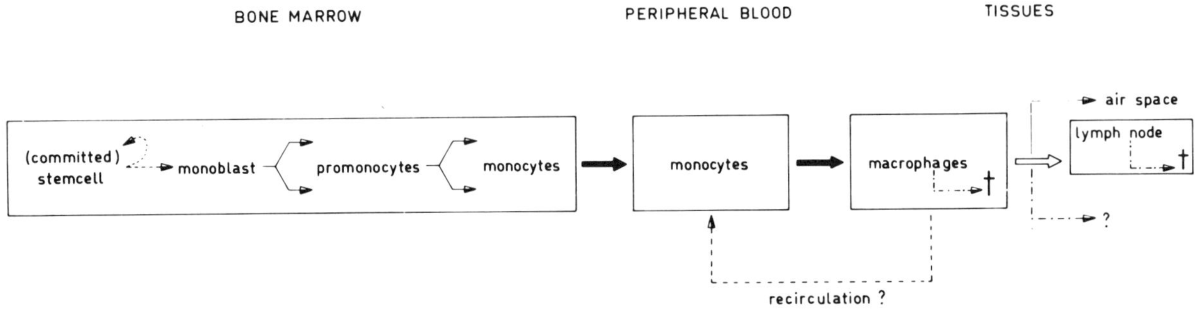

Fig. 1. Schematic representation of the origin, kinetics, and fate of the mononuclear phagocytes. Monocytes originate in the bone marrow from dividing precursor cells. Then they enter the peripheral blood, where they circulate until they leave the circulation to become macrophages in the tissues. The fate of these macrophages in the tissues is uncertain: they may die in the tissues, migrate via the lymphatics to local lymph nodes and die there, and/or migrate to other sites, eg the airspace in the lungs, other tissues, or the peripheral blood.

phages at various sites. Furthermore, it became clear that the mononuclear phagocytes in the tissues that label in vitro or are labeled in vivo, 1-2 hr after an IV injection of ^{3}H-thymidine, do not belong to the resident population of macrophages, but have recently (< 24–48 hr before harvesting) arrived in the tissues from the bone marrow. Kinetic studies with monocytes of normal and monocytopenic mice labeled in vivo and of mice irradiated with partial bone-marrow shielding proved that the monocytes migrate from the blood into the tissues, where they become macrophages [1,2].

A mathematical analysis of the kinetics of macrophages in a tissue compartment which takes into account the influx of monocytes, the local division of mononuclear phagocytes in the tissues, and the efflux of macrophages from the tissue compartment, showed that 75% of the pulmonary macrophage population is maintained by monocyte influx, and about 25% by local division of immature mononuclear phagocytes originating from the bone marrow. The calculated mean turnover time of pulmonary macrophages is then about 6 days, which is much shorter than the turnover time previously reported [3,4]. Similar calculations made for the Kupffer cells show that 90% of population of Kupffer cells is maintained by monocyte influx, and only 10% by a single local division of the mononuclear phagocytes in the liver. The calculated mean turnover time of Kupffer cells then amounts to about 4 days [5].

Quantitative studies further reveal that, of the monocytes leaving the circulation, about 56% become Kupffer cells [6], about 15% become pulmonary macrophages [3], and about 8% become peritoneal macrophages [7]; the remaining 21% will migrate to other tissues, such as the spleen and the GI tract.

In the normal, steady state the constant influx of monocytes into tissues, where they become macrophages, implies a constant efflux of cells from the tissue compartment and/or a constant cell death in the tissues. Nothing is known about this point, but various studies have shown that macrophages from the liver, lung, gut, and skin arrive in the local lymph nodes (Fig. 1). The absence of monocytes and macrophages in efferent lymph originating from lymph nodes suggests that the macrophages that remain in the nodes die there, but this would not hold for the lung macrophages, which can also leave the body via air spaces (Fig. 1). Firm information about recirculation of macrophages via the peripheral blood is lacking, but if such recirculation occurred at all, it would probably be on a very small scale.

HUMORAL REGULATION OF MONOCYTE PRODUCTION DURING INFLAMMATION

When a rather large number of macrophages are required at the site of inflammation, a regulatory mechanism acting at the level of the dividing mononuclear phagocytes in the bone marrow is needed to stimulate the formation of more monocytes.

Recent investigations have shown that plasma and sera sampled during the onset of an inflammatory reaction contain a factor that stimulated monocytopoiesis [8-11]. This factor, called factor-increasing monocytopoiesis (FIM), is synthesized and secreted by macrophages at the site of inflammation [12] and then transported via the circulation to the bone marrow, where it exerts its stimulatory action on monoblasts and promonocytes.

This factor has been fairly well characterized in mice and rabbits [9,13]. FIM is a small protein with a molecular weight of about 20 K dalton, has no carbohydrate moieties essential for its function, is cell-line specific (ie no effect on the formation of granulocytes and lymphocytes), is not species specific (ie rabbit FIM is active in mice and vice versa), is not related to complement or clotting factors, and has no chemotactic activity toward macrophages. Since FIM does not stimulate the formation of bone-marrow colonies in vitro, it is not identical with colony-stimulating factor.

Indications were obtained that in the second phase of an inflammatory response the increased monocyte production is reduced by a serum factor that inhibits monocytopoiesis. This factor, called monocyte-production inhibitor (MPI), is known to have a molecular weight of approximately 50 K dalton, but the site of its production has not yet been established [10].

It has been demonstrated that, in genetically well-defined mice, the resistance to an infection with Listeria monocytogenes is genetically controlled [14]. Listeria-susceptible (Lr^s) CBA mice show no increase in the number of monocytes during infection and only a small increase of the number of peritoneal macrophages after an inflammatory stimulus, whereas Listeria-resistant (Lr^r) C57B1/10 mice respond in the opposite way to the same challenges. It has been shown that the sera of both Lr^r and Lr^s mice contain FIM after an intraperitoneal injection of a saline extract of Listeria monocytogenes; the extract itself has no FIM activity. In both sera the peak levels of FIM were almost the same, but the course of FIM activity was not exactly synchronous. Further studies showed, however, that Lr^s mice did not respond to sera containing FIM by increased monocytopoiesis, whereas Lr^r mice responded even to highly diluted serum containing FIM [15]. These findings indicate that one of the mechanisms underlying the natural resistance to Listeria infection is not enhanced FIM synthesis, but rather the genetically controlled ability of monocyte precursors in the bone marrow to respond to FIM by increased monocyte production [15].

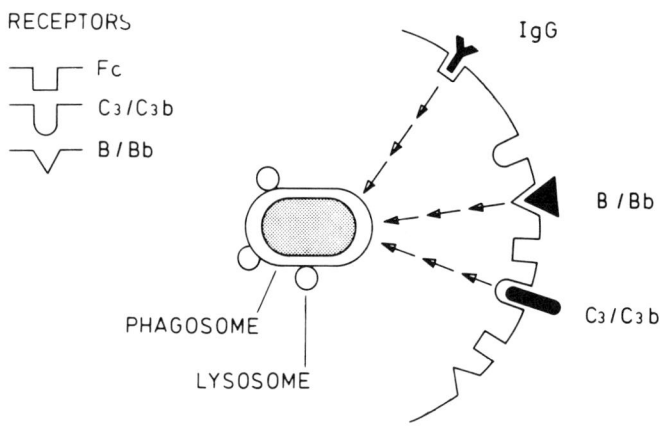

Fig. 2. Schematic representation of the stimulation of the intracellular killing by extracellular stimuli (IgG, C3/C3b, and B/Bb) via an interaction with their respective membrane receptors.

PHAGOCYTOSIS, INTRACELLULAR KILLING, AND DIGESTION OF MICROORGANISMS

When an infection occurs, the number of phagocytic cells already present in the tissue is not sufficiently high enough to permit elimination of all of the invading microorganisms. In such a situation, phagocytic cells migrate from the circulation to the site of infection. This process is governed not only by serum factors (eg complement component C5a [16]), but also by chemotactic stimuli derived from the microorganisms themselves [16], and has 2 phases: a) the site of infection is reached by granulocytes, and b) the number of exudate macrophages increase [16]. In addition, plasma proteins pass through the vascular wall and form the inflammatory exudate. This exudate contains Igs and complement components, the latter of which can be activated by the microorganisms present at the site of infection.

After the exudation of plasma proteins and migration of cells to the site of infection, opsonization of microorganisms is brought about by IgG antibodies, IgG antibodies plus complement (C3b), IgM antibodies plus complement (C3b), or complement (C3b) alone.

It has been demonstrated recently that, for optimal ingestion of particles, the latter must be entirely covered by equally distributed opsonins, because then specific receptors (ie Fcγ receptor and C3b receptors) can interact with the opsonins when the pseudopods of the cell surround the particles. This phenomenon of opsonin-receptor interaction has been called the zippering phenomenon [17].

Optimal intracellular killing also required interaction between plasma proteins (IgG, C3/C3b, and B/Bb) and membrane receptors [18-20], as illustrated in Figure 2. On this basis, it is conceivable that suboptimal intracellular killing may be the result of inadequate stimulation of the membrane of the phagocytes, or defective transmission of the membrane stimulation to the inside of the cell. It is not yet known exactly what mechanism is triggered by membrane stimulation, but proof that such stimulation is obligatory has been obtained by using nonphysiologic stimuli, namely, plant lectins, which interact with specific sugars in the cell membrane. These lectin-receptor interactions lead to the same stimulation of intracellular killing as the serum proteins induce [21].

After microorganisms are killed intracellularly, they are digested by

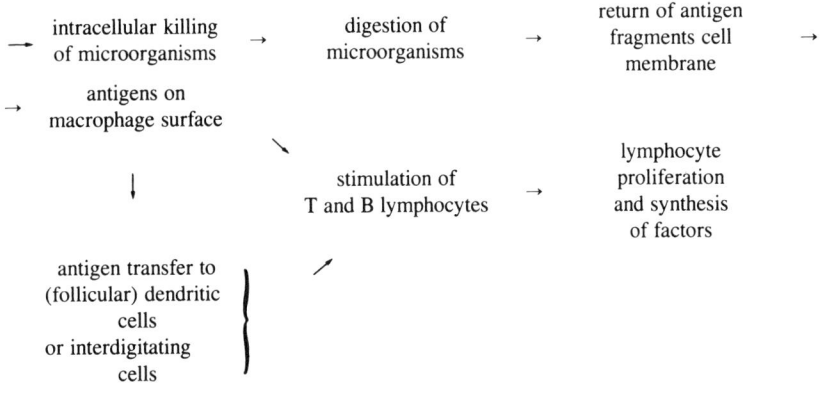

Fig. 3. Outline of the role of macrophages in the induction of an immune response by microorganisms. This scheme indicates that antigen fragments or molecules must first be released from microorganisms before they can serve as immunogen at the surface of macrophages, or after transfer, at the surface of (follicular) dendritic cells or interdigitating cells. Red blood cells, tumor cells, and antigen-antibody complexes may follow a similar pathway before they can induce an immune response.

lysosomal enzymes which come into contact with the microorganisms after phagosome-lysosome fusion. Granulocytes, which have a short life-span, disintegrate after they digest the microorganisms and have no function in antigen presentation, whereas macrophages, which live longer in the tissues, degrade microorganisms into small fragments. These fragments of microorganisms may be immunogens and induce an immune response, but to do so they must migrate from the phagolysosome to the surface of the macrophages (Fig. 3).

MACROPHAGES AND THE IMMUNE RESPONSE

There is still no consensus as to which cell presents antigens to lymphocytes. It is generally accepted that the antigen-presenting cell must also bear Ia antigens at the cell surface, and Ia antigens occur in macrophages, dendritic cells, Langerhans cells, and interdigitating cells [22–24]. In any case it is an obligatory condition that most of the biologically relevant antigens, eg particulate antigens, such as foreign red cells, bacteria, viruses, and protozoa, be killed and degraded to smaller fragments before they can induce a humoral or cellular immune reaction (Fig. 3). Since microorganisms are mainly killed and degraded intracellularly, the antigen fragments must reach the surface of the phagocytic cell before they become available for lymphocyte recognition. The mechanism involved here is not yet well understood. According to some investigators, it is the macrophages themselves that present antigens to the lymphocytes to induce antibody formation and cell-mediated immunity (CMI) [25–29], whereas others have put forward evidence that it is performed by dendritic cells localized in the follicles of spleen and lymph nodes [30, 31] (Fig. 3). However, the latter contention raises the question as to how, in vivo, antigen molecules or fragments are transferred from macrophages to dendritic cells and interdigitating cells (Fig. 3). Whatever the case may be, it is clear that, by antigen presentation, B lymphocytes and/or T lymphocytes are stimulated to proliferate and to secrete biologically active products, that result in a humoral or cellular immune response. The roles of, and interactions between, T-helper and T-suppressor lymphocytes and the events leading to generation of cytotoxic T lymphocytes and T lymphocytes involved in CMI (ie delayed-type hypersensitivity) will not be discussed here. It is of interest that the products formed during an adequate humoral immune response (ie antibodies by B lymphocytes and plasma cells) and a cell-mediated reaction (ie lymphokines by T (helper) lymphocytes,) promote a more efficient ingestion, intracellular killing, and digestion of foreign materials (eg microorganisms).

REFERENCES

1. Furth van R: Mononuclear phagocytes in inflammation. In Vane JR, Ferreira SH (eds): "Handbook of Experimental Pharmacology. Inflammation." Berlin, Heidelberg, New York: Springer-Verlag, 1978, vol 50/I, pp 68–108.
2. Furth van R, Meer van der JWM, Blussé van Oud Alblas A, Sluiter W: Development of mononuclear phagocytes. In Mizuno D, Cohn ZA, Takeya K, Ishida N (eds): "Self-defense Mechanisms. Role of Macrophages." Amsterdam, New York: University of Tokyo Press/Elsevier Biomedical Press, 1982, pp 25–41.
3. Blussé van Oud Alblas A, Furth van R: Origin, kinetics and characteristics of pulmonary macrophages in the normal steady state. J Exp Med 149:1504–1518, 1979.
4. Blussé van Oud Alblas A, Mattie H, Furth van R: A quantitative evaluation of pulmonary macrophage kinetics. Cell Tissue Kinet (In press).
5. Furth van R, Blussé van Oud Alblas A: New aspects on the origin of Kupffer cells. In Knook DL, Wisse E (eds): "Sinusoidal Liver Cells." Amsterdam: Elsevier Biomedical Press, 1982, pp 173–184.
6. Crofton RW, Diesselhoff-den Dulk MMC, Furth van R: The origin, kinetics and characteristics of the Kupffer cells in the normal steady state. J Exp Med 148:1–7, 1978.
7. Furth van R, Diesselhoff-den Dulk MMC, Mattie H: Quantitative study on the production and kinetics of mononuclear phagocytes during an acute inflammatory reaction. J Exp Med 138:1314–1330, 1973.

8. Waarde van D, Hulsing-Hesselink E, Sandkuyl LA, Furth van R: Humoral regulation of monocytopoiesis during the early phase of an inflammatory reaction caused by particulate substances. Blood 50:141-154, 1977.
9. Waarde van D, Hulsing-Hesselink E, Furth van R: Properties of a factor increasing monocytopoiesis (FIM) occurring in the serum during the early phase of an inflammatory reaction. Blood 50:727-724, 1977.
10. Waarde van D, Hulsing-Hesselink E, Furth van R: Humoral control of monocytopoiesis by an activator and an inhibitor. Agents Action 8:432-437, 1978.
11. Sluiter W, Waarde van D, Furth van R: Regulation of monocyte precursor cell proliferation by two endogenous factors. Immunobiology 161:219-226, 1982.
12. Sluiter W, Hulsing-Hesselink E, Furth van R: Synthesis and release of factor increasing monocytopoiesis (FIM) by macrophages. In Rossi F, Patriarca P (eds): "Biochemistry and Function of Phagocytes. Advances in Experimental Medicine and Biology." New York, London: Plenum Presss, 1982, pp 225-231.
13. Sluiter W, Elzenga-Claasen I, Hulsing-Hesselink E, Furth van R: Presence of the factor increasing monocytopoiesis (FIM) in rabbit peripheral blood during an acute inflammation. Submitted for publication.
14. Skamene E, Kongshaven PAL, Sachs DH: Resistance to Listeria monocytogenes in mice: Genetic control by genes that are not linked to the H-2 complex. J Infect Dis 139:228-231, 1979.
15. Sluiter W, Elzenga-Claasen I, Voort van de Kley van der van Andel, Furth van R: Genetic control of humoral regulation of monocyte production during inflammation. Submitted for publication.
16. Wilkinson PC: The adhesion, locomotion, and chemotaxis of leucocytes. Supra #1, pp 109-137.
17. Silverstein SC, Loike JD: Phagocytosis. In van Furth R (ed): "Mononuclear Phagocytes. Functional Aspects." The Hague, Boston, London: Martinus Nijhoff Publishers, 1980, pp 895-917.
18. Leijh PCJ, Barselaar van den MTh, Zwet TL, Daha MR, Furth van R: Requirement of extracellular complement and immunoglobulin for intracellular killing of microorganisms by human monocytes. J Clin Invest 63:772-784, 1979.
19. Leijh PCJ, Zwet TL, Furth van R: Effect of extracellular serum in the stimulation of intracellular killing of streptococci by human monocytes. Infect Immun 30:421-426, 1980.
20. Leijh PCJ, Barselaar MT, Daha MR, Furth van R: Participation of immunoglobulins and complement components in the intracellular killing of Staphylococcus aureus and Escherichia coli by human granulocytes. Infect Immun 33:714-724, 1981.
21. Leijh PCJ, Zwet van TL, Furth van R: Effect of some plant lectins on the intracellular killing of microorganisms. Submitted for publication.
22. Unanue ER: Symbiotic relationships between macrophages and lymphocytes. In Normann SJ, Sorkin E (eds): "Macrophages and Natural Killer Cells. Regulation and Function. Advances in Experimental Medicine and Biology." New York, London: Plenum Press, 1982, vol 155, pp 49-63.
23. Tew JG, Thorbecke GJ, Steinman RM: Dendritic cells in the immune response: Characteristics and recommended nomenclature (a report from the Reticuloendothelial Society Committee on Nomenclature). J Reticuloendothel Soc 31:371-380, 1982.
24. Dijkstra CD: Characterization of non-lymphoid cells in rat spleen, with special reference to strongly Ia-positive branched cells in T-cell areas. J Reticuloendothel Soc 32:167-178, 1982.
25. Unanue ER, Farr AG, Kiely J-M: Multiple interactions between Listeria-immune T lymphocytes and macrophages: Regulation by the major histocompatibility gene complex. Supra #17, pp 1837-1852.
26. Erb P, Feldmann M, Gisler R, Meier B, Stern A, Vogt P: Role of macrophages in the in vitro induction and regulation of antibody responses. Ibid, pp 1857-1883.
27. Rosenwasser LJ, Werdelin O, Braendstrup O, Rosenthal AS: Physical and functional macrophage-lymphocyte interactions in antigen recognition by T lymphocytes. Ibid, pp 1887-1904.
28. Unanue ER: Cooperation between mononuclear phagocytes and lymphocytes in immunity. N Engl J Med 303:977-985, 1980.
29. Rosenthal AS: Regulation of the immune response. Role of the macrophage. N Engl J Med 303:1153-1156, 1980.
30. Steinman RM, Chen LL, Witmer MD, Kaplan G, Nussenzweig MC, Adams JC, Cohn ZA: Dendritic cells and macrophages. Current knowledge of their distinctive properties and functions. Ibid, pp 1781-1799.
31. Steinman RM, Nussenzweig MC, Witmer MD, Nogueira N, Cohn ZA: A comparison of dendritic cells and macrophages. In Forster O, Landy M (eds): "Heterogeneity of Mononuclear Phagocytes." London, New York, Toronto, Sydney, San Francisco: Academic Press, 1981, pp 189-194.

The Identification and Function of T Cells, T-Cell Subsets, and Their Factors*

Raif S. Geha, MD

Division of Allergy and Immunology, Children's Hospital Medical Center, and the Department of Pediatrics, Harvard Medical School, Boston, MA 02115

The past few years have witnessed a greater understanding of the function of human T cells, of the surface antigenic markers expressed by these cells, and of the correlation between discrete surface markers and function. These new tools for studying T cells have been applied to the study of human immunodeficiency diseases. On one hand, this has resulted in a better understanding of these diseases. On the other hand, the study of these experiments of nature has permitted a better delineation of the importance and the in vivo relevance of various aspects of T-cell function. The present review will attempt to present some of the current concepts of human T-cell biology and illustrate them with the study of selected immunodeficiency diseases.

DEVELOPMENT OF T CELLS

As early as the 8th week of gestation, lymphoid tissue cells start migrating through the epithelial thymus where they undergo a process of differentiation to emerge as mature T cells. From studies of normal thymuses and from the study of patients with severe combined immunodeficiency (SCID) it appears that pre-T cells express the antigenic marker identified by the monoclonal antibody OKT10. In this regard, whereas normal bone marrow contains 5-10% OKT10+ cells, bone marrow from SCID with an epithelial thymus was found to contain as much as 40% OK10+ cells. During their passage through the thymus, T cells acquire a number of differentiation markers [1]. Some of these markers, such as the T6 antigen which is present on 80% of thymocytes, are lost prior to the emergence of the T cells from the thymus, whereas others, such as the T3, T4, and T8 antigens, remain expressed by the mature T cells that emerge into the periphery. A scheme for the development of T-cell markers intrathymically is shown in Figure 1.

A second important event which occurs during the maturation of T cells in the thymus is the education of T cells in the recognition of self. This is the process by which T cells are enabled to recognize foreign antigen in association with self determinants, which are products of the major histocompatibility complex. This will be discussed in detail later.

T-CELL FUNCTION: ITS PLACE IN THE IMMUNE RESPONSE

The scheme in Figure 2 illustrates the function of T cells in the immune response. These are divided into regulatory functions and effector functions.

Regulatory T cells can be helper (Th) cells or suppressor (Ts) cells. Th cells express the T4 antigenic marker and recognize antigen in association with HLA-DR or HLA-DR-linked (DC-1,DS,MB,MT,SB) determinants on the surface of macrophages and dendritic cells [2]. This results in Th-cell proliferation and in the exertion of helper effects (either directly or via soluble mediators) on a number of potential targets. These targets include B cells, cytotoxic effector T cells, macrophages, natural killer (NK) cells, as well as cells which do not belong to the immune system, ie erythrocyte precursors, mast cells, etc. The second category of regulatory T cells consists of Ts cells which express the T8 antigenic marker and appear to recognize antigen either directly or in association with I-J or I-J-like determinants. Little is known about specific suppressor cells in man. However, polyclonal suppressor cells have been described after stimulation of T cells with Concanavalin A (Con A) [3], and, in some instances, after stimulation with macrophages coated with anti-Ia antibodies [4]. In the tetanus toxoid (TT) system, antigen-specific suppressor cells appear to be idiotype positive and can be activated by anti-idiotypic antibodies [5].

Effector T cells include cytotoxic T cells. These T cells are under the regulation of Th and Ts cells and are important for the lysis of virally infected targets, cells bearing neoantigen, and allogeneic cells (HLA-A and B antigens). Like Ts cells they bear the T8 surface antigen. However, there is a minor subpopulation of cytotoxic cells which bears the T4 antigen and recognizes HLA-DR antigens [6].

ANTIGENIC MOIETIES RECOGNIZED BY T CELLS AND T-CELL RECEPTORS

As alluded to in the section above, the antigenic moieties recognized by

---

*Supported by USPHS grant AI-05877 and the March of Dimes Birth Defects Foundation. RSG is the recipient of an Allergic Diseases Academic Award K07-AI0440-01.

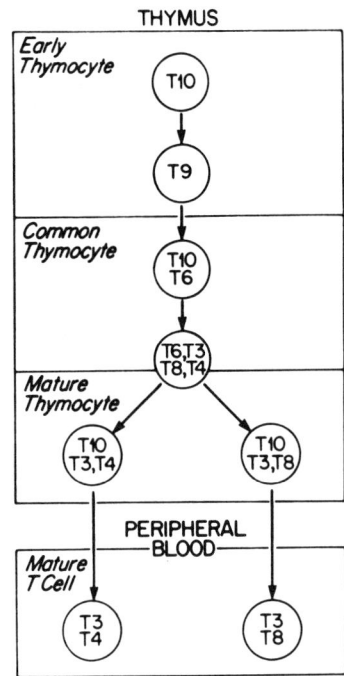

Fig. 1. Acquisition of T-cell surface antigenic markers during maturation.

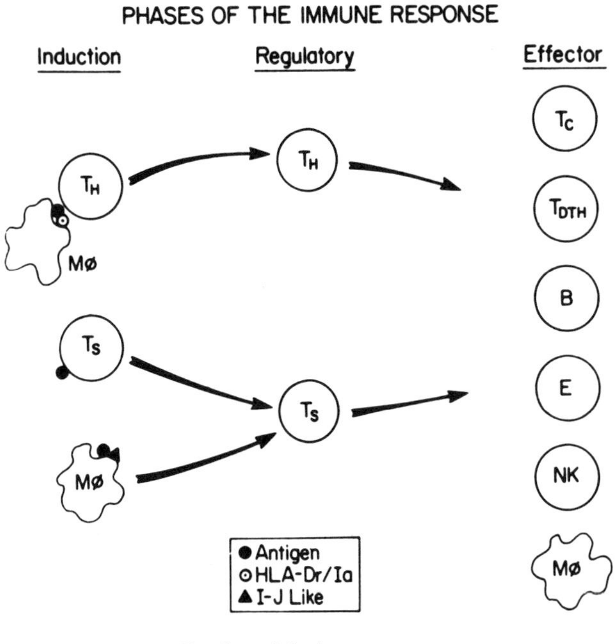

Fig. 2. T cells and the immune response.

TABLE 1. Effect of Antisera on Mo-Dependent T-Cell Proliferation to Tetanus Toxoid (TT)

Antiserum	cpm of ^{3}H-Thymidine Incorporated per Culture
—	46,211
Anti-TT	43,417
Anti-p 29, 34	6,358
Anti-B$_2$ microglobulin	39,420

Cultures contained 1×10^5 nylon wool purified T cells and 2×10^4 autologous Mo which have been pulsed for 18 hours with TT antigen (10 μg/ml). Cultures containing T cells and unpulsed Mo incorporated 1,000 cpm and were not affected by any of the antisera. Immunosorbent purified rabbit anti-TT was used at 10 μg/ml. Turkey antihuman p 29, 34 and turkey human B$_2$ microglobulin were used.

T cells differ with the function of the T cell. The following rules apply.

a) Th cells recognize antigen in association with Ia-like HLA-DR or HLA-DR-linked determinants. The antigenic determinants recognized by Th cells differ from those recognized by serum antibodies to the antigen.

The failure of immunosorbent purified antibody to T4 to inhibit T-cell proliferation in response to TT-pulsed autologous monocytes (Mo) is illustrated in Table 1. In contrast, turkey antihuman p 29,34, but not turkey antihuman B$_2$ microglobulin, inhibits T-cell recognition of antigen (Table 1). Interestingly, a urea-denatured preparation of TT, which has been depleted of antigenic determinants recognized by antibody to TT, elicits a very good response by the T cells [7]. This latter result indicates that the determinants recognized by the T cells are different from those recognized by the B cells. These determinants may be the result of the recognition of antigen processed by Mo, or may be the result of the recognition of determinants expressed on portions of the native molecule that do not elicit an antibody response. The data of Unanue and Ziegler [8] that chloroquine and NH$_4$Cl, which interfere with macrophage lysosomal activity, interfere with antigen recognition, are in favor of the former explanation. However, there is no clearcut evidence for Mo processing versus differences between B-and T-cell immunodominant epitopes.

b) Cytotoxic T T8+ cells recognize antigen in association with HLA-A/B determinants. The antigenic determinants recognized are similar to those recognized by serum antibodies.

A subpopulation of allocytotoxic T4+ cells has been described recently, and recognize HLA-DR (Ia-like) determinants [6].

c) The antigenic moiety recognized by human suppressor cells is not well defined. It may include soluble antigen with or without association with an I-J-like determinant, as in the case in some experimental animal systems and in the human system described by Ballieux (this volume).

The structure of the human T-cell receptor for antigen is not known. However, recent data in experimental animals suggest that the receptor consists of 2 chains. One chain has mol wt (MW) of ~70,000 and contains a V_H segment attached to a T-cell constant Igh-linked gene segment. A second chain is ~25,000 in MW and contains an I region encoded segment: I-J for suppressor cells, I-A for helper cells. To account for the dual recognition of self plus antigen, one model proposes a receptor for antigen with its own particular V_H segment coupled to a receptor for self with its own particular V_H segment, whereas another model proposes 2 separate receptors, one for self, Ia, and one for antigen.

MECHANISMS OF ANTIGEN RECOGNITION BY Th CELLS: MEDIATORS INVOLVED

Th-cell proliferation and mediator production in response to antigen is strictly monocyte/macrophage (Mo) dependent. This also holds true for the mitogens pokeweed and Concanavalin A (Con A). Figure 3 shows that Mo-depleted human T cells do not proliferate to TT antigen. This Mo-T cell interaction works mostly via soluble mediators. T cells recognizing antigen or mitogen induce Mo to secrete interleukin 1 (IL-1 15,000 in MW) which then interacts with an IL-1 receptor on T cells to induce initial proliferation and interleukin-2 (IL-2 18,000 MW) production. IL-2 will then interact with IL-2 receptors on T-cell blasts to cause further proliferation. The importance of these interactions to in vivo situations was recently illustrated by a case of immunodeficiency which presented with absent in vivo and in vitro responses to antigens and markedly decreased response to mitogens. Peripheral blood lymphocytes (PBL) from this child failed to produce IL-2 after PHA stimulation despite their normal capacity to make IL-1. Addition of IL-2 normalized the PHA response which was at 50% of normal at day 3 and at 2% of normal at day 6. Interestingly, the failure to make IL-2 after PHA stimulation could be bypassed by the addition of phorbol mycystic acetate (PMA) which mimics IL-1 activity but works at a different site on the T-cell membrane. Absorption studies suggested that this child had defective IL-1 receptors on his T cells. This resulted in deficiency to make IL-2 and in absent responses to antigen in vivo and in vitro.

MECHANISMS OF ANTIGEN RECOGNITION BY Th CELLS: ALLELIC EXCLUSION AT THE LEVEL OF THE RECEPTOR RECOGNIZING SELF PLUS ANTIGEN

Since Th cells recognize antigen in association with HLA-DR (or DR-linked) determinants, allelic exclusion would be expected at the level of the T-cell receptor for HLA-DR plus antigen recognition. This is shown in Table 2. In this experiment T-cell clones specific for TT antigens were tested for reactivity in the presence of autologous Mo, paternal Mo, and maternal Mo. Three types of clones were detected—one which responds to antigen in the presence of autologous Mo or paternal Mo, one which responds in the presence of autologous Mo or maternal Mo, and one which responds to autologous Mo only. The first 2 types of clones illustrate allelic exclusion, whereas the third type of clone probably represents a response to a hybrid association of maternal and paternal HLA-DR (or DR-linked) chains.

The learning of self-recognition is thought to occur in the thymus when T cells come in contact with HLA antigens of the thymic epithelium. However, it is possible that learning self-recognition might occur when T cells come in contact with bone marrow-derived elements which reside in the thymus, such as macrophages,

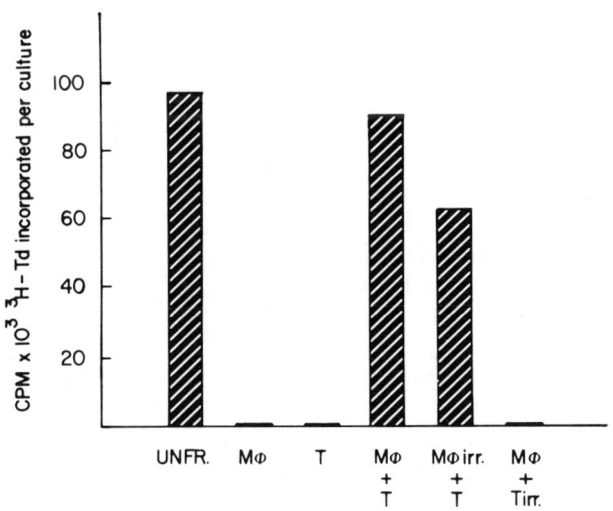

Fig. 3. Mo dependence of the T-cell proliferative response to TT antigen.

TABLE 2. Proliferation of Clones to TT

Clone	#	Source of Presenting Mo			
		F1	Paternal	Maternal	Allogeneic
MB7	300	11,000	18,000	400	400
MB10	200	3,000	150	3,700	220
MB21	230	4,000	370	280	210

Numbers show cpm of ^{3}H-thymidine incorporated by 2×10^4 cloned T cells in the presence of TT and 2×10^4 Mo.

TABLE 3. Presentation of Antigen by EBV-B Cells

TT-specific T cells	Stimulus	cpm of ^{3}H-Thymidine Incorporated per Culture Antigen presenting cells		
		—	Mo$_{irr}$	EBV-B$_{irr}$
T-cell line Bo	—	383 ± 72	517 ± 92	1,203 ± 132
	TT	434 ± 21	13,240 ± 518	15,660 ± 941
	DT	358 ± 55	482 ± 46	1,075 ± 278
Clone B 7	—	315 ± 32	506 ± 47	443 ± 27
	TT	297 ± 53	8,920 ± 865	13,426 ± 716
	DT	284 ± 24	463 ± 39	412 ± 60

2×10^4 T cells were cultured with 2×10^4 antigen presenting cells for 4 days then pulsed for 18 hours with ^{3}H-thymidine and harvested.
Bo - name of cell line
irr - irradiated
DT - diphtheria toxoid

nurse cells, etc. That this does indeed occur in man was illustrated by our recent observations on the behavior of a TT-specific T-cell line derived from the recipient of an HLA-mismatched bone marrow transplant recipient. The TT-specific cell line of this HLA-DR 3,4 recipient of HLA-DR 3-5 bone marrow responded vigorously to TT antigen in the presence of HLA-DR-5 bearing monocytes, and thus contained T cells which matured into an HLA-DR 5 environment which could not have been provided by the thymic epithelium of the HLA-DR 3,4 recipient. Hence, both thymic epithelium and bone marrow-derived cells appear to contribute to the education of T cells into self-recognition.

COOPERATIVE CELL INTERACTIONS: T-B AND TT

The cooperation of human T and B cells in the antibody response has been well established and will not be reviewed here. From data in experimental animals and in man up to 3 signals are required for specific antibody synthesis [9]: 1) B-cell binding of antigen; 2) a nonspecific T-cell helper factor, similar to IL-2; and 3) interaction between antigen-specific T and B cells either via cell-to-cell contact or via an antigen-specific helper factor.

One recently discovered interesting aspect of T-B-cell interaction is the capacity of activated B cells to present antigen to Th cells [10]. In this regard we have shown that Epstein-Barr virus-transformed human B-cell lines can present TT antigen to TT-specific T-cell clones in the total absence of detectable Mo contamination (Table 3). The implication of this finding is that there is 2-way traffic between T and B cells, and although Mo may be the primary trigger for T-cell expansions after antigenic stimulation, activated B cells may serve to amplify this T-cell activation.

Interaction between regulatory Th cells and cytotoxic T cells appears to follow the same general principles as T-B interactions. Thus, 3 signals appear to be required for the activation of cytotoxic T cells [11]: 1) target binding; 2) IL-2; and 3) a cytotoxic differentiation factor (CDF). In this regard it is interesting to note that children with atopic dermatitis have defective cell-mediated lympholysis (CML) [12]. On the basis of co-culture experiments of purified T4 and T8 cells from patients and healthy sibs this defect appears to be due to both a defect in T8+ cytotoxic cells, as well as to a defect in T4+ helper cells. Preliminary investigations suggest that the defect in helper function lies at the level of CDF production rather than at the level of IL-2 production.

The list of cooperative interactions between T cells and other cells is very long. A short list of interactions involving cells of the immune system is presented in Table 4. Recently accumulated evidence reveals that T cells secrete helper factors which are isotype specific. Some of these factors may act by switching Ig synthesis of activated B cells. Thus, we have found that supernatants of T cells from hyper IgE patients contain factors which enhance IgE but not IgG synthesis in normal B cells (Table 4). Dr. Fu Man Shu et al (this volume) report on a T-T hybridoma which secretes IgA-specific helper factors.

FUNCTIONAL T-CELL SUBSETS AND T-CELL ACTIVATION MARKERS

No review of T cells would be complete without a mention of the surface antigenic markers which in the past years have allowed a dissection of T cells into subsets with more or less discrete functions. The acquisition of maturation markers in the

TABLE 4. T-Cell Factors

Factor	Target	Action
IL-2	T	Expansion
CDF	T	Differentiation
BCGF, LMF	B	Expansion
Antigen-specific helper factor	B	Differentiation
Isotype-specific helper factors	B	Switching of isotype synthesis
Suppressor factors	T/B?	Suppression
MAF	Mo	Activation
MMIF	Mo	Inhibition of migration

BCGF - B-cell growth factor
LMF - lymphocyte mitogenic factor
MAF - macrophage activating factor
MMIF - macrophage migration inhibition factor

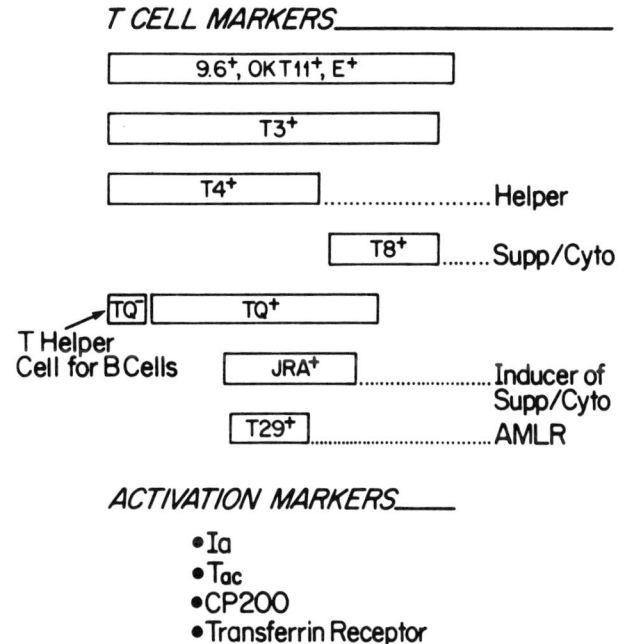

Fig. 4. Summary of markers expressed by peripheral blood T cells.

thymus has already been discussed and is summarized in Figure 1. Figure 4 attempts to summarize the present state-of-the-art of the most commonly used T-cell markers. Analysis of these markers in immunodeficiency diseases has provided important clues to their function. Thus, the deficiency of T8+ cells in the hyper-IgE syndrome gave the clue to the importance of this subset in the regulation of IgE synthesis [13].

Finally, a word should be said about T-cell activation markers since these markers should serve as clues for activated T cells in human disease. A number of markers for activated T cells have been described including Ia, the Tac antigen described by Waldmann which is the receptor for interleukin-2, and the transferrin receptor defined by the monoclonal antibody OKTG. Ia is usually expressed on <5% of peripheral blood T cells but on a number of higher proportions of T cells from subjects recently immunized or who are suffering from autoimmune diseases [14]. However, although Ia is a useful marker its presence does not always accompany T-cell activation. Thus, Tac rather than Ia appears on activated suppressor cells in the newborn.

CONCLUSION

Although by no means exhaustive, this review illustrates the benefits of applying modern concepts of T-cell function to the study of human immunodeficiencies, and the unique understanding of normal T-cell function that is provided by the study of these experiments of nature.

ACKNOWLEDGMENTS

The author thanks Miss Melissa Smith for excellent secretarial assistance, and Drs. Donald Leung, Martin Broff, and Edward Chu for carrying out various aspects of the work from our laboratory discussed herein.

REFERENCES

1. Reinherz EL, Kung PC, Goldstein G, Schlossman SF: Separation of functional subsets of human T cells by a monoclonal antibody. Proc Natl Acad Sci USA 76:4061, 1979.
2. Geha RS, Milgrom HF, Broff M, Alpert S, Martin S, Yunis EJ: Macrophage T cell interaction in man: A subpopulation of adherent accessory cells bearing DRw antigens is required for antigen specific human T lymphocytes proliferation. Proc Natl Acad Sci USA 76(8):4038, 1979.
3. Fineman SM, Rosen FS, Geha RS: Transient hypogammaglobulinemia, elevated IgE levels and food allergy. J Allergy Clin Immunol 64(8):216, 1979.
4. Muchmore AV, Blaese RM, Decker JM, Mann DL, Broder S: Inhibition of antigen specific proliferation by antisera recognizing antigens encoded by the human DR locus may be due to active suppression. Clin Res 25:506A, 1980.
5. Geha RS: Idiotypic determinants on human T cells. Clin Res 28(2):503A, 1980.
6. Krensky AM, Reiss CS, Mier JW et al: Long term human cytolytic T-cell lines allospecific for HLA-DR6 antigen are

OKT4+. Proc Natl Acad Sci USA 79:2365, 1982.
7. Broff MD, Jonsen ME, Geha RS: Nature of the immunologic moiety recognized by the human T cell proliferating in response to tetanus toxoid antigen. Eur J Immunol 11:365, 1981.
8. Ziegler HK, Unanue ER: Decrease in macrophage antigen catabolism caused by ammonia and chloroquine is associated with inhibition of antigen presentation to T cells. Proc Natl Acad Sci USA 79:175, 1982.
9. Andersson J, Melchers F: T cell-dependent activation of resting B cells: Requirement for both nonspecific unrestricted and antigen-specific Ia-restricted soluble factors. Proc Natl Acad Sci USA 78(4):2497, 1981.
10. Issekutz T, Ghus E, Geha RS: Antigen presentation by human B cells: T cell proliferation induced by Epstein Barr virus B lymphoblastoid cells. J Immunol (In press).
11. Raulet DH, Bevan MJ: A differentiation factor required for the expression of cytotoxic T-cell function. Nature 296:754, 1982.
12. Leung DYM, Wood N, Dubey D, Geha RS: Cellular basis for defective cell mediated lympholysis in atopic dermatitis. Clin Res 30(2):164A, 1982.
13. Geha R, Reinherz E, Leung D, Schlossman S, Rosen F: Suppressor T cell deficiency in the hyper IgE syndrome. J Clin Invest 68(3):783-791, 1981.
14. Yu DTY, Winchester RJ, Fu SM, Gibofsky A, Ko HS, Kunkel HG: Peripheral blood Ia-positive T cells: Increases in certain diseases after immunization. J Exp Med 151:91, 1980.

Suppressor T-Cell Circuit in Man*

Cobi J. Heijnen, PhD, and Rudy E. Ballieux, PhD

Department of Immunology, University Children's Hospital, 3512 LK Utrecht, The Netherlands (C.J.H.), Department of Clinical Immunology, University Hospital, 3500 CG Utrecht, The Netherlands (R.E.B.)

INTRODUCTION

The increasing sophistication of techniques and the discriminative power of monoclonal antibodies have provided the insight that control of the immune response is not an autonomous property of one cell type. The cells which are programmed to effect—positively or negatively—the intensity of the immune response need, most of the time, inducing signals from other, inducer-type cells which ultimately determine the regulating capacity of the effector cells. There is also growing evidence that these various interacting subsets can communicate via soluble macromolecular factors endowed with the ability to mediate the activity ascribed to the producer cell [1].

In this paper we describe such a chain of events leading to T-cell mediated regulation of the human plaque-forming cell (PFC) response. It has been demonstrated previously that human T cells bearing an FC receptor for IgM ($T\mu^+$), when properly primed in vitro by antigen, acquire the capacity of inducing a suppressor activity in unprimed human T cells [2]. The interaction of these primed T-suppressor-inducer (Tsi) cells with unprimed T cells leads to maturation of these T cells into T-suppressor effector (Tse) cells. The population of unprimed T cells therefore contains T-suppressor-precursor (Tsp) cells which can function as target for activated Tsi cells. The Tsp cells could be located in the T-cell fraction that does not bear Fc receptors for IgM or IgG ($T\mu\gamma^-$), and could be isolated by the fact that the $T\mu\gamma^-$ cells have affinity for autologous erythrocytes (Tar^+) [3]. The cellular components of this Ts circuit are related by a shared specificity of the antigen-receptors involved, as the transition process of Tsp cells to Tse cells, as well as the activation of Tsi cells, are clearly antigen-specific events [4].

The aim of this paper is to define the various T-cell subsets involved in this regulatory circuit and to investigate the mechanism that determines the intensity of the activity.

MATERIALS AND METHODS

All methods concerning isolation of PBL, T, B, AC, $T\mu^+$, $T\gamma^+$ and Tar^+ cells have been described extensively elsewhere [3,5,6].

Priming of $T\mu^+$ Cells

$T\mu^+$ cells isolated according to the method described [5] were cultured in the presence or in the absence of 10% AC and the antigen ovalbumin (OA) in the inserts of a Marbrook-Diener tube. The medium that was used in the inserts, as well as in the outer compartments of the tubes, consisted of RPMI-1640 that was supplemented with antibiotics, 2 mM glutamin and 5×10^{-5} M 2-mercaptoethanol and 10% human AB serum, that had been preabsorbed with SE [5]. After 5–6 days the cells were harvested, washed, and added to the various target cell cultures.

Isolation of Subsets by Complement-Induced Lysis With Monoclonal Antibodies of the OKT Series

T cells or T-cell subsets (10×10^6 cells/ml) were mixed with the relevant monoclonal antibodies. After an incubation period of 1 hr at room temperature, complement (low tox H rabbit complement, Cedarlane, Sanbio, The Netherlands) was added (250 μl/ml cell suspension), after which the cells were incubated for another period of 1½ hr at 37°C. After this treatment the cells were washed and incubated overnight at 37°C.

Complement-Induced Lysis of T Cells Reacting With Antibodies in a Serum From a Patient Suffering From Juvenile Rheumatoid Arthritis

10×10^6 T cells were incubated in 1 ml of JRA-serum (1:4 dilution) for 60 min at 4°C. After this period, 1 ml of complement was added and the cells were incubated again for 4 hr at

---

Abbreviations used in this paper: AC, adherent cells; OA, ovalbumin; SE, sheep erythrocytes; Tar^+, T cells rosetting with autologous erythrocytes; EAM, ox-erythrocytes coated with rabbit anti-ox-erythrocyte IgM; Tsi, T-suppressor-inducer cell; Tsp, T-suppressor-precursor cell; Tse, T-suppressor-effector cell; JRA, juvenile rheumatoid arthritis; PFC, plaque-forming cell; SLE, systemic lupus erythematosus; $T\mu^+$, T cells bearing an FC receptor for IgM; $T\mu\gamma^-$, T cells that do not bear Fc receptors for IgM or IgG.

---

*This work was supported in part by the Foundation for Medical Research (FUNGO), which is subsidized by the Netherlands Organisation for the Advancement of Pure Research (ZWO).

room temperature. After this treatment the cells were washed extensively and cultured overnight at 37°C before use in the target cell cultures.

Theophylline Treatment of Tμ⁺ Cells

Purified $T\mu^+$ cells were incubated in RPMI-1640 containing 2 mM theophylline. After 2 hr the cells were washed and rerosetted with ox-erythrocytes coated with rabbit anti-Eox IgM antibodies (EAM). The rosetting cells ($T\mu^+$ theo-resistant) and the nonrosetting cells ($T\mu^+$ theo-sensitive) were separated by density centrifugation over Ficoll-Isopaque (density = 1.077 g/cm³). The theo-resistant fraction, that had retained the capacity to rosette with the EAM-complexes, was freed of the erythrocytes by lysis with NH₄Cl.

Preparation of Tse Factors

The method for the production of the factor secreted by the in vitro generated Tse cells (Sup Tar*) is described below in Results.

The method for the production of the factor secreted by the in vivo generated FcγR⁺ Tse cell (TsF120) is described extensively in reference 7. Briefly, 15×10^6 $T\gamma^+$ cells or unseparated T cells were cultured for 4 days with a high dose of antigen (100 μg OA/ml) at 37°C. After this period the cells were washed and cultured for another 24 hr at 37°C in the presence of a low dose of antigen (3 μg OA/ml). After the incubation period, the supernatant was purified by immunoabsorption on a column containing insolubilized OA. As the Tse factor possesses a binding site for the antigen, the suppressive material could be located in the acid eluate fraction. After neutralization of the eluate, the material (TsF120-OA) was stored at −60°C until use.

RESULTS
Activation of Tsi Cells: Dependency of Adherent Cells

It has been shown previously that the presence of adherent cells (AC) is an absolute requirement for T-helper (Th) cells to become activated and to perform their helper function [8]. In contrast, Tsi cells can only be activated by antigen when the antigen is available in a soluble form. As shown in Figure 1b, no Tsi activity is generated if the antigen is presented at the surface of AC. As a consequence, AC, when present in the culture, interfere with the process of antigen-induced Tsi activation. As demonstrated in Figure 1a, Tsi cells can be activated by minute amounts (0.03 μg OA/ml) of antigen if AC are absent from the culture. However, when AC are present, a high amount of antigen (30–100 μg OA/ml) is needed for successful generation of Tsi cell activity. It is assumed that at these high concentrations of antigen, the AC can be bypassed by free antigen, resulting in Tsi activation.

Phenotypic Characterization of Tsi Cells

The results presented in the previous section establish that Th cells and Tsi cells differ in their demands for the mode of antigen presentation. Based on this observation, the possibility was considered that the two functionally defined subsets of Th and Tsi cells could be distinguished on the basis of a characteristic phenotype. We addressed this question by the use of monoclonal antibodies and allo-antibodies and by the analysis of theophylline-sensitivity in relation to rosette formation with EAM-complexes.

OKT-phenotype. It is clear from the data presented in Table 1 that the $T\mu^+$ subset is heterogeneous and contains T4⁺ as well as T8⁺ cells. In order to define the phenotype of the Th and the Tsi cells, we depleted the $T\mu^+$ fraction of T4⁺ or T8⁺ cells by complement-induced lysis of the cells, reactive with OKT4 or OKT8. After depletion the remaining $T\mu^+$ cells ($T8^+\mu^+$ and $T4^+\mu^+$, respectively) were analyzed for their potential regulating capacities. To test for the presence of Th activity, cells of either of the two $T\mu^+$ subfractions were cultured separately with B cells and 5% adherent cells in the presence of an optimum dose of OA. The capacity to induce suppressor activity was determined by investigating the effect of the T cells of the two fractions ($T8^+\mu^+$ and $T4^+\mu^+$), after prior priming with OA, on cultures of unseparated peripheral blood lymphocytes stimulated with an optimum dose of OA.

From the data depicted in Figure 2, we can deduce that Th and Tsi

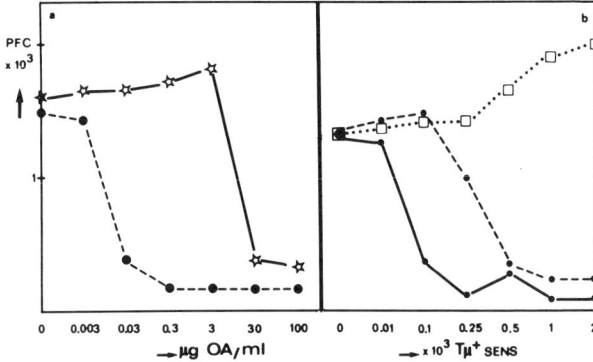

Fig. 1. Activation of Tsi cells: dependency of AC. a) $T\mu^+$ cells primed by various doses of OA (as indicated on the abscissa) were primed either in the absence of AC ●—● or in the presence of 10% AC ☆—☆. b) $T\mu^+$ cells, primed in the presence of 100 μg OA/ml ●——●; 100 μg OA/ml and 10% AC ●--●; 10% AC pulsed with OA □··□. After the priming period, the $T\mu^+$ cell fractions were washed and cultured with 5×10^6 PBL and 3 μg OA/ml for a period of 6 days. The AC pulsed with OA were capable of activating the PBL to generate PFC (1492 PFC/10⁶ ly).

TABLE 1. Phenotypic Characterization of T-Cell Subsets

Monoclonal antibodies	T total	$T\mu^+$	$T\mu\gamma^-$	Tar^+	$T\gamma^+$
OKT3	87 ± 1.8	86 ± 1.7	86 ± 3.1	84 ± 2.4	32 ± 2.0
OKT4	58 ± 2.0	69 ± 2.4	56 ± 1.8	50 ± 1.1	18 ± 1.6
OKT8	23 ± 2.0	15 ± 1.6	34 ± 1.8	42 ± 1.8	42 ± 2.0
OKM-1	18 ± 1.5	0.4 ± 0.1	1.0 ± 0.2	0.5 ± 0.3	65 ± 5.0

cells cannot be discriminated on the basis of OKT-phenotype: both functions are exerted by T lymphocytes bearing the T4 marker. Similar experiments using the monoclonal antibody 5/9 [9] also failed to discriminate between Th and Tsi cells: both functional subsets carry the 5/9 phenotype.

JRA-antibodies. It has been reported by Reinherz et al [10] that sera from patients with acute juvenile rheumatoid arthritis (JRA) may contain antibodies which react with approximately 30% of human peripheral T cells. These antibodies do not react with Th cells but have affinity for Ts cells which suppress the pokeweed mitogen-driven immunoglobulin synthesis [10].

In agreement with these data, we could show that the serum of a patient suffering from JRA contained antibodies that reacted with only 10% of normal peripheral blood $T\mu^+$ lymphocytes. When the reactive cells were lysed with complement, it appeared that the remaining T cells still contained functional Th cells but were completely devoid of cells expressing Tsi cell activity (Fig. 2).

Theophylline-sensitivity. In search of an additional difference between Th and Tsi cells, we separated $T\mu^+$ cells into two fractions on the basis of the differential sensitivity of the Fcμ receptor for theophylline [11]. To that end, the $T\mu^+$ cells were incubated with theophylline and rerosetted with EAM complexes (see Materials and Methods). The rosetting T cells (the theophylline-resistant fraction) were separated from the nonrosetting cells by density centrifugation. When the theophylline-resistant $T\mu^+$ cells (10–30%) were tested for their regulating capacities, it was found that they contained very active Th cells, but were devoid of Tsi cells (Fig. 2). In contrast, Tsi activity could only be detected in the theophylline-sensitive $T\mu^+$ fraction (Fig. 2). This last subset still contained T cells which could function as Th cells, but considerably less efficiently compared to the theophylline-resistant $T\mu^+$ fraction.

Phenotypic Characterization of the Tsp Cells

In the preceding sections and in reference 2 the Tsi cell has been defined as a cell that induces an unprimed Tsp cell to mature to a state in which it can directly suppress Th function. From previous studies [3] we knew that the unprimed Tsp cells are present in a T-cell subset that does not bear detectable Fc receptors for either IgM or IgG ($T\mu\gamma^-$), and form rosettes with autologous erythrocytes (Tar^+). Our next goal was to determine the phenotype of this subset by the use of monoclonal antibodies of the OKT series. Table 1 indicates that the $T\mu\gamma^-ar^+$ subset contains T4$^+$ as well as T8$^+$ cells. In order to investigate whether the Tsp cells did reside in one of these 2 subsets, we separated the Tar$^+$ fraction by complement-induced lysis of the reactive cells into T8$^+$ar$^+$ and T4$^+$ar$^+$ cells. When these fractions were cultured separately with Tsi cells, Th cells, B cells, and 5% AC in the presence of an optimum dose of OA, we obtained the following results (Table 2): T4$^+$ar$^+$ cells cannot function as Tsp cells; T8$^+$ar$^+$ cells have the capacity to mature to the effector stage under the influence

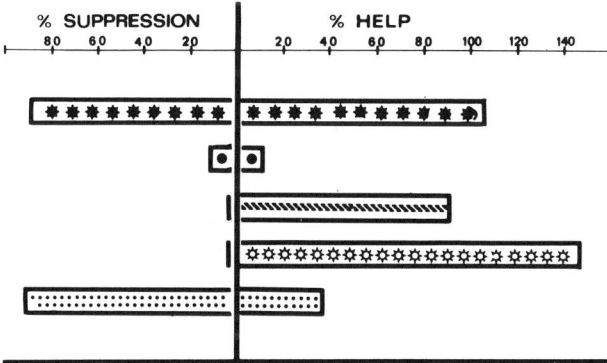

Fig. 2. Phenotypic characterization of Th- and Ts-inducer cells. $T\mu^+$ cells were incubated with either OKT8 ✱, OKT4 ●, or serum of a JRA patient ▨. After lysis of the reacting cells by complement, the remaining cells were washed, cultured overnight, and added to the various target cell cultures. The $T\mu^+$ fractions indicated by ✺ and ▦ were obtained by the separation of a $T\mu^+$ cell fraction into cells of which the FcμR was resistant to treatment with theophylline ✺ or sensitive to this drug ▦ (see Materials and Methods). The latter fractions were also tested for their capacity to induce Th- or Ts-activity. The helper activity of the fractions was determined by culturing the various $T\mu^+$ fractions separately with 1.5×10^6 B cells, 5% AC and 3 μg OA/ml. The PFC responses are expressed as the percentages of the PFC response generated in a culture of 3.5×10^6 $T\mu^+$ cells, 1.5×10^6 B cells, 5% AC, and 3 μg OA/ml (2134 ± 28; n=3). The Tsi-activity of the various $T\mu^+$ fractions determined by culturing the various primed T-cell subsets (0.5×10^6 cells) with 5×10^6 PBL, 5% AC, and 3 μg OA/ml. PFC responses are expressed as the percentages of suppression induced by 0.5×10^6 unfractionated primed $T\mu^+$ cells (234 ± 4; n=3) in cultures containing also 5×10^6 PBL, 5% AC, and 3 μg OA/ml.

TABLE 2. Phenotype of Ts-Precursor Cells in the Tar⁺ Subset

Possible Ts	% of control PFC response
—	100
1.0 Tar⁺	18
2.0 Tar⁺	21
1.0 T4⁺ar⁺	80
2.0 T4⁺ar⁺	97
1.0 T8⁺ar⁺	43
2.0 T8⁺ar⁺	38
0.5 T4⁺ar⁺ 0.5 T8⁺ar⁺	17

Assay system: 1.5 B cells, 2.0 Tar-depleted T cells, 0.5 OA-primed Tµ⁺ cells, and 3 µg OA/ml.

of primed Tµ⁺ suppressor-inducer cells. However, T4⁺ar⁺ cells have the capacity to amplify or to enhance this process, as optimum suppression could only be achieved in cultures when both types of Tar⁺ cells were present.

Phenotypic Characterization of the Tse Cells

The transition of precursor cells to the effector stage is often accompanied by a change in the phenotype of the precursor cell. Therefore, we tried to identify the Tse cells which develop from Tsp cells after the inductive activity of primed Tsi cells. As the activation of the Ts circuit by antigen is limited to antigen-specific T cells, the number of Tse cells generated in vitro was expected to be rather low. It was already known from previous experiments that the Tse cells, developed in vivo and present in peripheral blood of normal healthy individuals, express Fcγ receptors on their cell surface [5]. We wondered, therefore, whether generation of Tγ⁺ cells could be observed when Tar⁺ cells were cultured with primed Tsi cells. To address this issue, primed Tµ⁺ cells were cultured with Tar⁺ cells under conditions that both cell types were separated by a nucleopore membrane (0.22 µm). After an incubation period of 3 days, the Tar⁺ cell suspension was tested for the presence of Tγ⁺ cells. A low percentage (4.3% ± 1.2; n=6) of T cell expressing Fcγ receptors could be shown to be present. To investigate whether the few Tγ⁺ cells which appeared in the culture really represented the OA-specific Tse cells, these Tγ⁺ cells were removed by rosetting with EAG-complexes and subsequent density centrifugation (see Materials and Methods). The cultured Tar⁺ cells, after depletion of the generated Tγ⁺ cells, were checked again for the presence of OA-specific Tse cell activity. Such activity no longer could be demonstrated (Fig. 3). Since the cultured Tar⁺ cells had lost their capacity to rerosette with autologous erythrocytes, we could deduce from the data that the Tse cell generated in vitro expresses the T8⁺ar⁻γ⁺ phenotype.

Regulation of Tsi Cell Activity

Since previous results had established that the degree of Th activity does not primarily control the rate of Tsi cell activity [4], we investigated whether the latter activity might be influenced by a feedback mechanism exerted by its own end product: the Tse cell. To that end Tar⁺ cells were cultured for 4 days with OA-primed Tµ⁺ cells, but separated by a nucleopore membrane. After this period, the cells of the Tar⁺ compartment were washed and cultured with 3 µg OA/ml for 24 hrs in the absence of primed Tµ⁺ cells. The supernatant of these cells was then collected and tested for its capacity to suppress a PFC response of B cells, supplemented with Th cells, 5% AC, and an optimum dose of OA. As can be seen in Table 3, this supernatant (Sup Tar*) contained a soluble substance which suppressed the OA-induced PFC response. Since only Th cells were present and the OA-specific PFC response is T-dependent, it is reasonable to assume that the suppressive activity, like that produced by T8⁺ar⁻γ⁺ suppressor effector cells, blocked Th function. It is interesting that when this supernatant was added to the priming culture of Tµ⁺ cells, we could observe that

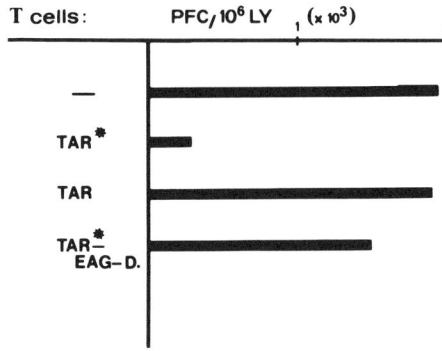

Fig. 3. Characterization of the Tse generated in vitro. 3.5 × 10⁶ Th T cells that have been irradiated (2,000 R), 1.5 × 10⁶ B cells, 5% AC were cultured with 3 µg OA/ml in the presence of the various T-cell fractions when indicated. Tar*: Tar⁺ cells cultured for 4 days with primed Tµ⁺ cells under conditions that both cell types were separated by a nucleopore membrane (0.22 µm). Both compartments of the culture vessel contained 3 µg OA/ml. Tar: Tar⁺ cells cultured for 4 days under the same conditions but in the absence of primed Tµ⁺ cells. Tar*-EAG-D: Tar⁺ cells cultured with the primed Tµ⁺ cells. After 4 days, however, the Tar* cells were depleted of cells bearing a FcγR before being added to the target cell culture.

TABLE 3. Suppressor Activity of Factors Secreted by Tse Cells

Factor	PFC/10⁶ ly
—	1984 ± 17
Sup Tar* 1%	1867 ± 12
Sup Tar* 5%	504 ± 11
Sup Tar* 10%	233 ± 4
TsF120-OA 10%	331 ± 4

The regulatory effect of the factors was tested by adding the factors to target cell cultures consisting of 3.5 × 10⁶ irradiated T cells (2,000 Rad), 1.5 × 10⁶ B cells, 5% AC, and 3 µg OA/ml. After 6 days the PFC assay was performed. SEM are given (n=3). For the preparation of the Tse factors, see Materials and Methods.

the generation of Tsi cells was very effectively inhibited also by this suppressive substance (Fig. 4). In addition, the generation of Tsi-activity could also be inhibited by a Tse-factor produced by the in vivo generated Tγ⁺ suppressor-effector cells (Fig. 4). The properties of this factor (TsF120) have been found to be identical to the properties of the factor

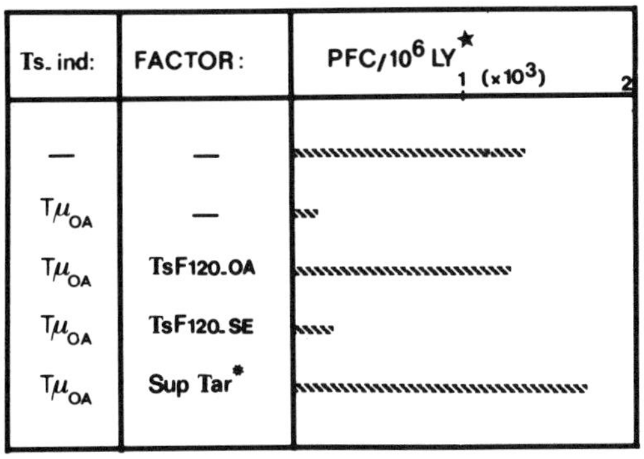

Ts. ind:	FACTOR:	PFC/10^6 LY*
		1 (×10^3) 2
—	—	~~~~~~~~~~~~~~~
Tμ_{OA}	—	~
Tμ_{OA}	TsF120.OA	~~~~~~~~~~
Tμ_{OA}	TsF120.SE	~~
Tμ_{OA}	Sup Tar*	~~~~~~~~~~~~~~~~~~~

Fig. 4. Tμ^+ cells were primed with 100 μg OA/ml in the presence or absence of Tse factors generated by (Tμ^+OA)-activated Tar$^+$ cells (Sup Tar*) or by Tγ^+ suppressor-effector cells (TsF120) either specific for the antigen OA or SE (see Materials and Methods). After the priming period, the Tμ^+ cells were washed and added to a target cell culture of PBL, 5% AC, and 3 μg OA/ml. After 6 days the PFC-assay was performed.

produced by the in vitro generated Tse cells (Sup Tar*) [7,12].

DISCUSSION

We have demonstrated here that on the basis of the dissection of the various T-cell subsets involved, the generation of Tse cells can be monitored in vitro.

We could show that Tsi cells, characterized by the phenotype T4$^+\mu^+$, can induce unprimed T8$^+$ar$^+\mu\gamma^-$ precursor cells to mature to T8$^+$ar$^-\gamma^+$ suppressor-effector cells.

As we know from a previous work [5] that the Tse cell which is present in the peripheral circulation of normal, healthy individuals carries the same phenotype, it is tempting to propose that these effector cells are identical to the Tse cells generated in vitro, and consequently may be derived from the same precursor cell: the T8$^+$ar$^+\mu\gamma^-$ cell.

The latter conclusion is supported by the data obtained in investigations of the regulatory capacities of T cells from SLE patients [3]. When the patients were in an active stage of the disease, we could show that their peripheral blood lymphocytes did not contain functional (Tar$^+$) Tsp cells. Moreover, the absence of the Tsp cells in the peripheral blood did always coincide with the phenotypic and functional absence of T8$^+$ar$^-\gamma^+$ suppressor-effector cells. On the basis of these data one may conclude that the Tγ^+ suppressor-effector cell is generated in vivo from Tar$^+$ precursor cells. This assumption stresses the importance of the in vitro findings reported in this paper.

An issue addressed in the present work relates to the following fundamental question: if suppression is a normal consequence of an ongoing immune response, is the activation of Tsi cells controlled by the activation state of the Th cell?

In order to solve this problem we tried to generate Tsi cell activity in the absence of T-cell help. This was achieved by omitting antigen-presenting cells from the priming culture. Figure 1 demonstrates that the generation of Tsi cells proceeds very efficiently under these circumstances. As Th cells can only be activated by antigen when adherent cells are present, the conclusion is warranted that the generation of Ts-inducer cells is not directly controlled by the state of activation of the Th cells.

Another aspect of the Ts-circuit concerns the possibility that the level of Ts-inducer cell activity might be regulated by a feedback mechanism by its own end product, namely, the Tse cell. Figure 4 clearly shows this to be the case. The soluble suppressor-effector molecules secreted by in vitro generated Tse cells and the soluble product of Tse cells present in vivo can both inhibit the activation of Tsi cells. This inhibition process can only happen when the Ts-effector molecule is added to the priming culture. The addition of a prosuppressor factor like TsF-24 [13] does not interfere with the generation of Tsi cells (manuscript in preparation).

Despite their antagonistic functions, the phenotypes of the Th cell and the Tsi cell display many similarities. The monoclonal antibodies used did not discriminate between the 2 subsets. Both cell types can be blocked in their function by the suppressor-effector factors, which might implicate that they both carry the same recognition-unit for these regulatory molecules.

However, antibodies present in the serum of a JRA patient were capable of dissecting the 2 functionally different subsets by their exclusive reaction with Tsi cells. Reinherz recently reported that the monoclonal antibody TQ1 defines a subset of T lymphocyte which includes the JRA$^+$ subset [14]. Since only TQ1$^-$ cells could exert Th function, the possibility is open that on the basis of the TQ1 antigen, Th and Tsi cells can be distinguished. Furthermore, we could show a difference between the sensitivity of the Fcμ receptor for the drug theophylline. It appeared that this receptor is resistant to theophylline treatment on most of the Th cells, whereas the receptor on the Tsi cells is not.

A clear-cut difference between Th and Tsi cells is their demands for antigen-presentation. Tsi cells cannot "see" the antigen present at the surface of the antigen-presenting cells, whereas Th cells do not "see" the antigen in its native form.

The independence of antigen-presenting cells of the activation of Tsi cells is in line with the earlier observation that the in vivo present T8$^+$ar$^-\gamma^+$ suppressor-effector cells can only be activated by antigen in its native form [15]. This observation suggests that a common pathway exists for the activation of cells of the suppressor lineage.

REFERENCES

1. Germain RN, Benacerraf B: Helper and suppressor T cell factors. Semin Immunopathol 3:93–127, 1980.
2. Heijnen CJ, UytdeHaag F, Pot CH, Ballieux RE: Feedback inhibition by human primed T helper cells. Nature 280:589–591, 1979.
3. Heijnen CJ, Pot KH, Kater L, Kluin-Nelemans HC, UytdeHaag F, Ballieux RE: Functional analysis of the defective T cell regulation of the antigen-specific PFC response in SLE-patients: Differentiation of suppressor precursor cells to suppressor effector cells. Clin Exp Immunol 47:359–367, 1982.
4. Heijnen CJ, UytdeHaag F, Pot KH, Ballieux RE: Regulatory mechanisms in the T-cell control of the antigen-induced PFC response in man. In Fauci AS, Ballieux RE (eds): "Human B Lymphocyte Function: Activation and Immunoregulation." New York: Raven Press, 1982, pp 239–251.
5. Heijnen CJ, UytdeHaag F, Gmelig-Meyling FHJ, Ballieux RE: Human B cell activation in vitro: Localization of antigen-specific helper and suppressor function in distinct T cell subpopulations. Cell Immunol 43:282–292, 1979.
6. Heijnen CJ, Pot KH, Ballieux RE: Characterization of human T suppressor-inducer, -precursor and -effector lymphocytes in the antigen-specific PFC response. Eur J Immunol 12:860–866, 1982.
7. UytdeHaag F, Heijnen CJ, Pot KH, Ballieux RE: Antigen-specific human T cell factors. II. T cell suppressor factor: Biologic properties. J Immunol 126:503–507, 1981.
8. Heijnen CJ, UytdeHaag F, Dollekamp I, Ballieux RE: Distinct human T-cell subpopulations regulating the antigen-induced antibody response. In Fauci AS, Ballieux RE (eds): "Antibody Production in Man: In Vitro Synthesis and Clinical Implications." New York: Academic Press, 1979, pp 231–254.
9. Corte G, Mingari MC, Moretta A, Damiani G, Moretta L, Bargellesi A: Human T cell subpopulations defined by a monoclonal antibody. I. A small subset is responsible for proliferation to allogeneic cells or to soluble antigens and for helper activity for B cell differentiation. J Immunol 128:16–19, 1982.
10. Reinherz EL, Strelkauskas AJ, O'Brien C, Schlossman SF: Phenotypic and functional distinctions between TH2+ and JRA+ T cell subsets in man. J Immunol 123:83–86, 1979.
11. Gupta S: Subpopulations of human T lymphocytes. XII. In vitro effect of agents modifying intracellular levels of cyclic nucleotides on T cells with receptors for IgM (Tμ), IgG (Tγ), or IgA (Tα). J Immunol 123:2664–2668, 1979.
12. Heijnen CJ, UytdeHaag F, Pot KH, Bentwich Z, Ballieux RE: Antigen-specific human T cell factors. III. T cell helper and suppressor factors: Immunochemical aspect. Ann Immunol (Paris) (In press).
13. UytdeHaag F, Heijnen CJ, Pot KH, Ballieux RE: T-T interactions in the induction of antigen-specific human suppressor T lymphocytes in vitro. J Immunol 123:646–653, 1979.
14. Reinherz EL, Morimoto C, Fitzgerald KA, Hussey RE, Daley JF, Schlossman SF: Heterogeneity of human T4+ inducer T cells defined by a monoclonal antibody that delineates two functional subpopulations. J Immunol 128:463–468, 1982.
15. UytdeHaag F, Heijnen CJ, Pot KH, Ballieux RE: Antigen-specific human T cell factors. V. Influence of adherent cells in the generation of T cell suppressor factor by Tγ cells. Supra #4, pp 253–262.

A Formula to Assess Lymphocyte Responsiveness In Vitro

Clifford S. Hosking, MD, FRACP, FRCPA, and Anne Balloch

Department of Immunology, Royal Children's Hospital, Parkville, Victoria 3052, Australia

INTRODUCTION

Lymphocyte response to mitogens has become the standard in vitro test for assessment of general lymphocyte function in suspected immune deficiencies [1]. Despite its popularity, many problems still exist in quantitation of the response. When lymphocyte responsiveness in vitro with PHA as the mitogen was introduced [2], the response was quantified by microscopy. The percentage of blast-transformed cells was used as a measure of lymphocyte reactivity.

In 1963, Michalowski [3] reported the incorporation of a radiolabeled DNA precursor into newly formed DNA as a marker of blastogenesis, and this has become the standard method.

To quantitate the response, authors have variously used the Stimulation Index (SI) (the ratio of mitogen stimulated to unstimulated responses), the absolute response, the net response (the difference between stimulated and unstimulated responses), the ratio at different concentrations of mitogens, and the ratio of the response at different days of culture with the mitogen. Some authors use counts per minute, and some use disintegrations per minute. Some relate the response back to the number of cells in culture, while others relate the response to the volume of blood used in the test. Some authors use untransformed counts, while others use log-transformed counts.

There is thus little agreement in expressing results. The reasons for this situation are not hard to find. The tests are difficult to perform, and there is no agreement or attempt at an agreement on standards. Minor technical differences between laboratories (or even within one laboratory on different days) can produce profound differences in the levels of response. This "within-laboratory" variation makes it difficult to separate "noise" from "message" in longitudinal studies or even in studies performed on similar patients at different times, and makes "between laboratory" comparisons virtually impossible except for the most gross abnormalities.

While the ultimate solution to these problems will require relating responses to some as-yet-to-be-defined generally agreed upon standard, this paper tackles the problem often faced by clinical immunologists both of reporting results to referring clinicians and of reporting results in the literature.

MATERIALS AND METHODS

Lymphocyte Response to Mitogens

The techniques used in this laboratory have been described in detail previously [4]. The mononuclear cells, previously separated from whole blood by a Ficoll-Isopaque discontinuous gradient, are platelet depleted by slow speed centrifugation and cultured in round bottomed microtiter trays in medium 199, containing 20% calf serum as a supplement. The mitogen phytohemagglutinin (PHA) was used as a stimulant at 0 and 60 µg/ml. The extent of mitosis was assessed by the uptake of tritiated thymidine into newly formed DNA over the last 2 hours of a 72-hour culture period. Lymphocyte cultures were set up in duplicate.

Patients and Controls

Patients used to demonstrate the formulae were a group of children with severe combined immunodeficiency (SCID). The results of 12 of these at the time of diagnosis were compared with the results of the control person's response on the day that the diagnosis of SCID was made. The mononuclear cultures of the controls and patients with SCID were established in batches of at least 6 (but more commonly 8) miscellaneous patients being investigated because of recurrent infections. The results from 4 of the patients who recovered immune function following bone marrow transplant were assessed at a time when the results and clinical course suggested that partial recovery had occurred.

Calculation of Lymphocyte Response

A total of 9 formulae were used in the graphing of results (Fig. 1) and for the calculations used in Table 1. They fell naturally into 2 groups. Formulae 1 to 4 use either the log counts per min or the absolute counts per min to determine net counts or the stimulation index. In these first 4 formulae, the results for the individual were compared with the mean of the results for the day and expressed as a percentage of this mean. In all of these determinations, an arbitrary cutoff was used to exclude patients whose response was less than 4 times

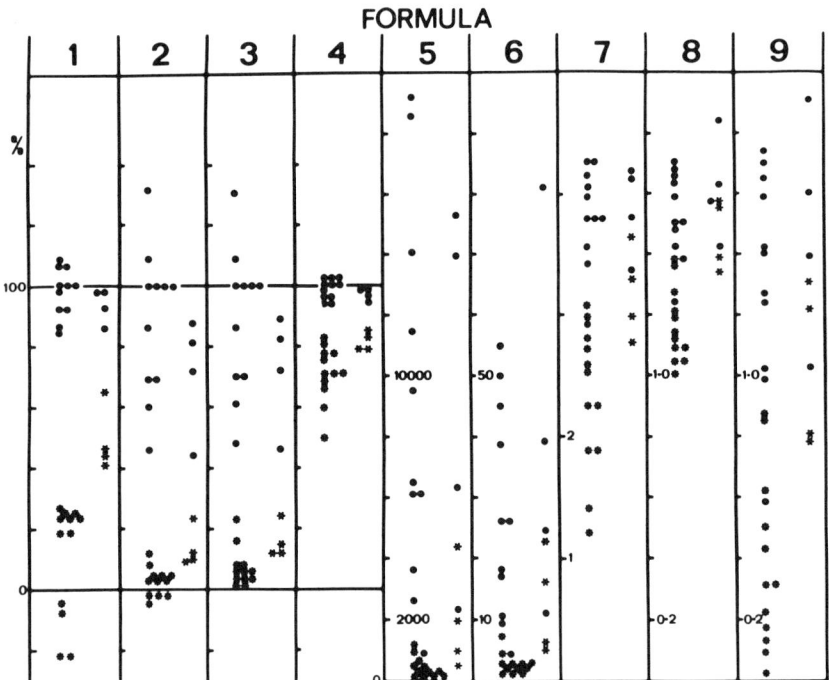

Fig. 1. Graphing of the results of lymphocyte responses to PHA using the 9 formulae shown in Table 1. ● controls, * patients with SCID at presentation, ✣ 4 of the patients with SCID after BMT.

TABLE 1. The Formulae That Were Used to Assess the Results of Lymphocyte Responsiveness to PHA

	FORMULA STIM = stimulation BG = background	Coefficient Variation Controls n = 11	Median Control − SCID n = 12
1	$\dfrac{\text{Log STIM cpm} - \text{Log BG cpm}}{[\Sigma\ (\text{Log STIM cpm} - \text{Log BG cpm})] \div n} \times 100\%$	8.2	76
2	$\dfrac{\text{STIM cpm} - \text{BG cpm}}{[\Sigma\ (\text{STIM cpm} - \text{BG cpm})] \div n} \times 100\%$	28.3	92
3	$\dfrac{\text{STIM cpm} / \text{BG cpm}}{[\Sigma\ (\text{STIM cpm} / \text{BG cpm})] \div n} \times 100\%$	27.3	84
4	$\dfrac{\text{Log STIM cpm} / \text{Log BG cpm}}{[\Sigma\ (\text{Log STIM cpm} / \text{Log BG cpm})] \div n} \times 100\%$	2.8	26
5	STIM cpm − BG cpm	69.1	8,929
6	STIM cpm / BG cpm	63.6	24.8
7	Log (STIM cpm − BG cpm)	10.5	1.3
8	Log STIM cpm / Log BG cpm	9.2	0.43
9	Log STIM cpm − Log BG cpm	26.3	1.03

the background count from being used in the calculation of the mean. This was to prevent distortion of the mean by grossly abnormal patients.

In formulae 5–9, the net counts or SI and the results when these figures were log-transformed were used without relating the results back to the other tests done in that run.

RESULTS AND DISCUSSION

These results span a 9-year period. The degree of variability is consistent with that reported in the literature [5–7]. Log-transformation of data was used in several of the formulae, as mitogenic responses of lymphocytes have been shown to be more normally distributed when log-transformed [8,9].

The results of the assays are graphed in Figure 1. Formula 5 and Formula 6 give the results of the most commonly used techniques for assessing responses—net counts and the SI, respectively.

The aim of this study was to produce a simple way of handling data that will allow one to legitimately compare the results obtained over a period of time. Few people working on lymphocyte proliferation assays would deny the wide variations that can occur in absolute counts per min in controls not only assessed in the one run but more importantly with time. Few also would claim to have a problem in distinguishing a patient with a SCID from a control. This is because the patient with a severe cellular deficiency is so different from a control that the signal can be seen clearly over (or under) the background noise.

However, lesser degrees of signal may well be lost. This is suggested with many of the formulae illustrated in Figure 1. To the right of each channel in the graph is the response of 4 of the patients with SCID taken post-BMT and the control on those days. The responses were assessed before PHA stimulation was back to control levels. With many of the formulae these intermediate values overlap either the "deficient" results or the "control" results, or both.

As yet, there are no accepted standard lymphocyte preparations that can be used to compare mitogenic responses of different groups of patients and controls that will eliminate the effects of both experimental and individual variations. The aim of assessing mitogenic responsiveness of lymphocytes is to allow one to make clinical assumptions about the cell-mediated immunity of the patient, or of a patient group. The better the discrimination that can be

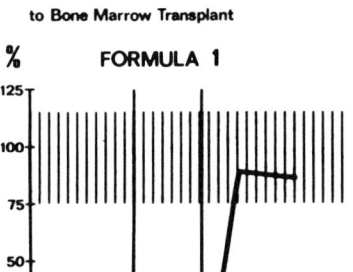

Fig. 2. Use of Formula 1 for estimating the lymphocyte responsiveness to PHA of a patient with SCID following successful BMT from a histocompatible sib. The response of the patient at different ages is shown by the solid line. The 5th to 95th%ile of the results from a group of controls is indicated by the vertical shading.

drawn between patient and control groups, the less likely is one to make type 2 errors (that no difference between groups is demonstrated when in fact a true difference exists).

To assess each of the formulae, the following questions should be asked: how wide is the control range? how different from the controls are the SCID patients on presentation? how different from both the controls and the SCID patients at presentation are the partially recovered patients?

Formula 1 would appear to be the most useful compromise. Formula 1 has been used for the graphing of the results over time of one of the patients with SCID following 2 BMTs from a histocompatible sib (Fig. 2). This shows reasonable robustness in that the response at diagnosis and until treatment is successful is well outside of the fairly narrow control range but improves until the response is within this range.

The difficulties with formulae 1 to 4 are that a number of patients must be tested in the one batch, and that if all the patients in the batch are abnormal, skewing of the results is possible. The first problem is a simple organizational one and requires that appointments be made for tests, or that a number of controls be included, if urgent tests are performed. The second, while potentially vexing, does not seem to have had much effect in practice. If this were to be a problem, one would expect the control range, ie that of the laboratory control in each run, to have a median well above 100%. In fact, the median for controls for formula 1 assessed over 68 runs was 98 with 75 to 115 being the 5th to 95th%ile range.

Thus, we would propose that of the formulae tested, formula 1, the difference between the log of the stimulated counts and the log of the background counts expressed as a percentage of the mean for the run, best fulfills the criteria for practical use in the assessment of lymphocyte responsiveness to mitogens.

REFERENCES

1. Hitzig WH, Kay HEM, Cottier H: Familial lymphopenia with agammaglobulinaemia. Lancet 2:151–154, 1965.
2. Nowell PC: Phytohaemagglutinin: An initiator of mitosis in cultures of normal human leukocytes. Cancer Res 20:462–466, 1960.
3. Michalowski A: Time course of DNA synthesis in human leucocyte cultures. Exp Cell Res 32:609–612, 1963.
4. Hosking CS, Fitzgerald MG, Shelton MJ: The immunological investigation of children with recurrent infections. Aust Paediatr J 13(Suppl):56–60, 1977.
5. Roberts NJ: Variability of results of lymphocyte transformation assay in normal human volunteers. Am J Clin Pathol 73:160–164, 1980.
6. Rees JC, Rossio JL, Wilson HE, Minton JF, Dodd MC: Cellular immunity in neoplasia. Cancer 36:2010–2015, 1975.
7. Merrin C, Han T: Immune response in bladder cancer. J Urol 111:170–172, 1974.
8. Fitzgerald MG: The establishment of a normal human population dose-response curve for lymphocytes cultured with PHA (phytohaemagglutinin). Clin Exp Immunol 8:421–425, 1971.
9. Ziegler JB, Hansen PJ, Davies WA, Penny R: The PHA dose-response curve: Validation of the use of logarithmic graph paper by computer analysis. J Immunol 113:2035–2039, 1974.

B-Cell Differentiation*

Max D. Cooper, MD

Departments of Pediatrics and Microbiology, and The Comprehensive Cancer Center, University of Alabama in Birmingham, Birmingham, AL 35294

The analysis of antibody deficiency diseases depends heavily upon an understanding of the normal life history of B cells, from their generation in hemopoietic tissues to their terminal differentiation in lymphoid tissues throughout the body. All normal individuals are genetically endowed with the capacity to generate millions of B-cell clones, each of which expresses a unique set of Ig genes determining antibody specificity. Heavy-chain isotype switching, on the other hand, is a common feature of all B-cell clones. Cells of B lineage are also marked by changing expression of a diverse assortment of nonimmunoglobulin proteins that are located on the cell surface and are involved in interactions between B cells and other cells. These interactions influence B-cell migration, growth, and differentiation into plasma cells.

OUTLINE OF STAGES IN B-CELL DIFFERENTIATION

Progression along the B-cell pathway can be roughly divided into antigen-independent and dependent phases. The antigen-independent phase includes the pre-B cell stage in differentiation during which Ig V_H, D_H, and J_H genes are selected for rearrangement and transcription along with the C_μ-gene [1-4]. The μ-chain products are expressed in the cytoplasm of pre-B cells, and usually do not reach the surface. Next a set of V_L and J_L genes is productively rearranged [5,6]. The subsequent expression of a complete membrane-bound IgM molecule marks the onset of B-cell differentiation and the potential for antigens to influence clonal behavior. Thus, while clonal diversity is generated among pre-B cells that lack antibody receptors, B-cell activation, proliferation, and terminal plasma cell differentiation are initiated through contact with antigens and helper T cells, or by polyclonal mitogens.

The precursors of B cells include a series of cell types that are generated first in the fetal liver and then in bone marrow as hemopoiesis shifts during development [7,8]. Multipotent hemopoietic stem cells give rise to immature pre-B cells that express neither Ig heavy or light chains, although they share surface antigen markers with more mature pre-B and B cells [1,9-12]. The large Ig negative pre-B cells divide to give rise to large pre-B cells with μ-chains in their cytoplasm. The latter in turn divide to produce small pre-B cells with cytoplasmic μ-chains. When postmitotic pre-B cells achieve functional V-J rearrangements of either the kappa- or lambda-gene families, this heralds their conversion into small immature B cells with membrane-bound IgM molecules.

Failure to achieve functional rearrangements of either the heavy- or light-chain genes would result in abortive development of pre-B cells, but the degree of cell wastage occurring within the normal pre-B cell compartment is unknown. We also know very little about mechanisms that regulate changes in transcription and translation of mRNA for the membrane and secretory forms of μ-chains as a function of B-cell differentiation.

Soon after B cells are formed in fetal liver or bone marrow, they enter the circulation and migrate to special areas of residence in spleen, lymph node, Peyer patches, and other secondary lymphoid tissues. In mice, large numbers ($> 10^8$) of B cells are generated each day in the bone marrow, but most live for only a few days after migration to the spleen [9,13]. The kinetics of B-cell generation and traffic appear to be similar in humans [1,14].

B cells display a variety of cell-surface components (Fig. 1), the expression of which can change as they mature, receive stimulation by antigen, and are influenced by T-cell signals to proliferate and differentiate into plasma cells.

The most immature B cells express surface IgM molecules. With further maturation, B cells begin to express surface IgD and other membrane-bound glycoproteins, such as receptors for complement components [7,15,16]. An important feature of newly formed B cells is their ease of inhibition by surface IgM cross-linkage [7,17], whereas the same stimulus can induce mature B cells to enter the cell cycle, enlarge, and proliferate [18-20]. The negative signal received through surface Igs by the immature B cell may represent an important mechanism by which self-antigens abort development of autoreactive clones of B cells. Anti-idiotype antibodies may also selectively abort clones of immature B cells and thus affect development of the B-cell repertoire.

---

*Supported by USPHS grants CA 16673, CA 13148, and RR32, and grant 1-608 from the March of Dimes Birth Defects Foundation.

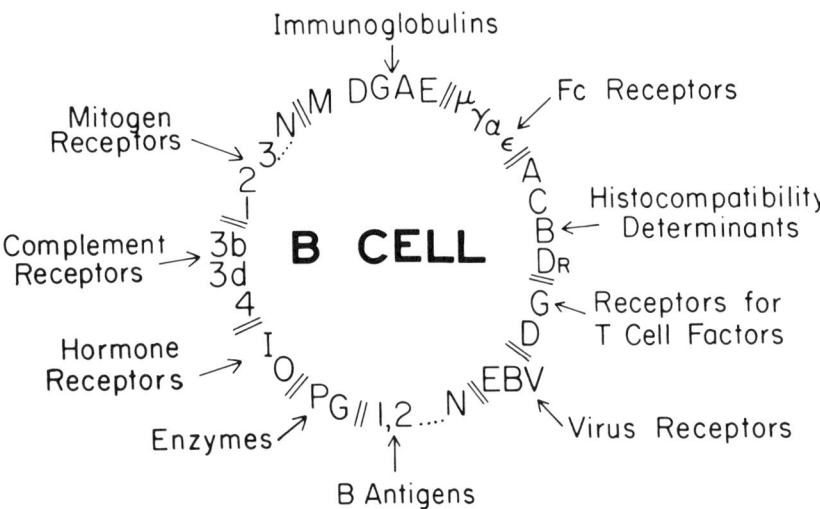

Fig. 1. Schematic model illustrating some of the membrane-bound protein molecules expressed by mature B cells. Symbols used: receptors for insulin (I) and other (O) hormones; phosphorylase (P) and glycosyltransferase (G) enzymes; and receptors for growth (G) and differentiation (D) factors of T-cell origin.

HLA-DR molecules, analogous to Ia in mice, are expressed on the surface of all pre-B and B cells in humans [8,21]. These genetically polymorphic glycoproteins serve as recognition elements in the interaction with activated T cells, a basic requirement for antigen activation of the resting B cell [22]. On antigen interaction with surface antibody molecules and autologous T-cell interaction with Ia, the resting B cell is induced to enlarge and to express receptors for nonantigen-specific T-cell factors that deliver signals for proliferation and differentiation into plasma cells (Fig. 2).

When mature B cells are activated to divide by antigenic stimulation and T-cell help, some members of the clone remain lymphoid and do not undergo terminal plasma cell differentiation. These are called memory B cells, are relatively long-lived, and can be more easily triggered than virgin B cells by subsequent contact with antigen. Memory B cells are responsible for the prompt, heightened antibody responses that occur with a second exposure to antigen. They may exhibit considerable heterogeneity in terms of size, surface Ig isotypes, and expression of other surface components. For example, surface IgD expression is lost by the majority of memory B cells late in the immune response [23]. Similarly, expression of Fc and C3 receptors may not persist on memory B cells [24,25].

The final step in B-cell differentiation is the plasma cell. The progression from activated B lymphocyte is marked by a gradual loss of HLA-DR and surface Ig along with conversion from synthesis of membrane-type to secretory Ig molecules. The capacity to produce and secrete several thousand Ig molecules per second comes with the expense of cell longevity. Plasma cells seldom divide, and they have an estimated lifespan of 2 to 3 days.

POKEWEED-RESPONSIVE B CELLS

One of the most widely used methods for study of human B-cell differentiation has involved the in vitro stimulation of blood mononuclear cells by an extract of the *Phytolacca americana* plant [26]. Pokeweed extract is a polyclonal B- and T-cell mitogen, which can induce differentiation of plasma cells of all isotypes [27-29]. Responsive B cells are present in newborn blood at low frequencies, increase in numbers during infancy, and require non-MHC restricted T-cell help for induction of plasma cell differentiation [30,31]. The T helper (Th) cells can be replaced by their soluble products [27] which include B-cell growth and differentiation factors. Th cells in the pokeweed response can be identified by the monoclonal antibodies, T4 and Leu 3 [32]. Pokeweed mitogen (PWM) responses are negatively

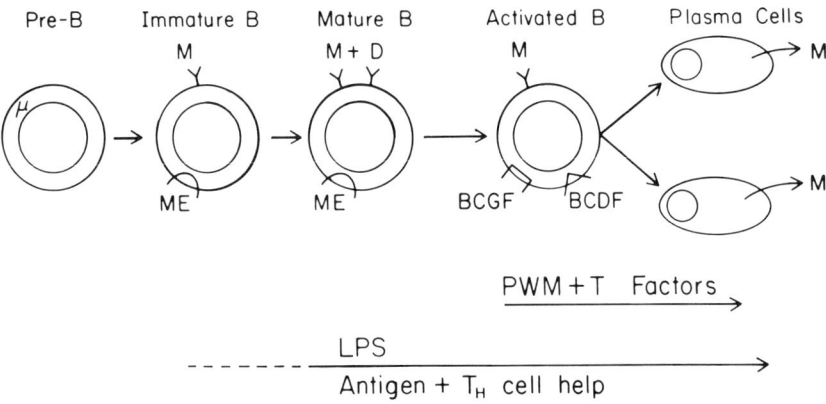

Fig. 2. Model of B-cell differentiation emphasizing some stage-specific features of cell activation. Symbols for receptors on B cells: ME, mouse erythrocyte; BCGF, B-cell growth factors; BCDF, B-cell differentiation factor; LPS, lipopolysaccharide; PWM, pokeweed mitogen.

regulated by suppressor T cells which express the T8 or Leu 2 antigen.

Ontogenetic studies suggest that immature B cells lack responsiveness to PWM [28]. Moreover, even mature B cells that are small resting lymphocytes lack the capacity to respond. B cells that are unresponsive to PWM can also be identified by their relatively high buoyant density and expression of receptors for mouse erythrocytes [33–35]. Many of them express surface IgD and IgM [20,34,35].

On the other hand, the B cells that can respond with plasma cell differentiation to PWM stimulation and T-cell help constitute a relatively small subpopulation of cells with features implying in vivo preactivation [20,33–36]. They are relatively large, buoyant B cells that no longer express surface IgD and receptors for mouse erythrocytes. Although representing many B-cell clones, the repertoire of PWM-responsive B cells reflects prior antigen exposure of the donor [36].

We have used antibodies specific for the human Ig isotypes to examine the surface Igs expressed by the PWM-inducible B-cell precursors of plasma cells [20,35,37,38]. Blood mononuclear cells were cultured with PWM in the presence of monoclonal anti-μ, -δ, -γ, or -α antibodies or they were selectively depleted of IgM, IgD, IgG or IgA B cells before culture and stimulation with PWM. Removal of IgD$^+$ B cells had no demonstrable effect. All of the other monoclonal anti-isotype specific antibodies inhibited PWM-induced differentiation of B cells, but each in a different way. Anti-μ antibody suppressed differentiation not only of IgM plasma cells, but also of IgG and IgA plasma cells in a dose-dependent fashion. Selective depletion of IgM B cells also diminished the number of IgM plasma cells induced by more than 90%, and of IgG and IgA plasma cells by approximately 50%. The addition of monoclonal anti-γ or anti-α antibodies, or removal of IgG or IgA B cells, selectively depleted the precursors of plasma cells producing the homologous IgG or IgA isotype.

Three major subpopulations of PWM-inducible B-cell precursors were thus identified: 1) SIgM$^+$ precursor of IgM plasma cells that do not express IgG or IgA, 2) SIgG$^+$ precursors of IgG plasma cells that may or may not express SIgM but do not express IgA, and 3) SIgA$^+$ precursors of IgA plasma cells that do not express IgG, but approximately half of which express functional IgM receptors. The IgA B-cell subpopulation is further divisible into 2 separate sublines of IgA$_1$ and IgA$_2$ B cells [38,39].

We have also used monoclonal antibodies to examine the IgG subclasses expressed in circulating B cells, their in vivo plasma cell progeny, and their in vitro plasma cell progeny generated in responses to PWM and to LPS [40]. The subclass distribution for circulating IgG B cells was IgG$_2$ (48%) > IgG$_1$ (40%) > IgG$_3$ (8%) > IgG$_4$ (1%), while that for IgG plasma cells in blood, marrow, tonsil, and spleen was IgG$_1$

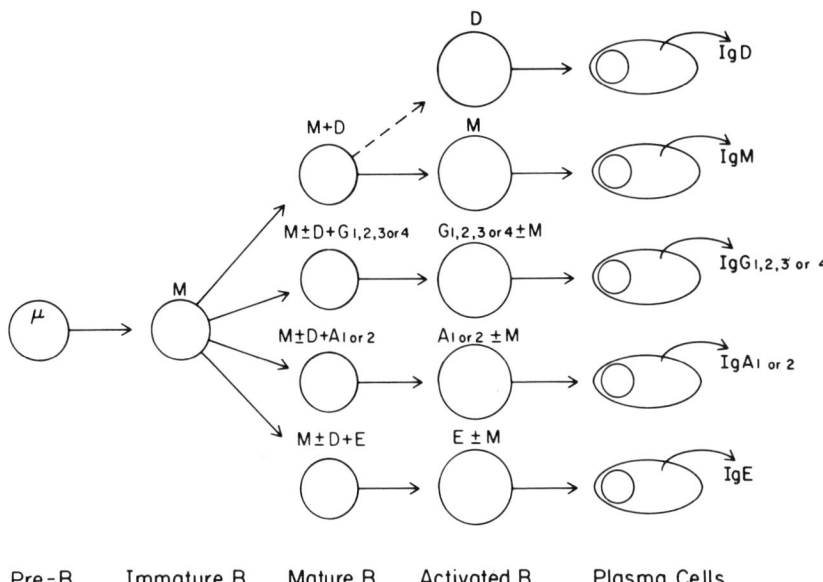

Fig. 3. Generation of Ig isotype diversity as a function of B-cell differentiation in a model clone.

(~64%) > IgG$_2$ (~24%) IgG$_3$ (~10%) > IgG$_4$ (~2%), a distribution pattern similar to that found in normal serum.

These differences in IgG subclass distribution patterns at the B-cell and plasma cell levels imply that regulatory control of the IgG subclass expression may vary according to the stage in B-cell differentiation. It has been shown in mice that T cells can selectively affect the subclass distribution of IgG plasma cells by either helper or suppressor influences [41, 42]. We examined the T-cell influence on human IgG plasma cell responses to both LPS and PWM. Although both polyclonal responses were T-cell dependent, there was a remarkable difference in IgG subclass expression among LPS-induced and PWM-induced plasma cells. In LPS-stimulated cultures, IgG$_2$ plasma cells were predominant (> 80%); IgG$_2$ plasma cells were much less frequent (<20%), and IgG$_3$ and IgG$_4$ plasma cells were rarely found. On the other hand, PWM induced all 4 subclasses of IgG plasma cells with a distribution pattern in perfect concordance with normal serum levels:

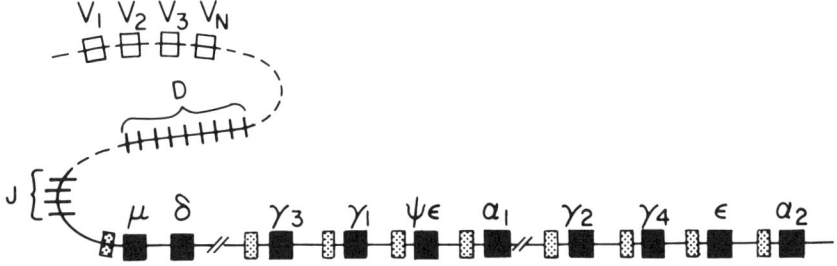

Fig. 4. Map of the Ig heavy-chain genes on chromosome 14 (after Flanagan and Rabbitts, ref. 43). Heavy-chain switch regions are indicated by shaded blocks (▨). Variable region, V; diversity, D; joining, J; constant region genes. ΨE = pseudo-epsilon gene.

$IgG_1 \sim 65\%$, $IgG2 \sim 25\%$, $IgG_3 \sim 8\%$ and $IgG_4 \sim 1\%$. Further analysis revealed that PWM induction of IgG_1 plasma cell differentiation is highly dependent upon T-cell help, while differentiation of IgG_2 plasma cell precursors was less T-cell dependent. We also found that T cells do not direct IgG subclass switching in this model system, but instead, preferentially enhance the differentiation of B-cell subpopulations precommitted to IgG subclass. The way in which T cells exert isotype-specific help is currently being pursued intensively in many laboratories.

MODEL OF IMMUNOGLOBULIN ISOTYPE SWITCHING

The foregoing results are consistent with the model of intraclonal generation of Ig isotype diversity shown in Figure 3. This model illustrates the view that most IgM/IgD cells which switch to the expression of another Ig isotype do so directly rather than by a sequential switch mechanism. The order of the heavy-chain constant region (C_H) genes has now been established for humans (see Fig. 4 and [39]).

The molecular basis for Ig isotype switching (reviewed in refs. [43-45]) involves the joining of a switch region of highly repetitive DNA sequences 5' to the μ-gene with a similar switch region 5' to a downstream C_H gene. The intervening DNA is deleted either by excision or by sister chromatid exchange. The mechanism responsible for regulating the isotype switches has not been elucidated yet. The X-linked inheritance of a defect in Ig-isotype switching ([46] and our unpublished observations) suggests that one important regulatory gene is on the X chromosome. Studies of the heavy chains expressed in pre-B cell leukemias suggest that heavy chain switching may occur in a stochastic fashion and that this is not a random process determined simply by the order of the C_H genes [47].

CONCLUSION

While the features of B-cell differentiation have been sufficiently well outlined to serve as a useful guide for the analysis of defects in antibody production, many important details of this complex process are still not understood. Studies of the defects in B-cell differentiation occurring in immunodeficient individuals should continue to provide important clues toward elucidation of normal features of B-cell clonal diversification, activation, growth, and differentiation.

ACKNOWLEDGMENTS

I thank my colleagues for sharing their ideas and data with me, Ann Brookshire for typing the manuscript, and Maxine Aycock for preparing the illustrations.

REFERENCES

1. Cooper MD: Pre-B cells: Normal and abnormal development. J Clin Immunol 1:81, 1981.
2. Davis MM, Calame K, Early PW, Livant DL, Joho R, Weissman IL, Hood L: An immunoglobulin heavy chain is formed by at least two recombinatorial events. Nature 283:733, 1980.
3. Sakano H, Maki R, Kurosawa Y, Roeder W, Tonegawa S: Two types of somatic recombination are necessary for the generation of complete immunoglobulin heavy chain genes. Nature 286:676, 1980.
4. Maki R, Kearney JF, Paige C, Tonegawa S: Immunoglobulin gene rearrangements in immature B cells. Science 209:1366, 1980.
5. Hieter PA, Korsmeyer S, Waldmann TA, Leder P: Human immunoglobulin light chain genes are deleted or rearranged in λ-producing B cells. Nature 290:368, 1981.
6. Coleclough C, Perry RP, Karjalainen K, Weigert M: Aberrant rearrangements contribute significantly to the allelic exclusion of immunoglobulin gene expression. Nature 290:372, 1981.
7. Gathings WE, Lawton AR, Cooper MD: Immunofluorescent studies of the development of pre-B cells, B lymphocytes, and immunoglobulin isotype diversity in humans. Eur J Immunol 7:804, 1977.
8. Owen JJT, Wright DE, Habu S, Raff MC, Cooper MD: Studies on the generation of B lymphocytes in fetal liver and bone marrow. J Immunol 118:2067, 1977.
9. Osmond DG: Production and differentiation of B lymphocytes in the bone marrow. In Battisto JR, Knight KL (eds): "Immunoglobulin Genes and B Cell Differentiation." New York: Elsevier/North-Holland, 1980, p 135.
10. Kamps WA, Cooper MD: Microenvironmental studies of pre-B and B cell development in human and mouse fetuses. J Immunol 129:526, 1982.
11. Landreth KS, Rosse C, Clagett J: Myelogenous production and maturation of B lymphocytes in the mouse. J Immunol 127:2027, 1981.
12. Kincade PW: Formation of B lymphocytes in fetal and adult life. Adv Immunol 31:177, 1981.
13. DeFreitas AA, Coutinho A: Very rapid decay of mature B lymphocytes in the spleen. J Exp Med 154:994, 1981.
14. Pearl ER, Vogler LB, Okos AJ, Crist WM, Lawton AR, Cooper MD: B lymphocyte precursors in human bone marrow. An analysis of normal individuals and patients with antibody deficiency states. J Immunol 120:1169, 1978.

15. Kearney JF, Cooper MD, Klein J, Abney ER, Parkhouse RME, Lawton AR: Ontogeny of Ia and IgD on IgM bearing lymphocytes in mice. J Exp Med 146:297, 1977.
16. Gelfand MC, Elfenbein GJ, Frank MM, Paul WE: Ontogeny of B lymphocytes. II. Relative rate of appearance of lymphocytes bearing surface immunoglobulin and complement receptors. J Exp Med 139:1128, 1974.
17. Raff MC, Owen JJT, Cooper MD, Lawton AR III, Megson M, Gathings WE: Differences in susceptibility of mature and immature mouse B lymphocytes to anti-immunoglobulin-induced immunoglobulin suppression in vitro: Possible implications for B-cell tolerance to self. J Exp Med 142:1052, 1975.
18. DeFranco AL, Raveche ES, Asofsky R, Paul WE: Frequency of B lymphocytes responsive to anti-immunoglobulin. J Exp Med 155:1523, 1982.
19. Chiorazzi N, Fu SM, Kunkel HG: Stimulation of human lymphocytes by antibodies to IgM and IgG: Functional evidence for the expression of IgG or B-lymphocyte surface membranes. Clin Immunol Immunopathol 15:301, 1980.
20. Kuritani T, Cooper MD: Human B cell differentiation. III. Enhancing effect of monoclonal anti-immunoglobulin D antibody on pokeweed mitogen-induced plasma cell differentiation. J Immunol 129:2490, 1982.
21. Winchester RJ, Fu SM, Wernet P, Kunkel HG, Dupont B, Jersild C: Recognition by pregnancy serums of non-HLA alloantigens selectively expressed on B lymphocytes. J Exp Med 141:924, 1975.
22. Melchers F, Anderson J, Lernhardt W, Schreier MH: Roles of surface-bound immunoglobulin molecules in regulating the replication and maturation to immunoglobulin secretion of B lymphocytes. Immunol Rev 52:89, 1970.
23. Black SJ, van der Loo W, Loken MR, Herzenberg LA: Expression of IgD by murine lymphocytes. Loss of surface IgD indicates maturation of memory B cells. J Exp Med 147:984, 1978.
24. Dickler H: Lymphocyte receptors for immunoglobulin. Adv Immunol 24:167, 1976.
25. Lewis GK, Ranken R, Nitecki DE, Goodman JW: Murine subpopulations responsive to T-dependent and T-independent antigens. J Exp Med 144:382, 1976.
26. Barker BE, Farnes P, Fanger H: Mitogenic activity in *Phytolacca americana* (pokeweed). Lancet 1:170, 1965.
27. Janossy G, Greaves M: Functional analysis of murine and human B-lymphocyte subsets. Transplant Rev 24:177, 1975.
28. Wu LYF, Lawton AR, Cooper MD: Differentiation capacity of cultured B lymphocytes from immunodeficient patients. J Clin Invest 52:3180, 1973.
29. Waldmann TA, Broder S, Blaese RM, Durm M, Blackman M, Strober W: Role of suppressor T cells in pathogenesis of common variable hypogammaglobulinemia. Lancet 2:609, 1974.
30. Wu LYF, Blanco A, Cooper MD, Lawton AR: Ontogeny of B-lymphocyte differentiation induced by pokeweed mitogen. Clin Immunol Immunopathol 5:208, 1976.
31. Keightley RG, Cooper MD, Lawton AR: The T cell dependence of B cell differentiation induced by pokeweed mitogen. J Immunol 117:1538, 1976.
32. Reinherz EL, Schlossman SF: Regulation of the immune response-inducer and suppressor T-lymphocyte subsets in human beings. N Engl J Med 303:370, 1980.
33. Dagg M, Levitt D: Human B lymphocyte subpopulations. I. Differentiation of density-separated B lymphocytes. Clin Immunol Immunopathol 21:3, 1981.
34. Lucivero G, Lawton AR, Cooper MD: Rosette formation with mouse erythrocytes defines a population of human B lymphocytes unresponsive to pokeweed mitogen. Clin Exp Immunol 45:185, 1981.
35. Kuritani T, Cooper MD: Human B cell differentiation. II. Pokeweed mitogen-responsive B cells belong to a surface immunoglobulin D-negative subpopulation. J Exp Med 155:1561, 1982.
36. Findlay GJ, Booth RJ, Marbrook J: Antibody responses of human lymphocytes in vitro. Specificity and physical properties of plaque-forming cell precursors. Aust J Exp Biol Med 57:587, 1979.
37. Lucivero G, Lawton AR, Cooper MD: Pokeweed mitogen-induced differentiation of human peripheral blood B lymphocytes. II. Suppression of plasma cell differentiation by heavy chain specific antibodies and development of immunoglobulin as class restriction. Human Lymphocyte Differentiation 1:27, 1981.
38. Kuritani T, Cooper MD: Human B cell differentiation. I. Analysis of immunoglobulin heavy chain switching using monoclonal anti-immunoglobulin M, G and A antibodies and pokeweed mitogen-induced plasma cell differentiation. J Exp Med 155:839, 1982.
39. Conley ME, Kearney JF, Lawton AR III, Cooper MD: Differentiation of human B cells expressing the IgA subclasses as demonstrated by monoclonal hybridoma antibodies. J Immunol 125:2311, 1980.
40. Mayumi M, Kuritani T, Kubagawa H, Cooper MD: IgG subclass expression by human B lymphocytes and plasma cells: B lymphocytes precommitted to IgG subclass can be preferentially induced by polyclonal mitogens with T cell help. J Immunol 130:671, 1983.
41. Mongini PKA, Stein KE, Paul WE: T cell regulation of IgG subclass antibody production in response to T-independent antigens. J Exp Med 155:839, 1982.
42. Lowy I, Joskowicz M, Theze J: Characterization of suppressor cells regulating in vitro expression of IgG_{2a} and IgG_{2b} antibody responses. J Immunol 128:768, 1982.
43. Flanagan JG, Rabbitts TH: Arrangement of human immunoglobulin heavy chain constant region genes implies evolutionary duplication of a segment containing γ, ϵ and α genes. Nature 300:709, 1982.
44. Honjo T: The molecular mechanisms of the immunoglobulin class switch. Immunol Today 3:214, 1982.
45. Marcu KB, Cooper MD: New views of the immunoglobulin heavy-chain switch. Nature 298:327, 1982.
46. Geha RS, Hyslop N, Alami S, Farah F, Schneeberger EE, Rosen FS: Hyper immunoglobulin M immunodeficiency (dysgammaglobulinemia). Presence of immunoglobulin M-secreting plasmacytoid cells in peripheral blood and failure of immunoglobulin M-immunoglobulin G switch in B cell differentiation. J Clin Invest 64:385, 1979.
47. Kubagawa H, Mayumi M, Crist WM, Cooper MD: Immunoglobulin heavy chain switching in pre-B leukemias. Nature 301:340, 1983.

The Regulation of the Human Humoral Immune Response and Functional Assays for Its Assessment

Thomas A. Waldmann, MD

National Cancer Institute, NIH, Bethesda, MD 20205

The application of the techniques of molecular biology, the functional assays for B-cell, helper T-cell, and suppressor T-cell activity and the phenotypic analysis of T-cell surface antigens using monoclonal antibodies to the study of patients with primary immunodeficiency diseases and to those with lymphocytic leukemias has led to major insights concerning the molecular events and cellular interactions that control the human immune response and the disorders in these processes that occur in disease. These studies have led to a more rational classification of the Ig deficiency diseases and have provided the scientific basis for more effective therapeutic approaches to these diseases. The regulation of Ig synthesis can be divided conveniently into 2 broad phases: 1) the control of the maturation of stem cells into B cells, and 2) the regulation of the terminal maturation of B lymphocytes into Ig-secreting plasma cells, a process controlled by a complex network of regulatory T cells. In the first phase, there is a carefully orchestrated series of rearrangements of Ig genes that occur as an uncommitted stem cell matures into a B cell that has a specific commitment to respond to a particular antigen [1-7]. Human Ig genes in their embryonic or germ-line state exist as discontinuous gene segments. For example, Ig heavy-chain genes are separated in the germ line into variable (V_H), diversity (D_H), and joining (J_H) regions as well as distinguishing constant region genes [2-4]. During differentiation, as a cell matures from a pluripotent stem cell into a terminally differentiated plasma cell, there is an initial rearrangement of DNA to combine a D_H region with a specific J_H region and then with a V_H gene to form an active heavy-chain gene. Subsequently, there is a corresponding joining of a light-chain variable (V_L) region gene with an appropriate joining (J_L) region gene to activate a light-chain gene [1,5-7]. This system of gene rearrangements provides great versatility and represents one of the mechanisms for generating antibody diversity. However, it is a very error prone system; frequently, there are nonproductive rearrangements that do not code for an effective long-lived Ig chain.

We have applied radiolabeled probes complementary to the constant, joining, and diversity region genes of heavy chains and the constant and joining region genes of kappa and lambda light-chains to the analysis of the Ig gene rearrangements that occur in lymphocytic leukemias and cloned cultured lines of normal and leukemic B-cell, T-cell and non-T, non-B-cell phenotypes [6,7]. All B-cell populations studied had at least one effective rearrangement of the heavy-chain genes and, in 80% of cases, a nonproductive rearrangement as well. In addition, all kappa expressing B-cell populations had cells with an effective kappa gene rearrangement on chromosome 2. Lambda expressing B cells not only had a rearrangement of the lambda genes on chromosome 22 but also had a nonproductive rearrangement or deletion of all kappa constant region genes on chromosome 2 in all cases as well [5-7]. In contrast to the gene rearrangements that occurred in all B cells, the human T-cell leukemias and lines examined displayed no rearrangements of their light-chain genes and, in 90% of cases, had germ-line configurations of their heavy-chain constant and joining region genes as well [6,7]. In order to obtain more information on the order of gene rearrangements, we analyzed the arrangement of Ig genes in leukemias of precursor cells, that is non-T, non-B acute lymphocytic leukemia cells that did not bear surface immunoglubulin (SIg), that did not form rosettes with sheep red blood cells (SRBC) and that did not react with anti-T-cell antibodies [6,7]. All 25 of these acute non-T-cell lymphocytic leukemia populations had Ig gene rearrangements suggesting that these cells were in the B-cell precursor series. Eleven of the 25 cases had rearrangements of heavy-chain genes but not of the light-chain genes. Since there were no cases with rearrangements of light-chain genes without rearrangements of heavy-chain genes, it appears that heavy-chain gene rearrangements precede those of light-chain genes. A few of these leukemic cell populations had rearrangements of both sets of heavy-chain genes without producing heavy-chain proteins. These cells may have had aberrant rearrangements of V_H, D_H, and J_H genes on both relevant chromosomes and may have deleted the required D segment material and the flanking recombinational sequences and spaces required

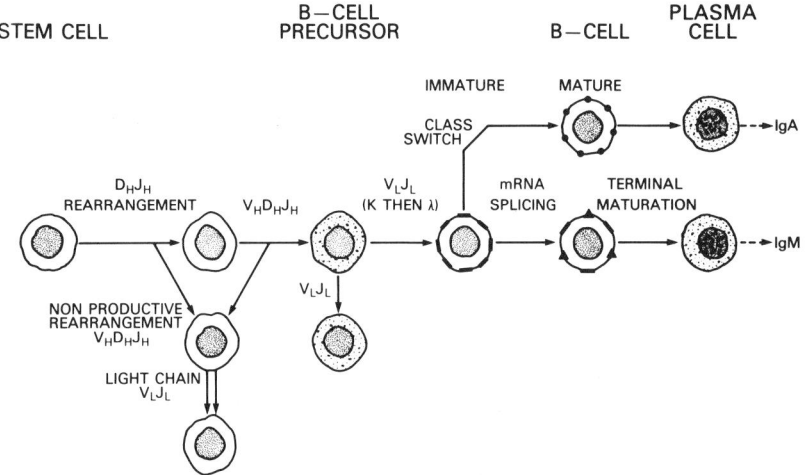

Fig. 1. The gene rearrangements that occur as a stem cell matures into a plasma cell. Cells with effective gene rearrangements on the pathway toward the development of plasma cell, as well as those with aberrant rearrangements on both relevant chromosomes that are unable to mature further along the B-cell pathway, are outlined.

to produce an Ig molecule and, therefore, may be "frozen" in the B-cell precursor stage of maturation. The patterns of gene rearrangements that we have observed in leukemic B cells and B-cell precursors suggest a hierarchy of gene rearrangements with heavy-chain gene rearrangements always preceding light-chain gene rearrangements and kappa-gene rearrangements, and deletions preceding lambda-gene rearrangements. The gene rearrangements that occur in the development of a plasma cell from a stem cell are reviewed in Figure 1. The first gene rearrangement committing a stem cell to the B-cell series occurs on chromosome 14 and brings together a D_H and a J_H segment. The subsequent gene rearrangement brings a V_H segment in contact with the joined D_H and J_H segments. Following such effective heavy-chain gene rearrangements, the cell can develop into a classic pre-B cell with μ-chains demonstrable in its cytoplasm. Subsequently, there is a rearrangement of the V_L and J_L light-chain gene segments to activate a light-chain gene and permit the production of a complete Ig molecule, and thus lead to the development of an immature B cell with IgM on its cell surface. To develop further along the pathway toward an IgA-producing plasma cell, there is a switch of heavy-chain isotype by one of a number of genetic mechanisms leading to the development of a mature B cell with IgA among other isotypes on its surface. Such IgA-bearing B cells can be induced to terminal maturation into IgA-producing plasma cells. This maturation is accompanied by the conversion of the cell from one that synthesizes the membrane form of IgA with a transmembrane hydrophobic peptide sequence into the secretory form of IgA that has another nonhydrophobic carboxyterminus. This conversion involves an alteration in the site of splicing of messenger RNA for the IgA heavy-chain peptide.

The terminal maturation of immature B cells into Ig-synthesizing plasma cells is a process that is very carefully regulated by different sets of T cells, as outlined in Figure 2. One set of T cells, termed switch T cells, may play a role in the final switch of a B cell with membrane IgM into a cell with another isotype, such as IgA, on its surface [8]. In addition, at least 2 subsets of helper or inducer T cells exist that facilitate the terminal maturation of B cells [9]. These 2 helper cells differ in terms of their radiosensitivity, in terms of their binding to nylon wool columns, and in terms of their manifestation of certain antigens such as the inducible receptor for T-cell growth factor or interleukin-2 (TCGF or IL-2) on their cell surface following activation [9]. A distinct population of T cells that emerges from the thymus as prosuppressor cells that can be induced to mature into effectors of suppression following interaction with a radiosensitive inducer population acts to inhibit B-cell maturation and Ig synthesis [10–11].

Theoretically, one may have a defect of Ig synthesis due to an intrinsic B-cell defect, due to a deficiency of Th cells or due to excessive activity of a cell in the suppressor series. Many approaches have been used to analyze these defects. In our own studies we have emphasized short-term in vitro culture techniques where we quantitate Ig synthesis by mononuclear cells stimulated by polyclonal activators of B cells that differ in terms of their requirements for Th cells and monocytes, and in terms of their propensity to activate prosuppressor cells into effectors of suppression [12–15]. I would like to start by considering the use of assays for detecting helper cell deficiency. The criteria that we use to conclude that a helper cell deficiency is the cause of a primary immunodeficiency disease include: 1) absence or markedly reduced helper cell activity by purified T cells of the patient when they are co-cultured with normal B cells and a T-cell-dependent polyclonal activator such as PWM; 2) normal Ig synthesis by the patient's B cells and normal T cells when they are cultured with a T-cell-dependent polyclonal activator such as PWM and normal Ig synthesis of the patient's B cells when they are cultured alone with a Th-cell-independent activator, such as the Epstein-Barr virus (EBV). We have seen such a pattern in pa-

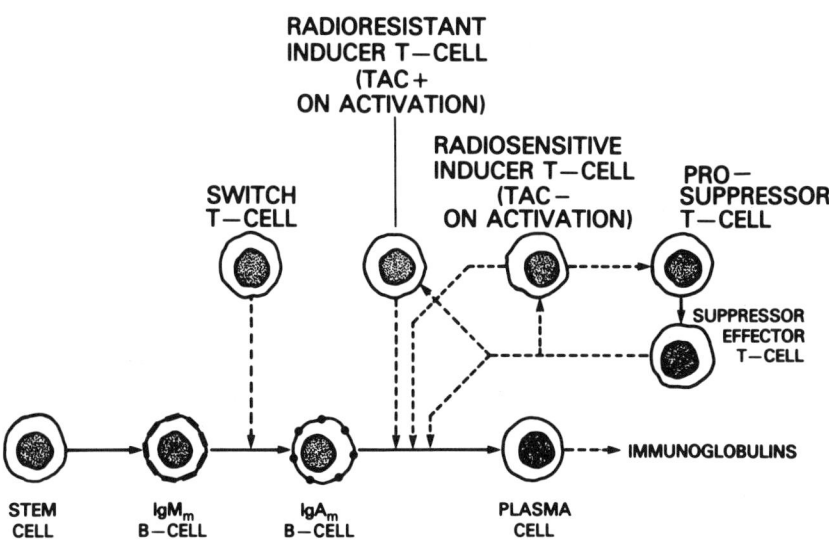

Fig. 2. The regulatory network of T cells that control B-cell isotype switching and the terminal maturation of B lymphocytes into Ig synthesizing and secreting plasma cells.

tients who have SCID with normal numbers of B cells. Ig deficiency may also occur due to an intrinsic defect of B cells. Our criteria for concluding that a B-cell defect is the sole cause of an immunodeficiency are: 1) rigorously T-cell and monocyte-depleted B cells of the patient should be unable to produce Ig molecules normally when cultured with a Th-cell-independent activator such as the EBV, and 2) that the B cells of the patient should not produce Igs normally when cultured with normal T cells, monocytes, and a Th-cell-dependent polyclonal activator.

Patients with ataxia telangiectasia (AT) have a complex defect that includes a defect of Th cells as well as a B-cell defect [16]. The analysis of these defects may aid in illustrating the approaches for detecting Th-cell and intrinsic B-cell defects. The majority of patients studied with AT had T cells that provided diminished Th-cell activity when co-cultured with normal B cells with helper cell activity equal to 22% of that provided by normal allogeneic T cells [16]. The peripheral blood cells of each of the patients had at least some helper cell activity. To clarify the role of the potential Th-cell defect further, we determined the effect of the addition of irradiated normal T cells to the PWM-stimulated unseparated cells from patients with AT. In the majority of cases, the addition of normal T cells to the mononuclear cells from AT patients led to an augmentation of IgG and IgM synthesis, and for those patients who had detectable serum IgA for IgA as well. However, there was no IgA synthesis, either before or after the addition of the normal T cells, by the cultures of unseparated mononuclear cells of patients with AT who had no demonstrable serum IgA. On the basis of these results we conclude that a Th- cell defect contributes to the immunoglobulin deficiency seen in AT but is clearly not the sole defect, and that another defect contributes to the immunodeficiency. We showed that such patients have a B-cell defect that plays a role in their Ig deficiency [16]. As noted above, patients with AT with no serum IgA did not synthesize IgA in the presence of normal T cells and PWM. Furthermore, these patients with a profound IgA deficiency were unable to make IgA molecules in vitro when stimulated with a relatively Th-cell-independent activator, Nocardia water-soluble mitogen, or with the completely Th-cell-independent activator, EBV. EBV-induced B-cell lines from such patients did not synthesize IgA molecules. Thus, the patients with AT appear to have both a Th- and B-cell defect that underlie their IgA deficiency. Such a broad defect of lymphocyte maturation, taken in conjunction with the demonstration of immaturity of the thymus, ovaries, and testes [17–19], and our demonstration that patients with AT have the persistent production of alpha-fetoprotein [20], supports our view that they have a generalized defect in organ maturation.

Before leaving the Th-cell system entirely, I would like to present our criteria for concluding that certain neoplastic T cells have Th-cell activity. Helper activity for B-cell maturation should be demonstrable when the neoplastic T cells are co-cultured with rigorously T-cell-depleted normal B cells and a Th-cell-dependent activator. These co-cultures should be performed at low neoplastic T-cell to normal B-cell ratios to rule out potential helper activity provided by nonneoplastic normal T cells that could contaminate the neoplastic T-cell preparations. As we have shown previously, Sezary cells from some, but not all, patients frequently fulfill these criteria [13]. These leukemic T-cell populations should be examined for their capacity to synthesize B-cell growth factor, B-cell differentiation factor, and T-cell replacing factors in light of the fact that they can help B cells in a genetically unrestricted polyclonal fashion.

Another potential cause of immunoglobulin deficiency is excessive suppressor cell activity. Minimal criteria to define excessive suppressor T-cell activity as a cause of immunodeficiency include: 1) there should be suppression of Ig synthesis by the patient's mononuclear cells when co-cultured with normal B cells and T cells at physiologic T-cell to B-cell ratios; 2) the patient's B cells depleted of suppressor cells should produce Igs when co-cultured with polyclonal activators and normal T cells or autologous Th cells; and 3) suppression of Ig synthesis should be observed when the patient's unseparated T cells are reintroduced into these latter cultures of the patient's B cells and autologous Th cells. We have seen these minimal criteria fulfilled in the 6 patients examined who represent a subset of patients with common variable hypogammaglobulinemia with increased suppressor cell activity [12,21].

I would like to continue the discussion of suppressor T cells by considering a very instructive leukemia, the adult T-cell leukemia initially described in Japan by Uchiyama, Takatsuki, and co-workers [22]. This is a leukemia of mature T cells with pleomorphic nuclei that infiltrate the skin. The adult T-cell leukemia has been associated with a new unique type C retrovirus described by Gallo and co-workers [23], whereas, in most cases, patients with the Sezary T-cell leukemia do not have circulating antibodies to this virus [24]. In contrast to the Sezary leukemic T cells, the adult T-cell leukemic cells do not provide helper activity when co-cultured with normal B cells. Furthermore, the cells of 6 of the 9 patients examined suppressed the Ig synthesis of normal indicator PWM-stimulated B cells and irradiated T cells when co-cultured with them. Furthermore, culture supernatants from lines from some such leukemic populations suppressed Ig synthesis without affecting T-cell proliferation.

Over the past few years, great advances have been made in the correlation of cell surface phenotypes as identified by monoclonal antibodies with the functions of T-cell populations [25–30]. Most of the leukemic T-cell populations with retained functions have reacted with an antibody termed T3 that defines mature T cells. Certain leukemic cells that were not discussed, which suppress immune responses, react with an antibody termed T8, whereas helper leukemic cells react with an antibody termed T4. However, when we applied these monoclonal antibodies to the study of the Sezary leukemic cells and the adult T-cell leukemic cells, these antibodies were not of value in differentiating these 2 types of leukemias with different immunoregulatory functions. Both of these functional leukemic cell populations bore the maturation antigen T3. In addition, both of the cell populations bore the T4 antigen that has usually been associated with Th-cell activity, and neither of the leukemic cell populations manifested the T8 antigen that is usually associated with suppressor activity. Clearly the use of monoclonal antibodies for the definition of T-cell surface phenotypes in patients with these immunodeficiency diseases or with leukemias has been of great value, but such reactivity with monoclonals is not sufficient to predict the regulatory T-cell defects or functions that are associated with these diseases. For example, the data that I have just presented, as well as data emerging from many laboratories [28–30], support the view that cells defined by the T4 and T8 antibodies are quite complex populations that are not solely inducer or suppressor/cytotoxic populations, respectively [28–30]. This body of data supports the alternative view that these cells may differ, not in terms of function per se, but in terms of the class of antigen with which the T cells interact; that is, T8 cells appear to be involved in those cellular interactions and functions that are controlled by class I molecules (HLA-A or B molecules), whereas T4-positive cells appear to be involved in interactions that are concerned with class II molecules (ie HLA-DR). In this scheme T4 cells would not only be helper cells in their interactions with other lymphoid cells but would also act as suppressor or cytotoxic cells when HLA-DR type molecules are involved. Thus, the use of reactivity of lymphoid cells with monoclonal antibodies such as T4 or T8 antibodies to define the functional status of the immunoregulatory circuit may lead to erroneous interpretations unless functional assays are performed as well.

I would like to conclude by discussing a monoclonal antibody termed anti-Tac which we have developed that reacts with a 55,000 dalton glycosylated membrane protein that appears to be the receptor for T-cell growth factor (TCGF or IL-2), and that appears to differentiate the Sezary helper from the adult T-cell suppressor leukemic cells [9,31,32]. The evidence that supports the view that anti-Tac reacts with the TCGF receptor includes: 1) both anti-TAC and TCGF bind to activated T cells and TCGF-dependent T-cell lines but not to monocytes, resting T cells or TCGF-independent T-cell lines; 2) anti-Tac inhibits the proliferation of TCGF-dependent T-cell lines but not that of TCGF-independent T-cell lines or EBV-induced B-cell lines; and 3) anti-Tac inhibits the binding of radiolabeled TCGF to its receptor on TCGF-dependent cultured T-cell lines. The human T-cell leukemia/lymphoma virus (HTLV) associated adult T-cell leukemia cells differed from the HTLV-negative Sezary cells in terms of their reactivity with anti-Tac antibodies. The leukemic cells of all 11 patients with the adult T-cell leukemia studied reacted with the anti-Tac antibody, whereas the leukemic cells of 9 of the 10 HTLV-negative Sezary patients were not reactive with this monoclonal. Thus, the ATL cells that react with the anti-Tac antibody appear to have an activated receptor for TCGF. The fact that the ATL cells have an active receptor for TCGF may have implications for our understanding of the pathogenesis of this leukemic transformation and the continued proliferation of these T cells. The infection of mature T cells with HTLV appears to lead to the production of TCGF and to the activation of a receptor for this growth factor. This production of TCGF, and the activation of a receptor for this factor, may play an important role in the pathogenesis of the uncontrolled growth of these neoplastic cells. When anti-Tac was added to cultured leukemic cells from ATL patients in the presence of complement the cells were killed; in the absence of complement there was an inhibition of the growth of those leukemic cell lines that still required exogenous TCGF. In light of these observations, we have initiated trials to determine the efficacy of intravenously administered anti-Tac antibodies in the treatment of patients with Tac-positive adult T-cell leukemia. The anti-Tac antibodies have greater specificity for the leukemic cells than do most monoclonals used in the therapy of T-cell leukemia since the leukemic cells are Tac-antigen-positive, whereas normal resting T cells are Tac-antigen-negative. Furthermore, should the anti-Tac monoclonal lead to the modulation of the TCGF receptor from the leukemic cells, these cells would no longer bear this receptor that may be required for the growth of these cells.

CONCLUSION

The development of an antigen-committed B cell from a pluripotent stem cell involves a hierarchical series of Ig gene rearrangements with heavy-chain gene rearrangements preceding light-chain gene rearrangements, and kappa gene rearrangements preceding lambda light-chain gene rearrangements. A series of assay systems using polyclonal activators of B cells as well as antigen-specific antibody systems have been developed to aid in defining the regulatory network that controls the terminal maturation of B cells and to categorize Ig deficiencies as disorders of the B cells, helper T cells or as abnormalities of the suppressor T-cell network.

REFERENCES

1. Hieter PA, Max EE, Seidman JG, Maizel JV, Leder P: Cloned human and mouse kappa immunoglobulin constant and J region genes conserve homology in functional segments. Cell 22:197–207, 1980.
2. Early P, Huang H, Davis M, Calame K, Hood L: An immunoglobulin heavy chain variable region gene is generated from three segments of DNA V_H, D_H and J_H. Cell 22:918–920, 1980.
3. Kataoka T, Kawakami T, Takahashi H, Honjo T: Rearrangement of immunoglobulin gamma 1-chain gene and mechanism for heavy-chain class switch. Proc Natl Acad Sci USA 77:919–923, 1980.
4. Sakano H, Maki R, Kunsawa Y, Roeder W, Tonegawa S: Two types of somatic recombination are necessary for the generation of complete immunoglobulin heavy-chain genes. Nature 286:676–683, 1980.
5. Hieter PA, Korsmeyer SJ, Waldmann TA, Leder P: Human immunoglobulin kappa light chain genes are deleted or rearranged in lambda producing B-cells. Nature 290:368–372, 1981.
6. Korsmeyer SJ, Hieter PA, Ravetch JV, Poplack DG, Waldmann TA, Leder P: A development hierarchy of immunoglobulin gene rearrangements in human leukemic pre-B-cells. Proc Natl Acad Sci USA 78:7096–7100, 1981.
7. Korsmeyer SJ, Arnold A, Bakhshi A, Ravetch JV, Siebenlist U, Hieter PA, Sharrow SO, LeBien TW, Kersey JH, Poplack DG, Leder P, Waldmann TA: Immunoglobulin gene rearrangement and cell surface antigen expression of acute lymphocytic leukemias of T-cell and B-cell precursor origin. J Clin Invest 71(2):301–313,1983.
8. Kawanishi H, Saltzman LE, Strober W: Characteristics and regulatory function of murine Con A-induced, cloned T cells obtained from Peyer's patches and spleen: Mechanisms regulating isotype-specific immunoglobulin production by Peyer's patch B cells. J Immunol 129:475–483, 1982.
9. Uchiyama T, Nelson DL, Fleisher T, Waldmann TA: A monoclonal antibody (anti-Tac) reactive with activated and functionally mature T cells. II. Expression of Tac antigen on activated cytotoxic T cells, suppressor cells and on one of two types of helper T cells. J Immunol 126:1398–1403, 1981.
10. Gershon RK: T cell control of antibody production. In Cooper MD, Warner NL (eds): "Contemporary Topics in Immunobiology." New York, London: Plenum Press, 1974, vol 3, pp 1–40.
11. Waldmann TA, Broder S: Suppressor cells in the regulation of the immune response. In Schwartz RS (ed): "Progress in Clinical Immunology." New York: Grune & Stratton, 1977, vol 3, pp 155–199.
12. Waldmann TA, Broder S, Blaese RM, Durm M, Blackman M, Strober W: Role of suppressor T cells in pathogenesis of common variable hypogammaglobulinemia. Lancet 2:609–613, 1976.
13. Broder S, Edelson RL, Lutzner MA, Nelson DL, MacDermott RP, Durm ME, Goldman CK, Meade BD, Waldmann TA: The Sezary syndrome: A malignant proliferation of helper T cells. J Clin Invest 58:1297–1306, 1976.
14. Broder S, Poplack D, Whang-Peng J, Durm M, Goldman C, Muul L, Waldmann TA: Characterization of a suppressor cell leukemia: Evidence for the requirement of an interaction of two T cells in the development of human suppressor effector cells. N Engl J Med 298:66–72, 1978.
15. Waldmann TA, Broder S: Polyclonal activators in the study of the regulation of immunoglobulin synthesis in the human system. In Kunkel H, Dixon FJ (eds): "Advances in Immunology." New York: Academic Press, 1982, vol 32, pp 1–63.
16. Waldmann TA, Broder S, Goldman CK, Frost K, Korsmeyer SJ, Medici MA: Disorders of B cells and helper T cells in the pathogenesis of the immunoglobulin deficiency of patients with ataxia-telangiectasia. J Clin Invest 71(2):282–295, 1983.
17. Peterson RDA, Kelley WD, Good RA: Ataxia-telangiectasia: Its association with a defective thymus, immunological-deficiency disease, and malignancy. Lancet 1:1189–1193, 1964.
18. Boder E: Ataxia-telangiectasia: Some historic, clinical, and pathologic observations. In Bergsma D, Good RA, Finstad J (eds): "Immunodeficiency in Man and Animals." Sunderland, Massachusetts: Sinauer for the National Foundation–March of Dimes, BD:OAS XI(1):255–270, 1975.
19. McFarlin DD, Strober W, Waldmann TA: Ataxia-telangiectasia. Medicine 51:281–314, 1972.
20. Waldmann TA, McIntire KR: Serum-alpha-fetoprotein levels in patients with ataxia-telangiectasia. Lancet 2:1112–1115, 1972.
21. Waldmann TA, Broder S, Goldman CK, Marshall S, Muul L: Suppressor cells in common variable immunodeficiency. In Seligmann M, Hitzig W (eds): "Primary Immunodeficiencies. Inserm Symposium Series No. 16." Amsterdam: Elsevier North-Holland Biomedical Press, 1980, pp 119–128.

22. Uchiyama T, Yodoi J, Sagawa K, Takatsuki K, Uchino H: Adult T cell leukemia: Clinical and hematologic features of 16 cases. Blood 50:481–492, 1977.
23. Gallo RC, Popovic M, Ruscetti FW, Wainberg MA, Royston I, Reitz MS Jr, Broder S, Robert-Guroff M: Interaction of T cell growth factor and a new retrovirus (HTLV) with human T cells. In Fox CF (ed): "Differentiation and Function of Hematopoietic Cell Surfaces." New York: Alan R. Liss, 1982, pp 231–246.
24. Gallo RC, Wong-Staal F: Retroviruses as etiologic agents of some animal and human leukemias and lymphomas and as tools for elucidating the molecular mechanism of leukemogenesis. Blood 60:545–557, 1982.
25. Reinherz EL, Kung PC, Goldstein G, Schlossman SF: Separation of functional subsets of human T cells by a monoclonal antibody. Proc Natl Acad Sci USA 76:4061–4065, 1979.
26. Reinherz EL, Kung PC, Goldstein G, Schlossman SF: A monoclonal antibody reactive with the human cytotoxic/suppressor T cell subset previously defined by hetero-antiserum termed TH_2. J Immunol 124:1301–1307, 1980.
27. Reinherz EL, Kung PC, Goldstein G, Levy RH, Schlossman SF: Discrete stages of human intrathymic differentiation: Analysis of normal thymocytes and leukemic lymphoblasts of T-cell lineage. Proc Natl Acad Sci USA 77:1588–1592, 1980.
28. Biddison WE, Rao PE, Talle MA, Goldstein G, Shaw S: Possible involvement of the OKT4 molecule in T cell recognition of class II HLA antigens: Evidence from studies of cytotoxic T lymphocytes specific for SB antigens. J Exp Med 156:1065–1076, 1982.
29. Krensky AM, Reiss CS, Mier JW, Strominger JL, Burakoff SJ: Long-term human cytolytic T cell lines allospecific for HLA-DR6 antigen are $OKT4^+$. Proc Natl Acad Sci USA 79:2365–2369, 1982.
30. Meuer SC, Hussey RE, Hodgdon JC, Hercend T, Schlossman SF, Reinherz EL: Surface structures involved in target recognition by human cytotoxic T lymphocytes. Science 218:471–473, 1982.
31. Uchiyama T, Broder S, Waldmannn TA: A monoclonal antibody (anti-Tac) reactive with activated and functionally mature human T cells. I. Production of anti-Tac monoclonal antibody and distribution of Tac^+ cells. J Immunol 126:1393–1397, 1981.
32. Leonard WJ, Depper JM, Uchiyama T, Smith KA, Waldmann TA, Greene WC: A monoclonal antibody, anti-Tac blocks the membrane binding and action of human T-cell growth factor. Nature 300:262–264, 1982.

Human T-Cell Hybridomas Secreting Factors for B-Cell Differentiation and Proliferation*

Shu Man Fu, MD, PhD, Lloyd Mayer, MD, and Henry G. Kunkel, MD

Oklahoma Medical Research Foundation, Oklahoma City, OK 73104 (S.M.F.), Rockefeller University, New York, NY 10021 (L.M., H.G.K.)

Accumulated evidence indicates that non-antigen specific T-cell derived factors play important roles in B-cell proliferation and maturation. The investigation of these factors has been facilitated by the developments of T-cell clones and T-T hybridomas. In man, recent investigations reported some results with human T-T hybridomas [1–3]. We have utilized this methodology to obtain T-cell factors for B-cell maturation and differentiation [4].

GENERATION OF T-T HYBRIDOMAS

HGPRT (hypoxanthine guanine phosphoribosyl transferase)-deficient mutants of 2 human T-cell leukemia cell lines (Jurkat and KE37) were generated according to the method described by Epstein et al [5]. These mutant lines were used to fuse with Con A activated OKT4$^+$ T cells from normal individuals with polyethylene glycols. The hybridomas were selected in hypoxanthine (10^{-4}M), thymidine (1.6×10^{-5}M), and aminopterin (3×10^{-8}M). Details of the procedure have been reported elsewhere [4].

Fusion of activated T cells with a nonmutagenized T-cell line—Jurkat—was performed in a similar manner except that no selective medium (HAT) was used. The normal T cells were positive for HLA B27. To favor fusion between normal T blasts and leukemic T cells, fusions were carried out at a ratio of 100:1 (normal T blasts:leukemic cells). The fusion products were cloned on soft agarose and the resulting clones were selected by their staining with an anti-B27 monoclonal antibody.

Supernatants from the fusion resultant clones were screened for their ability to support T-cell depleted tonsillar B cells or peripheral blood B cells to proliferate and to mature to Ig-secreting cells. Four clones of interest will be discussed. J1.3 secreted a factor specific for the generation of IgA plaque-forming cells (PFC). J2S1 supernatant was able to induce polyclonal B-cell activation to generate IgM, IgG, and IgA PFC. K1 and K8 induced B-cell proliferation. HLA and other phenotype studies indicated that these 4 clones were indeed fusion products between normal T cells and leukemic cells (Table 1). Thus, J1.3 was a fusion product between a Jurkat cell and normal T blasts because it expressed HLA A2, B7 from the Jurkat cell line and HLA A1 and B11 from the normal donor. J2S1 expressed HLA B27 from its donor parent while K1 and K8 expressed HLA A1 and B17 from the donor T cells.

B-CELL DIFFERENTIATION

Supernatants from hybrid cultures were added to a purified tonsillar B-cell population which was depleted of T cells by a sheep red cell rosetting method. As shown in Table 2, the supernatant from J1.3 hybridoma induced 700 IgA PFC/well. In contrast, no IgA PFC were detected in the control culture. Similar data were obtained using different B-cell preparations from tonsils and peripheral blood. Occasionally, some increases

TABLE 1. HLA and Other Surface Phenotypes of Parental and Hybrid Cells

Cell Lines	Normal Donors	Hybridomas
Jurkat HLA A2, A4, B7 Fcμ$^-$	Donor 1 HLA A1, A30, B35, B17 Fcμ$^+$	J1.3 HLA A1, A2, B7, B11 Fcμ$^+$
Jurkat HLA B27$^-$	Donor 2 HLA B27$^+$	J2S1 HLA B27$^+$
KE 37 HLA A11, AW30, B35, B44 OKT4$^-$	Donor 1 HLA A1, A30, B35, B17 OKT4$^+$	K1 and K8 HLA A1, A11, B17 OKT4$^+$

J1.3: IgA PFC helper factor.
J2S1: Polyclonal B-cell helper factor.
K1 and K8: B-cell growth factor.

*Supported by NIH grant CA24338, American Cancer Society grant 1M255, and March of Dimes Birth Defects Foundation grant 1-819; work was performed at the Rockefeller University.

TABLE 2. Induction of Immunoglobulin Secretion by Hybrid Supernatants*

	B Cells	Media Control			Supernatant[c]			+ Autologous T Cells		
		G	A	M[a]	G	A	M	G	A	M
T-cell hybridoma J1.3	Tonsil B[b]	0	0	100	200	700	0	0	100	800
	Tonsil B	0	300	0	0	2400	0	—		
	Tonsil B	20	0	0	90	600	20	—		
	Tonsil B	20	0	0	10	260	0[d]		+ T + PWM	
	PB non-T	0	0	0	100	700	0	3420	880	1220
	PB MNC	0	0	0	0	500	0	—		
T-cell hybridoma J2S1	Tonsil B	40	0	90	520	80	450	190	30	20
			GAM			GAM			GAM	
	Tonsil B		50			1170			—	
	Tonsil B		50			170[e]			+ T + PWM	
	PB non-T		100			700			1600	
Hybrids K1	Tonsil B		0			0			—	
K8	Tonsil B		0			0			—	
Parent line Jurkat 3	Tonsil B		0			0			—	

*From Mayer L, Fu SM, Kunkel HG: Human T cell hybridomas secreting factors for IgA-specific help, polyclonal B cell activation, and B cell proliferation. J Exp Med 156:1860–1865, 1982, by copyright permission of The Rockefeller University Press.
[a]PFC/10⁶ cells at initiation of culture. Ig isotypes measured by reverse plaque assay at day 6.
[b]Each B-cell preparation represents a different experiment.
[c]Supernatant at 1/3 dilution.
[d]Supernatant at 1/100 dilution.
[e]Supernatant at 1/200 dilution.

in IgM and IgG PFC were observed. However, these increases were always less than the increases in IgA PFC. The action of the J1.3 supernatant was independent of T cells or mitogens such as pokeweed mitogen (PWM), Con A or phorbol ester. The magnitude of the responses were 40–80% of that seen with autologous T cells and PWM. Variability in the responsiveness of several B-cell preparations was noted. The nature of the responding cells was also investigated. Depletion of IgA-bearing cells from the B-cell population abolished its responsiveness to the supernatant of J1.3. Thus, it appears that the factor is specific for IgA⁺ B cells to mature to IgA PFC.

In contrast, the supernatant of J2S1 induced PFC of all Ig isotype classes tested (IgM, IgG, and IgA) (Table 2). The action of J2S1 supernatant was also T-cell and mitogen independent. The T-cell and mitogen independence of J1.3 and J2S1 was further supported by their ability to induce IgA⁺ leukemic cells to mature to plasma cells and IgA PFC [4]. Both supernatants from J1.3 and J2S1 could be diluted to a considerable degree before losing their activity.

B-CELL PROLIFERATION

³H-Thymidine uptake of purified tonsil B cells incubated with supernatants were measured at day 2 to 5. Supernatants from hybrids K1 and K8 induced B-cell proliferation with stimulatory indices of 20.4 and 35.4, respectively, on day 3. This proliferation was not associated with B-cell maturation (Table 2). Supernatants from J1.3 and J2S1 induced only modest increases in ³H-thymidine uptake (stimulatory indices 4–6) while the parental line KE37 gave a stimulatory index of 3.

CONCLUSION

Four human T-T hybridomas were studied. They secrete an IgA PFC-helper factor, a polyclonal B-cell activation factor, and a B-cell growth factor. The chemical nature of these factors is being investigated. Whether these factors are similar to those reported previously [1,6–8] remains to be ascertained. The ability to obtain a large amount of these factors would aid their purification. However, caution must be taken to clone repeatedly these hybridomas because of their unstable nature. The availability of purified factors will permit further studies regarding the receptor studies of B cells in normal and disease states. In particular, a B-cell receptor defect for these factors might be found in patients with immunodeficiency of the B-cell type.

REFERENCES

1. Irigoyen O, Rizzolo PV, Thomas Y, Rogozinski L, Chess L: Generation of functional human T cell hybrids. J Exp Med 154:1827–1837, 1981.
2. Grillot-Courvalin C, Brouet JC, Berger R, Berheim A: Establishment of a human T-cell hybrid line with suppressive activity. Nature 292:844–845, 1981.
3. Okada M, Yoshimura N, Kaieda T, Yamamura Y, Kishimoto T: Establishment and characterization of human T hybrid cells secreting immunoregulatory molecules. Proc Natl Acad Sci USA 78:7717–7721, 1981.
4. Mayer L, Fu SM, Kunkel HG: Human T cell hybridomas secreting factors for IgA-specific help, polyclonal B cell activation, and B cell proliferation. J Exp Med 156:1860–1865, 1982.
5. Epstein LA, Kelley WN, Littlefield JW: Mutagen-induced diploid human lymphoblast variants containing altered hypoxanthine guanine phosphoribosyl transferase. Somatic Cell Genet 3:135–148, 1977.
6. Endoh M, Sakai H, Nomoto Y, Tomino Y, Kaneshige H: IgA-specific helper activity of T cells in human peripheral blood. J Immunol 127:2612–2613, 1981.
7. Sredni B, Sieckman DG, Kumagai S, House S, Green I, Paul WE: Long-term culture and cloning of nontransformed human B lymphocytes. J Exp Med 154:1500–1516, 1981.
8. Andersson J, Melchers F: T cell dependent activation of resting B cells: Requirement of both nonspecific unrestricted and antigen-specific Ia restricted soluble factors. Proc Natl Acad Sci USA 78:2497–2501, 1981.

Specific In Vitro Anti-Mannan Antibody Production by Human Blood Lymphocytes

Anne Durandy, MD, Alain Fischer, MD, and Claude Griscelli, MD

Unité d'Immunologie et d'Hématologie Pédiatriques, Département de Pédiatrie, INSERM U 132, Hôpital des Enfants Malades, 75730 Paris Cedex 15, France

Several systems have been described for the generation of specific antibody production in vitro in primary responses to particulate antigens like sheep red blood cells (SRBC) and trinitrophenyl (TNP) polyacrylamide beads, or to soluble antigens such as ovalbumin (OA). Secondary in vitro responses to influenza viruses, tetanus toxoid (TT) or keyhole limpet hemocyanin (KLH) have also been described allowing studies of the regulation of the specific antibody production in humans. We report here a new system of in vitro antibody production using an antigen prepared from Candida albicans cell wall and containing more than 96% pure mannan. Blood lymphocytes from Candida albicans immune donors have been tested for in vitro antibody production. The assay involves identification of specific antibody-containing cells by radioautography with tritiated mannan together with measurement of anti-mannan antibody in culture supernatants using an enzyme-linked immunoassay (ELISA).

MATERIALS AND METHODS

The antigen used was extracted from Candida albicans strain by a technique previously reported by Summers et al [1]. It contained >96% mannan and 3.6% protein. Mannan antigen was tritiated by L. Pichat (Centre d'Energie Atomique, France) by catalyzed exchange in solution with tritium (^{3}H) as described by Evans et al [2].

Samples were obtained from healthy adult volunteers or from cord blood on preservative-free heparin (100 IU/ml). Donors were tested for the presence of anti-Candida antibody in serum.

Peripheral blood lymphocytes (PBL) were cultured in flat or round bottom microtiter wells (Falcon) at 2×10^5 in 0.2 ml RPMI 1640 culture medium supplemented with 10% heat-inactivated fetal calf serum (FCS), antibiotics, amphotericin B (4 µg/ml), and glutamine (0.3 mg/ml). Cultures were stimulated by varying amounts of either mannan or mannan extemporaneously absorbed with methylated bovine serum albumin (MBSA) (5–250 µg/ml). Some cultures were initiated with MBSA alone (1–100 µg/ml). In control experiments, 2 other antigens were used: pneumococcal polysaccharide SIII (10–100 µg/ml), and influenza A/X31 virus antigen (courtesy of Dr. Skehel) 0.5 µg/ml. At day 4, the culture medium was replaced by 0.2 ml of fresh medium (RPMI 1640 + FCS) without further addition of antigen or mitogen. Cultures were stopped at day 7 except when otherwise stated.

Smears of harvested cells were fixed in ethanol, covered with labeled antigen (1:100 dilution of stock solution) for 30 minutes, and then fixed again in ethanol. Intracytoplasmic binding of labeled antigen (^{3}H mannan or ^{3}H SIII) was revealed by radioautography after an 8-day exposure in emulsion. Smears were then stained with methyl green pyronin.

Specific anti-mannan antibody content of culture supernatants was determined by a solid ELISA. The supernatants were harvested at day 7.

RESULTS

Generation of Anti-Mannan Antibody-Containing Cells by Human Lymphocytes

PBL obtained from most normal Candida albicans-sensitized volunteers (ie 35/40 subjects who exhibited antibodies) matured in 7 days into anti-mannan antibody-containing cells (ACC) in cultures initiated with 50 µg/ml mannan absorbed on MBSA (Mannan-MBSA) (Table 1). The number of ACC generated in 7-day cultures varied around $16,300 \pm 4,200$ for 10^6 input cells. Besides these results with 50 µg/ml mannan-MBSA which appeared to be the optimal concentration, ACC were also obtained when cultures were initiated with 10 µg/ml (mean of ACC $7,800 \pm 2,300/10^6$ cells) and with 100 µg/ml (mean of ACC $8,900 \pm 2,800/10^6$ cells) of mannan-MBSA. Mannan or MBSA alone, whatever the doses used and the duration of the culture (3–10 days), was unable to induce anti-mannan ACC generation. Mannan-MBSA was also able to elicit the generation of immunoglobulin containing cells (ICC) of the IgM or the IgG class, but not of the IgA class.

Anti-mannan-containing cells were easily detectable on radioautography smears after staining with methyl green pyronin as large pyronino-

TABLE 1. Generation of Anti-Mannan Antibody-Containing Cells by Human Lymphocytes Stimulated by Mannan-MBSA

Cultures Stimulated With	Number of Experiments Performed	Proliferative Response* Number of Recovered Cells ($\times 10^{-3}$)	Number of Anti-Mannan Antibodies Containing Cells† ($\times 10^{-3}$)	Number of Cells Containing IgM‡ ($\times 10^{-3}$)	IgG(3) ($\times 10^{-3}$)
0	35	150 ± 86	< 0.1	0.4 ± 0.5	0.3 ± 0.4
Mannan-MBSA (50 µg/ml)	35	707 ± 135	16.3 ± 4.2	11.7 ± 5.7	8.5 ± 6.6
Mannan (40 µg/ml)	6	277 ± 80	< 0.1	0.3 ± 0.1	0.4 ± 0.2
MBSA (10 µg/ml)	6	170 ± 103	< 0.1	0.2 ± 0.1	0.3 ± 0.2
PWM (25 µl/ml)	20	985 ± 236	< 0.5	218.2 ± 46.3	214.7 ± 39.9

Results, means ± 1 SD of responses obtained with PBL from 35 responders among 40 *Candida albicans* (CA)-sensitized donors (positive serum antibodies to CA) are given for 10^6 input cells.
*Proliferative response was also evaluated by ^{3}H thymidine incorporation: △cpm of 40,000 ± 4,000 for 50 µg mannan:MBSA.
†Number of anti-mannan antibody-containing cells was evaluated by enumeration of cells fixing ^{3}H mannan, and revealed by radioautography.
‡IgM- or IgG-containing cells were detected by intracytoplasmic immunofluorescence.

TABLE 2. Production of Anti-Mannan Antibodies Measured by ELISA in Cultures Stimulated With Mannan-MBSA

Cultures Stimulated With	Number of Experiments Performed	Specific Antibody Concentration IgM (U/ml)	IgG (U/ml)
0	15	1.7 ± 1.4	2.3 ± 2.9
MBSA-Mannan (50 µg/ml)	15	17.1 ± 10.3	18.8 ± 17.8
Mannan (40 µg/ml)	5	1.8 ± 2.4	1.4 ± 1.6
MBSA (10 µg/ml)	5	2.2 ± 1.9	0.8 ± 0.8
PWM (25 µλ/ml)	5	2.8 ± 1.8	3.2 ± 3.1

Results, means ± 1 SD with PBL of CA-sensitized responder donors, are expressed in U/ml by comparison with the 1:10,000 dilution of a reference serum from a CA-sensitized donor. Supernatants were harvested from day 4 to 7 of cultures initiated with 10^6 cells.

philic cells. Analysis of labeled cells showed that they were negative for OKT3 and OKM1 monoclonal antibodies and unable to phagocyte latex beads. Moreover, they bore surface Igs (IgM or IgG) and contained intracytoplasmic Igs.

PBL from most *Candida albicans*-sensitized subjects were differentiating in vitro into ACC in the presence of mannan-MBSA. However, PBL from unsensitized subjects, ie blood donors without detectable serum anti-Candida antibodies, or isolated from cord blood, never matured into ACC, indicating that mannan-MBSA did not induce a nonspecific polyclonal Ig production. The specificity of the intracytoplasmic labeling by ^{3}H mannan of mannan-MBSA stimulated cells was studied in different ways. First, cell smears were incubated with a large excess (30–100-fold) of cold mannan before the addition of ^{3}H mannan. In this condition, ACC were not detectable by radioautography. On the contrary, addition of a large excess of an unrelated cold polysaccharide SIII before incubation with ^{3}H mannan did not inhibit intracytoplasmic binding of ^{3}H mannan. Second, PBL from recently immunized subjects (15–30 days after immunization) and stimulated by pneumococcal polysaccharide SIII proliferated and generated specific anti-SIII-ACC of both IgM and IgG classes, as revealed by the use of ^{3}H SIII which were not labeled by ^{3}H mannan. Conversely, mannan-MBSA stimulated blast cells that were able to bind ^{3}H mannan were not labeled by ^{3}H SIII.

Detection of Anti-Mannan Antibodies in Culture Supernatants

In cultures of PBL from sensitized donors, stimulated with mannan absorbed on MBSA immediately before being added to cultures, IgM and IgG anti-mannan antibodies were easily detected by a solid phase ELISA. Table 2 shows results observed with PBL from different sensitized subjects. In unstimulated or mannan-stimulated (5–250 µg/ml) cultures, antibody titer was very low for IgM as well as for IgG. With mannan-MBSA for concentrations ranging from 10–100 µg/ml (with the optimal dose of 50 µg/ml), a significantly higher titer ($\times$ 8) of both IgM anti-mannan antibodies or IgG anti-mannan antibodies was found.

The production of anti-mannan antibody was shown to be specific. Indeed, in cultures of PBL isolated from A/X31 influenza-virus sensitized donors stimulated with A/X31 virus, no anti-mannan antibodies were detected in supernatants, while large amounts of IgG anti-A/X31 were found. Conversely, when PBL from the same donors were cultured

TABLE 3. Cellular Requirements for T-Cell Dependency of Anti-Mannan Antibody Production in 50 µg/ml Mannan-MBSA Stimulated Cultures

Cultured Cells	Antibody-Containing Cells ($\times 10^{-3}$)	Supernatant Antibody Concentrations (U/ml)	
		IgM	IgG
Unseparated PBL:	13.0	14	10
E(+)	<0.1	2	1
E(−)	0.1	3	2
Co-Cultures:			
E(+) and autologous E(−)*	12.0	23	17
Irradiated E(+)† and autologous E(−)*	≤0.1	4	3
E(+) and allogeneic E(−)*	0.1	2	1
E(+) and autologous AC‡ + allogeneic E(−)*	7.5	ND	ND
E(+) and autologous AC‡	<0.1	ND	ND
E(+) and semi-identical E(−)*	8.6	ND	ND

Results of a representative experiment with total or separated PBL from a responder donor and E(−) cells isolated from either an unrelated HLA-different or an HLA semi-identical responder control.
E(−) preparations were treated with OKT3 and complement. Similar results were obtained after partial depletion of monocytes by 3 successive steps of adherence on plastic.
*E(+) lymphocytes were added to E(−) cells at ratio 1:1.
†E(+) lymphocytes were irradiated at 1,000 rads.
‡Around 15×10^3 AC were added to 100×10^3 E(+) lymphocytes. Similar results were obtained with 30×10^3 AC added, or with irradiated (3,000 rads) AC. E(+) and E(−) cells were added to flat-bottom microwells in which AC had been previously isolated.

with mannan-MBSA, no antibodies to A/X31 were detected, while both IgM and IgG anti-mannan antibodies were produced.

T-CELL DEPENDENCY OF ANTI-MANNAN ANTIBODY PRODUCTION

T-cell dependency of specific anti-mannan antibody production was studied by performing E-rosette fractionation of PBL. As shown in Table 3, E(+) preparations were neither able to differentiate into anti-mannan ACC nor to produce antibodies when cultured for 7 days in presence of 50 µg/ml of mannan-MBSA. Likewise, E(−) cell populations, prepared by a depletion of T lymphocytes using OKT3 in the presence of complement, did not produce any anti-mannan ACC or specific anti-mannan antibody supernatants. These negative results were still observed after depletion of E(−) preparations of the excess of monocytes by 3 successive steps of adherence to plastic. However, addition of autologous E(+) lymphocytes to E(−) cells allowed the generation of anti-mannan ACC and of supernatant antibodies. This helper effect appeared at a low E(+):E(−) ratio of 1:4, was maximal at a ratio of 1:1, but decreased at higher ratios. Irradiation from 1,000 rads of the E(+) lymphocytes before being added to autologous E(−) cells completely abolished the production of anti-mannan ACC and anti-mannan antibodies in supernatants. In culture mixing E(+) and E(−) cells from 2 unrelated HLA-different donors (ratio 1:1) no helper activity was observed. However, addition of adherent cells (AC) autologous to E(+) lymphocytes restored a normal generation of specific anti-mannan ACC. This effect was constantly observed, whatever the ratio AC:E(+) (from 0.15:1 to 0.3:1) and was resistant to irradiation (3,000 rads) of the AC. The control culture, mixing E(+) and autologous AC, was negative, indicating the absence of a sufficient contamination by B lymphocytes of AC. In co-cultures mixing E(+) lymphocytes from one donor, and E(−) plus AC isolated from a second donor, no production of ACC could be detected. Finally, a production of ACC could be detected in mannan-MBSA stimulated cultures mixing E(+) and E(−) cells from related HLA semi-identical donors (mother and daughter).

DISCUSSION

In the present study, we have developed an in vitro assay that detects human B cells producing antibodies to mannan, a polysaccharide from *Candida albicans*. This system provides a new way of testing specific in vitro antibody production in humans. Cultures of PBL obtained from sensitized donors were stimulated with purified mannan absorbed with MBSA. In our system, the proportion of anti-mannan ACC among immunoglobulin-containing-cells (ICC) was remarkably high when compared to that observed in previously published in vitro antibody production assays [3–5], but was comparable to that observed in the KLH system [6]. However, mannan is known to be a strong immunogen [7] and the radioautographic method used to detect the ACC can be more sensitive than hemolytic plaque-forming cell (PFC) assay and than the immunofluorescence technique used to detect the ICC. The radioautographic technique takes a longer time for detecting in vitro production of antibodies than other techniques, but it gives a direct identification of the antibody-producing cells. The detection of anti-mannan antibodies by an ELISA method confirmed that mannan truly triggered B cells to produce specific antibodies. A relatively high concentration of mannan was necessary for the first step of the ELISA suggesting a low-binding affinity of mannan for plastic. However, the mannan binding was stable enough to allow the titration of specific antibodies.

Two major issues about our assay need more discussion in order to delineate its significance, that is, the nature of the antigen and the specificity of the antibody response. The antigen preparation we used contained above all mannan. However, there is a tiny contamination with protein. One could thus envisage a possible anti-proteomannan response in this system, especially since relatively high concentrations of antigen were required for the induction of antibody production. However, this hypothesis appears unlikely since the protein contaminant was < 4% of the antigen preparation. Furthermore, we showed that the antigen preparation alone did not trigger proliferation and maturation into ACC. On the contrary, other *Candida albicans* antigen preparations like Candida metabolic antigen that contains higher amounts of protein (> 10%) induced a proliferation of sensitized PBL [8].

The generation of anti-mannan antibodies appears to be a specific immune response and not a mitogen-induced polyclonal Ig production like that observed with purified protein derivatives (PPD) [9] or different bacterial cell walls containing peptidoglycans [10], since nonresponder B cells were not induced to differentiate into ICC. Evidence of the specificity of the response was given in experiments in which it was possible to obtain anti-SIII antibody-containing cells by using cells from donors recently immunized with the SIII pneumococcal polysaccharide. As measured by ELISA, mannan-MBSA did not induce anti-influenza A antibody production by B cells from influenza A-primed donors and, conversely, influenza A virus did not induce a detectable anti-mannan antibody production. On the other hand, a polyclonal stimulation of B cells by pokeweed mitogen (PWM) resulted in a very low percentage of anti-mannan ACC among ICC, showing that ICC were not nonspecifically stained by ^{3}H mannan. It was surprising to observe that PWM did not induce a higher number of anti-mannan ACC or anti-mannan antibodies in culture supernatants as previously observed for other antigenic systems [6,11]. Since PWM acts only on a given B-cell subset [12], one can envision that the mannan-responding B cells mostly belong to another population. It would be interesting to know if B cells specific for other polysaccharides behave in the same manner.

One interesting aspect was the possibility of raising the question of the T-cell dependency of anti-mannan antibody responses in humans. Indeed, in the mouse, antibody production to most polysaccharides is thymo-independent. Our results clearly show that the generation of anti-mannan ACC required the presence of T cells (even in small number) since a preparation of B lymphocytes and monocytes completely depleted of T cells failed to mature into anti-mannan ACC. However, one cannot distinguish between the existence of T helper (Th) cells for mannan itself or an equivalent of a hapten-carrier help in which T cells would recognize MBSA and help B cells to produce anti-mannan antibodies. A genetic restriction has been shown already in the in vitro antibody assay for tetanus toxoid (TT) [13] and influenza virus [14]. In our system the results show that addition of autologous adherent cells to T lymphocytes permits a normal help to allogeneic B cells, which favors the hypothesis of a restriction located to T-macrophage cell interaction, as already suggested in another antigenic system.

The development of an in vitro system for specific antibody production by human PBL to a polysaccharide antigen opens the way for studies, which have not yet been possible, about the fine regulation of antibody production to polysaccharides in humans, as most adults have already been primed to mannan from *Candida albicans*. On the other hand, such a study should also provide information in pathologic conditions like the chronic mucocutaneous candidiasis or the Wiskott-Aldrich syndrome in which an impairment of antibody production to polysaccharides has been found.

REFERENCES

1. Summers DF, Grollman AP, Hasenclever HF: Polysaccharide antigens of candida cell wall. J Immunol 92:491–499, 1964.
2. Evans EA, Scheppard HC, Turner JC, Warrel DC: A new approach to specific labelling of organic compounds with tritium gas. J Labelled Compounds 10:569–575, 1974.
3. Dosch HM, Gelfand EW: Generation of human plaque forming cells in culture: Tissue distribution, antigenic and cellular requirements. J Immunol 118:302–308, 1977.
4. Heijnen CJ, Uytdehaag F, Dollekamp I, Ballieux RE: Distinct human T cell subpopulations regulating the antigen induced antibody response. In Fauci AS, Ballieux RE (eds): "Antibody Production in Man." New York: Academic Press, 1979, pp 231–252.
5. Delfraissy JF, Galanaud P, Dormont J, Wallon C: Primary in vitro antibody response from human peripheral blood lymphocytes. J Immunol 118:630–635, 1977.

6. Lane HC, Volkman DJ, Whalen G, Fauci AS: In vitro antigen-induced, antigen specific antibody production in man. Specific and polyclonal components, kinetics and cellular requirements. J Exp Med 154:1043-1057, 1981.
7. Axelsen NH: Analysis of human candida precipitins by quantitative immunoelectrophoresis. A model for analysis of complex microbial antigen-antibody systems. Scand J Immunol 5:177-187, 1976.
8. Fischer A, Ballet JJ, Griscelli C: Specific inhibition of in vitro Candida induced lymphocyte proliferation by polysaccharide antigens present in the serum of patients with chronic mucocutaneous candidiasis. J Clin Invest 62:1005-1013, 1978.
9. Banck G, Forsgren A: Many bacterial species are mitogenic for human blood B lymphocytes. Scand J Immunol 8:347-354, 1978.
10. Ringden O, Rynnel-Dagoo R, Waterfield EM, Moller E, Moller G: Polyclonal antibody secretion in human lymphocytes induced by killed staphylococcal bacteria and by lipopolysaccharide. Scand J Immunol 6:1159-1169, 1977.
11. Geha RS, Schneeberger E, Rosen F, Merler E: Interaction of human thymus-derived and non-thymus derived lymphocytes in vitro. Induction of proliferation and antibody synthesis in B lymphocytes by a soluble factor released from antigen-stimulated T-lymphocytes. J Exp Med 138:1230-1247, 1973.
12. Kuritani T, Cooper MD: Human B cell differentiation. II. Pokeweed mitogen-responsive B cells belong to a surface immunoglobulin D-negative subpopulation. J Exp Med 155:1561-1566, 1982.
13. Geha RS, Mudawwar FR: Antigen specific and antigen non-specific triggering of human B lymphocytes. Supra 4:101-114.
14. Callard R, Smith CM: Histocompatibility requirements for T cell help in specific in vitro antibody responses to influenza virus by human blood lymphocytes. Eur J Immunol 11:206-211, 1981.

Appearance of Antibody-Producing Cells in the Peripheral Blood in Response to Immunization With a Specific Antigen*

Hans D. Ochs, MD, John Bohnsack, MD†, Samuel R. Heller, MS, and Ralph J. Wedgwood, MD

Department of Pediatrics, University of Washington, Seattle, WA 98195

In vitro antibody synthesis by human peripheral blood mononuclear cells (PBM) can be initiated by adding to the cultures a polyclonal B-cell activator [1-4] or a specific antigen to which the cell donor has been previously exposed either through natural infection (eg influenza, varicella, herpes simplex) or immunization with a specific antigen (eg keyhole limpet hemocyanin [KLH], tetanus toxoid [TT]) [5-10]. Because of our long-standing interest in the in vivo antibody responses of normal and immune deficient individuals to bacteriophage ϕX 174, a T-cell dependent neoantigen [11-14], we have developed an in vitro system to study spontaneous and antigen-induced antibody production to this antigen by PBM from normal individuals previously immunized with bacteriophage.

Normal adult subjects (4 female, 4 male) were immunized with bacteriophage ϕX 174 intravenously twice, 6 weeks apart, at the standard dose of 2×10^9 PFU/kg body weight. Serum was collected at weekly intervals for antibody determination using a phage-neutralizing assay. The antibody titer was expressed as the rate of phage inactivation or K value (Kv) as derived by a standard formula [13]. Antibody of the IgG class is 2-mercaptoethanol (2-ME) resistant; IgM is 2-ME sensitive [15].

ANTIBODY RESPONSE IN VIVO

All subjects studied showed a primary antibody response consisting of IgM and a secondary response with typical amplification and switch from IgM to IgG. The 4 female subjects had higher antibody titers during the secondary response than the male subjects.

ANTIBODY SYNTHESIS IN VITRO

Following immunization, 2 functionally distinct cell populations were identified in the peripheral blood: cells which produced spontaneous antibody when placed in culture, and antigen-reactive cells which synthesized antibody only after in vitro antigen stimulation.

Spontaneous antibody synthesis was observed in cultures of PBM from 6 of 8 individuals after primary immunization with phage (Fig. 1). The spontaneously antibody-secreting cells appeared in the circulation as early as 1 week after the first phage injection. By 4 weeks these cells were either no longer present or, when demonstrable, the amount of antibody synthesized had markedly diminished. Spontaneous antibody-secreting cells could not be detected in the 2 individuals with the lowest serum antibody titers. Following secondary immunization, cells spontaneously secreting antibody in vitro appeared in the circulation as early as 3 days, producing significantly more antibody than during the primary response (Fig. 2). With 2 exceptions, spontaneous antibody-secreting cells were no longer detectable at 4 weeks, and by 6 weeks none of the subjects had circulating cells that produced antibody spontaneously. There was a positive correlation between the magnitude of spontaneous in vitro antibody synthesis and the antibody titer of the serum. Spontaneously synthesized antibody was detected only in cultures containing B lymphocytes. Autologous T cells neither suppressed nor augmented the antigen independent antibody synthesis. Addition of puromycin to the cell cultures or irradiation of the cells with 1,000 R abrogated spontaneous antibody production, indicating de novo in vitro antibody synthesis rather than release of antibody synthesized in vivo. Spontaneously synthesized antibody could be demonstrated in the supernate of the cultures at 36 hours, and was maximal at 72 hours; net synthesis was no longer demonstrable thereafter.

Antigen-stimulated in vitro antibody synthesis, as measured by the increment of antibody synthesized in antigen-stimulated wells compared to nonstimulated wells, was present in cultures of PBM in 7 of 8 subjects at 2 weeks, and in all subjects studied at 4 weeks and 6 weeks after primary immunization (Fig. 1). Following secondary immunization, antigen-reactive antibody-producing cells appeared in the circulation in 3 of 5

---

*Supported by grants from NIH (AI-07073) and from the March of Dimes Birth Defects Foundation (6-273). A portion of this work was conducted through the Clinical Research Center facility at the University of Washington supported by NIH grant RR-37.

†Supported by training grant 5-T32-HDO7171-02.

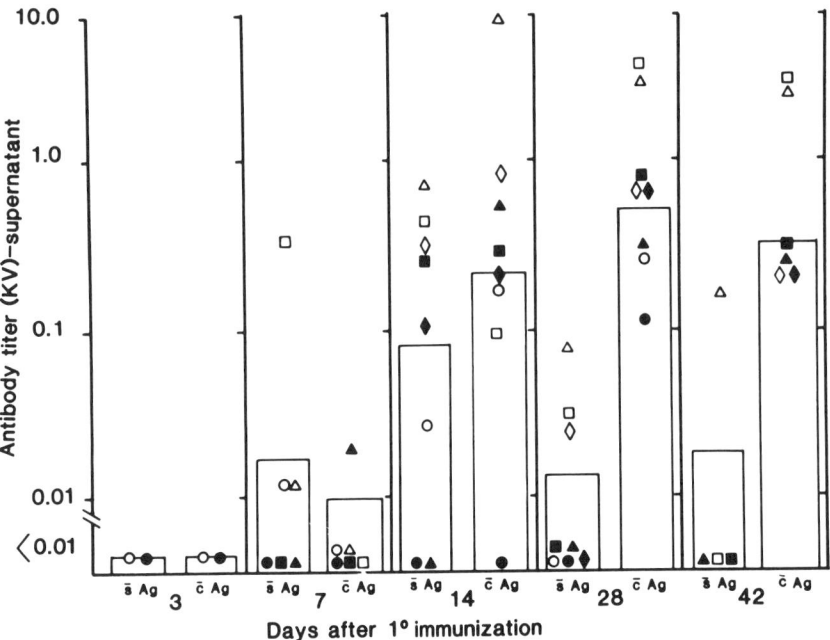

Fig. 1. In vitro antibody synthesis by PBM following primary (1°) immunization with φX 174. The columns designated s̄ Ag indicate spontaneous antibody synthesis; those designated c̄ Ag indicate antigen-induced antibody synthesis. PBM were collected from individuals (solid symbols = males, open symbols = females) at various times after immunization as shown on the abscissa and cultured at 2×10^6 PBM/ml in round-bottom microtiter plates (total volume 0.2 ml), without (s̄) or with (c̄) antigen (Ag) (1×10^6 PFU/ml). Supernatants were harvested on day 12 and antibody titers determined by a neutralizing assay. All antibody during 1° immunization was IgM. Antigen-induced antibody was determined by subtracting the amount of spontaneous antibody produced in wells without added antigen.

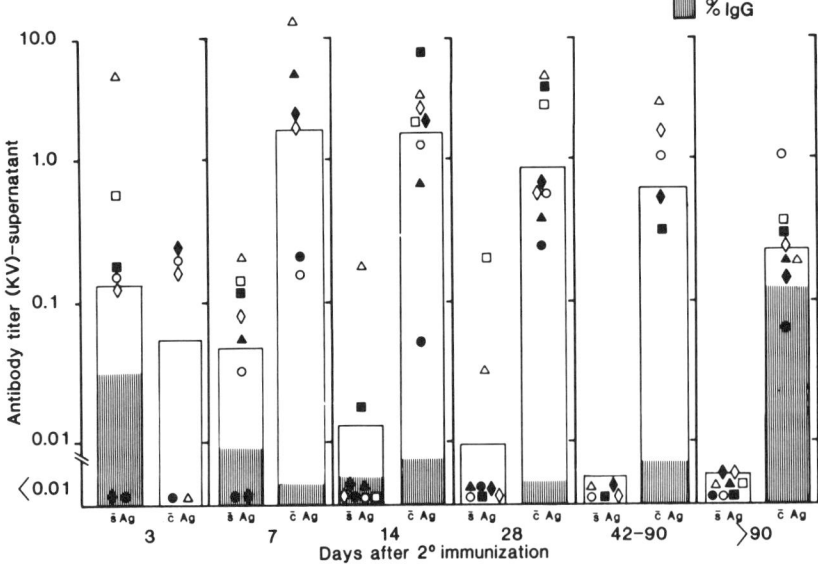

Fig. 2. In vitro antibody synthesis by PBM following secondary (2°) immunization with φX 174. (For details see legend of Fig. 1.) Percent IgG, determined as antibody resistant to 2-ME treatment, is shown as the shaded part of each column.

subjects at day 3, and in all by day 7 (Fig. 2). Antigen-reactive cells have persisted in the circulation in all 8 subjects during the 10 months of observation after immunization.

To assess the long-term persistence of antibody-synthesizing PBM, we studied 7 individuals who had been multiply immunized 2 to 16 years previously. Although all had significant serum antibody titers of the IgG class, none had spontaneous antibody-producing cells in the circulation. When cultured with antigen, PBM of all individuals immunized years previously showed demonstrable in vitro antibody synthesis. However, the antibody titers were much lower and the amount of antibody produced in quadruplicate wells from a single individual varied significantly, reflecting a very low number of circulating antigen-reactive or memory cells.

ISOTYPE SWITCH

Following primary immunization with bacteriophage φX 174, the majority of antiphage antibody in vivo was IgM; at 4 weeks small amounts of IgG antibody could be detected in the serum of all subjects. Following secondary immunization the rapid rise in antibody titer was largely due to the production of IgG antibody. In vitro spontaneous antibody-synthesizing cells produced the same isotype of antibody found in vivo: during primary immunization, in vitro synthesized antibody was entirely IgM; during secondary immunization, the in vitro synthesized IgG antibody was proportional to the percentage of IgG (approximately 50%) found in serum (Figs. 2 and 3). Antigen-induced antibody synthesis after primary immunization was IgM; following secondary immunization, PBM from recently immunized individuals (within 3 months) produced predominantly IgM antibody (Fig. 2), at a time when IgG synthesis in vivo was at its peak and spontaneous antibody-synthesizing cells produced

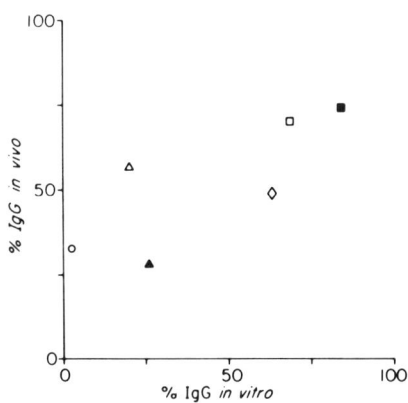

Fig. 3. Serum samples obtained 2 weeks following secondary immunization with φX 174 and supernatants from 12-day-old (antigen free) cultures of PBM obtained simultaneously from the same subjects were analyzed for specific IgG antibody. The percent IgG found in the serum is proportional to the percent IgG produced spontaneously by PBM (correlation coefficient, r = 0.60).

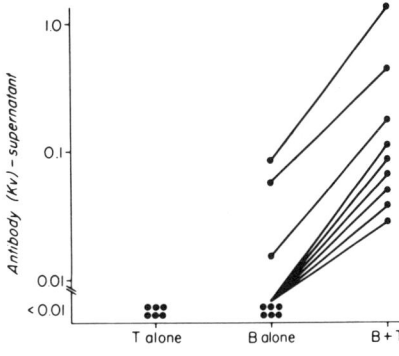

Fig. 4. T-cell dependence of antigen-induced antibody synthesis in vitro. T-enriched (T) and T-depleted (B) cells were obtained after secondary immunization and cultured alone or together at a ratio of 3:1 (total cell number 1×10^6/ml) in the presence of antigen. Supernatants were harvested at day 12 of culture and antibody titers determined. Recently immunized individuals and subjects immunized two or more years ago are included.

considerable amounts of IgG (50–60%). In contrast, antigen-induced antibody synthesis by PBM obtained from individuals reimmunized more than 3 months before the in vitro studies produced mainly IgG antibody (63–100%), reflecting the isotype present in the circulation (Fig. 2).

T-CELL DEPENDENCE

Antigen-induced in vitro antibody synthesis required both B and T cells: B cells alone, obtained from immunized subjects at a time when cells spontaneously secreting antibody were no longer detectable, synthesized only minute amounts of antibody or none at all when cultured with antigen (Fig. 4). Addition of autologous T cells at a T:B ratio of 3:1 significantly increased the amount of antibody. Cultures of T cells alone failed to synthesize any demonstrable antibody.

COMMENT

The initiation of an antibody response to a specific antigen requires the interaction of antigen-recognizing and -presenting cells, modulating lymphocytes, and antibody-producing cells [16]. We have studied in vitro the production of specific antibody by PBM from human subjects after immunization with bacteriophage φX 174. Following primary immunization, cells that spontaneously synthesize antibody in vitro are regularly found in the circulation by 2 weeks and disappear by 4 weeks. Following secondary immunization, spontaneous antibody-producing cells appear as early as 3 days and disappear by 2 weeks. The intensity of spontaneous in vitro antibody synthesis reflects the magnitude of the individual serum antibody response. De novo synthesis, rather than release of antibody by these cells during culture, is demonstrated by the sensitivity to puromycin and irradiation. Cells synthesizing antibody spontaneously without the need of antigen have been described in the circulation of humans following booster immunization with TT [17] or killed salmonella vaccine [18]. These antibody-synthesizing cells appear in the peripheral blood 3–10 days after booster immunization, similar to our observation in the phage system.

A second type of cell capable of synthesizing in vitro specific antibody was found in the circulation during the primary and secondary immune response to phage. In contrast to the cells that spontaneously produce antibody, "memory" cells have to be induced to synthesize antibody in vitro by antigen, a process that takes several days and is T-cell dependent. During the primary antibody response, circulating memory cells when cultured in the presence of antigen will produce mainly IgM; during the first 3 months of the secondary response, most antibody synthesized in vitro is of the IgM class although approximately 50% of the serum antibody activity is IgG. Thereafter, in vitro synthesized antibody is predominantly IgG and years after repeated phage injections all of the antibody produced in vitro consists of IgG; the in vivo situation at that time is similar—all of the serum antibody is of the IgG class.

Cells that synthesize antibody spontaneously or in response to in vitro antigenic stimulation were not detected in individuals who had not been immunized with φX 174, a finding in accord with Volkman et al who did not detect circulating KLH-reactive cells in subjects without prior immunization to KLH [7]. Others have noted a difference in antibody class synthesized by circulating B cells activated in vitro and the class of serum antibody being synthesized simultaneously in vivo. PWM-stimulated PBM produced mainly IgM anti-KLH antibody in vitro early after secondary in vivo immunization when serum anti-KLH antibody was both IgG and IgM. At an interval of 1 year after in vivo immunization, PWM-stimulated PBM synthesized mainly IgG anti-KLH antibody suggesting a delayed appearance in the circulation of cells committed to this isotype; alternatively, further in vivo antigenic stimulation may be required before cells that can produce IgG upon activation in vitro appear in the circulation [19].

In vitro studies of human B-cell activation and cellular interactions involving the control of antibody synthesis have focused primarily on systems using polyclonal activators without regard to recent antigenic exposure. However, studies of the interaction of cellular phenotypes involved in the in vitro antibody response to a specific antigen should produce a more exact understanding of the actual role of these cells in the human immune response, and may define more precisely the defect responsible for abnormal antibody responses of patients with primary immune deficiency disorders.

REFERENCES

1. Waldmann TA, Broder S, Blaese RM et al: Role of suppressor T cells in pathogenesis of common variable hypogammaglobulinemia. Lancet 2:609, 1974.
2. Ginsburg WW, Foukleman FD, Lipsky PE: Circulating and mitogen-induced immunoglobulin-secreting cells in human peripheral blood. Evaluation by a modified reverse hemolytic plaque assay. J Immunol 120:33, 1978.
3. Stevens R, Saxon A: Immunoregulation in humans. Control of antitetanus toxoid antibody production after immunization. J Clin Invest 62:1154, 1978.
4. Möller G (ed): Activation of antibody synthesis in human B lymphocytes. Immunol Rev 45:3–305, 1979.
5. Mudawware F, Yunis E, Geha RS: Antigen-specific helper factor in man. J Exp Med 148:1032, 1978.
6. Brenner MK, Munro AJ: Human antitetanus antibody response in vitro: Autologous and allogeneic T cells provide help by different routes. Clin Exp Immunol 46:171, 1981.
7. Volkman D, Lane HD, Fauci AS: Antigen-induced in vitro antibody production in humans: A model for B cell activation and immunoregulation. Proc Natl Acad Sci USA 78:2528, 1981.
8. Souhamii RL, Babbage J, Callard RE: Specific in vitro antibody response to varicella zoster. Clin Exp Immunol 46:98, 1981.
9. Callard RE: Specific in vitro antibody response to influenza virus by human blood lymphocytes. Nature 282:734, 1979.
10. Froelich TL, Lum LG: Immunoglobulin secretion by human B lymphocytes exposed to Herpes simplex type I antigen. Immunobiology 162:94, 1982.
11. Ching YC, Davis SD, Wedgwood RJ: Antibody studies in hypogammaglobulinemia. J Clin Invest 45:1593, 1966.
12. Ochs HD, Davis SD, Wedgwood RJ: Immunologic responses to bacteriophage ϕX 174 in immunodeficiency diseases. J Clin Invest 50:2559, 1971.
13. Wedgwood RJ, Ochs HD, Davis SD: The recognition and classification of immunodeficiency diseases with bacteriophage ϕX 174. In Bergsma D, Good RA, Finstad J (eds): "Immunodeficiency in Man and Animals." Sunderland MA: Sinauer Associates for the National Foundation–March of Dimes, BD:OAS XI(1): 331–338, 1975.
14. Jackson CG, Ochs HD, Sieber OF, Jones JF, Wedgwood RJ: Interaction of T- and B-lymphocytes in the immune response to a thymus-dependent antigen. (Abstract) Clin Res 25:155A, 1977.
15. Grubb R, Swahn B: Destruction of some agglutinins but not others by two sulfhydryl compounds. Acta Pathol Microbiol Scand 43:305, 1958.
16. Jerne NK: Towards a network theory of the immune system. Ann Immunol (Paris) 125 C:373, 1974.
17. Stevens RH, Macy E, Morrow C, Saxon A: Characterization of a circulating subpopulation of spontaneous antitetanus toxoid antibody producing B cells following in vivo booster immunization. J Immunol 122:2498, 1979.
18. Thomson P, Harris N: Detection of plaque forming cells in the peripheral blood of actively immunized humans. J Immunol 118:1480, 1974.
19. Lane HD, Volkman DJ, Whalen G, Fauci AS: In vitro antigen-induced, antigen-specific antibody production in man. Specific and polyclonal components, kinetics and cellular requirements. J Exp Med 154:1043, 1981.

The Regulatory Role of Human Neonatal Monocytes in the In Vitro Antigen-Specific Plaque-Forming Cell Response*

M.J.D. van Tol, PhD, J. Zijlstra, B.J.M. Zegers, PhD, and R.E. Ballieux, PhD

Department of Immunology, University Children's Hospital, Het Wilhelmina Kinderziekenhuis (M.J.D.v.T., J.Z., B.J.M.Z.); and Department of Clinical Immunology, University Hospital (R.E.B.), Utrecht, The Netherlands

INTRODUCTION

Most studies which address the immature nature of the B-cell response in human newborns are based on stimulation of cord blood mononuclear cells (CBMC)** in vitro using polyclonal activators such as PWM, Epstein-Barr virus, and Nocardia water soluble mitogen [1]. Few data have been published regarding antigen-specific responses of neonatal B lymphocytes in vitro. It has been reported by Pascal et al [2] that a TNP-specific plaque-forming cell (PFC) response can be generated in CBMC in vitro. However, the presence of lipopolysaccharide (LPS) as co-stimulator in the culture system is required. Dosch and Gelfand [3], and more recently Misiti and Waldmann [4], and Lane et al [5], have described techniques for the antigen-specific induction in vitro of IgM-PFCs in peripheral blood mononuclear cells (PBMC) of adults in the absence of nonspecific stimulating agents. None of these methods has been applied to analyze a (primary) antigen-specific response of neonatal blood lymphocytes.

It was the object of the present study to investigate the capacity of human cord blood B cells to develop into IgM-PFCs after antigenic stimulation in vitro. The results obtained establish that the human newborn can respond to the 2 T-cell-dependent antigens employed: OA and SE. However, the antigen dose required to obtain optimal PFC responses in CBMC is a 2 log magnitude lower than the corresponding dose in adult PBMC. The data presented in this paper indicate that the different antigen-dose dependency of the PFC response in CBMC is related to characteristic properties of neonatal antigen-presenting cells.

MATERIALS AND METHODS

Antigen-specific induction and enumeration of PFCs. The technique, originally described by Dosch and Gelfand [3], has been used. The methodologic aspects have been extensively reviewed [6-8]. The antigens used were OA and SE.

Isolation of (subsets of) cells from blood. All methods concerning the isolation of mononuclear cells, the depletion and isolation of adherent cells (AC), and the isolation, depletion and identification of T and B cells have been described elsewhere [9].

Production of OA-induced T-helper factor: ThF120. The method has been published previously [10]. In short, purified human adult T lymphocytes were cultured in the inserts of Marbrook tubes in the presence of 5% autologous AC and 3 μg OA/ml. After 96 hours, the cells were collected, washed, and cultured for an additional 24 hours in tissue culture tubes with antigen. After this period the cell-free culture fluid was collected. It contains OA-specific ThF. The biologic properties and mode of action of this factor (after purification) have been reported by Heijnen et al [10]. In this study the ThF was not further purified, but the cell-free culture fluid was used as a source of the OA-specific helper factor. It will be referred to as ThF120. Furthermore, neonatal T cells were cultured under similar conditions in the presence of autologous neonatal or semiallogeneic parental AC with various doses of antigen. Supernatants obtained after 120 hours of culture were tested for OA-specific helper activity as described earlier [10].

RESULTS

Dose-response profile of the PFC response. As shown recently [11], CBMC are able to mount an antigen-specific IgM-PFC response after stimulation in vitro with either a soluble antigen of protein nature (OA) or a corpuscular antigen (SE). The PFC responses to both antigens are dependent on the presence of T cells and monocytes in the cell cultures (data not shown) [see ref. 11]. The results depicted in Figure 1 show

---

*This work was supported in part by the Foundation for Medical Research (FUNGO), which is subsidized by the Netherlands Organization for the Advancement of Pure Research (ZWO).

**Abbreviations used in this paper: OA, ovalbumin; SE, sheep erythrocytes; CBMC, cord blood mononuclear cells; PBMC, peripheral blood mononuclear cells; PFC, plaque-forming cell; AC, adherent cells; Th, T helper; Ts, T suppressor; PGE-2, prostaglandin E2; PWM, pokeweed mitogen; AET, 2-aminoethylisothiouronium bromide hydrobromide.

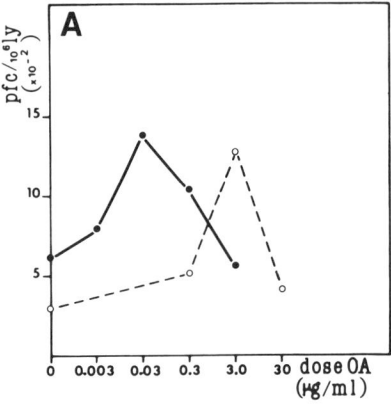
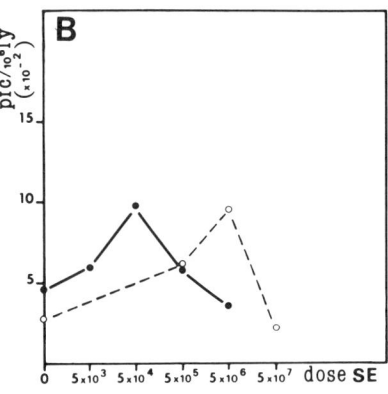

Fig. 1. Antigen dose-PFC-response profile of CBMC (●——●) and adult PBMC (○--○). 5×10^6 Mononuclear cells were cultured for 6 days in the presence of the concentration indicated A) OA or B) SE. The antigen-specific PFC-assay was performed at day 6. The results are expressed as PFC/10^6 lymphocytes and are the mean of 5 experiments.

TABLE 1. Antigen-Dose Dependency of the Stimulation of Neonatal B Cells Cultured in the Presence of 5% Autologous AC and 10% (v/v) Adult ThF120

OA-dose (μg/ml)	PFC-response (PFC/10^6 B ly*)
0.003	450 ± 437
0.03	756 ± 510
0.3	638 ± 300
3.0	574 ± 388

*Mean ± SD (n=4).

Fig. 2. Generation of Ts cells at supraoptimal antigen doses. Neonatal and adult T cells or non-T cells were cultured for 24 hr in the presence of 5% autologous AC and the OA-dose indicated. 5×10^6 Primed cells were added to cultures of 5×10^6 autologous mononuclear cells stimulated with the optimal OA-dose for the induction of a PFC response. The data shown are the mean of 3 experiments.

that optimal responses are obtained at an OA-concentration of 0.03 μg/ml and at a SE-CBMC ratio of 1:100. The magnitude as well as the bell-shaped dose-response profile of the PFC response of CBMC are comparable to those found for adult PBMC. However, PFCs are optimally generated in CBMC at antigen-concentrations which are a hundredfold lower than the optimal concentration of antigen for PBMC.

A search for the cause of the decrease of the PFC response at supraoptimal antigen doses. Isolated B cells can be tolerized by interaction with antigen at high concentrations. This is true in particular for immature B lymphocytes [1]. The decrease of the PFC response of CBMC at supraoptimal antigen doses therefore could be due to the induction of B-cell unresponsiveness. This possibility was investigated by stimulation of isolated cord blood B cells with various doses of OA in the presence of 5% autologous monocytes and OA-induced T-cell-derived helper factor (ThF120) produced by allogeneic adult human T lymphocytes in vitro. It was found that neonatal B cells in these experimental conditions respond with an adequate PFC response (Table 1), even when stimulated at a concentration of 3.0 μg OA/ml. As shown in Figure 1A, this dose of antigen is supraoptimal for the induction of a PFC response in unfractionated CBMC. It can be concluded, therefore, that the decline in the PFC response of CBMC at 3.0 μg OA/ml is not caused by B-cell unresponsiveness induced at this particular concentration of antigen.

Since after the substitution of T cells by ThF120 the decrease of the PFC response at supraoptimal doses could no longer be demonstrated, it was reasonable to assume that the reduced number of PFCs generated in CBMC at 3.0 μg OA/ml is due to a suppressive activity induced in the neonatal T-cell population. This assumption is strongly supported by earlier reports on the existence in adult PBMC of antigen-specific T suppressor (Ts) effector cells, which are activated at supraoptimal antigen doses (100 μg OA/ml) [12]. To test whether Ts cells were generated in cultures of cord blood cells at 3.0 μg OA/ml, CBMC were separated in a T-cell-enriched (T-cell fraction) and a T-cell-depleted population (non-T-cell fraction) by rosetting with AET-treated SE. Cells from both fractions were cultured for 24 hours in vitro in the presence of 5% autologous AC and 3.0 μg OA/ml. After this period, the cells were washed twice and added to cultures of autologous, non-separated CBMC, containing 0.03 μg OA/ml (which is the optimal dose, see Fig. 1). After 6 days, the PFC responses were measured. The results show that antigen-induced suppressive activity can be generated in neonatal T cells at 3.0 μg OA/ml (Fig. 2). This is in contrast to adult PBMC where a concentration of 3.0 μg OA/ml in the culture leads to optimal responses and suppressor T-cell activity is only generated at OA-concentrations of 30–100 μg/ml [12].

What causes CBMC to develop a PFC response at a hundredfold lower dose of antigen? The ability to mount a PFC response to T-cell-dependent antigens depends on the presence of antigen-reactive B cells, of functionally active Th cells, and of antigen-processing AC. It was considered feasible that differences in functional properties of neonatal cells in each of these 3 cell populations (B, T, and AC) could contribute to the characteristic dose-response relationship of the PFC response of CBMC. This issue was addressed in experiments in which CBMC of a newborn and PBMC of the mother were depleted of AC, and reconstituted in a reciprocal manner with the semiallogeneic* AC of the mother and the newborn, respectively. The data given in Figure 3 clearly show that the optimal dose of antigen for AC-depleted CBMC shifted toward an adult value of 3.0 μg OA/ml if the cells were reconstituted with parental AC. In a reciprocal type of experiment it was found that optimal PFC responses in adult AC-depleted PBMC were obtained at 0.03 μg OA/ml when neonatal AC were added to the cultures. These results strongly suggest that AC play a crucial role in determining the antigen dose-response relationship in this in vitro system.

The following series of experiments focused on the role of AC in the activation of Th cells, because the differences in antigen-dose dependency of the PFC response in CBMC and adult PBMC suggest that neonatal Th cells need less antigen to be activated compared to adult Th cells (Fig. 1). To that end, neonatal T cells were cultured in presence of autologous neonatal AC or semiallogeneic parental AC after addition of various doses of antigen. After a culture period of 120 hours, the supernatants, obtained from the different cell combinations stimulated with OA in various concentrations, were tested for the presence of ThF120 activity.

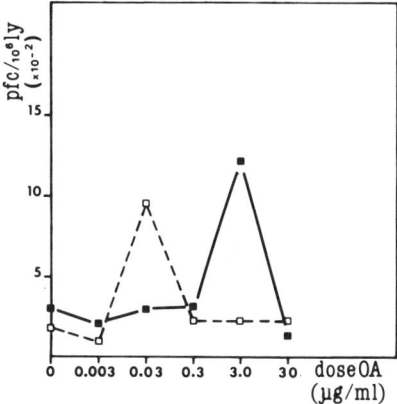

Fig. 3. Effect of the reconstitution of neonatal lymphocytes with semi-allogeneic parental AC (■——■) and of parental lymphocytes with semi-allogeneic neonatal AC (□----□) on the antigen dose-response relationship. CBMC and parental PBMC were completely depleted of AC and reconstituted with 10% parental AC and 10% neonatal AC, respectively. 5×10^6 Cells were stimulated with the OA-dose indicated. The results of one representative experiment out of 2 are given.

Adult B cells supplemented with 5% autologous AC and stimulated with 3 μg OA/ml were used as assay system. The results, summarized in Figure 4, show that the antigen-dose dependency for the generation of ThF120 activity in neonatal T cells is closely linked to the origin of the antigen-presenting AC in the cultures.

Next, the role of the AC in the activation of B lymphocytes was investigated. Therefore, neonatal B cells were cultured with a dose range of antigen after addition of 5% semi-allogeneic parental AC and ThF120 produced by allogeneic adult T cells. As shown in Figure 5, B cells from cord blood can adequately be activated at concentrations of antigen (0.003 μg OA/ml) which are suboptimal for induction of a PFC response in unseparated CBMC. The antigen-dose dependency for the activation of cord blood B cells in the presence of parental AC is not changed compared to the dose-response relationship obtained when autologous neonatal AC are present. It is noteworthy that adult B cells need higher concentrations of antigen (lower level 0.3 μg OA/ml) to become responsive to ThF120.

The results described so far indicate that the AC play a crucial role in determining the antigen dose-response relationship in the culture sys-

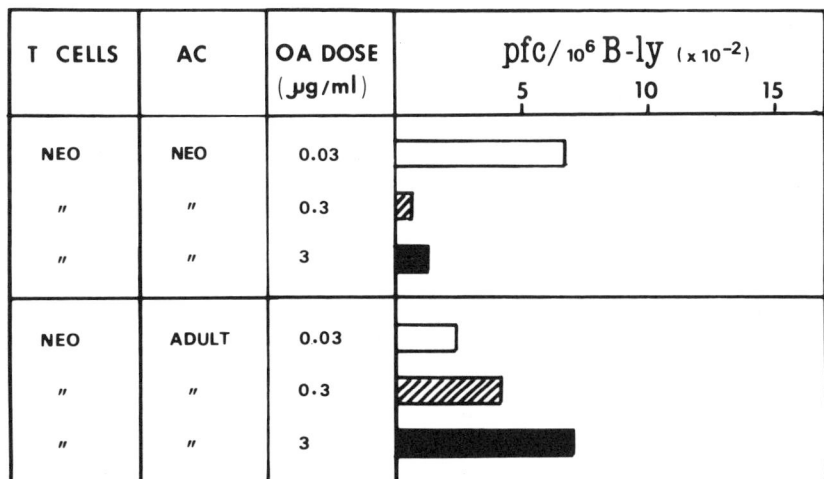

Fig. 4. Role of AC in the activation of neonatal Th cells. Neonatal T cells were cultured in the presence of 5% autologous neonatal AC or semi-allogeneic parental AC after addition of the dose of OA indicated. After 120 hr of culture, the supernatants obtained were tested for ThF120 activity by adding them to cultures of $3-5 \times 10^6$ adult B cells supplemented with 5% adult AC and stimulated with 3.0 μg OA/ml. The results (expressed as PFC/10^6 B ly) of one representative experiment out of 2 are given.

---

*Antigen presentation by AC to Th and to B cells is HLA-D(R) restricted. However, semi-allogeneic AC can adequately function as antigen-presenting cells [see ref. 13 and also Zegers et al, this volume].

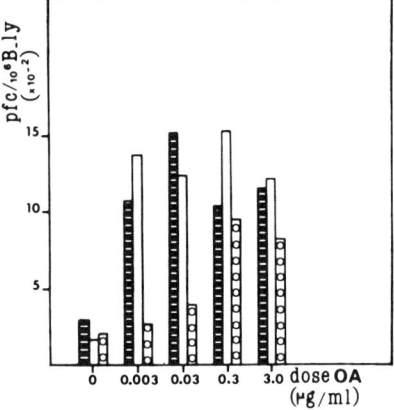

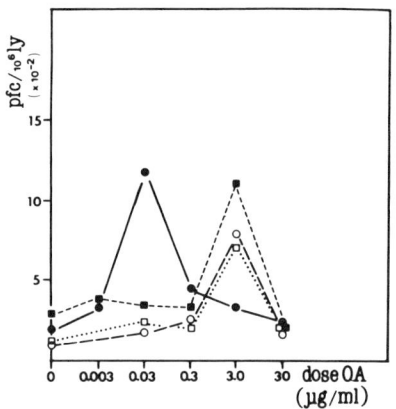

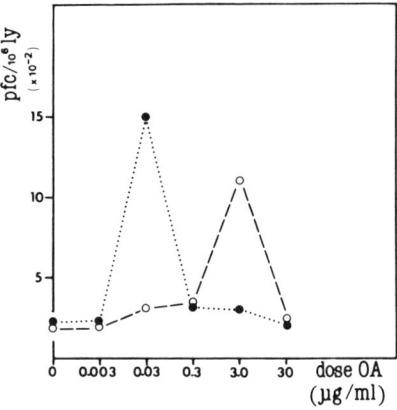

Fig. 5. Role of AC in the activation of neonatal B cells. 3×10^6 Neonatal B cells were supplemented with 5% autologous neonatal AC (■) or semi-allogeneic parental AC (□) and stimulated with the various doses of OA indicated in the presence of adult ThF120. The same type of experiment was performed with adult B cells supplemented with 5% autologous adult AC (⊡). The results (expressed as PFC/10^6 B ly) of one representative experiment out of 2 are shown.

Fig. 6. Effect of indomethacin on the antigen dose-response relationship for CBMC and adult PBMC.
Indomethacin (5 µg/ml) was added at the initiation of cultures containing 5×10^6 CBMC (■----■) or adult PBMC (□----□) stimulated with the OA-doses indicated. In control cultures of CBMC (●——●) or adult PBMC (○----○) indomethacin was absent. The results of one representative experiment out of 3 are given.

Fig. 7. Effect of PGE-2 on the antigen dose-response relationship for adult PBMC.
5×10^6 Adult PBMC were cultured with (●----●) or without (○----○) the addition of 1 µM PGE-2 at culture initiation. The results of one representative experiment out of 2 are given.

tem used. This regulatory activity becomes apparent at the level of interaction with Th cells rather than with the B cell.

Effect of indomethacin and PGE-2 on the antigen dose-response relationship. It has been reported recently that prostaglandins may have a negative influence on the expression of Ia at the cell surface of murine macrophages [14]. Since antigen presentation to Th cells in man shows allogeneic restriction and most probably involves HLA-D-related structures [15], the effect of blocking PGE-2 synthesis by indomethacin was studied. The addition of 5 µg indomethacin/ml to cell cultures of CBMC and adult PBMC, stimulated with various doses of antigen, resulted in an impressive shift in antigen-dose requirement for optimal PFC responses in CBMC (Fig. 6). In fact, the antigen-dose dependency of the PFC response of CBMC in the presence of indomethacin became very similar to that found for adult PBMC. No effect was noticed in cultures of adult PBMC.

In the next series of experiments we addressed the issue whether the addition of PGE-2 to cultures of adult PBMC would change the antigen-dose requirements to that of CBMC type. Adult PBMC were stimulated with various doses of OA with or without the addition of 1 µM PGE-2. As can be seen from the results presented in Figure 7, the addition of PGE-2 to the cultures of adult PBMC resulted in a neonatal type of antigen-dose requirement for the induction of optimal PFC responses.

DISCUSSION

The results presented in this paper confirm the observation made previously [11] that neonatal human B lymphocytes can be stimulated by antigen to mature into IgM-secreting PFCs. The responses to OA and SE have been described to be T-cell dependent in adults [9] as well as in newborns [11]. In addition, the presence of AC in the culture is required for the successful generation of a PFC response.

Three aspects of the present findings need further comment. It has been reported by a number of investigators, using polyclonal B-cell activators, that the response of human neonatal B lymphocytes is limited to IgM synthesis in relatively low amounts. It has been suggested that the lack of an adult type of antibody response was due to an intrinsic immaturity of the neonatal B-cell compartment [1]. The present data establish, however, that the magnitude of the specific IgM response of CBMC is of the same order as that of adult PBMC. This suggests that the pool size and the functional properties of anti-OA and anti-SE PFC-precursors in neonates do not differ significantly from those in adults.

A second aspect, related to the former, regards T-cell regulation of B-cell responses in the newborn. Various levels of Th activity have been measured in neonatal blood cells by different investigators. These data were obtained in cultures of CBMC, stimulated with mitogens such as PWM [1]. The results presented in this paper indicate that, at least for the antigens OA and SE, Th function is adequately developed at neonatal age. In a separate investigation, which will be reported elsewhere, this assumption has been confirmed.

Many investigators have reported that T-cell-mediated suppression dominates Th activity in responses of CBMC, stimulated in vitro with mitogens [1]. In accordance with these observations we found that a dominant Ts activity is induced in CBMC when the cells are stimulated with antigen doses which give rise to optimal responses in adult PBMC. However, at a hundredfold lower antigen concentration good PFC responses could be obtained in CBMC. This finding implies that a) antigen specific Ts-cell activity can adequately be induced in CBMC, and b) the dominance of Ts function over Th emerges at much lower antigen concentration in cultures of newborn mononuclear blood cells.

This brings us to the last important aspect to be discussed: the role of the AC in determining the antigen-requirement in the PFC system used. It has been reported previously [15] that antigen presentation to Th cells involves AC and that Th-AC interaction is restricted at HLA-D(R) level. Hoffman et al [13] established that histocompatibility for one haplotype suffices to allow for adequate stimulation of Th cells. This is also illustrated in the present study by the finding that neonatal Th activity could be generated in vitro after activation of cord blood T cell with antigen presented by parental AC.

Piguet et al [16] and Snijder et al [14] recently reported that PGE-2, produced by cells of monocyte-macrophage nature, may have a negative influence on the in vitro immune response of neonatal murine lymphoid cells. Therefore, the possible involvement of PGE-2 in determining the antigen dose requirements for optimal PFC responses was investigated. It was found that the antigen-dose dependency of the neonatal PFC response became very similar, if not identical, to that found for adult PBMC if indomethacin had been added to the cultures of CBMC (Fig. 6). In a reversed type of experiment it could be shown that the addition of physiologic amounts of PGE-2 to cultures of adult PBMC resulted in a change of antigen-dose requirement to that of the neonatal type (Fig. 7). Studies are underway which analyze this phenomenon in more detail. However, the present results establish an important regulatory role of human neonatal monocytes in the in vitro antigen-specific PFC response.

ACKNOWLEDGMENT

The secretarial assistance of Ms. T. Matze is gratefully acknowledged.

REFERENCES

1. Möller G (ed): Ontogeny of human lymphocyte function. Immunol Rev 57:5-161, 1981.
2. Pascal C, Galanaud P, Dormont J, Wallon C: Primary in vitro antibody response in human cord blood lymphocytes. J Reprod Immunol 1:275-283, 1980.
3. Dosch HM, Gelfand EW: Generation of human plaque-forming cells in culture: Tissue distribution, antigenic and cellular requirements. J Immunol 118:302-308, 1977.
4. Misiti J, Waldmann TA: In vitro generation of antigen-specific hemolytic plaque-forming cells from human peripheral blood mononuclear cells. J Exp Med 154:1069-1084, 1981.
5. Lane HC, Volkman DJ, Whalen G, Fauci AS: In vitro antigen-induced, antigen-specific antibody production in man: Specific and polyclonal components, kinetics and cellular requirements. J Exp Med 154:1043-1057, 1981.
6. Fauci AS, Ballieux RE (eds): "Antibody Production in Man. In Vitro Synthesis and Clinical Implications." New York: Academic Press, 1979.
7. Ballieux RE, Heijnen CJ, UytdeHaag F, Zegers BJM: Regulation of B cell activity in man: Role of T cells. Immunol Rev 45:3-39, 1979.
8. Dosch HM, Gelfand EW: Specific in vitro IgM responses of human B cells: A complex regulatory network modulated by antigen. Immunol Rev 45:243-274, 1979.
9. Heijnen CJ, UytdeHaag F, Gmelig-Meyling FHJ, Ballieux RE: Localization of human antigen-specific helper and suppressor function in distinct T-cell subpopulations. Cell Immunol 43:282-292, 1979.
10. Heijnen CJ, UytdeHaag F, Pot KH, Ballieux RE: Antigen-specific human T cell factors. I. T cell helper factor: Biologic properties. J Immunol 126:497-502, 1981.
11. Tol MJD v, Zijlstra J, Heijnen CJ, Kuis W, Zegers BJM, Ballieux RE: Antigen-specific plaque-forming cell response of human cord blood lymphocytes after in vitro stimulation by T cell-dependent antigens. Eur J Immunol (in press).
12. UytdeHaag F, Heijnen CJ, Ballieux RE: Induction of antigen-specific human suppressor T lymphocytes in vitro. Nature 271:556-557, 1978.
13. Hoffman AA, Hayward AR, Kurnick JT, Defreitas EC, McGregor J, Harbeck RJ: Presentation of antigen by human newborn monocytes to maternal tetanus toxoid-specific T-cell blasts. J Clin Immunol 1:217-221, 1981.
14. Snijder DS, Lu CY, Unanue ER: Control of macrophage Ia expression in neonatal mice-role of a splenic suppressor cell. J Immunol 128:1458-1465, 1982.
15. Rees A, Feldmann M, Woody JN, Erb P: Genetics of human T cell-monocyte interaction in helper cell induction. Clin Exp Immunol 44:445-452, 1981.
16. Piguet PF, Irle C, Vassalli P: Immunosuppressor cells from newborn mouse spleen are macrophages differentiating in vitro from monoblastic precursors. Eur J Immunol 11:56-61, 1981.

Immune Regulation in the Hyper-IgE/Job Syndrome*

Hans D. Ochs, MD, Michael J. Kraemer, MD, Catherine G. Lindgren, BS, Clifton T. Furukawa, MD, and Ralph J. Wedgwood, MD

Department of Pediatrics, University of Washington, Seattle, WA 98195

The hyperimmunoglobulinemia E (hyper-IgE) syndrome, or Job syndrome, is a disorder characterized by recurrent staphylococcal infections, including deep skin abscesses, lymphadenopathy, and lung abscesses; severe eczema; and markedly elevated levels of serum IgE [1, 2]. Many patients with this disorder have characteristic coarse features, growth retardation, and hyperkeratotic fingernails. Laboratory abnormalities include very high serum IgE levels—a large proportion being specific IgE antibody against staphylococcal and *Candida albicans* [3, 4] antigens—eosinophilia, abnormal antibody responses to some antigens, depressed in vitro proliferative responses to specific antigens, large quantities of spontaneous in vitro IgE synthesis by peripheral blood B lymphocytes, and a variable chemotactic defect [5–9]. Several families with more than one affected member have been reported; an autosomal recessive mode of inheritance with incomplete penetrance [5] or an autosomal dominant mode of inheritance [10] has been suggested.

The pathophysiology of this syndrome is unknown. Recently, it was proposed that these patients lack T-suppressor (Ts) cells which normally inhibit excess synthesis of IgE [6, 7]. This hypothesis was based on the observation that in vitro IgE synthesis by B cells from hyper-IgE patients was suppressed by Ts (OKT8$^+$) cells from normal controls but not by autologous Ts cells from the hyper-IgE patient.

To explore the possibility that an allogeneic suppressor defect was responsible for these observations, we have studied the interaction between allogeneic hyper-IgE T cells and IgE-synthesizing B cells obtained from 2 nonrelated hyper-IgE patients. Furthermore, the functions of B cells, T helper (Th) cells and Ts cells were tested in a pokeweed mitogen (PWM)-driven hemolytic plaque assay system.

METHODS

Patients

Eight patients with serum IgE levels exceeding 3,000 IU/ml were included in the study. Clinical details are summarized in Table 1. None of the patients was treated systemically with steroids at the time of the study. Five patients (*Cases 1–5*) with recurrent staphylococcal infections were previously shown to have depressed neutrophil and/or monocyte chemotaxis [9–11]. *Patients 2, 3, 5,* and *8* had many of the clinical features of the syndrome described by Davis et al [1] and Buckley et al [2]; *Patient 3* is one of the original cases described in reference 1. These patients had more severe infections, including recurrent deep staphylococcal infections associated with few inflammatory reactions ("cold" abscesses), and the 3 older patients (*cases 3, 5,* and *8*) had presented with lung abscesses resulting in pneumatoceles. Three of these patients had developed characteristic hyperkeratotic fingernail changes. Five young adults with normal serum IgE levels and no evidence of atopic disease served as controls.

Cell Separation

Peripheral blood mononuclear cells (PBM) were separated by Ficoll-Hypaque gradient centrifugation. Adherent cells were removed by incubating PBMs in plastic Petri dishes for 30 minutes at 37°C. Nonadherent cells were removed by several washes with RPMI 1640 and the cells were further separated in T- and B-lymphocyte-enriched cell populations by a rosetting technique [12] using 2-amino-ethyl-isothiouronium bromide, hydrobromide- (Sigma Chemical Co., St. Louis, Missouri) treated sheep red blood cells (AET-SRBC). The B-cell-enriched interface (B cells) contained <5% SRBC-receptor positive lymphocytes; approximately 44% of these cells were myeloperoxidase positive. The pellet, containing T lymphocytes, was incubated with buffered NH$_4$Cl to lyse the SRBCs. This T-cell-enriched preparation (T cells) was monocyte free as defined by myeloperoxidase staining, and 98% of the cells show T-cell characteristics by rerosetting with SRBC. Viability of both T-cell and B-cell fractions was >96%.

T-Lymphocyte Surface Markers

Monoclonal antibodies of the OKT series (Ortho Pharmaceutical Corp., Raritan, New Jersey) were used to identify T cells (OKT3$^+$), Th cells (OKT4$^+$), and Ts cells (OKT8$^+$). The percentage of fluorescent cells

---

*Supported by grants from NIH (AI-07073) and from the March of Dimes Birth Defects Foundation (6-273). A portion of this work was conducted through the Clinical Research Center facility at the University of Washington supported by NIH grant RR-37. MJK was supported by training grant 1-T32-HD-07172-02.

TABLE 1. Clinical Features of Study Patients*

						Recurrent Infections	
Patient No.	Age	Sex	IgE (IU/ml)	Eczema	Skin	Pulmonary Abscesses, Empyema, Pneumatocele	Comment
1	11	F	50,000	+++	+		—
2	3	M	21,200	+++	+++		Job syndrome
3	29	F	10,500	+	+++	++ (Staph)	Job syndrome (mother of Patient 2)
4	12	M	6,200	++	+		—
5	21	M	24,000	+	+++	++ (Staph)	Job syndrome
6	12	M	9,200	++	+		—
7	16	M	3,600				—
8	11	F	27,800	+	++	+++ (Pneumococci Staph)	Job syndrome
Controls (n = 5)	19–24	3F, 2M	12–49				

*The severity of the clinical findings is indicated by + (mild) to +++ (extensive).

was determined by counting 400–500 cells with immunofluorescence and phase contrast microscopy [8].

Preparation of T-Cell Subsets

Selective depletion of Ts or Th cells was accomplished by incubation of T lymphocytes with the appropriate monoclonal antibodies and complement as previously described [8]. Cell killing was determined by trypan blue dye uptake. Cell mortality was 20–69% if treated with OKT4, 13–34% with OKT8.

IgE Measurement

A double antibody RIA (Prist^R, Pharmacia, Piscataway, New Jersey) was used to estimate IgE. Preformed IgE was defined as the average amount of IgE present in puromycin-treated culture supernatants of B cells and autologous T cells. Preformed IgE was subtracted from the total IgE of an untreated culture to estimate de novo IgE synthesis.

Co-Culture System to Assess Regulation of In Vitro IgE Synthesis

Two to 4 replicate cultures were established for each experimental combination using flat bottom microtiter plates. Each well contained 2.5×10^5 B cells, 2.5×10^5 T cells in RPMI 1640 with 10% heat inactivated fetal calf serum (FCS), penicillin (100 U/ml), streptomycin (100 μg/ml), and l-glutamine (2 mM). To determine preformed IgE, puromycin (10 μg/ml) was added at day 0. Plates were incubated at 37°C in 5% CO_2 for up to 10 days, freeze-thawed 5 times, centrifuged at 650 g for 10 minutes, and the supernatant was harvested for IgE assay. The effect of T-cell subsets on IgE synthesis was studied by assessment of IgE synthesis in various cell mixtures. Suppression was expressed as the percentage decrease in de novo IgE synthesis of cell mixtures compared to de novo IgE synthesis by B cells alone.

In Vitro Functional Assessment of B Lymphocytes, Th Cells, Ts Cells

Under certain conditions, antibody-producing PBMs can be identified by hemolytic plaques, formed within a monolayer of SRBC after addition of complement [13]. The system requires B cells, adherent cells (activated macrophages), Th cells, and the presence of either a polyclonal activator, eg PWM or specific antigen [14]. PBMs are incubated in Petri dishes at 37°C and the nonadherent cells are washed off. The adherent population is harvested by scraping them off mechanically and the suspended adherent cell population is kept on ice until added to the culture system. OKT8-treated T cells (OKT8$^+$ depleted) are designated as Th cells. Optimal numbers of plaques are formed in the following cell culture system: 0.5×10^6 B cells; 1.5×10^6 OKT4$^+$ enriched Th cells and 0.1×10^6 activated adherent cells incubated in RPMI 1640 in a total volume of 2 ml with the addition of PWM 1:100, 10% SRBC-absorbed AB serum, penicillin/streptomycin and l-glutamine. The cells are harvested after 7 days of culture and cell aliquots are incubated on SRBC monolayers which have been fixed to plastic with poly-L-lysine for 30 minutes. Plaques are developed with fresh frozen (SRBC absorbed) guinea pig serum and counted under an inverted microscope.

RESULTS

Percentages of OKT3$^+$ (T cells), OKT4$^+$ (Th cells), and OKT8$^+$ (Ts cells) lymphocytes were not different between patients with the hyper-IgE/Job syndrome and normal controls. The percentages were the same if peripheral blood mononuclear cells or if E-rosette positive cells were studied.

In vitro IgE synthesis was observed in cultures from all hyper-IgE/Job syndrome patients. Concentrations of de novo synthesized IgE and of preformed IgE determined in

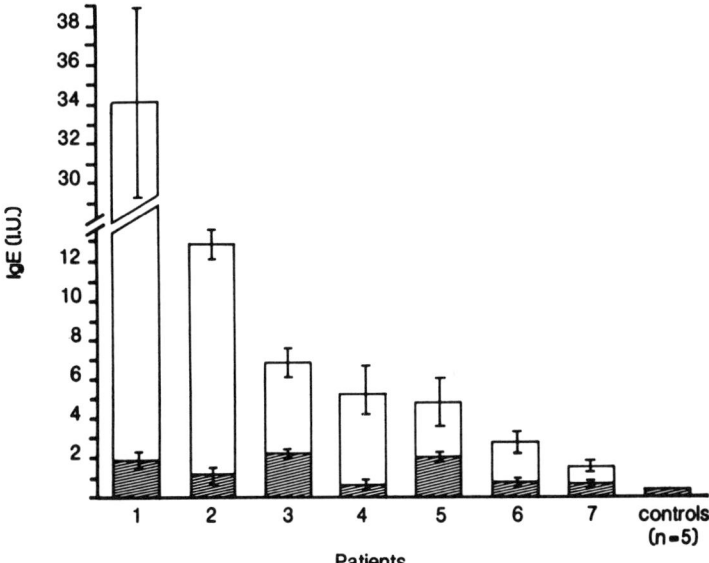

Fig. 1. IgE produced by 10-day cultures of B cells in the presence of autologous T cells is shown for 7 hyper-IgE/Job syndrome patients and 5 normal controls. Each bar represents mean ± SD total IgE from 4 replicate assays. The shaded portions define mean ± SD preformed IgE determined by treating cultures with puromycin. The difference between total and preformed IgE represents de novo synthesized IgE (open position of the bar). (Figs. 1–3 reprinted from Clin Immunol Immunopathol 25:157–164, 1982, with permission.)

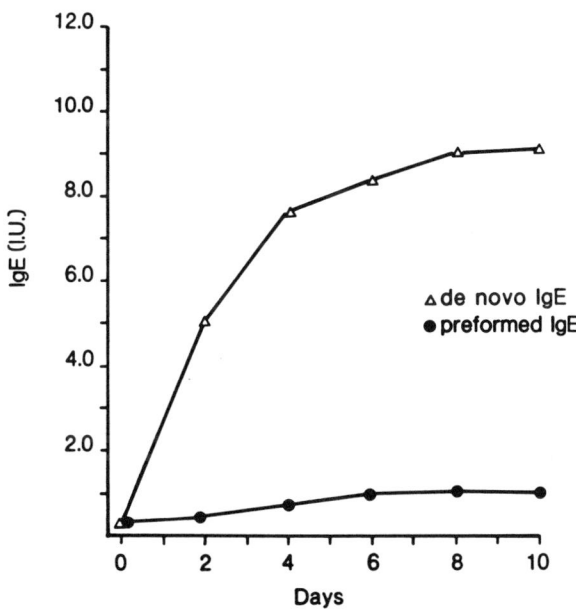

Fig. 2. Cultures of hyper-IgE B cells and autologous T cells were analyzed at 2-day intervals for cumulative IgE synthesis. Preformed IgE (●) and de novo synthesized IgE (△) are illustrated. Each point represents the geometric mean of duplicate observations from 4 patients (*Patients 1, 2, 4, 6*).

10-day cultures of B cells cultured together with autologous T cells are shown for each patient in Figure 1. Cultures from normal controls showed small amounts of preformed but no measurable de novo synthesis of IgE. Cumulative IgE synthesis of hyper-IgE/Job B cells co-cultured with autologous T cells is shown in Figure 2. Rapid de novo synthesis of IgE occurred during the first 6 days, and then leveled off.

The effect of autologous and allogeneic T cells or T-cell subsets on IgE synthesis by hyper-IgE/Job B cells is shown in Figure 3. Allogeneic T cells from either hyper-IgE patients or normal controls suppressed IgE synthesis in a similar fashion. The effect appeared related to Ts cells (OKT8$^+$); Ts-enriched mixtures showed suppression; Ts-depleted cultures did not. Thus, in the allogeneic system, cells from hyper-IgE patients were as capable of in vitro suppression of IgE synthesis as normal control cells.

Function of lymphocyte subsets of 4 patients (*Patients 2, 3, 5, 8*) with the characteristic findings of Job syndrome were studied in the PWM-dependent direct hemolytic plaque assay. Results are shown in Figure 4. Control B cells, if co-cultured with macrophages and autologous or allogeneic control Th cells, formed hemolytic plaques, and allogeneic T suppression was not observed. However, B cells from patients did not form hemolytic plaques if co-cultured with autologous patient Th cells; if co-cultured with allogeneic control Th cells, 2 of 4 patients were able to generate a small number of hemolytic plaques. Patient helper cells could not provide help if cocultured with control B cells. Furthermore, patient T cells, if added to a culture of control B cells plus control T cells, suppressed plaque formation in 3 of 4 instances, suggesting the presence of suppressor cells.

DISCUSSION

As others have shown, all hyper-IgE/Job syndrome patients synthesized measurable amounts of IgE. Spontaneous de novo IgE synthesis was greatest during the first 6 days and slower thereafter. As has been shown by a number of investigators, addition of allogeneic control lym-

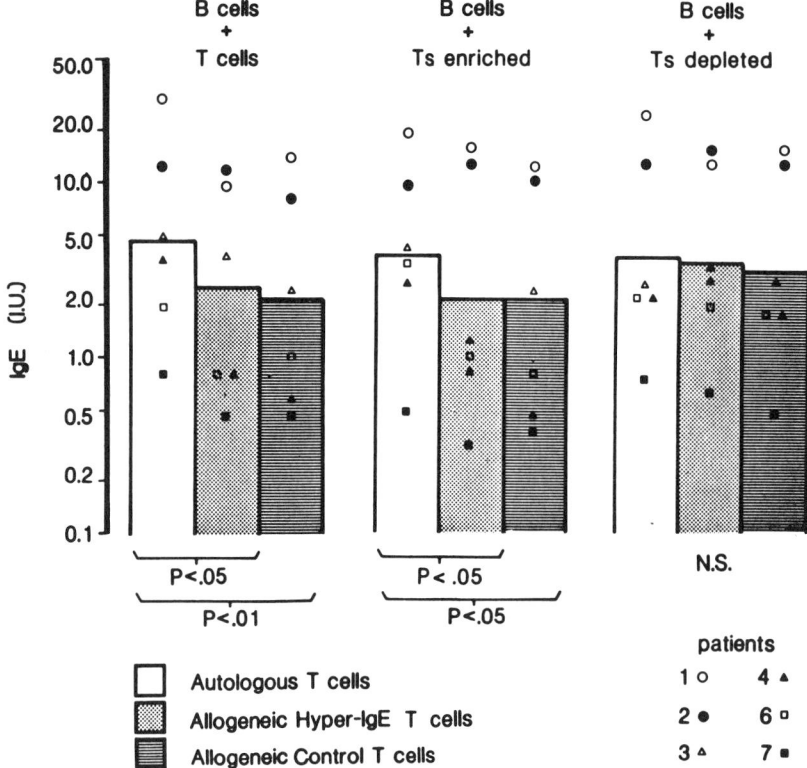

Fig. 3. Shown are statistical comparisons of the geometric means of B- and T-cell subset mixing experiments performed in 6 of the hyper-IgE/Job syndrome patients. Compared to cultures of B cells with autologous T cells, a significant suppression (p < .05) occurred when T cells were from allogeneic hyper-IgE/Job syndrome patients or normal controls. The same allogeneic suppression occurred in Ts-enriched co-cultures (p < .05). When (OKT8$^+$) Ts cells were depleted, no allogeneic suppression occurred.

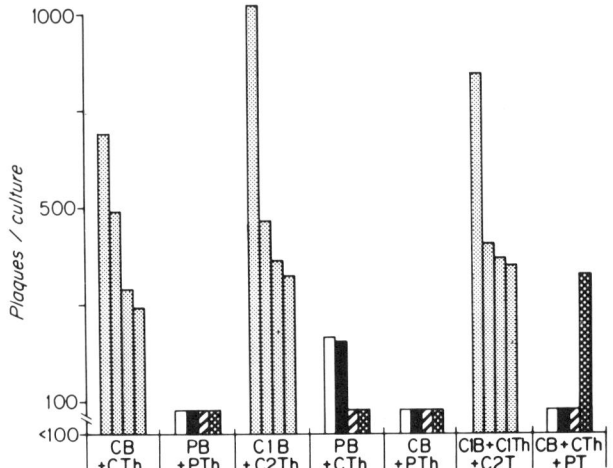

Fig. 4. Assessment of the function of lymphocyte subsets of 4 patients with hyper-IgE/Job syndrome. Control B cells (CB) always formed hemolytic plaques if co-cultured with macrophages and autologous or allogeneic Th cells (CTh); allogeneic T suppression was not observed. Patient B cells (PB) did not form hemolytic plaques if co-cultured with autologous patient Th cells (PTh), but in 2 of 4 patients, B cells formed plaques if co-cultured with allogeneic control Th cells. None of the patients could provide help if PTh were co-cultured with CB. Patient T cells (PT), if added to cultures of CB + CTh, suppressed plaque formation in 3 of 4 instances suggesting the presence of suppressor cells in 3/4 patients.

phocytes to hyper-IgE B cells has resulted in suppression of spontaneous IgE synthesis [6, 7, 15]. On the other hand, addition of autologous lymphocytes did not significantly suppress spontaneous IgE synthesis by B cells from patients with the hyper-IgE/Job syndrome. These data have been interpreted as evidence for the absence of Ts cells in the hyper-IgE/Job syndrome disorders. However, the studies reported here have demonstrated that IgE-producing B cells from hyper-IgE patients were equally suppressed by adding allogeneic hyper-IgE T cells from another nonrelated hyper-IgE patient. Therefore, it would appear that the regulatory defect responsible for hyper-IgE is more complex than the mere presence or absence of Ts cells, or nonresponsiveness of committed hyper-IgE B cells. We therefore studied individually, in a T-cell-dependent PWM-driven direct hemolytic plaque assay, the function of lymphocyte subsets. This is possible because the system is not HLA restricted. Using this system, peripheral blood lymphocytes of patients with the hyper-IgE/Job syndrome showed defective B-cell function in 2 of 4 patients, defective Th function in all, and the presence of excessive suppressor activity in 3 of 4 patients studied. These findings clearly indicate that patients with hyper-IgE/Job syndrome have a more generalized immune deficiency involving T-cell subsets and possibly B cells, and that impaired immune regulation may not be restricted to IgE synthesis.

REFERENCES

1. Davis SD, Schaller J, Wedgwood RJ: Job's syndrome: Recurrent, "cold" staphylococcal abscesses. Lancet 1:1013–1015, 1966.
2. Buckley RH, Wray BB, Belmaker EZ: Extreme hyperimmunoglobulinemia E and undue susceptibility to infections. Pediatrics 49:59–70, 1972.
3. Schopfer K, Baerlocher K, Price P, Krech U, Quie PG, Douglas SD: Staph-

ylococcal IgE antibodies, hyperimmunoglobulinemia E and staphylococcus aureus infections. N Engl J Med 300:835–838, 1979.
4. Berger M, Kirkpatrick CH, Goldsmith PK, Gallin JI: IgE antibodies to *Staphylococcus aureus* and *Candida albicans* in patients with the syndrome of hyperimmunoglobulin E and recurrent infections. J Immunol 125:2437–2443, 1980.
5. Buckley RH: Disorders of the IgE system. In Stiehm ER, Fulginiti VA (eds): "Immunologic Disorders in Infants and Children." Philadelphia: WB Saunders, 1980, pp 274–285.
6. Buckley RH, Fiser PM, Becker WG: In vitro studies of IgE synthesis by human blood mononuclear cells. Fed Proc 40:2167–2170, 1981.
7. Geha RS, Reinherz E, Leung D, McKee KT Jr, Schlossman S, Rosen FS: Deficiency of suppressor T cells in the hyperimmunoglobulin E syndrome. J Clin Invest 68:783–791, 1981.
8. Kraemer MJ, Ochs HD, Furukawa CT, Wedgwood RJ: In vitro studies of the hyper-IgE disorders: Suppression of spontaneous IgE synthesis by allogeneic suppressor T lymphocytes. Clin Immunol Immunopathol 25:157–164, 1982.
9. Hill HR, Ochs HD, Quie PG, Clark RA, Pabst HF, Klebanoff SJ, Wedgwood RJ: Defect in neutrophil granulocyte chemotaxis in Job's syndrome of recurrent "cold" staphylococcal abscesses. Lancet 1:616–619, 1974.
10. Kraemer MJ, Ochs HD, Klebanoff SJ, Altman LC, Wedgwood RJ: The inheritance of Job syndrome. (Abstract) Clin Res 29:122A, 1981.
11. Furukawa CT, Altman LC: Defective monocyte and polymorphonuclear leukocyte chemotaxis in atopic disease. J Allergy Clin Immunol 61:288–293, 1978.
12. Pellegrino MA, Ferrone S, Dierich MP, Reisfeld RA: Enhancement of sheep red blood cell human lymphocyte rosette formation by the sulfhydryl compound 2-amino ethylisothiouronium bromide. Clin Immunol Immunopathol 3:324–333, 1975.
13. Jerne NK, Nordin AA, Henry C: The Agar plaque technique for recognizing antibody producing cells. In Amos B, Koprowski (eds): "Cell Bound Antibodies." Philadelphia: The Wistar Institute Press, 1963, p 103.
14. Ballieux RE, Heijnen CJ, UytdeHaag F, Zegers BJM: Regulation of B cell activity in man: Role of T cells. Immunol Rev 45:3, 1979.
15. Fiser PM, Buckley RH: Human IgE biosynthesis in vitro: Studies with atopic and normal blood mononuclear cells and subpopulations. J Immunol 123:1788–1794, 1979.

SECTION 2
SEVERE COMBINED IMMUNODEFICIENCIES (SCID)

Diagnosis and Classification of Severe Combined Immunodeficiency Disease

Erwin W. Gelfand, MD, FRCP(C), and Hans-Michael Dosch, MD

Division of Immunology, The Hospital for Sick Children, Toronto, Ontario, Canada M5G 1X8

INTRODUCTION

Severe combined immunodeficiency disease (SCID) represents a spectrum of disorders characterized by the inability to manifest normal cell-mediated and humoral immunity. During the first workshop held in 1967 [1], there were perhaps more names for this disease than actual patients described. Even at this early stage, the descriptions of individual cases showed considerable heterogeneity in inheritance pattern and clinical and laboratory features. The first workshop spawned the exciting prospects for immunologic reconstitution which formed the basis for a large part of the discussion of the second workshop held in 1972 [2]. Many laboratories presented their successful attempts at immunologic reconstitution and cure of this fatal condition following bone marrow transplantation (BMT).

The last decade has witnessed a significant expansion in our knowledge of this disease entity. The heterogeneity of this condition, previously suspected on clinical and genetic grounds, has now been supported by studies characterizing lymphoid precursor cell development and circulating lymphocyte subpopulations. The advent of cell surface marker studies and new ways for assessing lymphocyte function have further identified important differences in individual patients. The demonstration of circulating B cells and T cells or T-cell precursors in many of them argues against the concept of a primary stem-cell defect underlying the disease in these patients.

Patients with SCID have played a major role in our understanding of normal lymphocyte ontogeny. Because of the heterogeneity of the disease, it is not easy to adopt simple criteria for diagnosis or classification. Despite this heterogeneity, SCID is appropriately named, since the majority of affected infants die before their first birthday. In addition, regardless of the complexity of laboratory findings, they all manifest a profound impairment of functional activity in both the T- and B-cell compartments.

DIAGNOSIS OF SCID (Table 1)
Clinical Features

Inheritance. The majority of cases occur as isolated events, although some families have been reported with autosomal recessive or X-linked inheritance. Consanguinity has been observed in more than half of our families. Initial descriptions suggested major differences between autosomal recessive and X-linked forms of SCID. These differences are likely not tenable today. Males outnumber females (4:1).

Clinical Features. The single most common presenting feature of SCID is failure to thrive. These infants are often below the 3rd % for weight, whereas linear growth may not be impaired at all. Significant failure of weight gain generally presents between 3–6 months of age; rarely, an infant may thrive for up to 10–12 months of age. Despite normal caloric intake, weight gain is poor, even when the calories are provided by other than the gastrointestinal route.

Recurrent infections generally begin between 3 and 6 months of age, at a time when maternally endowed humoral immunity has virtually disappeared; problems in the neonatal period are the exception. Bacterial otitis media, pneumonitis, and sepsis have all been described but, perhaps due to the liberal use of antibiotics, may not be the major problem. Recurrent and persistent oral and perianal candidiasis are frequent. Diarrhea and malabsorption, commonly secondary to one of the enteric viruses (mini-reo-, orbi-, or rotavirus), are common. In a survey of more than 20 infants with SCID, 11 presented with one or more of these enteric viruses and watery diarrhea [3]. Often, these viruses may be hospital acquired.

Pulmonary infections are also common. Pneumocystis carinii pneumonitis is often seen in SCID at the time of presentation. Because of the relatively rapid response to pentamidine isethionate or trimethoprim-sulfa, it is now rarely fatal. More devastating has been pneumonitis secondary to parainfluenza, type III [3, 4].

A variety of skin rashes have been associated with SCID—many are bizarre in appearance and location and not easily diagnosed. Others range from mild seborrheic dermatitis to a desquamative exfoliative dermatitis as seen in the Letterer-Siwe or Omenn syndromes (see be-

TABLE 1. Major Clinical and Laboratory Features in SCID

Parameter	Relative Frequency
History	
Positive family history	++
Physical examination	
Absence of lymphoid tissue	+++
Laboratory	
General	
ADA deficiency	++
Lymphopenia	++
CMI (T-cell)	
Low numbers (<10%) E-rosettes	+++
Absent lymphocyte proliferation-PHA	++++
Absent lymphocyte proliferation-MLR	+++
Absent delayed hypersensitivity	++++
Failure to reject allogeneic skin graft	++++
Thymus biopsy showing absence of cortico-medullary demarcation and Hassall corpuscles	+++
Humoral (B-cell) immunity	
Hypogammaglobulinemia-IgG	+++
Hypogammaglobulinemia-IgM	+++
Hypogammaglobulinemia-IgA	++++
Absence of specific antibodies	++++
Presence of circulating B lymphocytes	+++
Experimental	
Presence of T-cell precursors	+++

+: A few patients with SCID.
++: Some but not all patients with SCID.
+++: Majority of SCID.
++++: Virtually all patients with SCID.

low). Some of these skin manifestations may herald graft-versus-host disease (GVHD) as a consequence of intrauterine acquired maternal lymphocytes [5].

On physical examination, in addition to being scrawny, there is a marked absence of palpable lymphoid tissue and tonsillar buds. Rarely, lymphoid tissue may be present and even hyperplastic. On biopsy, these nodes show little organization, are lymphocyte-depleted, and large sheets of macrophages are observed.

Laboratory Features

In keeping with the absence of functional T cells, patients with SCID fail to manifest delayed cutaneous reactivity to any injected antigens or to reject a third-party skin graft. Their susceptibility to GVHD further attests to the absence of functional T cells.

In the majority of patients, lymphopenia is not a prominent feature. In our experience with more than 30 patients, adequate numbers of circulating lymphocytes (> 1500/mm^3) were found in more than 75% of cases. A proportion of these may be large, blast-like, or atypical in appearance, suggesting an immature state. Most patients with SCID have < 5% E-rosetting T cells and often < 2%. When the sheep erythrocytes (SEs) are modified (eg pretreated with neuraminidase or aminoethylisothiouronium bromide) a larger number may be identified [6]. In keeping with the paucity of circulating T cells and their immaturity, few cells stain as T cells with alpha-naphthyl-acetate esterase [7].

As increasing numbers of patients have been studied, a small but distinct group has been observed with normal numbers and proportions of circulating T cells. These may have a mature phenotype by a variety of assays, including pharmacologic manipulation or antigenic markers.

In vitro lymphoproliferative responses to plant lectins (eg phytohemagglutinin [PHA], specific antigens or allogeneic cells (mixed lymphocyte reaction, [MLR]) are profoundly depressed, often with marginal incorporation of radioisotope over background levels. Rarely, near-normal PHA or MLR responses have been documented.

Whereas proportions of T lymphocytes are markedly reduced in most patients, numbers of circulating B cells are often normal or increased. The surface immunoglobulin (Ig)-staining pattern of these cells may be normal, restricted to IgM, or express only IgD [8]. Since these B cells express Ia, those patients with high percentages of B cells may express "extraneous reactions" during HLA typing [9]. The extra reactions of the HLA typing sera can be attributed to Ia antibody in the typing sera.

Most patients are profoundly hypogammaglobulinemic with very low or undetectable levels of IgG, IgA, and IgE. Levels of circulating IgM are more variable, ranging from a complete absence to normal levels. As discussed below, there are several variants with normal levels of all Ig classes or paraproteinemia.

Regardless of the level of serum Ig, there is little evidence for specific antibody formation. Attempts to demonstrate antibodies to routine antigens such as tetanus, polio, diphtheria, or bacteriophage ϕX 174 are generally unsuccessful.

It is of interest that many of the circulating lymphocytes cannot be easily assigned to B- or T-cell lineage. These so-called "null" cells probably represent precursor cells of both lineages. With the advance in membrane antigen and receptor technology and monoclonal antibodies, these cells will likely be assigned a rightful place in ontogeny.

VARIANTS OF SCID WITH PARTICULAR DISEASE ASSOCIATIONS

A number of syndromes or concomitant conditions or abnormalities have been observed in some patients with SCID. In many, the association seems unrelated; in others, clues to the pathogenesis of the underlying immunodeficiency (ID) may be present.

SCID Associated With Short-Limbed Dwarfism

Several instances of SCID associated with a distinctive form of short-limbed dwarfism have been reported [10–12]. The dwarfism can be distinguished from achondroplasia. They do share certain features with cartilage hair hypoplasia, particularly combined developmental abnormalities of the skeletal and immunologic systems.

SCID With Ig

A hereditary primary ID syndrome presenting with gradual onset, variable course, and prolonged survival has been distinguished from SCID. However, these patients share many features with SCID patients including recurrent infections, failure to thrive, absence or paucity of lymphoid tissue, lymphopenia, abnormal thymus structure, and impaired lymphocyte proliferative responses [13]. Despite the presence of normal or elevated Ig levels, specific antibodies are not synthesized in response to antigenic challenge. Originally described by Breton and further characterized by Nezelof [1], it has been excluded from the usual classifications of SCID. Although the etiology may be entirely distinct from other forms of SCID, at the present time all evidence points to it being some variant of the more "classical" variety.

SCID With Paraproteinemia

Many immunodeficient states are associated with quantitative and qualitative changes in serum Ig levels. Paraproteinemia has been described in SCID as well and includes IgG and IgE as well as the predominating abnormalities of IgM [14–16]. It is of particular interest that similar paraproteins have arisen in SCID following attempted reconstitution with transfer factor and thymic epithelial grafts [17,18, and E.W. Gelfand unpublished data].

SCID Associated With Adenosine Deaminase (ADA) Deficiency

Approximately 15% of all patients with SCID have an associated deficiency of the enzyme adenosine deaminase (see Hirschhorn, this volume). The majority of these infants are profoundly lymphopenic, without detectable lymphocytes in either peripheral blood or bone marrow.

SCID Presenting as a Proliferative Abnormality of the Reticuloendothelial System

Two related or identical conditions can present with a laboratory picture indistinguishable from SCID. These are the Letterer-Siwe syndrome [19] and malignant reticuloendotheliosis (Omenn syndrome) [20]. In both conditions, the onset is in the first weeks to months; death often occurs in less than 12 months. The presenting features include a diffuse skin rash, hepatosplenomegaly, eosinophilia, and lymphadenopathy. The laboratory findings vary significantly from patient to patient but in some there are hypogammaglobulinemia, an absence of specific antibody formation, and failure of all aspects of T-cell immunity. In almost all cases, biopsy or necropsy of thymus has revealed marked lymphocyte depletion and the absence of Hassall corpuscles. In 3 patients with malignant reticuloendotheliosis, we also noted markedly elevated serum IgE levels and an absence of lymphocyte ecto-5′-nucleotidase activity [21, 22]. Because this syndrome was observed in a patient with a lymphoproliferative disorder, one with cartilage hair hypoplasia, and one with a combined immunodeficiency (CID), we suggested that some extrinsic process (eg viral infection) may impose itself on an immunodeficient host resulting in this syndrome [22].

SCID and the Bare Lymphocyte Syndrome

This syndrome is characterized by CID associated with the lack of expression of HLA-A, -B, and -C antigens and β_2-microglobulin on the lymphocyte surface (see Touraine, this volume).

SCID as a Consequence of Lymphocyte Membrane Abnormalities

Despite the presence of normal numbers and proportions of T and B lymphocytes, normal levels of serum Igs, and normal thymus histology, a 5-month-old infant failed to show any evidence of T-cell or B-cell immunity [23]. In searching for a specific membrane abnormality, we examined the lateral mobility of the cell-surface receptor for concanavalin A (Con A). In both T and B lymphocytes, an unusually high accumulation of Con A receptors in surface caps was observed. This capping abnormality was exaggerated by colchicine, an inhibitor of microtubule assembly, suggesting that plasma membrane-cytoskeleton interactions were impaired in this patient, preventing the normal expression of lymphocyte function.

A second syndrome has been described where, in the face of normal T-cell numbers and thymus histology, circulating lymphocytes were unresponsive to antigenic or mitogenic stimuli. The lymphocytes were responsive to the calcium ionophore A23187, an agent which facilitates calcium uptake into lymphocytes, triggering cell proliferation [24]. The bypassing of normal physiologic mechanisms by the ionophore suggests some defect in membrane function. Since calcium uptake and cytoskeleton functions are linked, the 2 syndromes may suggest a common etiology for the failure of immune function in the presence of adequate lymphocyte numbers.

SCID Associated With α_1-Antitrypsin Deficiency

We have observed one patient with SCID in whom a serum cellulose acetate electrophoresis indicated an abnormally low peak in the α_1 region. Further study revealed that the patient was Pi type ZZ and both parents were MZ [45]. We estimated that SCID and α_1-antitrypsin deficiency together would be expected by chance in about 1 in 700 million individuals. We do not know if the association is causal or fortuitous, since abnormal immune function is not characteristic in α_1-antitrypsin deficiency.

B-CELL DIFFERENTIATION AND FUNCTION IN SCID

The demonstration of circulating B cells in normal or elevated numbers in many of the patients with SCID argues against the concept of a primary stem-cell defect underlying the disease in these patients. Since T cells are required for the terminal differentiation of B cells to an antibody-secreting stage, the CID may be the consequence of abnormalities of T-cell differentiation and function. Several independent pieces of evidence support the concept that B cells in SCID may be intrinsically normal but fail to function in vivo (Table 2).

In the presence of functional T cells, SCID B cells can generate normal Ig responses as well as specific antibodies in vitro. In several labo-

TABLE 2. Evidence That Circulating B Cells in SCID are Functionally Intact

1. In vitro antibody responses to PWM or specific antigen.
2. Proliferative response to B-cell mitogens.
3. Host B-cell function following immune reconstitution or GVHD.
4. B-cell lymphoproliferative disorders following attempted immune reconstitution.

ratories, B cells from some (but not all) patients have been shown to undergo terminal differentiation in vitro in the presence of normal T cells and pokeweed mitogen (PWM) [25-28]. Similarly, specific IgM antibody responses to T-cell-dependent antigens could be observed when SCID B cells were co-cultured with normal T cells [29-32]. The failure of B-cell function in these patients appears to be secondary to a lack of T-cell help. An excess of T-suppressor (Ts) cells is at best rarely a means of explaining the CID [28].

Additional studies have compared the capacity of SCID B cells to proliferate when incubated with either "T-independent" or "T-dependent" mitogens. Formalinized *S. aureus*, Cowan I strain serves as a reliable T-independent, B-cell mitogen. SCID B cells are capable of normal proliferation to this mitogen but not to the T-dependent mitogen PHA [33].

Perhaps the best evidence for the functional integrity of SCID B cells comes from experience following attempted immune reconstitution. In several cases following donor T-cell engraftment, host B cells have become functional. This has been described following bone marrow and fetal liver transplantation [27, 34, 35], as well as during GVHD [32, 36]. In addition, as noted above, following attempts at immune reconstitution, there have been several instances of the development of a B-cell lymphoproliferative disorder, including the synthesis of specific an-

tibody [17, 18, and E.W. Gelfand, unpublished data].

ABNORMALITIES OF T-CELL DIFFERENTIATION IN SCID

If the defect in many patients with SCID is not at the stem-cell level and the B-cell abnormalities may be explained by the lack of T-cell help, then some of the heterogeneity of the disease must be examined in light of what is known about T-cell differentiation. The role of the thymus in the acquisition and expression of immunity is well documented. Thymus histology at biopsy or necropsy in the majority of SCID patients is surprisingly uniform. The main features are marked lymphocyte depletion, absence of corticomedullary demarcation, and absence of Hassall corpuscles. Our studies have therefore focused on identifying distinct stages of T-cell differentiation in man as a means of understanding the defects in different patients with SCID.

In attempting to develop a model for T-cell differentiation in man, we utilized 4 regimens to induce T-cell differentiation [30-32]. Induction was monitored by an increase in E-rosetting T cells and the generation of T-helper cell activity in an antigen-specific plaque-forming cell (PFC) response [37]. The induction regimens included incubation of bone marrow or peripheral blood (often enriched for T-precursor cells by discontinuous gradient centrifugation) directly in contact with monolayers of cultured human thymic epithelial cells; thymic epithelial cell conditioned medium [38, 39]; the calf thymus extract, Thymosin fraction V; and theophylline [40].

Precursor T cells, responsive to all 4 inductive regimens, could be identified in normal bone marrow, peripheral blood, and fetal liver. The induction of increased numbers of E-rosetting cells and augmented PFC responses is interpreted as evidence for T-cell differentiation. However, this precursor cell response to the 4 regimens does not permit any conclusions regarding the identity of the target cell(s) for these treatments, whether all treatments act on the same or different T-precursor cell pools, or what is the ontogenic sequence of events.

A similar controversy concerning the nature of the target cell exists in analogous studies carried out in mice [reviewed in reference 41]. A variety of thymic humoral factors or drugs which increase intracellular levels of cyclic AMP have been shown to induce T-cell markers or function in thymectomized or nude mice [42]. Even with the most purified thymic humoral factors, it has not been regularly possible to induce the generation of competent T cells from early precursors, or immune reconstitute in the absence of the animals' thymic stroma [41].

Patients with SCID provide a good opportunity to resolve these issues since these disorders generally present as discrete blocks in normal maturation. Analysis of the response of SCID cells to the 4 inductive regimens has identified several patterns of responsiveness (Table 3). In the first group of patients with normal ADA activities, there is a failure to induce T-cell differentiation by any means. In our laboratory, this is infrequent and has been observed only in patients with few, if any, circulating T or B lymphocytes. This may suggest a true deficiency of T- (and possibly B-) precursor cells. A subset of this group comprises the patients with ADA deficiency where induction of T-cell differentiation can be achieved in vitro, but only if a suitable source of the enzyme is provided [43].

Patients in the second group, the largest in our experience, have precursor cells responsive only to incubation directly in contact with the thymic epithelial monolayers [32, 44]. In the third group, precursor cells responsive to the cell-free epithelial conditioned medium are detectable as well. Only one patient has been responsive to the first 2 regimens and thymosin in vitro (group 4) [45], suggesting a hierarchy of differentiation steps. As discussed above, we have identified a patient with SCID and normal numbers of T cells who was responsive to all inductive regimens (group 5). His defect was localized to an abnormality of plasma membrane–cytoskeleton interaction [23].

Taken together, these studies in SCID suggest that the normal ontogenic sequence of T-precursor cell maturation is characterized by the progressive acquisition of responsiveness to distinct triggering agents (Fig. 1). We propose that the earliest cells, prethymic precursor T cells, require direct contact with epithelial stroma for further differentiation. Subsequently, postthymic precursor T cells which have interacted with the epithelial cells, now acquire responsiveness to a variety of influences, including epithelial cell–derived factors, thymosin and then theophylline (or other drugs resulting in increased intracellular levels of cyclic AMP) [40]. In the thymus or peripheral lymphoid tissues, further maturation of T cells may be triggered by nonspecific factors, or antigen and be further regulated by a variety of lymphokines, particularly the "interleukins" [46, 47]. Failure to normally express receptors for these factors or interleukins may be shown to give rise to another group of SCID patients (group 6, Fig. 1).

Studies from several laboratories have confirmed the requirement for thymic epithelial cell contact in most patients with SCID before differentiation is observed, and the rarity of patients responsive to thymic factors alone [48–50]. Recent work in the rat, using thymic epithelial cell lines, has similarly suggested that the initial stage of differentiation can only be accomplished following direct contact of precursor cells with epithelium [51]. Several studies of patients following transplantation support this sequence of T-lymphocyte differentiative events [50, 52].

It would be naive to consider that the defects in SCID all reside primarily at the level of abnormal thymus epithelial cell function. The arrest of T-cell maturation at different stages in SCID, identified by the response to different triggering agents or by monoclonal antibody analysis [53], may reflect a variety of abnormalities. These would include the specific functions of thymic epithelial cells themselves (eg the synthesis or secretion of several polypeptides which act in a specific cascade or sequence), the absence of receptors on precursor cells or secretion of factors

TABLE 3. Identification of T-Cell Precursors in SCID Response to Inducing Regimen

Group	Thymic epithelial contact	Epithelial-derived factors	Thymosin	Theophylline
Normals	+	+	+	+
ADA-deficient	−*	−	−	−
ADA-normal				
1	−	−	−	−
2	+	−	−	−
3	+	+	−	−
4	+	+	+	−
5	+	+	+	+

*No differentiation observed in the absence of ADA.

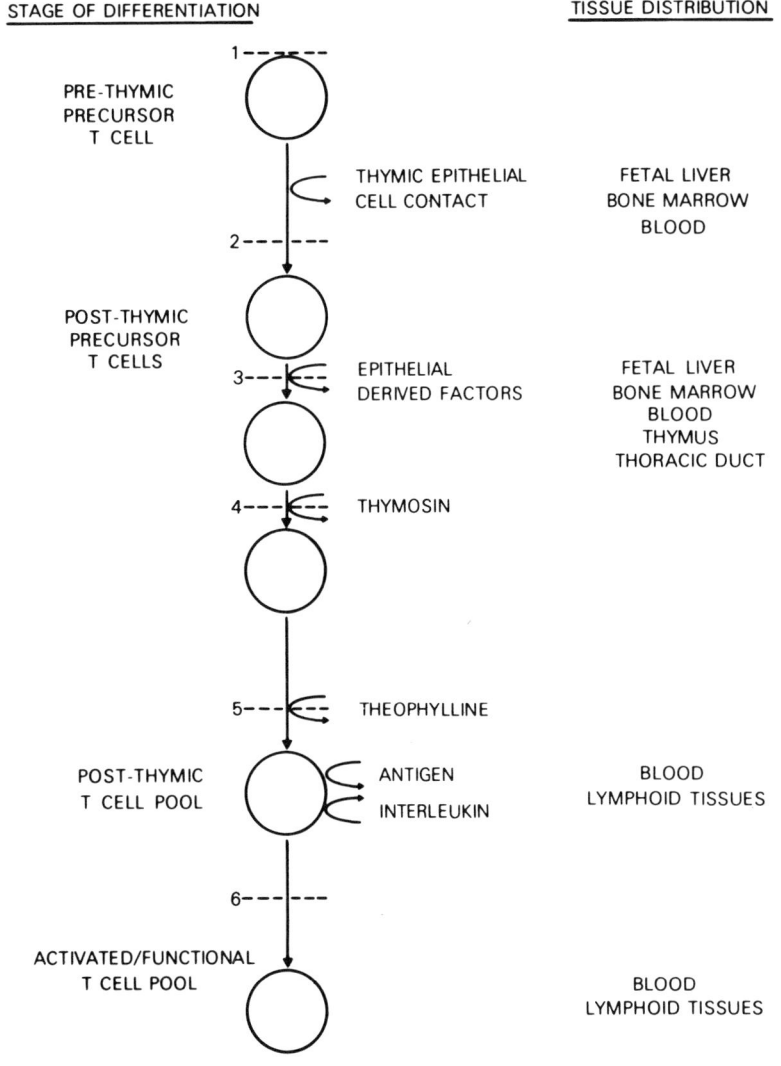

Fig. 1. Proposed model of human T-cell differentiation. Dotted lines identify blocks in T-cell differentiation which may give rise to SCID.

required for migration or chemotaxis to the thymus [54], or appropriate inducer cell interactions. As noted, thymic histology is surprisingly uniform regardless of the level of the defect [55, and E.W. Gelfand, unpublished data]. Only in the patient with normal numbers of T and B cells was there a normal biopsy. Surprisingly, thymus tissue from all groups obtained at biopsy or necropsy grew normally in culture with the development of confluent monolayers of epithelial cells, Hassall bodies, and the synthesis and secretion of functional conditioned medium [44, 49]. This may indicate the presence of antagonistic factors in the host environment which are not conducive to normal epithelial cell development.

CLASSIFICATION OF SCID

Any attempt at simple classification of SCID is difficult and necessarily incomplete. With the rapid advancement in technology and further analysis of these patients, new groupings, divisions, and subdivisions will result. A general classification may group them according to the mode of inheritance of the disease, the presence or absence of an associated enzymopathy or other disorders, or may be based on a framework of T-lymphocyte differentiation, such as illustrated in Table 3. The latter types of studies performed in concert with monoclonal antibodies may provide the best basis for understanding the heterogeneity of SCID as a disorder of lymphocyte differentiation. Certainly any attempt to classify the syndrome on the basis of Ig levels or standard T- or B- cell markers does not accommodate the complexity or heterogeneity of the syndrome. It is hoped that the definition of other enzyme disorders and membrane and receptor abnormalities can be linked to the failure of normal maturation, providing further insight into the pathogenesis of the disease.

ANTENATAL DIAGNOSIS OF SCID

Until quite recently, the antenatal diagnosis of SCID has been limited to those infants who had an associated absence of ADA [56]. With the recent advances in fetoscopy and fetal blood sampling, new opportunities for the antenatal diagnosis of this condition appear possible [57].

SUMMARY

The failure to demonstrate normal humoral and cell-mediated immunity (CMI) in patients diagnosed as SCID is seen to reflect the varied pathogenesis of this syndrome. Two major groups of patients have been described, those with or without an associated absence of the enzyme ADA. The heterogeneity of the syndrome is expressed in variable inheritance patterns (particularly defined X-linked or autosomal recessive modes of inheritance), differing clinical presentations, and significant variability in laboratory findings. Some of this heterogeneity of laboratory findings may in fact be contributed to by the high incidence of infection or engraftment of maternal cells in utero. Common to all, however, is the profound deficiency of functional attributes of humoral and cell-mediated immunity.

Insight into the biology of this immunodeficiency has advanced steadily in the last decade. Although initially hypothesized to represent a primary lymphoid stem-cell defect, newer technologies to identify and enumerate lymphocyte subpopulations and precursor lymphocytes have revealed the complexity of the disorder. This complexity may now be attributable to a number of abnormalities in the quantitative and qualitative differentiation of these lymphoid stem cells. Functional differentiation of lymphocytes is the result of a progressive and orderly sequence of events. In SCID, lymphocytes of both lineages may be arrested at specific and identifiable stages of maturation, leading to a deficiency of cell-mediated and humoral immunity. In many patients with SCID, the combined immune deficiency may be linked solely to a failure in the stepwise progression of T-cell differentiation.

ACKNOWLEDGMENTS

The authors are grateful to the many physicians and nurses responsible for the care of the patients in the Special Isolation Unit, and to the Medical Research Council of Canada for grant support.

REFERENCES

1. Bergsma D, Good RA (eds): "Immunologic Deficiency Diseases in Man." New York: The National Foundation-March of Dimes, BD:OAS 4(1), 1968.
2. Bergsma D (ed): "Immunodeficiency in Man and Animals." Sunderland, MA: Sinauer for the National Foundation-March of Dimes, BD:OAS 11(1), 1975.
3. Jarvis WR, Middleton PJ, Gelfand EW: The significance of viral infections in severe combined immunodeficiency disease. J Pediatr Infect Dis (In press).
4. Jarvis WR, Middleton PJ, Gelfand EW: Fatal parainfluenza pneumonia in severe combined immunodeficiency disease. J Pediatr 94:423–425, 1979.
5. Parkman R, Mosier D, Umansky I, Cochran W, Carpenter CB, Rosen FS: Graft-versus-host disease after intrauterine and exchange transfusions for hemolytic disease of the newborn. N Engl J Med 290:359–363, 1974.
6. Gelfand EW, Shore A, Green B, Lin MT, Dosch H-M: The E-rosette assay: A cautionary note. Clin Immunol Immunopathol 12:119–123, 1979.
7. Kulenkampf J, Janossy G, Greaves MF: Acid esterase in human lymphoid cells and leukemic blasts: A marker for T lymphocytes. Br J Haematol 36:231–240, 1977.
8. Preud'homme JL, Clauvel JP, Seligmann M: Immunoglobulin D-bearing lymphocytes in primary immunodeficiencies. J Immunol 114:481–485, 1975.
9. Falk JA, Gelfand EW, Ing P, Dosch H-M, Falk RE: Expression of Ia antigens in severe combined immunodeficiency disease. Transplant Proc 11:767–769, 1979.
10. McKusick VA, Cross HE: Ataxia-telangiectasia and Swiss-type agammaglobulinemia. JAMA 195:739–741, 1966.
11. Davis JA: A case of Swiss-type agammaglobulinemia and achondroplasia. Br Med J 2:242–243, 1967.
12. Gatti RA, Platt N, Pomerance HH, Hong R, Langer LO, Kay HEM, Good RA: Hereditary lymphopenic agammaglobulinemia associated with a distinctive form of short-limbed dwarfism and ectodermal dysplasia. J Pediatr 75:675–684, 1969.
13. Lawlor GJ, Ammann AJ, Wright WC, La Franchi SH, Bilstrom D, Stiehm ER: The syndrome of cellular immunodeficiency with immunoglobulins. J Pediatr 84:183–192, 1974.
14. DeFazio SR, Criswell BS, Kimzey SL, South MA, Montgomery JR: A para-protein in severe combined immunodeficiency disease detected by immunoelectrophoretic analysis of plasma. Clin Exp Immunol 19:563–570, 1975.
15. Kikkawa Y, Kamimura K, Hamajima T, Sekiguchi T, Kawai T, Takenaka M, Tada T: Thymic alymphoplasia with hyper-IgE-globulinemia. Pediatrics 51:690–696, 1973.
16. Geha RS, Schneeberger E, Gatien J, Rosen FS, Merler E: Synthesis of an M component by circulating B lymphocytes in severe combined immunodeficiency. N Engl J Med 290:726–728, 1974.
17. Gelfand EW, Baumal R, Huber J, Crookston MC, Shumak K: Polyclonal gammopathy and lymphoproliferation following transfer factor in severe combined immunodeficiency disease. N Engl J Med 289:1385–1389, 1973.
18. Borzy MS, Hong R, Horowitz SD, Gilbert E, Kaufman D, DeMendonca W, Oxelius V-A, Dictor M, Pachman L: Fatal lymphoma after transplantation of cultured thymus in children with combined immunodeficiency disease. N Engl J Med 301:565–568, 1979.
19. Cederbaum SD, Niwayama G, Stiehm ER, Neerhout RC, Ammann AJ, Berman W: Combined immunodeficiency presenting as the Letterer-Siwe syndrome. J Pediatr 85:466–471, 1974.
20. Omenn GS: Familial reticuloendotheliosis with eosinophilia. N Engl J Med 273:427–430, 1965.
21. Cohen A, Mansour A, Dosch H-M, Gelfand EW: Absence of lymphocyte ecto-5'-nucleotidase in familial reticuloendotheliosis and combined immunodeficiency. Clin Immunol Immunopathol 15:245–250, 1980.
22. Gelfand EW, Rao CP, McCurdy D, Sigal NH, Cohen A: Absence of lymphocyte ecto-5'-nucleotidase in infants with reticuloendotheliosis and immunodeficiency. In DeBruyn CHMM, Simmonds H, Muller MM (eds): "Proceedings of the International Symposium on Human Purine and Pyrimidine Metabolism, Maastricht, The Netherlands." New York: Plenum Press (In press)
23. Gelfand EW, Oliver JM, Schuurman RK, Matheson DS, Dosch H-M: Abnormal lymphocyte capping in a patient with severe combined immunodeficiency disease. N Engl J Med 301:1245–1249, 1979.
24. Gehrz RC, McAuliffe JJ, Linner KM, Kersey JH: Defective membrane function in a patient with severe combined immunodeficiency disease. Clin Exp Immunol 39:344–348, 1980.
25. Buckley RH, Gilbertsen RB, Schiff RI, Ferreira E, Sanal SO, Waldmann TA: Heterogeneity of lymphocyte subpopulations in severe combined immunodeficiency. J Clin Invest 58:130–136, 1976.
26. Seeger RC, Robins RA, Stevens RH, Klein RB, Waldmann DJ, Zeltzer PM, Kessler SW: Severe combined immunodeficiency with B lymphocytes: In vitro correction of defective immunoglobulin production by addition of normal T lymphocytes. Clin Exp Immunol 26:1–10, 1976.
27. Griscelli C, Durandy A, Virelizier JL, Ballet JJ, Daguillard F: Selective defect of precursor T cells associated with apparently normal B lymphocytes in severe combined immunodeficiency disease. J Pediatr 93:404–411, 1978.
28. Pahwa S, Pahwa RN, Good RA: Heter-

ogeneity of B lymphocyte differentiation in severe combined immunodeficiency disease. J Clin Invest 66:543–550, 1980.
29. Dosch H-M, Lee JWW, Gelfand EW, Falk JA: Severe combined immuno-deficiency disease: A model of T-cell dysfunction. Clin Exp Immunol 34:260–267, 1978.
30. Gelfand EW, Dosch H-M, Shore A: The role of the thymus and thymus microenvironment in T-cell differentiation. In Golde DW, Cline MJ, Metcalfe D, Fox CF (eds): "Hematopoietic Cell Differentiation." New York:Academic Press, 1978, pp 277–293.
31. Gelfand EW, Dosch H-M, Shore A, Limatibul S, Lee JWW: The role of the thymus in human T-cell differentiation. In Gelfand EW, Dosch H-M (eds): "The Biological Basis for Immunodeficiency Disease." New York:Raven Press, 1980, pp 39–56.
32. Gelfand EW, Dosch H-M: Differentiation of precursor T lymphocytes in man and delineation of the selective abnormalities in severe combined immunodeficiency disease. Clin Immunol Immunopathol 25:303–315, 1982.
33. Schuurman RKB, Gelfand EW, Dosch H-M: Polyclonal activation of human lymphocytes in vitro: I. Characterization of the lymphocyte response to a T-cell independent, B-cell mitogen. J Immunol 125:820–826, 1980.
34. Vossen JM, deKoning J, van Bekkum DW, Dicke KA, Ejsvoogel VP, Hijmans W, van Loghem E, Radl J, van Rood JJ, van der Waay D, Dooren LJ: Successful treatment of an infant with severe combined immunodeficiency by transplantation of bone marrow cells from an uncle. Clin Exp Immunol 13:9–20, 1973.
35. O'Reilly RJ, Pahwa R, Dupont B, Good RA: Severe combined immunodeficiency: Transplantation approaches for patients lacking an HLA genotypically identical sibling. Transplant Proc 10:187–199, 1978.
36. Daguillard F, Garneau R, Deschenes L, Chouinar DC, Fudenberg HH, Schanfield M: Hyperactive production of antibody in a boy with thymic dysplasia undergoing graft-versus-host reaction. Clin Immunol Immunopathol 2:52–61, 1973.
37. Dosch H-M, Gelfand EW: Specific in vitro IgM responses of human B-cells: A complex regulatory network modulated by antigen. Immunol Rev 45:243–274, 1979.
38. Pyke KW, Gelfand EW: Morphological and functional maturation of human thymic epithelium in culture. Nature 251:421–423, 1974.
39. Pyke KW, Gelfand EW: Detection of T-precursor cells in human bone marrow and fetal liver. Differentiation 5:189–191, 1976.
40. Limatibul S, Shore AH, Dosch H-M, Gelfand EW: Theophylline modulation of E-rosette formation: An indicator of T-cell maturation. Clin Exp Immunol 33:503–513, 1978.
41. Stutman O: Intrathymic and extra-thymic T cell maturation. Immunol Rev 42:138–184, 1978.
42. Schied MP, Hoffman MK, Komuro K, Hammerling U, Abbott J, Boyse EA, Cohen GH, Hooper JA, Schulof RA, Goldstein AL: Differentiation of T cells induced by preparations from thymus and by non-thymic agents. J Exp Med 138:1027–1032, 1973.
43. Shore A, Dosch H-M, Gelfand EW: Role of adenosine deaminase in the early stages of precursor T-cell maturation. Clin Exp Immunol 44:152–155, 1981.
44. Pyke KW, Dosch H-M, Ipp MM, Gelfand EW: Demonstration of an intrathymic defect in a case of severe combined immunodeficiency disease. N Engl J Med 293:424–428, 1975.
45. Gelfand EW, Cox DW, Lin MT, Dosch H-M: Association of severe combined immune deficiency disease and α_1 antitrypsin deficiency. Lancet 2:202, 1979.
46. Gillis S, Baker PE, Ruscetti FW, Smith KA: The in vitro generation and sustained culture of nude mouse cytolytic T-lymphocytes. J Exp Med 149:1460–1476, 1979.
47. Wagner H, Hardt C, Heek K, Rollinghoff M, Pfizenmaier K: T-cell derived helper factor allows in vivo induction of cytotoxic T-cells in nu/nu mice. Nature 284:278–280, 1980.
48. Pahwa RN, Pahwa SG, Good RA: T-lymphocyte differentiation in severe combined immunodeficiency: Defects of the thymus. Clin Immunol Immunopathol 11:437–444, 1978.
49. Pahwa RN, Pahwa SG, Good RA: T-lymphocyte differentiation in vitro in severe combined immunodeficiency. Defects of stem cells. J Clin Invest 64:1632–1641, 1979.
50. Touraine JL: Human T-lymphocyte differentiation in immunodeficiency diseases and after reconstitution by bone marrow or fetal thymus transplantation. Clin Immunol Immunopathol 12:228–237, 1979.
51. Itoh T, Kasahara S, Mori T: A thymic epithelial cell line, IT-45R1, induces the differentiation of pre-thymic progenitor cells into post-thymic cells through direct contact. Thymus 4:69–75, 1982.
52. Gelfand EW, Dosch H-M, Cohen A, McClure PD: Post-transplant immunodeficiency: Secondary to thymic epithelial cell dysfunction? In Gale PP, Fox CF (eds): "Biology of Bone Marrow Transplantation. ICN-UCLA Symposia on Molecular and Cellular Biology." New York:Academic Press, 1980, vol 17, pp 97–117.
53. Reinherz EL, Cooper MD, Schlossman SF, Rosen FS: Abnormalities of T-cell maturation and regulation in human beings with immunodeficiency disorders. J Clin Invest 68:699–705, 1981.
54. Pyke KW, Bach JF: The in vitro migration of murine fetal liver cells to thymic rudiments. Eur J Immunol 9:317–323, 1979.
55. Borzy MS, Schulte-Wisserman H, Gilbert E, Horowitz SO, Pellett J, Hong R: Thymic morphology in immunodeficiency diseases. Results of thymic biopsies. Clin Immunol Immunopathol 12:31–51, 1979.
56. Hirschhorn R, Beratis W, Rosen FS, Stern R, Polmar S: Adenosine deaminase deficiency in a child diagnosed prenatally. Lancet 1:73–74, 1975.
57. Durandy A, Griscelli C, Dumez Y, Oury JF, Henrion R, Briard ML, Frezal J: Antenatal diagnosis of severe combined immunodeficiency from fetal cord blood (letter). Lancet 1:852–853, 1982.

Genetic Deficiencies of Adenosine Deaminase and Purine Nucleoside Phosphorylase: Overview, Genetic Heterogeneity and Therapy*

Rochelle Hirschhorn, MD

Department of Medicine, New York University School of Medicine, New York, NY 10016

INTRODUCTION

Immunodeficiency disorders have traditionally been classified within the conceptual framework that these disorders represent defects at different stages of differentiation of a common stem cell into either the humoral or cellular arms of the immune system [1]. During the past decade, the discovery of at least 3 specific inherited molecular defects, each of which gives rise to a different immunodeficiency syndrome, provides a further basis for diagnosis, classification, and delineation of primary immune disorders. These 3 disorders are inherited absence of adenosine deaminase (ADA), which usually results in the clinical syndrome of severe combined immunodeficiency (SCID); genetic absence of purine nucleoside phosphorylase (PNP), which results in a cellular immunodeficiency syndrome; and absence of transcobalamin II, which results in agammaglobulinemia (as well as defects of other hematopoietic stem cells). Eventually, it can be expected that a specific molecular defect will be found for every inherited immunodeficiency disorder. Although such specific molecular defects would then form the basis of specific diagnosis, the current conceptual framework can be expected to remain useful in differential diagnosis. By analogy, one can consider the subdivision of infections into pneumonia, meningitis, septicemia, etc and the further subdivision to etiologic agents, eg pneumococcal pneumonia, etc.

The finding of specific molecular defects with toxicity essentially limited to the lymphoid system can also be expected to provide tools for further insight into the normal differentiation and interaction of the components of the lymphoid system, the metabolic pathways involved, and for development of selective chemotherapeutic and immunomodulatory modalities.

I will briefly review our current state of knowledge, and, in more detail, discuss genetic heterogeneity and aspects of therapy in ADA deficiency.

ADENOSINE DEAMINASE DEFICIENCY
Clinical, Genetic, and Pathologic Aspects

In 1972, Giblett and co-workers described 2 unrelated female children who presented with autosomal recessive SCID and who also lacked the enzyme ADA [2]. Several lines of evidence demonstrated that the enzyme deficiency was genetically determined and thus bore a primary and causal relationship to the immunodeficiency [2-9]. Consistent with an autosomal recessive mode of inheritance, family studies demonstrated that the healthy parents of affected children (ie obligate heterozygotes) and one of each set of grandparents had approximately one half of normal activity of ADA in their erythrocytes and lymphocytes. Approximately 90% of obligate heterozygotes for the enzyme deficiency have erythrocyte ADA which is < 2 SD of the logarithmic mean of normal activity (Fig. 1). (Although approximately 10% of obligate heterozygotes have RBC ADA within 2 SD of the normal mean, this could reflect a wide variation in ADA similar to the wide variation seen in normals.) An additional marker for the presence of a deficiency allele for ADA is available because ADA is genetically polymorphic, with 2 common co-dominant alleles (ADA1 and ADA2) segregating in the normal population [10]. In several families of children with ADA deficiency and SCID, abnormal segregation of the common allelic forms of ADA has been demonstrated, compatible with segregation of a deficiency allele in addition to the 2 normal alleles. For example, in one family, a grandmother of an affected ADA⁻-SCID was phenotypically ADA 1 and her husband was phenotypically ADA 2-1. They had a daughter who was phenotypically ADA 2. This can be explained if the grandmother was genotypically ADA1-0, giving her daughter the null allele while the grandfather gave the daughter his ADA 2 allele. In this family, both the grandmother and daughter also had ADA activity in the heterozygous range consistent with the presence of a null allele. The daughter married a man who was also heterozygous for ADA and she gave birth to a child with ADA⁻-SCID [2-9]. Finally, determination of ADA in amniotic cells

---

*Supported by NIH grant AI 10343, and grant 6-4 from the March of Dimes Birth Defects Foundation.

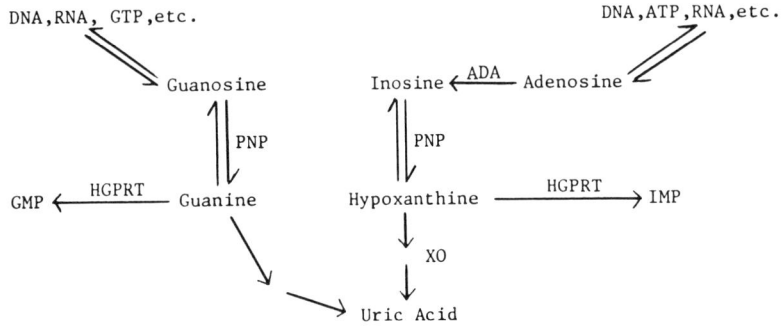

Fig. 1. Purine metabolism by adenosine deaminase (ADA) and purine nucleoside phosphorylase (PNP).

has allowed for the prenatal diagnosis of both ADA deficiency and immunodeficiency at birth. Over a dozen pregnancies at risk have been monitored and at least 2 affected children diagnosed correctly [9,11].

ADA deficiency has been found to account for between one-third and one-half of SCID cases, where the mode of inheritance is not obviously X-linked. In studies of 7 families where SCID is definitely transmitted as an autosomal recessive trait, the incidence of ADA deficiency has been found to be 57% with 95% confidence limits of 18-90%. It would therefore appear that a substantial proportion of autosomal recessive SCID is due to deficiency of ADA. Indeed, an informal survey of 130 patients with SCID, including both autosomal recessive and X-linked, revealed 22% with ADA deficiency [12-14].

Over 30 families with ADA deficiency and immunodeficiency have been described in the literature, and many more cases have been found [15]. Approximately 80-90% of the patients are indistinguishable clinically, as well as by in vitro tests of immune function, from other patients with SCID. Normal numbers of lymphocytes and T lymphocytes, as well as the presence of a response to PHA (albeit reduced), may be found at birth. Although this is unusual, it suggests that the diagnosis can most reliably be made at birth in a family at risk by determination of ADA activity in red cells. The disease is progressive, and any residual T-cell function found at birth rapidly disappears. Clinical manifestations usually develop in the first months of life; humoral immunity does not develop.

In 10-15% of the cases, onset of disease may occur later than 3-6 months. Thus, one of the first recorded patients, followed closely because of the prior death of a sib with SCID, was known to be immunocompetent and healthy until over 2 years of age, which is the latest known age of onset to date [2]. The outstanding feature in this group is the retention of Igs and the presence of specific antibody. However, Ig levels eventually fall, and in one case there was a preterminal monoclonal IgG [16]. Unless treated, death occurs by 3 years of age, but usually earlier. It is logical to expect that if all patients with primarily cellular immune defects were to be tested, even later age of onset and a more insidious course would be found. Indeed, such a child has been recently ascertained (see below).

During the initial studies of patients with ADA deficiency, it appeared that 2 features might discriminate between ADA-deficient and non-ADA-deficient SCID patients. The first of these was bony abnormalities, originally appreciated radiologically [17] and subsequently studied pathologically [18]. This bony abnormality (8 of 13 families) is evident on physical examination as prominence of the costochondral rib junction, similar to a rachitic rosary. On x ray, cupping and flaring of the costochondral junctions are seen, as well as a dysplastic pelvis. As initially noted, these changes are not pathognomonic. Similar radiologic changes, including cupping of the anterior rib ends, can be observed in nonimmunodeficient patients who are severely malnourished, as well as in ADA-normal immunodeficient patients [12,19]. Although the radiologic and physical changes may not be specific, these bony alterations have served to alert physicians to the possibility of ADA-deficient SCID and are extremely useful clinically. It was initially proposed that thymic pathology differed in the ADA-deficient cases with the retention of some Hassall corpuscles, suggesting secondary atrophy of a previously differentiated thymus [19]. However, on a practical level, in patients examined from 7 kindred, with and without ADA deficiency, we could find no such consistent correlation between thymic pathology and the presence or absence of ADA deficiency [12].

Neurologic abnormalities have been reported in 3 cases [15,20,21]. The most striking was in a patient admitted to the hospital primarily because of neurologic abnormalities, including nystagmus, spasticity, and choreoathetoid movements [12,21]. It is obvious that these neurologic manifestations could reflect a viral disease in these immunodeficient patients rather than specific pathology secondary to the enzyme deficiency. However, in 2 patients the neurologic abnormalities cleared completely, concomitant with red cell therapy and lowering of metabolites. In one of the patients, resolution of neurologic abnormalities occurred concomitant with reduction in metabolite concentrations brought about by partial red cell exchange transfusion.

TABLE 1. Enzyme Activity and Metabolites in ADA-Deficient Individuals

		% Normal Enzyme Activity		Metabolites				
		RBCs	Mononuclear Cells	RBC dATP[a]	Urinary dAr[b]	Urinary Ar[b]	Plasma dAr[c]	Plasma Ar[c]
ADA⁻-SCID untreated	(n=5)	<1.0	<1.0	950	960	25	0.3–3.9	3.0
Partial ADA⁻ healthy	(n=5)	<1.0	5–100	5–12	<4	4–18	—	—
ADA⁻-SCID post bone marrow	(n=2)	<1.0	~25.0	66	~30	8	<0.25	2.4
ADA⁻-SCID post RBC tx	(n=5)	~40.0	<1.0	70	~30	15	<0.25	3.0
Normals		100.0	100.0	3.0 ± 2.0	<0.1	4.0 ± 1	<0.05	0.3

[a] = nmoles/ml packed RBCs
[b] = nmoles/mg C
[c] = μMolar
Key: tx = transfusion, dAr = deoxyadenosine, Ar = adenosine

In addition, the neurologic improvement preceded by several months any alteration in immune function and occurred in the face of persistent diarrhea and malnutrition. These observations suggest that the neurologic manifestations may be an integral part of the syndrome, reflecting interaction of accumulated purines with purinergic receptors on brain cells [21]. More recent studies demonstrating an apparently dose-related incidence of neurologic abnormalities in patients treated with deoxycoformycin, an inhibitor of ADA, would support this hypothesis [22]. An in vitro defect in platelet aggregation has also been reported [23,24]. It is of interest that one patient had severe GI bleeding, albeit presumably from an ulcer (E. Gelfand, personal communication).

Abnormal Metabolites and Pathophysiologic Mechanisms in ADA Deficiency

Adenosine deaminase is an enzyme of the purine salvage pathway which catalyzes the irreversible deamination of adenosine and 2′-deoxyadenosine as well as of several naturally occurring modified adenine nucleosides (Fig. 1) [reviewed in 25,26].

Affected children accumulate and/or excrete markedly increased amounts of the substrates adenosine and deoxyadenosine in plasma, red cells, and urine. In addition, they accumulate enormous quantities of the phosphorylated metabolite deoxy ATP in erythrocytes and lymphocytes [21,27-37]. Affected children also uniquely excrete the modified adenine nucleoside 2′-0-methyladenosine and excrete fivefold increased amounts of another as yet unidentified modified adenine nucleoside [37] (Table 1). A two- to threefold increase in lymphocyte cyclic AMP has also been reported.

Several pathophysiologic mechanisms have been proposed whereby deficiency of ADA and the resulting accumulation of metabolites could result in immunodeficiency disease. Initial studies focused on adenosine since this compound was first reported to be increased in plasma, and because earlier studies had already shown that adenosine was toxic for lymphoid cells. Following the demonstration of the marked increase in deoxyadenosine excretion and increases in intracellular deoxy ATP, attention focused upon mechanisms involving deoxyadenosine toxicity. The mechanisms proposed have included adenosine-mediated pyrimidine starvation, adenosine-mediated increase in cyclic AMP (a known modulator of immune response), adenosine (and deoxyadenosine)-mediated increase in S-adenosyl homocysteine (SAH), an inhibitor of methylation reactions and deoxy ATP-mediated inhibition of ribonucleotide reductase [28,29,31,38,39]. Currently, the most favored pathophysiologic mechanism is one involving deoxyadenosine-mediated increases in deoxy ATP, since both in vivo as well as in vitro evidence support the hypothesis. Thus, enormous amounts of deoxy ATP are found in patients' cells at concentrations sufficient to be capable of inhibiting the enzyme ribonucleotide reductase. The normal functioning of ribonucleotide reductase is essential to provide deoxy nucleotides for normal DNA synthesis. In vitro experiments indicate that accumulation of deoxy ATP could account for the lymphospecific toxicity and the initially greater impairment of cellular versus humoral immunity. Thus, the thymus in man, compared with other tissues, has high activity of an enzyme which converts deoxyadenosine to deoxy ATP and lower capacity to degrade deoxy ATP. In vitro experiments have also shown preferential accumulation of deoxy ATP by T-derived cells as compared with B-derived cells [40]. Attractive as this hypothesis is, we must inject a note of caution in extrapolating from in vitro to in vivo events. Similar enzymatic and metabolic studies in mice predict that these animals will not preferentially accumulate deoxy ATP in their thymus. Nevertheless, we have found that mice, rendered artificially ADA deficient by injection with the ADA inhibitor deoxycoformycin, preferentially accumulate deoxy ATP in the thymus [41]. The next most attractive hypothesis is that of inhibition of methylation reactions. Children with ADA⁻-SCID have indeed been shown to have markedly diminished activity of the enzyme SAH-hydrolase, presumably as a result of "suicide inactivation" by deoxyadenosine of the SAH-hydrolase [31]. Inactivation of SAH hydrolase in vitro would lead to accumulation of SAH and reversal of the SAH/SAM (S-adenosyl methionine) ratio. The ratio of SAH to SAM is thought to determine the rate of SAM-dependent methylation reactions crucial for normal cellular functions. In vitro, such alterations have been found to interfere with methylation reactions in the whole cell. While elevations in SAH have yet to be demonstrated in genetically ADA-deficient patients, elevations of SAH have been found in cells of patients rendered artificially ADA deficient by treatment with deoxycoformycin, a potent inhibitor of ADA (see below).

There is, however, increasing in vitro data to indicate that deoxyadenosine toxicity may act at a site other than, or additional to, inhibition of ribonucleotide reductase. Finally, we should like to suggest that modified adenine nucleosides, which we have found to be inhibitory for in vitro lymphocyte responses and to be excreted uniquely or in increased amounts by ADA-deficient children, may also play a role in toxicity [37,42].

Therapy in ADA Deficiency

Bone marrow transplantation is the therapy of choice [3]. At least 7 children with ADA deficiency have been successfully transplanted. The oldest of these is over 12 years of age, and is clinically and immunologically normal. Bony changes originally noted have disappeared. Apparently, in addition to providing stem cells, the normal engrafted donor lymphocytes have sufficient ADA activity and transport sites to take up and degrade deoxyadenosine and adenosine, and thus prevent accumulation of toxic metabolites in host cells which still do not contain ADA. Chen et al [43] have demonstrated that bone marrow transplanted cells provided sufficient enzyme to lower red cell deoxy ATP to concentrations no longer detectable by high performance liquid chromatography (HPLC). Interestingly, in this patient only T lymphocytes were engrafted yet metabolites appeared to have been lowered sufficiently so that the recipient's own B lymphocytes became functional. We have similarly determined metabolites in 2 bone marrow transplanted ADA-deficient children. We have found that the engrafted lymphoid cells have sufficient transporting and deaminating capacity to almost, but not completely, lower metabolites in several body compartments. Although all metabolites are markedly diminished compared to concentrations in untreated ADA-deficient patients (Table 1), the 2 children still have slightly elevated erythrocyte deoxy ATP, excrete increased amounts of deoxyadenosine, have apparently increased plasma adenosine, and have diminished SAH hydrolase activity. However, deoxy ATP content of the engrafted donor lymphocytes appears normal [34].

Unfortunately, over half of affected children will not have a suitable donor. Alternative approaches to therapy have therefore been sought. It was found that addition of ADA in vitro to cultured lymphocytes from an ADA-deficient child (who had been diagnosed prenatally and was therefore in isolation and disease free), partially restored the ability of the lymphocytes to respond to mitogens [44]. Based upon these experiments (which may have been unique for this specially treated child), numerous children with ADA⁻-SCID have been partially exchanged, and transfused with normal frozen, irradiated RBCs. These erythrocytes, in addition to containing normal ADA, also have sites for intracellular transport of the accumulated substrates adenosine and 2'-deoxyadenosine [20], thus providing in theory an internal "dialysis machine" or an "enzyme loaded substrate trap."

Various children with ADA⁻-SCID have been treated with varying degrees of thoroughness with respect to amounts of red cells given, frequency of transfusion, and length of time. Following vigorous erythrocyte multiple partial exchange transfusions, it is clear that both erythrocyte deoxy ATP content and urinary deoxyadenosine excretion fall to approximately the same levels as seen in transplanted patients (Table 1). In some patients there has been an initial partial restoration of immune function, manifested by increased lymphocyte responses to mitogens, appearance of an MLR, increases in total lymphocyte count, appearance of a thymic shadow, and increases in serum Igs. Such children have most strikingly achieved normal growth and development. Two children survived at home attending school until about 5 years of age, one to die of varicella, and the other of an IgM-mediated autoimmune hemolytic anemia. At least 4 children are still alive after approximately 3–5 years of treatment. However, it is clear that even with equivalent therapy, many children do not show any clinical or immunologic response; in others, the response is less dramatic than that initially reported. In at least one case, marked diminution in metabolite concentrations did not result in clinical response and thus, the degree of response does not obviously correlate with degree of alterations in the concentrations of any of the proposed toxic metabolites. The presence or absence of response may correlate with the severity of clinical disease at the onset of therapy [reviewed in 45]. The lack of response in some children may reflect the loss of stem cells capable of being rescued or the lack of thymic factors needed for terminal differentiation due to irreversible toxic involution.

Indeed, several but not all of the children who have shown an immunologic and/or clinical response have also received either fetal thymus or cultured thymic epithelium. There also have been limited attempts at therapy with uridine and deoxycytidine, in attempts to reverse postulated "pyrimidine starvation." These attempts have been too limited in duration to allow for evaluation.

"Partial" ADA Deficiency and Genetic Heterogeneity

Almost simultaneous with the initial description of ADA⁻-SCID, Jenkins described an apparently healthy 10-year-old !Kung child who lacked ADA in his erythrocytes [46]. Subsequent studies demonstrated that although this !Kung child had only 2% of normal RBC ADA, he retained at least 10% of normal activity in white cells, and his cultured lymphoid line cells exhibited at least 50% of normal ADA activity. Population studies revealed that the gene for partial ADA deficiency was present in the !Kung tribe with a gene frequency of approximately 0.1% (the frequency of homozygotes = 1%). In addition to 2 other !Kung tribesmen, 4 additional children from 3 families have been reported who have "partial" ADA deficiency. Including the !Kung, they currently range in age from 3–20 years [47–49]. All are immunocompetent both clinically and in terms of laboratory tests. We have also studied 4 additional children with partial ADA deficiency ascertained as part of the New York State neonatal screening program for ADA deficiency. These latter 4 children are also all immunologically normal, but they are all still less than one year of age and eventual immunologic attrition cannot be excluded. All of these children have 1–2% or less of normal RBC ADA, but have substantial ADA in their lymphoid cells (unpublished observations). In contrast, children with ADA⁻-SCID have virtually undetectable ADA in their lymphocytes when assays are performed so as to eliminate possible contribution of a second isozyme of ADA (ADA2) which is not deficient in ADA⁻-SCID [47].

In addition to having substantial residual ADA activity in their peripheral blood mononuclear cells (PBMC), children with partial ADA deficiency do not accumulate, or only barely accumulate, the toxic metabolite deoxy ATP in their erythrocytes and excrete barely detectable amounts of deoxyadenosine in urine (Table 1). This contrasts with the 500–1,000-fold elevation in erythrocyte dATP content and urinary deoxyadenosine excretion by ADA⁻-SCIDs. Thus, total body adenosine deaminating activity is sufficient in these partially ADA-deficient children to prevent accumulation of deleterious nucleoside and nucleotide compounds [47 and unpublished observations].

Several different mechanisms could result in genetic absence of ADA in erythrocytes but its presence in lymphoid cells. These include 1) the presence of 2 different ADA isozymes controlled by separate genetic loci in the 2 types of cells; 2) a mutation at a regulatory locus controlling expression of ADA in erythrocytes; or 3) mutation(s) at the structural locus resulting in an unstable enzyme. The first possibility is unlikely since several studies have previously documented that the major ADA catalytic activity in all tissues, including both erythrocytes and lymphocytes, is coded for by a single genetic locus on chromosome 20. Several pieces of evidence do support the existence of a regulatory locus-controlling expression of ADA. Thus, Valentine et al have reported autosomal dominant inheritance of a 50-fold increase in ADA activity of erythrocytes, but normal activity in lymphocytes and fibroblasts [50]. Siciliano et al [51] have reported reexpression of human ADA in hybrids between a human tumor line not expressing ADA and a murine cell line suggesting a regulatory locus. Finally, a mutation at a structural locus coding for an unstable enzyme could result in absent or markedly diminished activity in erythrocytes. Thus, erythrocytes are incapable of synthesizing new protein and have a relatively long lifespan, during which time an unstable enzyme could be expected to diminish markedly in activity.

We have examined long-term cultured lymphoid line cells from 4 partially ADA-deficient children and have found evidence for at least 3 different structural mutations [49]. One child has an enzyme which is unstable at 56°C and has a more basic than normal isoelectric point; one child has an enzyme with normal heat stability but a more acidic than normal isoelectric point; while the third (!Kung) has an enzyme with normal isoelectric point but diminished stability at 56°C. Thus, partial ADA deficiency is a genetically heterogeneous defect (Table 2).

It was to be expected that a child would be found with "partial" ADA deficiency such that the activity in lymphoid cells and other body tissues was insufficient to clear metabolites to nontoxic levels. From the clinical picture of ADA⁻-SCID it could also be expected that such a child would have a predominantly cellular immune deficit, and based upon other genetic disorders, that onset of illness would be at a later age, reflecting attrition of the immune system. Such a child has been reported at this meeting by Drs. Ammann and Cowan (this volume).

I would like to suggest that determination of concentrations of toxic metabolites (ie deoxyadenosine in urine and deoxy ATP in erythrocytes) will more clearly correlate with the presence of impaired immune function than will determination of "apparent residual activity of ADA" in PBMC. There are several factors which suggest that test tube determinations of ADA activity in PBLs may not correlate with in vivo deaminating capacity. In immunodeficient patients, most of the PBMC are monocytes with possibly some immature T cells. Monocytes normally have higher ADA activity than do lymphocytes, while immature T cells have almost tenfold higher ADA activity than do mature T cells. Thus, any residual ADA activity may appear factitiously high when compared to normal mononuclear cells. Additionally, ADA is assayed in the test tube at concentrations markedly higher (approximately tenfold) than that found in plasma even of ADA deficients, and often at temperatures lower than that found in the body. Thus, both a mutation resulting in an ADA protein with abnormal avidity for adenosine (K_m mutation) or abnormal stability at body temperature, both of which could be important in vivo, would not be detected by a straightforward test tube determination of ADA activity. Finally, unstimulated PBLs have a low rate of protein synthesis, so that an unstable mutant could show lower enzyme activity in PBLs than in other body cells which are more actively synthesizing new ADA. Determinations of metabolite concentrations and ADA activity together may be a better prognostic indicator of eventual immune function than either alone.

PURINE NUCLEOSIDE PHOSPHORYLASE DEFICIENCY

Deficiency of purine nucleoside phosphorylase (PNP), the next enzyme in the purine salvage pathway, was initially discovered in a 5-year-old girl with a history of recurrent infection [52]. At least 9 children with PNP deficiency in 6 families have been found to date. It is apparent that all the patients have had severe T-cell dysfunction as measured by marked reduction in T-cell numbers, and response to mitogens and allogeneic cells. In marked contrast to ADA deficiency, humoral immunity has been quantitatively normal or increased as measured by normal numbers of B cells in the blood and of plasma cells in lymphoid tissue, normal-to-elevated Ig content in vivo and normal antibody response to antigens in vivo. Several patients have had excessive and abnormal antibody production, including Coombs-positive hemolytic anemia, positive antinuclear antibody (ANA), rheumatoid factor, and monoclonal gammopathy, all suggesting abnormalities in T-suppressor function.

In several patients, the disease has shown a course of immunologic attrition. Clinical onset of disease has varied from 6 months to 6 years of age. Nonimmunologic abnormalities have included anemia in 5 patients (4 of the 6 families). Three patients (2 families) have had neurologic abnormalities of spastic tetraplegia or ataxia and tremor, reminiscent of the abnormalities in ADA deficiency [52-58].

PNP deficiency would appear to be a rarer disorder than ADA deficiency. It is inherited in an autosomal recessive fashion, and obligate heterozygotes have usually been found to have half-normal PNP activity in their red cells. The disorder is clearly genetically heterogeneous, with several different mutant alleles at the PNP locus. Thus, in one of the families (Toronto) the 2 affected brothers have detectable residual PNP activity, albeit with an abnormal K_m. Correlating with the presence of residual enzyme activity, the 2 brothers are the oldest survivors, at over 10 years of age; one of the brothers was the oldest at age of onset. The 2 brothers, who are products of a nonconsanguineous mating, would appear to be doubly heterozygous for 2 different mutant PNP alleles. Thus, the father has an electrophoretically abnormal PNP which is also detectable with anti-PNP antibodies as excess cross-reacting material (CRM), while the mother has reduced enzyme and reduced CRM, and no electrophoretic aberrations of the enzyme molecule. Another patient has been shown to have yet another mutation, resulting in an electrophoretically altered enzyme but different from that seen in the brothers [3,59-63].

PNP reversibly catalyzes the phosphorylysis of guanosine, inosine, deoxyguanosine, and deoxyinosine (Fig. 1). Although the equilibrium of the reaction favors nucleoside synthesis, the availability of ribose-1-phosphate and 2'-deoxyribose-1-phosphate is minimal and thus, in vivo the direction is toward the generation of the free purine base from the corresponding ribo- or 2'-deoxyribonucleoside. The enzyme is a homotrimer with a subunit size of

TABLE 2. Genetic Heterogeneity in Partial ADA Deficients

	% Normal ADA activity	% Normal heat stability*	Electrophoretic mobility**	Isoelectric point
Normals	100.0	100.0	Normal	4.9
Partial ADA deficients (Healthy)				
1)	5.0	50.0	Increased	4.8
2)	10.0	10.0	Normal	5.0
3)	20.0	65.0	Normal	–
4)	70.0	16.0	Normal	4.9
Complete ADA deficients (SCID) n=4	0.3	–	–	–

*Percent of normal time for 50% loss of activity at 56°C
**Anodal mobility compared to the common normal ADA-1 allozyme, starch gel electrophoresis, pH 6.5

30,000 and is not genetically polymorphic [64-67]. Several secondary isozymes are generated by posttranslational modifications following "aging" either in vitro or, as in the erythrocyte, in vivo. The enzyme shows an "age-dependent decline" being higher in reticulocytes than in old erythrocytes. The enzyme is coded for by a locus on the long arm of chromosome 14 (20q13.2--1ter) [68].

Patients with PNP deficiency accumulate large amounts of all 4 substrates (inosine, guanosine, deoxyinosine, and deoxyguanosine) in their urine. Because the block is near the terminal portion of the major common pathway to uric acid, patients have low serum uric acid and excrete diminished amounts of uric acid. However, excretion of total purine precursors of uric acid is increased, indicating purine overproduction. Of the 4 substrates, only deoxyadenosine has been reported to be directly phosphorylated, while the other 3 substrates require prior conversion to hypoxanthine or guanine, a reaction which is blocked in PNP deficiency. Therefore, it is not surprising that deoxy GTP is the major phosphorylated metabolite accumulated by PNP-deficient children [53,69-71]. Deoxy GTP, like deoxy ATP, is also an allosteric inhibitor of ribonucleotide reductase albeit not as potent or all encompassing. It has been hypothesized that accumulation of deoxy GTP accounts for the lymphospecific and T-cell specific effects of PNP deficiency. In vitro enzymatic and metabolic studies, similar to those described for deoxy ATP, also support this hypothesis. Interestingly, Dosch and co-workers have demonstrated that in vivo administration of deoxyguanosine, but not of guanosine, results in loss of T-suppressor cells in mice [72].

REFERENCES

1. Belohradsky BH, Finstad J, Fudenberg HH, Good RA, Kunkel HG, Rosen F: Meeting report of the second international workshop on primary immunodeficiency diseases in man. Clin Immunol Immunopathol 2:281, 1974.
2. Giblett ER, Anderson JE, Cohen F, Pollara B, Meuwissen HJ: Adenosine-deaminase deficiency in two patients with severely impaired cellular immunity. Lancet 2:18, 1972.
3. Parkman R, Gelfand EW, Rosen FS, Sanderson A, Hirschhorn R: Severe combined immunodeficiency and adenosine deaminase deficiency. N Engl J Med 292:714, 1975.
4. Scott CR, Chen S-H, Giblett ER: Detection of the carrier state in combined immunodeficiency disease associated with adenosine deaminase deficiency. J Clin Invest 53:1194, 1974.
5. Chen S-H, Scott CR, Giblett ER: Adenosine deaminase: Demonstration of a "silent" gene associated with combined immunodeficiency disease. Am J Hum Genet 26:103, 1974.
6. Chen S-H, Scott CR, Giblett ER, Levin AS: Adenosine deaminase deficiency: Another family with a "silent" ADA allele and normal ADA activity in two heterozygotes. Am J Hum Genet 29:642, 1977.
7. Hirschhorn R: Prenatal diagnosis and heterozygote detection in adenosine deaminase deficiency. In Guttler F, Seakins JWT, Harkness RA (eds): "Inborn Errors of Immunity and Phagocytosis." Lancaster, England: MTP Press Ltd, 1979, p 121.
8. Hirschhorn R: Adenosine deaminase deficiency and immunodeficiencies. Fed Proc 36:2166, 1977.
9. Hirschhorn R, Beratis N, Rosen FS, Parkman R, Stern R, Polmar S: Adenosine-deaminase deficiency in a child diagnosed prenatally. Lancet 1:73, 1975.
10. Hopkinson DA, Cook PJL, Harris H: Further data on the adenosine deaminase (ADA) polymorphism and a report of a new phenotype. Ann Hum Genet 32:361, 1969.
11. Rubinstein A, Hirschhorn R, Sicklick M, Murphy RA: In vivo and in vitro effects of thymosin and adenosine deaminase on adenosine-deaminase-deficient lymphocytes. N Engl J Med 300:387, 1979.
12. Hirschhorn R, Vawter GE, Kirkpatrick JA Jr, Rosen FS: Adenosine deaminase deficiency: Frequency and comparative pathology in autosomally recessive severe combined immunodeficiency. Clin Immunol Immunopathol 14:107, 1979.
13. Hirschhorn R: Incidence and prenatal detection of adenosine deaminase deficiency and purine nucleoside phosphorylase deficiency. In Pollara B, Pickering RJ, Meuwissen HG, Porter I (eds): "Inborn Errors of Specific Immunity." New York: Academic Press, 1979, p 5.
14. Ackeret C, Pluss HJ, Hitzig WH: Hereditary severe combined immunodeficiency and adenosine deaminase deficiency. Pediatr Res 10:67, 1976.
15. Hirschhorn R: Clinical delineation of adenosine deaminase deficiency. Ciba Found Symp 68:35, 1978.
16. Hitzig WH, Landolt R, Muller G, Bodmer P: Heterogeneity of phenotypic expression in a family with Swiss-type agammaglobulinemia: Observations on the acquisition of agammaglobulinemia. J Pediatr 78:968, 1971.
17. Wolfson JJ, Cross VF: The radiographic findings in 49 patients with combined immunodeficiency. In Meuwissen HJ, Pickering RJ, Pollara B, Porter IH (eds): "Combined Immunodeficiency Disease and Adenosine Deaminase Deficiency: A Molecular Defect." New York: Academic Press, 1975, p 255.
18. Cederbaum SD, Kaitila I, Rimoin DL, Stiehm ER: The chondro-osseous dysplasia of adenosine deaminase deficiency with severe combined immunodeficiency. J Pediatr 89:737, 1976.
19. Huber J, Kersey J: Pathologic features. Supra #17, p 279.
20. Polmar SH, Stern RC, Schwartz AL, Wetzler EM, Chase PA, Hirschhorn R: Enzyme replacement therapy for adenosine deaminase deficiency and severe combined immunodeficiency. N Engl J Med 295:1337, 1976.
21. Hirschhorn R, Papageorgiou PS, Kesarwala HH, Taft LT: Amelioration of neurologic abnormalities after "enzyme replacement" in adenosine deaminase deficiency. N Engl J Med 303:377, 1980.
22. Siaw MFE, Mitchell BS, Koller CA, Coleman MS, Hutton JJ: ATP depletion as a consequence of adenosine deaminase inhibition in man. Proc Natl Acad Sci USA 77:6157, 1980.
23. Schwartz AL, Polmar SH, Stern RC, Cowan DH: Abnormal platelet aggregation in severe combined immunodeficiency disease with adenosine deaminase deficiency. Br J Haematol 39:189, 1978.
24. Lee CH, Evans SP, Rozenberg MC, Bagnara AS, Ziegler JB, Van der Weyden MB: In vitro platelet abnormality in adenosine deaminase deficiency and severe combined immunodeficiency. Blood 53:465, 1979.
25. Hirschhorn R, Ratech H: Isozymes of adenosine deaminase. In "Isozymes: Current Topics in Biological and Medical Research." New York: Alan R Liss, 1980, vol 4, p 131.
26. Zielke CL, Suelter CH: Purine, purine nucleoside and purine nucleoside aminohydrolases. In Boyer PD (ed): "The

Enzymes," 3rd Ed. New York: Academic Press, 1971.
27. Miles GC, Schmalsteig FC, Trimmer KB, Goldman AS, Goldblum RM: Purine metabolism in adenosine deaminase deficiency. Proc Natl Acad Sci USA 73:2866, 1976.
28. Cohen A, Hirschhorn R, Horowitz SD, Rubinstein A, Polmar SH, Hong R, Martin DW: Deoxyadenosine triphosphate as a potentially toxic metabolite in adenosine deaminase deficiency. Proc Natl Acad Sci USA 75:472, 1978.
29. Coleman MS, Donofrio J, Hutton JJ, Hahn L, Daoud A, Lampkin B, Dyminski J: Identification and quantitation of adenine deoxynucleotides in erythrocytes of a patient with adenosine deaminase deficiency and severe combined immunodeficiency. J Biol Chem 253:1619, 1978.
30. Simmonds HA, Watson JG, Hugh-Jones K, Perrett D, Sahota A, Potter CF: Deoxynucleotide excretion in adenosine deaminase deficiency and purine nucleoside phosphorylase deficiency. Supra #13, pp 377.
31. Hershfield MS, Kredich NM, Ownby DR, Ownby H, Buckley R: In vivo inactivation of erythrocyte S-adenosylhomocysteine hydrolase by 2'-deoxyadenosine in adenosine deaminase deficient patients. J Clin Invest 63:807, 1979.
32. Hirschhorn R, Roegner V, Rubinstein A, Papageorgiou P: Plasma deoxyadenosine, adenosine and erythrocyte deoxy ATP are elevated at birth in an adenosine deaminase-deficient child. J Clin Invest 65:768, 1980.
33. Donofrio J, Coleman MS, Hutton JJ, Daoud A, Lampkin B, Dyminski J: Overproduction of adenine deoxynucleotides and deoxynucleotides in adenosine deaminase deficiency with severe combined immunodeficiency disease. J Clin Invest 62:884, 1978.
34. Hirschhorn R, Roegner-Maniscalco V, Kuritsky L, Rosen F: Bone marrow transplantation only partially restores purine metabolites to normal in adenosine deaminase-deficient patients. J Clin Invest 68:1387, 1981.
35. Kuttesch JF, Schmalstieg FC, Nelson JA: Analysis of adenosine and other adenine compounds in patients with immunodeficiency diseases. J Liq Chromatogr 1:97, 1978.
36. Mills GC, Goldblum RM, Newkirk KE, Schmalstieg FC: Urinary excretion of purines, purine nucleosides and pseudouridine in adenosine deaminase deficiency. Biochem Med 20:180, 1978.
37. Hirschhorn R, Ratech H, Rubinstein A, Papageorgiou P, Kesarwala H, Gelfand E, Roegner-Maniscalco V: Increased excretion of modified adenine nucleosides by children with adenosine deaminase deficiency. Pediatr Res 16:362, 1982.
38. Ishi K, Green H: Lethality of adenosine for cultured mammalian cells by interference with pyrimidine biosynthesis. J Cell Sci 13:429, 1973.
39. Hirschhorn R, Grossman J, Weissmann G: Effect of cyclic 3', 5'-adenosine monophosphate and theophylline on lymphocyte transformation. Proc Soc Exp Biol Med 133:1361, 1970.
40. Mitchell BS, Mejias E, Dadonna PE, Kelley WN: Purinogenic immunodeficiency diseases: Selective toxicity of deoxyribonucleosides for T cells. Proc Natl Acad Sci USA 75:5011, 1978.
41. Ratech H, Thorbecke GJ, Hirschhorn R: Metabolic abnormalities of human adenosine deaminase deficiency reproduced in the mouse by 2'-deoxycoformycin, an adenosine deaminase inhibitor. Clin Immunol Immunopathol 23:119, 1981.
42. Ratech H, Kuritsky L, Thorbecke GJ, Hirschhorn R: Suppression of human lymphocyte DNA and protein synthesis in vitro by adenosine and eight modified adenine nucleosides in the presence or in the absence of adenosine deaminase inhibitors, 2'-deoxycoformycin (DCF) and erythro-9-(2-hydroxy-3-nonyl) adenine (EHNA). Cell Immunol 68:244, 1982.
43. Chen SH, Ochs HD, Scott CR, Giblett ER, Tingle AJ: Adenosine deaminase deficiency: Disappearance of adenine deoxynucleotides from a patient's erythrocytes after successful bone marrow transplantation. J Clin Invest 62:1386, 1978.
44. Polmar SH, Wetzler EM, Stern RC, Hirschhorn R: Restoration of in vitro lymphocyte responses with exogenous adenosine deaminase in a patient with severe combined immunodeficiency. Lancet 2:743, 1975.
45. Polmar SH: Enzyme replacement and other biochemical approaches to the therapy of adenosine deaminase deficiency. In Elliot K, Whelan J (eds): "Enzyme Defects and Immune Dysfunction." Ciba Foundation Symposium 68. New York: Excerpta Medica, 1979, p 213.
46. Jenkins T: Red blood cell adenosine deaminase deficiency in a "healthy" !Kung individual. Lancet 2:736, 1973.
47. Hirschhorn R, Roegner V, Jenkins T, Seaman C, Piomelli S, Borkowsky W: Erythrocyte adenosine deaminase deficiency without immunodeficiency: Evidence for an unstable mutant enzyme. J Clin Invest 64:1130, 1979.
48. Perignon JL, Hamet M, Cartier P, Griscelli C: Complete adenosine deaminase (ADA) deficiency without immunodeficiency, and with primary hyperoxaluria in a 12-year-old boy. J Clin Chem Biochem 17:406, 1979.
49. Hirschhorn R, Martiniuk F, Roegner-Maniscalco V, Ellenbogen A, Perignon J-L, Jenkins T: Genetic heterogeneity in partial adenosine deaminase deficiency. J Clin Invest (In press).
50. Valentine WN, Paglia DE, Tartaglia AP, Gilsanz F: Hereditary hemolytic anemia with increased red cell adenosine deaminase (45-70 fold) and decreased adenosine triphosphate. Science 195:783, 1977.
51. Siciliano MJ, Bordelon MR, Kohler PO: Expression of human adenosine deaminase after fusion of adenosine deaminase-deficient cells with mouse fibroblasts. Proc Natl Acad Sci USA 75:936, 1978.
52. Giblett ER, Ammann AJ, Wara DW, Sandman R, Diamond LK: Nucleoside phosphorylase deficiency in a child with severely defective T-cell immunity and normal B-cell immunity. Lancet 1:1010, 1975.
53. Stoop JW, Zegers BJM, Hendricks GFM, Siegenbeek van Heukelom LH, Staal GEJ, DeBree PK, Wadman SK, Ballieux RE: Purine nucleoside phosphorylase deficiency associated with selective cellular immunodeficiency. N Engl J Med 296:651, 1977.
54. Biggar WD, Giblett ER, Ozere RI, Grover BD: A new form of nucleoside phosphorylase deficiency in two brothers with defective T-cell function. J Pediatr 92:354, 1978.
55. Virelizier JL, Hamet M, Ballet JJ, Reinert P, Griscelli C: Impaired defense against vaccinia in a child with T-lymphocyte deficiency associated with inosine phosphorylase defect. J Pediatr 92:358, 1978.
56. Carapella de Luca E, Aiuti F, Lucarelli P, Bruni L, Baroni CD, Imperato C, Roos D, Astaldi A: A patient with nucleoside phosphorylase deficiency, selective T-cell deficiency, and autoimmune hemolytic anemia. J Pediatr 93:1000, 1978.
57. Rich KC, Arnold WJ, Palella T, Fox IH: Cellular immune deficiency with autoimmune hemolytic anemia in purine nucleoside phosphorylase deficiency. Am J Med 67:172, 1979.
58. Ammann AJ: Immunologic aberrations in purine nucleoside phosphorylase deficiencies. Supra #45, p 55.
59. Fox IH, Andres CM, Gelfand EW, Biggar D: Purine nucleoside phosphorylase deficiency: Altered kinetic properties of a mutant enzyme. Science 197:1084, 1977.

60. Wortmann RL, Andres CM, Kaminska J, Gelfand EW, Arnold W, Rich K, Fox IH: Biochemical heterogeneity in purine nucleoside phosphorylase deficiency. Arthritis Rheum 21:603, 1978.
61. Osborne WR, Chen S-H, Giblett ER, Biggar WD, Ammann AJ, Scott CR: Purine nucleoside phosphorylase deficiency. Evidence for molecular heterogeneity in two families with enzyme deficient members. J Clin Invest 60:741, 1977.
62. Gudas LJ, Zannis VI, Clift SM, Ammann AJ, Staal GE, Martin DW JR: Characterization of mutant subunits of human purine nucleoside phosphorylase. J Biol Chem 255:5606, 1980.
63. McRoberts JA, Martin DW Jr: Submolecular characterization of a mutant purine-nucleoside phosphorylase. J Biol Chem 255:5605, 1980.
64. Agarwal RP, Parks RE Jr: Purine nucleoside phosphorylase from human erythrocytes. IV. Crystallization and some properties. J Biol Chem 244:644, 1969.
65. Zannis V, Doyle D, Martin DW Jr: Purification and characterization of human erythrocyte purine nucleoside phosphorylase and its subunits. J Biol Chem 253:504, 1978.
66. Osborne WR: Human red cell purine nucleoside phosphorylase. Purification by biospecific affinity chromatography and physical properties. J Biol Chem 255:7089, 1980.
67. Edwards YH, Hopkinson DA, Harris H: Inherited variants of human nucleoside phosphorylase. Ann Hum Genet 34:395, 1971.
68. Creagan RP, Tan YH, Chen S-H, Tischfield JA, Ruddle FJ: Mouse/human somatic cell hybrids utilizing human parental cells containing a (14;22) translocation: Assignment of the gene for nucleoside phosphorylase to chromosome 14. In Bergsma D (ed): "Human Gene Mapping." Miami: Symposia Specialists for The National Foundation-March of Dimes, BD:OAS X(3):83, 1974.
69. Cohen A, Doyle D, Martin DW Jr, Ammann AJ: Abnormal purine metabolism and purine overproduction in a patient deficient in purine nucleoside phosphorylase. N Engl J Med 295:1449, 1976.
70. Simmonds HA, Watson JG, Hugh-Jones K, Perreti D, Sahota A, Potter CF: Deoxynucleotide excretion in adenosine deaminase deficiency and purine nucleoside phosphorylase deficiency. Supra #13, p 377.
71. Edwards NL, Gelfand EW, Biggar D, Fox IH: Particle deficiency of purine nucleoside phosphorylase: Studies of purine and pyrimidine metabolism. J Lab Clin Med 91:736, 1978.
72. Dosch HM, Mansour A, Cohen A et al: Inhibition of suppressor T-cell development following deoxyguanosine administration. Nature 285:494, 1980.

The Bare Lymphocyte Syndrome: Immunodeficiency Resulting From the Lack of Expression of HLA Antigens

Jean-Louis Touraine, MD, and Hervé Bétuel, MD

Transplantation and Immunobiology Unit, Hôpital Edouard Herriot, 69374 Lyon Cedex 2, France

In early 1974, we identified a new form of combined immunodeficiency (CID), characterized by the lack of cellular expression of HLA A and B antigens. We suggested that the immunodeficiency resulted from the absence of cell-surface HLA antigens, and we named this condition the bare lymphocyte syndrome (BLS) [1]. In the following years, 2 other patients from a Turkish family [2], a second patient from the initial Algerian family [3], and several other patients have been found with a similar syndrome [4,5]. The first 9 cases have been reported recently [6] and 4 additional patients have been partially reported to the BLS Registry (Table 1). This registry has been set up in Lyon where the syndrome was described, under the sponsorship of the World Health Organization, in order to elucidate the important relationship between surface HLA antigens and lymphocyte differentiation and functions [7].

The important biologic significance of HLA antigens in the development of immunity has only been studied by comparing cell interactions in cases of HLA identity and in cases with slightly different HLA molecules. The existence of a condition characterized by the lack of expression of class I HLA antigens represents an "experiment of nature" which provides direct evidence for the importance of these antigens in lymphocyte development. The analysis of this syndrome demonstrates that the lack of expression of HLA antigens hinders not only most effector functions of T lymphocytes but also their intrathymic differentiation and possibly homing in secondary lymphoid organs. Our studies in these patients have shown a blockage of differentiation at an early stage in the T-lymphocyte lineage (but at a stage where normal cells clearly express HLA antigens).

TABLE 1. Registry of the Bare Lymphocyte Syndrome (1978–1982)

13 cases in 8 families
In all cases:
1) Abnormality of T-lymphocyte differentiation and/or function
2) Hypo𝛾globulinemia
3) Absence of $\beta 2m$, HLA A, B, and C on lymphocytes.
↑Infections
The ID is either very severe (death in infancy) or relatively more moderate (diagnosis during childhood).

MAIN CHARACTERISTICS OF THE IMMUNODEFICIENCY

Clinical manifestations have included oral candidiasis, bacterial pneumonia, pneumocystis, and herpes virus infections, gastroenteritis, and septicemia. Respiratory infections have been responsible for the death of 3 of the first 4 patients. The 4th patient died of extreme malabsorption, with marasmus, hypoglycemia, and very poor general condition. Attempts at treatment have involved a fetal thymus transplant which had little effect, and a bone marrow transplant which resulted in a transient immunologic improvement but was unable to restore a correct normal condition in the marasmic infant [1,3,8].

TABLE 2. CID in BLS

Moderate lymphopenia
Number of T lymphocytes: ↘↘
Number of B lymphocytes: normal
Plasma cells: absent
Delayed hypersensitivity skin reactions: ↘↘
Proliferative responses
  to mitogens: ↘↘
  to allogeneic cells: ↘↘
IgM: ↘↘ IgA: ↘↘
Allohemagglutinins: absent
Antibody production: absent
FTS: ↘↘
Inducible marrow prothymocytes: ↘↘
Thymus and lymphoid organs: severely hypoplastic
Complement, zinc, platelet counts, karyotype: normal

Immunologic findings in the various patients have been characteristic of a partial CID (Table 2). Lymphopenia was moderate. Numbers of T lymphocytes were usually reduced. B lymphocytes were present but plasma cells were either absent or very few. Delayed hypersensitivity skin reactions were very weak. Proliferative responses to phytomitogens, allogeneic cells, and antigens were usually decreased. In one child with a virtually normal lymphocyte proliferative response to mitogens, the lymphocytes were also able to exert a cytotoxic effect against unrelated lymphoblasts [4]. Pokeweed mitogen (PWM)-induced B-cell differentiation was impaired [2,9]. Serum levels of IgM and IgA were very low. When IgG of maternal origin disappeared from the infant's serum, levels of IgG were also found below normal. Allohemagglutinins were virtually absent. Antibody production was not demonstrable. Serum thymic factor activity was below normal. Marrow prothymocytes able to acquire the HTLA+ phenotype were very few. C2 and C4 complement levels, karyotype analysis, platelet counts, and zinc levels were normal. At necropsy, the thymus and the other lymphoid organs were hypoplastic and contained few lymphocytes.

Using an in vitro plaque-forming cell (PFC) assay to study cells from one patient with the BLS, Dr. R.E. Ballieux et al demonstrated that a) the patient's T lymphocytes could not produce functional antigen-specific helper or suppressor factors, b) the patient's monocytes could not bind helper factor or present the factor to B cells, and c) the patient's B cells could not be activated by helper factor from normal T cells, in the presence of normal, HLA-DR identical monocytes and antigen.

MAIN CHARACTERISTICS OF THE IMMUNOGENETIC DEFECT

HLA A, B, and C antigens were shown to be absent from the lymphocyte surface by cytotoxicity and immunofluorescence methods. These antigens were also absent from the platelet surface, as demonstrated by a complement fixation test. HLA antigens were, however, detected by absorption techniques in the patients' serum and on fibroblasts cultured from the skin [1,10,11]. Similarly, β2-microglobulin was present at a normal level in the serum but was not found at the lymphocyte surface by cytotoxicity and immunofluorescence assays. In some patients β2-microglobulin was absent from both T and B cells, while in other patients it was not found on T lymphocytes in suspension but was detected, in reduced amounts, on B lymphocytes [2,3,6]. β2-microglobulin and HLA antigens were also virtually absent from the surface of EVB-transformed B-lymphoblastoid cells (Fig. 1) but became detectable after several weeks of culture and several passages [7]. HLA D/DR determinants

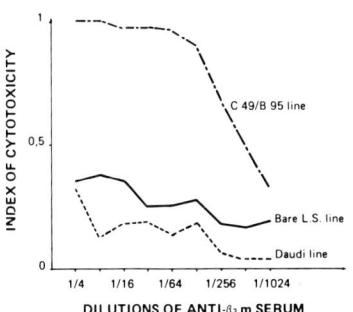

Fig. 1. Virtual absence of β2 m detected by a cytotoxicity assay on B-lymphoblastoid cells of a line derived from a BLS patient. Similar results were obtained with immunofluorescence. (From Touraine JL et al: The bare lymphocyte syndrome. I. Immunological studies before and after bone marrow transplantation. Blut 41:198–202, 1980, with permission.)

were detected in virtually all reported patients and their expression is therefore not as much altered as that of β2-microglobulin and HLA A, B, and C antigens. It is, however, still uncertain whether the expression of HLA DR antigens is completely normal or relatively reduced as suggested by a positivity with only some anti-HLA DR antisera [2]. Other surface antigens, of a different nature (eg immunoglobulins, differentiation antigens of T lymphocytes) were demonstrated on the surface of lymphocytes from the various subsets, suggesting that the defect is relatively specific.

Family analysis, including investigations of sibs with this syndrome and normal sibs from the same family, suggests that the BLS is an autosomal recessive condition associated with genes different from those of the MHC region [6]. In one family, 2 patients had different HLA genotypes and each had normal "HLA identical" sibs (Fig. 2). In another family, 2 affected brothers did not share the same HLA genotype [2]. The BLS and its genetic transmission therefore reveal the presence of gene(s) not borne by the no. 6 chromosome but controlling the expression of β2-microglobulin and class I HLA antigens.

DISCUSSION

In man, as in other animal species, the selective pressure of evolution has favored development of resistance mechanisms against the major cause of death before the age of reproduction: infection with a variety of organisms. In this regard, the HLA system is likely to play an important role, especially in defense against facultative intracellular parasitic organisms [12]. It may appear surprising that, despite numerous associations reported between various diseases and certain HLA phenotypes, no clear association has been found between congenital immunodeficiencies and such phenotypes. The association between the lack of expression of class I HLA antigens and a congenital immunodeficiency demonstrates, however, even better than a difference in any antigen frequency, that HLA molecules are of crucial importance in the development of immunity.

Several lines of evidence link MHC determinants and differentiation of functional lymphocytes [12,13]. Our investigations in BLS patients showed both impairment of T-lymphocyte functions and blockage of T-lymphocyte differentiation. Determinants coded for by genes of the MHC region may thus be necessary for several types of cell interactions, eg those mediating in T-lymphocyte differentiation; cytotoxic, helper and suppressor T-cell

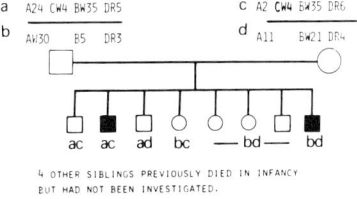

Fig. 2. HLA genotypes in one family with BLS. The 2 investigated patients had inherited different no. 6 chromosomes from their parents. (From Touraine JL: The bare lymphocyte syndrome: Report on the Registry. Lancet 1:319–321, 1981, with permission.)

functions; lymphocyte homing, and self-recognition.

When the first patient was described it was predicted "that various forms and degrees of immunodeficiency may be associated with the absence of cell surface HLA A and B antigens," hence the word "syndrome" rather than "disease" [1]. The analysis of several patients with BLS has confirmed some variation in the degree of clinical severity and immunologic deficiency. It is, however, remarkable that all patients have CID, severe in some cases but more moderate in others, with certain T-lymphocyte functions being totally absent in all reported patients, while antibody production is also severely altered. It is possible that the mild variations in expressivity of the immunologic alterations are associated with comparable variations in the immunogenetic defect.

The analysis of families with BLS has shown that it is transmitted independently of the no. 6 chromosome. Genes of a different region thus control the expression of β2-microglobulin and class I HLA antigens, especially at the surface of cells of hematopoietic origin. Studies in progress on lymphocytes of the patients and their family members may identify the chromosome bearing these genes and clarify the nature of this regulation (eg synthesis of a molecule needed for optimal expression of β2-microglobulin and HLA antigens at the membrane level). An improved understanding of factors controlling this antigenic expression may provide us with means to modulate the surface concentration of HLA antigens, with a capability either to decrease it or to increase it as interferon does.

ACKNOWLEDGMENTS

We thank Drs. R.K.B. Shuurman, J.J. Van Rood, C. Griscelli, F. Touraine, G. Souillet, G. Lenoir, N. Philippe, H. Renaud, W. Kuis, and R.E. Ballieux for the studies that they have done to improve the understanding of the Bare Lymphocyte Syndrome; and the World Health Organization for encouragement and financial support in the setting up of the Registry.

REFERENCES

1. Touraine JL, Bétuel H, Souillet G, Jeune M: Combined immunodeficiency disease associated with absence of cell-surface HLA-A and B antigens. J Pediatr 93:47–51, 1978.
2. Schuurman RKB, Van Rood JJ, Vossen JM, Schellekens PThA, Felkamp-Vroom ThM, Doyer E, Gmelig-Meyling F, Visser HKA: Failure of lymphocyte-membrane HLA-A and B expression in two siblings with combined immunodeficiency. Clin Immunol Immunopathol 14:418–434, 1979.
3. Touraine JL, Bétuel H, Philippe N: The bare lymphocyte syndrome. I. Immunological studies before and after bone marrow transplantation. Blut 41: 198–202, 1980.
4. Kuis W, Roord J, Zegers BJM, Schuurman RKB, Heijnen CJ, Balddwin WM, Goulmy E, Claas F, Van de Griend RJ, Rijkers GT, Van Rood JJ, Vossen JM, Ballieux RE, Stoop JW: Clinical and immunological studies in a patient with the "Bare Lymphocyte" Syndrome. In Touraine JL, Gluckman E, Griscelli C (eds): "Bone Marrow Transplantation in Europe." Amsterdam: Excerpta Medica, 1981, vol 2, pp 201–208.
5. Griscelli C, Durandy A, Virelizier JL, Grospierre B, Oury C, De Saint-Basile G, Couillin P, Niaudet P, Bétuel H, Hors J, Lepage V, Colombani J: Impaired cell to cell interaction in partial combined immunodeficiency with defective synthesis and membrane expression of HLA antigens. Ibid, pp 194–200.
6. Touraine JL: The bare lymphocyte syndrome: Report on the Registry. Lancet 1:319–321, 1981.
7. Touraine JL: An informal registry for the "Bare Lymphocyte Syndrome." Thymus 1:133, 1979.
8. Philippe N, Touraine JL, Renaud H, Evrard A, Bétuel H, Monnet P: The Bare Lymphocyte Syndrome. II. Clinical course before and after bone marrow transplantation. Blut 41:202–206, 1980.
9. Schuurman RKB, Gelfand EW, Touraine JL, Van Rood JJ: Lymphocyte-membrane abnormalities associated with primary immunodeficiency disease. In Seligmann M, Hitzig WH (eds): "Primary Immunodeficiencies." Amsterdam: Elsevier, 1980, pp 87–99.
10. Bétuel H, Touraine JL, Souillet G, Jeune M: Absence of cell-membrane HLA antigens in an immunodeficient child. Tissue Antigens 11:68–70, 1978.
11. Touraine JL, Bétuel H: Immunodeficiency diseases and expression of HLA antigens. Hum Immunol 2:147–153, 1981.
12. Zinkernagel RM, Callahan GN, Klein J, Dennert G: Cytotoxic T cells learn specificity for self H-2 during differentiation in the thymus. Nature 271:251–253, 1978.
13. Dausset J, Contu L: Is the MHC a general self-recognition system playing a major unifying role in an organism? Hum Immunol 1:5–17, 1980.

Combined Immunodeficiency With Defective Expression of HLA: Modulation of an Abnormal HLA Synthesis and Functional Studies

Barbara Lisowska-Grospierre, MD, Anne Durandy, MD, Jean-Louis Virelizier, MD, Alain Fischer, MD, and Claude Griscelli, MD

Unité d'Immunologie et d'Hématologie Pédiatriques, Département de Pédiatrie, INSERM U 132 Hôpital des Enfants Malades, 75730 Paris Cedex 15, France

A CID associated with a defective expression of membrane HLA antigens now has been reported by several groups [1–6]. There are apparently two different types, one in which HLA A, B, and C antigens and β_2 microglobulin (β_2m) are only poorly expressed [1–3], and a second in which HLA DR antigens are also not normally detected on B- and activated T-cell membranes [4–6].

The main immunologic abnormalities observed in this syndrome are: 1) an absence of delayed skin reactivity to antigens which correlated with defective in vitro proliferative responses to antigens, 2) a hypogammaglobulinemia, variable from one patient to another, and a constant absence to antibody formation after vaccination. The immunodeficiency syndrome has a severe course. Several patients died from infections in early childhood [1–4].

Studies performed in 10 patients with a defective membrane expression of HLA antigens with special reference to their modulation by treatment with interferon (IFN) and to their in vitro biosynthesis are reported here. We also performed functional in vitro studies of Ig and antibody production in some patients.

CASE REPORTS

We observed 10 patients with CID associated with a defective expression of HLA antigens. The 10 patients (in 7 families) had the first symptoms 1 to 5 months after birth, dominated by a diarrhea (7 patients). The main clinical symptoms were then a chronic diarrhea associated with bronchitis (9 of 10 patients). A peculiar susceptibility to viral infections was noted since, in our series, we observed a poliomyelitis (Wild virus type II or III) in 3 patients, one of them with encephalomyelitis, a diffuse Coxsackie virus (untyped) infection with neurologic impairment in another patient. Six of the 10 patients died between 9 to 33 months of age. The 4 others (aged 6 mos, 3 yrs, 3 yrs, and 10 yrs) are alive but in poor clinical condition.

The usual immunologic characteristics showed a normal number of blood lymphocytes with a percentage of T cells, normal in 2 patients and decreased (13–46%) in the others. Percentage of blood B lymphocytes which varied from 7–80% was increased in 3 patients (26, 44, and 80%). Delayed skin reactions to antigens and proliferative responses to antigens were negative in all patients, whereas mitogen-induced proliferations as well as response in MLR were in the normal range. Generation of cytotoxicity activity during the MLR was normal in the 3 patients tested. A hypogammaglobulinemia, variable in intensity and from class to class, was observed in all patients. Postvaccinal antibody formation was constantly profoundly impaired. Allohemagglutinins to blood group substances were normal in 3 patients and defective in the others.

DEFECT OF MEMBRANE EXPRESSION OF HLA AND β_2M DETERMINANTS

We have already shown, in previous reports on 7 of our 10 patients [4, 5] that, using different methods of detection, HLA A, B, and β_2m were poorly expressed on the membrane of PBL, separated T and B lymphocytes, monocytes, and platelets (Table 1). We showed that HLA DR was absent or hardly detectable on the membrane of fresh B lymphocytes, and variably expressed on monocytes. In contrast with these observations, we observed the presence of serum HLA A and B in 4 of 6 patients tested, and a normal level of serum β_2m in all patients. Finally, we showed that patients' leukocytes used as stimulators in a MLR were generally unable to normally stimulate allogeneic cells.

We now report more extensive studies on the expression of HLA antigens and β_2m on the membrane of cultured lymphoid cells (Table 1). Three-day PHA-induced T blasts as well as PHA-induced blasts obtained after a two-week culture maintained with Interleukin 2 (Il2) did not express common HLA DR antigens normally detected in 50–90% to control blasts with a monoclonal anti-DR (Ortho-Pharm, Raritan, New Jersey). Common HLA antigens and β_2m (revealed by a corresponding monoclonal antibody from Sera Lab, Sussex, England and a specific hetero anti-β_2 antiserum raised in rab-

TABLE 1. Membrane Expression of HLA Antigens and β_2m on Fresh or Culture Lymphocytes

	Fresh lymphocytes						PHA-induced blasts			EBV-transformed cells		
	+ 0			+ IFN								
	HLA	β_2m	DR	HLA	β_2m	DR	HLA	β_2m	DR	HLA	β_2m	DR
Controls	100	100	10	100	100	10	98	97	89*	100	100	100
							100	100	50**			
Patients												
AC	40	5	1	92	90	1	20	10	0**	NT	NT	NT
JB	45	2	0	74	48	0	NT	NT	NT	100	100	0†
										100	100	100‡
RA	7	7	1	75	48	1	37	13	0**	NT	100	0
DA	53	6	0	68	51	0	23	16	0**	NT	100	0
NH	67	58	1	82	79	1	96	78	0*	NT	NT	NT
OT	62	51	15	85	72	13	98	84	0*	NT	NT	NT
RA	80	75	0	NT	77	0	NT	NT	NT	NT	NT	NT

*3-day culture.
** ≥ 15 day-culture + Il 2.
†2-week culture.
‡ ≥ 4-week culture.
Results are expressed as the percentage of immunofluorescent cells.
NT = not tested.

bits from Nordic Lab, Tilburg, The Netherlands) were only partially deficient on PHA-induced blast membrane. It is striking to note that if T-cell blasts with undetectable DR antigens could normally proliferate in presence of Il 2 for 2 to 3 weeks, they could not be maintained longer. In contrast to fresh B lymphocytes, EBV-transformed B-blast cells did normally express common HLA A and B antigens and β_2m. Furthermore, a B-cell line obtained from PBL of *Patient JB* did also express common DR antigens after 4 weeks of culture (Table 1).

BIOSYNTHESIS OF HLA ANTIGENS AND β_2m

Preliminary experiments had been performed with cells of 4 of the 10 patients by incubating 3 days-PHA, PWM, or UCHT$_1$ (M. Feldmann, London) induced blasts in presence of either ^{3}H-leucine (Amersham, 40–60 Ci/mm, 25 µc/ml) for 6 hours, or ^{35}S methionine (Amersham, 600 Ci/mmol, 100 µc/ml) for 2 hours. HLA antigens were then precipitated from NP40 cell lysates by incubating with different monoclonal or rabbit antisera followed by Sepharose-Protein A: rabbit anti-α and anti-β chains of HLA DR (B. Mach, Geneva), rabbit anti-β_2m (C. Vincent, Lyon), monoclonal anti-HLA DR (B 8.12), anti-common HLA A and B (B 9.12) (B. Mallissen, Marseille), monoclonal anti-HLA A, B, and C (W 6/32 HLK), anti-HLA DR (E 15/4 HLK from Sera Lab). Washed precipitates were analyzed by SDS-acrylamide gel electrophoresis. This protocol was applied 3 times for 2 patients (*AC* and *NH*) and once for 2 other patients (*JB* and *RA*).

Biosynthetic activity of cells, if expressed by ratio of cpm of incorporated isotope to number of cells, was 2 to 5 times lower for patients' cells, as compared to control cells. This cannot be explained in all cases by lower percentage of blasts although, in some experiments, lymphoblastic response of patients' lymphocytes was decreased. HLA A and B antigens were detected in 3 (*AC, RA, NH*) out of 4 patients studied, and absent in *Patient JB* cell lysate (Fig. 1B). However, as judged by the intensity of 44 K daltons band, the amount of HLA A and B polypeptides was always inferior to control and could vary quantitatively from one experiment to the other for the same patient (Fig. 2B). HLA DR antigens were absent in PHA-induced blast cells obtained from patients *AC* and *JB* (Fig. 1A), and present in very faint amounts in blasts from *Patient RA*. Patient *NH*'s blast-cell apparently contained the α, β, and I DR chains in amounts similar to control (Fig. 2A). On the contrary, β_2m was present in cell lysates of all patients in amount comparable or very close to controls (Figs. 1B and 2C). A family study was performed for *Patient JB*. Cells from mother, father, and sister contained HLA DR, and β_2m and no abnormal migration of those determinants was observed (Fig. 1).

These results clearly indicate that HLA antigens, already shown not to be normally expressed on the cell membranes, are not normally produced. Indeed, in *Patient JB*, for instance, a complete absence of HLA A, B, and DR was observed, indicating that those molecules were absent in cell-cytoplasm. A variability was, however, observed since similarly to the surface immunofluorescence study, HLA A and B can be variably detected by biosynthetic studies in blast cells from other patients.

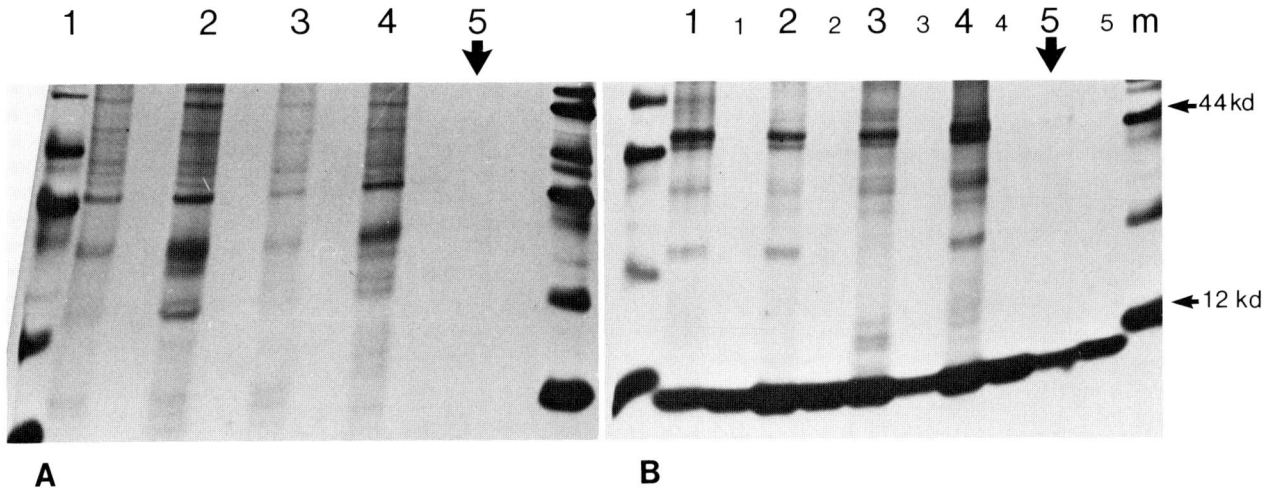

Fig. 1. SDS polyacrylamide gel (12.5%) electrophoresis of immune precipitates from blast lyastes of *Patient JB* and his family members. Lysates from 1) normal control, 2) father, 3) sister, 4) mother, and 5) Patient PHA blasts. Precipitates obtained with A) monoclonal anti-HLA DR (1–5); B) molecular weight standards.

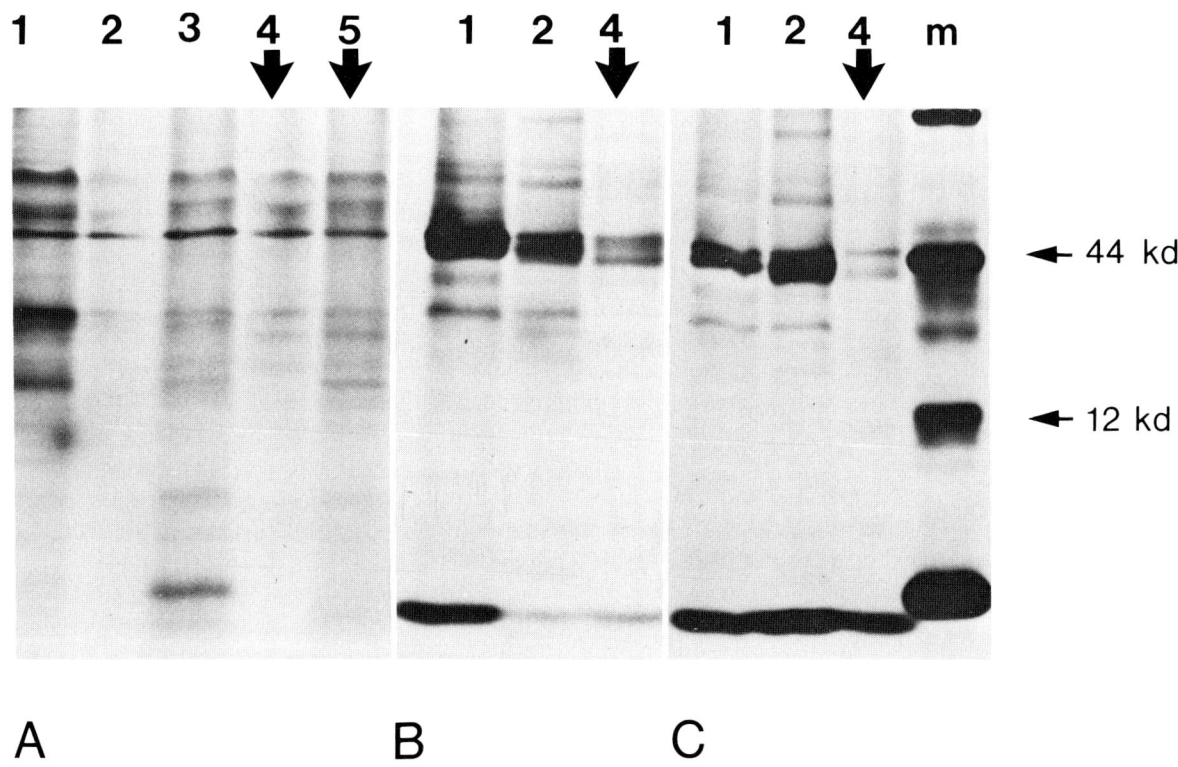

Fig. 2. SDS polyacrylamide gel (12.5%) electrophoresis of immune precipitates from blast lysates of *Patient NH* and controls. Lysates from Raji cells (1), normal control (2, 3) and *Patient NH* (4, 5) PHA blasts. Precipitates obtained with A) rabbit anti-α DR (A2, A4), anti-β DR (A3, A5) or mixture of both (A1); B) monoclonal anti-common HLA (ABC) antigens; C) rabbit anti β_2. M = molecular weight standards.

TABLE 2. In Vitro Ig and Antibody Production

	PWM-induced ICC generation*			Mannan-MBSA-induced ACC generation**		Specific anti-mannan supernatant antibodies		Specific anti(A/X 31) Supernatant antibodies
	IgM $\times 10^{-3}$	IgG $\times 10^{-3}$	IgA $\times 10^{-3}$	IgM $\times 10^{-3}$	IgG $\times 10^{-3}$	IgM (U/ml)	IgG (U/ml)	IgG (ng/ml)
Controls	100 ± 45	96 ± 31	65 ± 31	10 ± 6	6 ± 4	17 ± 10	19 ± 18	36 ± 25
AC	68	30	1	NT	NT	NT	NT	NT
	<1	<1	<1	0	0	0	0	0
JB	<1	<1	<1	17	0	8	0	0
RA	<1	<1	<1	3	3	5	10	NT
OA	<1	<1	<1	0	0	0	0	NT
NH	NT	NT	NT	1.9	0	1	0	NT
OT	1	1	1	NT	NT	NT	NT	NT
AR	100	41	25	1	3	NT	NT	NT

Results are expressed for 1×10^6 input cells.
*Number of IgM, IgG, or IgA containing cells (cc).
**Number of anti-mannan antibody cc revealed by radioautography [10].
†Solid phase enzyme immunoassay [10,11].

MODULATION OF EXPRESSION OF HLA ANTIGENS AND β_2m BY IFN

Since IFN is known to enhance HLA A and B, but not DR antigen expression on cell membranes [7–9], we have tested the in vitro effect of α (Institut Pasteur, Paris) or β (Rega Institute, Leuwen, Belgium) IFN on HLA expression on various cells. We observed that α or β IFN treatment significantly enhanced HLA A, B, and β_2m antigen expression on freshly drawn lymphocytes (Table 1). On the contrary, there was no enhancement of HLA DR expression. This effect was truly due to IFN since it was completely abolished by a specific anti-β IFN antiserum (Rega Institute). IFN was shown to act at the level of HLA-antigen synthesis since cycloheximide also inhibited its effect.

In a different set of experiments, blast cells were used as targets of IFN. Incubation of PHA-induced blast cells with α IFN for the last 18 hours of a 6-day culture also resulted in an increased percentage of β_2m-bearing cells. In parallel, the ability of these IFN-treated blasts to be destroyed by specific cytotoxic T cells increased. In fact, untreated blasts which did not express detectable β_2m at all were not destroyed significantly more than unrelated target cells. In contrast, a positive specific cytotoxicity correlated with clear detectability of β_2m on a patient's blast cells.

IN VITRO FUNCTIONAL STUDIES OF Ig AND ANTIBODY PRODUCTION

In the PWM-driven system, studied before any treatment by γ-globulins, results were variable from one patient to another, and variable in the same subject *(AC)* (Table 2). Similar observations were made for both T-helper and B-cell functions in co-culture assays. Whether the variation paralleled the observation in HLA A, B, DR antigen expression was a tentative but unproven hypothesis.

Production and secretion of Ig by patient's PWM blasts was also studied. Using a biosynthetic labeling, cells from patient *RA* normally synthesized and secreted IgM molecules in amounts comparable to control cells, but IgA and IgG were absent. Blast lysate from patient *AC* contained very small amount of IgG, A, and M, but corresponding molecules were absent from extracellular medium.

In antibody assay for mannan of *Candida albicans* [10], we were surprised to observe, a production of specific anti-mannan antibody (Table 2) in 4 out of 6 patients. These results are in apparent discordance with the observation made by Kuis et al [6] in a patient who had defective in vitro production of antibody to ovalbumin or to SRBC. A similar defect was found in 2 of our patients tested for the ability of their PBL to produce in vitro specific antibody to influenza virus proteinic antigen (A/X31) (Table 2) [11].

CONCLUSION

We have reported new data about the CID associated with a defective expression of HLA determinants, also called "bare lymphocyte syndrome." Our results indicate a variability (from one patient to another and for a given patient tested sequentially) of the membrane expression of these determinants. Biosynthetic labeling, which studies the membrane as well as the intracellular molecules, confirmed the variability of the defective expression. However, β_2m appeared to be comparable in amount to control cells in all patients tested, and production, as well as membrane expression of HLA DR, was more profoundly defective in mitogen-induced blasts. HLA DR was not found on the membrane of PHA-induced-T blasts and of EBV-transformed B cells (when tested before 2 to 3 weeks of culture) and a biosynthetic labeling showed that α, β, and I-DR chains were equally affected in 3 out of 4 patients. In one patient *(NA)*, however, α, β, and I-DR chains were normally detected in the cell lysates, while HLA DR was poorly expressed on membrane. This last observation shows again the variability from patient to patient, and possibly the heterogeneity of the syndrome.

That incubation with IFN enhanced the membrane expression of HLA A, B, and β_2m is another evidence for the hypothesis that their abnormal expression does not result from a lack of genetic information for the synthesis, but rather from an abnormal regulation of either synthesis, intracellular transport, membrane insertion, or shedding of these molecules. Furthermore, enhancement of HLA A and B expression and thus, the ability of target cells to be recognized by specific cytotoxic T cells may have important consequence if IFN may also increase the T-cell mediated anti-viral host defense. It is in fact striking to note the frequency and severity of viral infections in the syndrome.

Data obtained by us and others [6] about T-B-macrophage cooperation for in vitro Ig and antibody production are controversial (see Table 2). It is thus still impossible to assume a role for the HLA DR expression deficiency in the in vivo abnormal antibody production and delayed type hypersensitivity.

REFERENCES

1. Schuurman RKB, Van Rood JJ, Vossen JM, Schellekens PT, Feltkamp-Vroom TM, Visser HKA: Hypogammaglobulinemia and HLA gene products. (Abstract) Pediatr Res 12:71, 1978.
2. Schuurman RKB, Van Rood JJ, Vossen JM, Schellekens PT, Feltkamp-Vroom TM, Doyer E, Gmelig-Meyling F, Visser HKA: Failure of lymphocyte-membrane HLA-A and -B expression in two siblings with combined immunodeficiency. Clin Immunol Immunopathol 14:418, 1979.
3. Touraine JL, Bétuel H, Souillet G, Jeune M: Combined immuno-deficiency disease associated with absence of cell surface HLA-A and -B antigens. J Pediatr 93:47, 1978.
4. Griscelli C, Durandy A, Virelizier JL, Hors J, Lepage V, Colombani J: Impaired cell to cell interaction in partial combined immunodeficiency with variable expression of HLA antigens. In Seligmann M, Hitzig WH (eds): "Primary Immunodeficiencies." Amsterdam: Elsevier/North Holland Biomedical Press, 1980, p 499.
5. Griscelli C, Durandy A, Virelizier JL, Grospierre B, Oury C, de Saint-Basile G, Couillin P, Niaudet P, Bétuel H, Hors J, Lepage V, Colombani J: Impaired cell to cell interaction in partial combined immunodeficiency with defective synthesis and membrane expression of HLA antigens. In Touraine JL, Gluckman E, Griscelli C (eds): "Bone Marrow Transplantation in Europe." Amsterdam: Excerpta Medica, 1981, p 194.
6. Kuis W, Roord J, Zegers BJM, Schuurman RKB, Heijnen CJ, Baldwin WM, Goulmy E, Claas F, Van de Griend RJ, Rijkers GT, Van Rood JJ, Vossen JM, Ballieux RE, Stoop JW: Clinical and immunological studies in a patient with the "Bare lymphocyte" syndrome. Ibid, p 201.
7. Lindahl P, Leary P, Gresser I: Enhancement by interferon of the expression of surface antigens on murine leukemia L 1210 cells. Proc Natl Acad Sci USA 70:2785, 1972.
8. Lindahl P, Leary P, Gresser I: Enhancement of the expression of histocompatibility antigens of mouse lymphoid cells by interferon *in vitro*. Eur J Immunol 4:799, 1974.
9. Vignaux F, Gresser I: Differential effects of interferon or the expression H-2K, H-2D and Ia antigens on mouse lymphocytes. J Immunol 118:721, 1977.
10. Durandy A, Fischer A, Griscelli C: Specific in vitro anti-mannan antibody production by human blood lymphocytes. This volume.
11. Callard RE: Specific *in vitro* antibody response to influenza virus by human blood lymphocytes. Nature 282:734–736, 1979.

Defective Expression of Mononuclear Cell Membrane HLA Antigens Associated With Combined Immunodeficiency: Impaired Cellular Interactions*

B.J.M. Zegers, PhD, **C.J. Heijnen,** PhD, **J.J. Roord,** MD, **W. Kuis,** MD, **R.K.B. Schuurman,** MD, **J.W. Stoop,** MD, and **R.E. Ballieux,** PhD

Department of Immunology, University Children's Hospital (B.J.M.Z., C.J.H., J.J.R., W.K., J.W.S.); Department of Clinical Immunology, University Hospital (R.E.B.), Utrecht; Department of Immunohematology, University Hospital, Leiden (R.K.B.S.), The Netherlands

INTRODUCTION

Combined immune deficiency (CID)** associated with defective expression of HLA-A, -B, -C and -β_2m on mononuclear cells was first described by Schuurman et al [1] and Touraine et al [2]. Additional patients have since been found; some of them also showed defective expression of DR antigens [3,4]. The most striking similarity in the patients described concerns the absence of immunologic reactivity toward exogenous antigens [5]. This is not unexpected as it is well established that antigens coded for by genes of the major histocompatibility complex (MHC) play an important role in cellular interactions of T cells, B cells, and macrophages in afferent and efferent phases of the immune response.

We recently described a Dutch infant with CID and defective expression of HLA-A, -B, -C, -DR and -β_2m [4]. It could be shown that interactions between lymphocytes and monocytes in the patient were disturbed, leading to defective helper and suppressor cell functions [4]. Using a cell culture system which allows for the induction and measurement of an antigen-specific PFC response of human peripheral blood lymphocytes in vitro [6], we analyzed in more detail the role of HLA-antigens in the humoral immune response in this child.

CASE REPORT

Patient T.F., a male, was born in 1980 as the first child of healthy consanguineous parents of Dutch origin. From the age of 4 months he suffered from recurrent respiratory tract infections and oral candidiasis. At the age of 6 months, pneumocystis carinii was diagnosed and treated successfully. The absolute number of peripheral blood lymphocytes was normal, as was the T/B ratio (Se$^+$/SIg$^+$). In the serum, only trace amounts of IgG and IgM were present, and IgA was not demonstrable. The bone marrow contained a normal number of Ig-bearing B cells (with a normal distribution of isotypes), but a few IgM-containing plasma cells were present, and IgG and IgA-containing cells were absent. Following immunization, no antibodies against diphtheria toxoid, tetanus toxoid, and poliomyelitis virus were detectable in serum. Lymphocyte proliferative responses to PHA and Con A were variable; proliferative responses to anamnestic antigens like tetanus toxoid and *Candida albicans* were completely negative, as was the delayed type skin reaction to Candida antigen. HLA-typing of peripheral blood mononuclear cells disclosed a lack of HLA-A, -B, -C, -DR and β_2m. It could be concluded that the patient suffered from a CID associated with defective expression of HLA antigens. More detailed clinical and immunologic data, as well as the results of HLA-typing, were published previously [4].

MATERIALS AND METHODS
Antigen-Specific Induction and Enumeration of PFCs

The technique, originally described by Dosch and Gelfand [6], has been used. The methodologic aspects have been extensively reviewed [7]. The antigens used were OA and Se.

Isolation of (Subsets of) Cells From Blood

All methods concerning the isolation of mononuclear cells, the depletion and isolation of macrophages (Mϕ) by adherence to plastic and the isolation, depletion and identification of T and B cells have been described elsewhere [8].

Production of OA-Induced T Helper Factor: ThF120

The method has been published previously [9]. In short, purified T lymphocytes, of normal human adults

---

*This study was supported in part by the Foundation for Medical Research (FUNGO), which is subsidized by the Netherlands Organization for the Advancement of Pure Research (ZWO).

**Abbreviations used in this paper: HLA, Human leukocyte antigen; β_2m, $\beta_2$microglobulin; MHC, Major histocompatibility complex; CID, Combined immunodeficiency; Mϕ, mononuclear phagocytosing cells (monocytes) isolated by adherence to plastic; OA, Ovalbumin; PHA, Phytohemagglutinin; Con A, Concanavalin-A; ThF, T helper factor; Se, Sheep erythrocytes; SIg, Surface immunoglobulin; PFCs, plaque forming cells.

or of Patient T.F., were cultured in the inserts of Marbrook tubes in the presence of 3 μg OA/ml and 5% autologous or allogeneic Mφ of different HLA haplotype. After 96 hours the cells were collected, washed, and cultured for an additional 24 hours in tissue culture tubes with antigen. After this period, the cell-free culture fluid was collected. It contained OA-specific ThF. The biologic properties and mode of action of this factor (after purification) have been reported by Heijnen et al [9]. In this study, the ThF was not further purified, but the cell-free culture fluid was used as a source of the OA-specific helper factor. It will be referred to as ThF120.

Measurement of ThF120 Activity

Isolated B cells, either of normal human adults or of our patient were stimulated in culture with 3 μg OA/ml in the presence of OA-induced T-cell derived helper factor (ThF120) and 5% autologous Mφ or allogeneic Mφ of different HLA haplotypes. After 6 days, the generation of PFCs was measured in the PFC assay as described earlier [6,7].

RESULTS
Macrophage—T-Helper Cell Interaction

It has been reported earlier that in cultures of peripheral blood lymphocytes the activation of T-helper cells by antigen requires the presence of Mφ [7]. The latter cells present antigen, most probably in conjunction with MHC-coded structures, to the T-helper cell. This is reflected in the observation that antigen-pulsed Mφ can adequately stimulate T-helper cells (Heijnen and Ballieux - this volume; Van Tol et al - this volume) and by the fact that antigen-presenting function shows allogeneic restriction. In previous studies we could show that T-helper cells when properly stimulated in vitro for 120 hours with OA in the presence of Mφ, produce antigen-specific helper factor (ThF120) which is secreted in the culture fluid. This factor can substitute for OA-specific T-helper cells in the process of B-cell activation by OA. To identify the allospecificity of the restricting antigen in the interaction of Mφ with T-helper cells, ThF120 was prepared from T-helper cells which were stimulated with OA in the presence of autologous Mφ or Mφ compatible either at the HLA-A-B-C loci or at the HLA-DR locus. The results presented in Figure 1 clearly show that ThF120, and thus T-helper function, is only generated if the antigen-presenting Mφ and the T-helper cells are identical at the

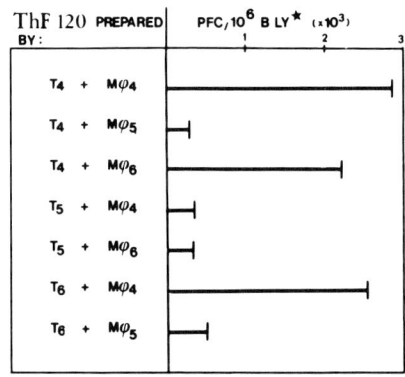

Fig. 1. *B cells from unrelated normal donor were cultured with the various batches of ThF prepared by the cells mentioned above. 4 = normal donor; 5 = normal donor, HLA-A,B,C, = D ≠ to donor 4; 6 = normal donor, HLA-A,B,C ≠ D = to donor 4.

HLA-DR locus (combination 4 and 6). Data obtained by Rees et al [10] (see also Van Tol et al, this volume) establish that DR identity of only one haplotype is sufficient to obtain adequate stimulation of T-helper cells. In analogous studies using isolated T cells and Mφ of our patient, it was found that the child's T cells do not produce functional ThF120 after presentation of the antigen by HLA-DR identical Mφ of a normal donor (Fig. 2, combination T_1 + $M\phi_2$). The results of the reciprocal combination (T_2 + $M\phi_1$) show that the Mφ of our patient are not able to present antigen adequately to HLA-DR identical T-helper cells of a normal donor. In control experiments, the T cells of this donor 2 respond normally to stimulation with OA presented by Mφ of donor 3 identical at the HLA-DR locus.

Macrophage—B-Cell Interaction

Heijnen et al [9] recently found that purified human peripheral blood B cells can be stimulated in culture with antigen to develop into PFCs, provided antigen-specific ThF120 and Mφ are present. It was reported by these authors that ThF120 is not genetically restricted in its action, but that for successful activation of B cells the Mφ had to be HLA-identical. To analyze which loci of the MHC complex code for the restricting alloantigen in the B cell - Mφ interaction, B lymphocytes were

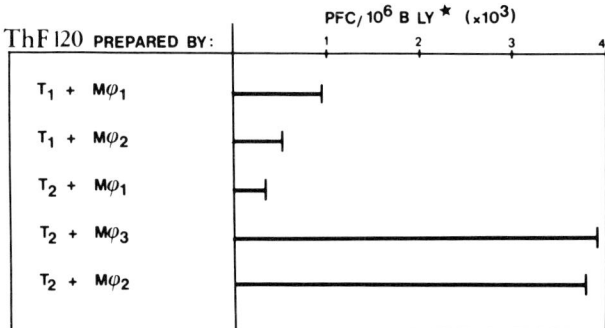

Fig. 2. *B cells from an unrelated normal donor were cultured with the various batches of ThF prepared by the cells mentioned above. 1 = to Patient T.F.; 2 = normal donor, HLA-A,B,C ≠ D = to Patient T.F.; 3 = normal donor, HLA-A,B,C ≠ D = to Patient T.F.

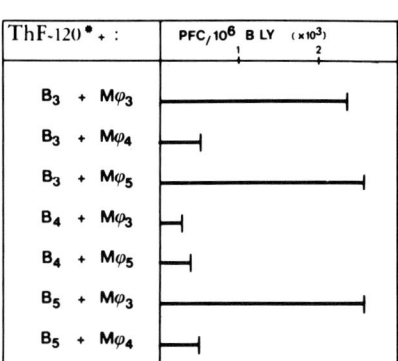

Fig. 3. *ThF120, prepared from the cells of a nonrelated normal donor, was cultured with the various B cells and Mφ mentioned above. 3 = normal donor; 4 = normal donor, HLA-A,B,C= D≠ to donor 3; 5 = normal donor, HLA-A,B,C≠ D= to donor 3.

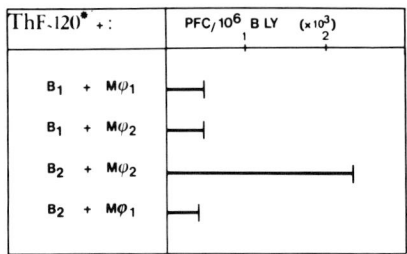

Fig. 4. *ThF120, prepared from the cells of a nonrelated normal donor, was cultured with the various B cells and Mφ mentioned above. 1 = *Patient T.F.*; 2 = HLA-A,B,C≠ D=.

stimulated with OA in the presence of ThF120 and Mφ in various allogeneic combinations. The results shown in Figure 3 establish that identity at the HLA-DR locus (combination 3 and 5) is required for effective B-cell activation. These studies were extended using purified B cells and Mφ of *Patient T.F.* It can be seen in Figure 4 (combination B1 + Mφ2) that the lack of HLA-DR antigen at the B-cell surface apparently interferes with effective presentation of antigen and/or ThF120 by normal, DR-identical Mφ. From the results in the reciprocal situation (B2 + Mφ1) it is clear that the absence of HLA-DR antigens at the surface of Mφ of *Patient T.F.* prevents effective presentation of antigen and/or ThF120 to the B cells of a normal DR-identical donor 2.

DISCUSSION

The present study was undertaken to analyze in more detail the role of HLA antigens in cellular interactions which take place in a humoral immune response. It is accepted nowadays that T-cell activation involves recognition by T cells of class I or class II type HLA molecules [11]. Stimulation of $T4^+$ helper lymphocytes by antigen, presented by Mφ is linked to recognition of class II (HLA-DR) molecules on the antigen-presenting cell [11]. The absence of HLA antigens at the surface of the Mφ of our patient coincides with the inability of the Mφ to present OA adequately to HLA-DR identical T-helper cells of normal adult donors (Fig. 2). In addition, however, the experiment of nature which we could study allowed us to observe another aspect, ie the presumed absence of HLA-antigens of T-helper cells coincides with the failure of the T cells to exert antigen-specific helper function after proper stimulation with antigen in the presence of normal HLA-DR identical Mφ. This observation may indicate that T cells lacking HLA-DR antigens cannot be stimulated by antigen even if the antigen-presenting cell carries the relevant HLA-DR antigen. This would imply that for effective interaction between T-helper cells and antigen-presenting cells and/or recognition and binding of antigen the concomitant presence of identical HLA-DR structures at the cell surfaces of both cell types is required [11,12]. In addition, the absence of measureable T-helper activity might also be brought on by the absence of HLA-DR or Ia-like structures in the antigen-specific helper factor which mediates helper function. As reported earlier [13,14], human antigen-specific T-cell derived helper factors do contain Ia-like moieties which may dictate the effective interaction with Mφ and/or B cells. The absence of such a stretch in the helper factor may lead either to a defective function or may even prevent the production and/or secretion of such factor.

A second aspect concerning the role of HLA-DR antigens in cellular interactions is shown by the data given in Figures 3 and 4. These results clearly establish that B cells lacking HLA-DR antigens at their cell surface cannot be activated by antigen presented in concert with antigen-specific ThF by adherent cells which are histocompatible at the HLA-DR locus and do carry the corresponding DR-alloantigen at the cell surface. In addition, B lymphocytes which carry a given HLA-DR alloantigen at their cell surface cannot be activated by antigen, presented in concert with antigen-specific ThF by adherent cells which are potentially histocompatible at the HLA-DR locus but lack the corresponding DR-alloantigen at the cell surface. It can be concluded, therefore, that the activation of B lymphocytes in vitro by antigen in concert with antigen-specific ThF requires not only the presence of adherent cells in the culture but also the concomitant presence of compatible HLA-DR structures at the surfaces of both cell types. The study of this "experiment of nature" confirms that the expression of the DR-alloantigens on the cell surface is a prerequisite for cells of the immune system to interact. The mechanisms involved, however, are not yet fully understood. We assume that it not only involves antigen-presentation and recognition, but also the production and processing of regulatory factors.

REFERENCES

1. Schuurman RKB, van Rood JJ, Vossen JM, Schellekens P, Feltkamp-Vroom Th, Doyer ThM, Gmelig-Meyling F, Visser HKA: Failure of lymphocyte-membrane HLA-A and B expression in two siblings

1. with combined immunodeficiency. Clin Immunol Immunopathol 14:418–434, 1979.
2. Touraine JL, Betuel H, Souillet G, Jeune M: Combined immunodeficiency disease associated with absence of cell-surface HLA-A and B antigens. J Pediatr 93:47–51, 1978.
3. Griscelli C, Durandy A, Virelizier JL, Hors J, Lepage V, Colombani J: Impaired cell to cell interaction in partial combined immunodeficiency with variable expression of HLA-antigens. In Seligmann M, Hitzig WH (eds): "Primary Immunodeficiencies." Amsterdam: Elsevier, 1980, pp 499–504.
4. Kuis W, Roord JJ, Zegers BJM, Schuurman RKB, Heijnen CJ, Baldwin WM, Goulmy E, Claas F, van de Griend RJ, Rijkers GT, van Rood JJ, Vossen JM, Ballieux RE, Stoop JW: Clinical and immunological studies in a patient with the "bare lymphocyte" syndrome. In "Bone Marrow Transplantation in Europe." Amsterdam: Excerpta Medica, 1981, vol 2, pp 201–208.
5. Touraine JL: The bare lymphocyte syndrome: Report on the registry. Lancet 1:319–320, 1981.
6. Dosch HM, Gelfand EW: In vitro induction of hemolytic plaque forming cells (PFC) in man. J Immunol Methods 11:107–113, 1976.
7. Ballieux RE, Heijnen CJ, UytdeHaag F, Zegers BJM: Regulation of B cell activity in man: Role of T cells. Immunol Rev 45:3–39, 1979.
8. Heijnen CJ, UytdeHaag F, Gmelig-Meyling FHJ, Ballieux RE: Localization of human antigen-specific helper and suppressor function in distinct T cell populations. Cell Immunol 43:282–292, 1979.
9. Heijnen CJ, UytdeHaag F, Pot KH, Ballieux RE: Antigen specific human T cell factors. I. T cell helper factor: Biologic properties. J Immunol 126:497–502, 1981.
10. Rees A, Feldmann M, Woody JN, Erb P: Genetics of human T cell monocyte interaction in helper cell induction. Clin Exp Immunol 44:445–452, 1981.
11. Engleman EG, Benike CJ, Grumet C, Evans RL: Activation of human T lymphocyte subsets: Helper and suppressor/cytotoxic T cells recognize and respond to distinct histocompatibility antigens. J Immunol 127:2124–2129, 1981.
12. Lonai P, Steinman L: Physiological regulation of antigen-binding to T cells: Role of a soluble macrophage factor and of interferon. Proc Natl Acad Sci USA 74:5662–5666, 1977.
13. Feldmann M, Kontiainen S: The role of antigen-specific T cell factors in the immune response. In Pick E, Landy M (eds): "Lymphokines." New York: Academic Press, 1981, vol 2, pp 87–123.
14. Heijnen CJ, UytdeHaag F, Pot KH, Bentwich Z, Ballieux RE: Antigen-specific human T cell factors. III. T cell helper and suppressor factors: Immunochemical aspects. Ann Immunol (Paris) 133D:221–234, 1982.

GPL-115 Deficiency: A New Class of Immunodeficiencies*

Robertson Parkman, MD, Eileen Remold-O'Donnell, PhD,
Dianne M. Kenney, PhD, and Fred S. Rosen, MD

Divisions of Immunology and Hematology-Oncology, Children's Hospital Medical Center, Division of Pediatric Oncology, Sidney Farber Cancer Institute (R.P.), Center for Blood Research (E.R.-O., D.M.K.), and Division of Immunology, Children's Hospital Medical Center (F.S.R.), Boston, MA 02115

T-lymphocyte immunodeficiencies can be classified as diseases due to intrinsic metabolic defects (adenosine deaminase (ADA) deficiency, nucleoside phosphorylase (NP) deficiency, etc) or to the absence of thymus-derived differentiating hormones (DiGeorge syndrome) [1,2]. We report here T-lymphocyte immunodeficiencies due to abnormalities of a lymphocyte glycoprotein, GPL-115. GPL-115 deficiency may represent the first of a new class of immunodeficiency (ID) diseases due to membrane glycoprotein abnormalities. Defects in membrane glycoproteins may be the basis for multisystem ID diseases such as the Wiskott-Aldrich syndrome (WAS), ataxia telangiectasia (AT), etc which involve both lymphoid and nonlymphoid cells.

Following the initial observation of Lum et al [3] that the size and function of platelets from WAS patients normalized following splenectomy, we investigated the effect of splenectomy on the size of lymphocytes from WAS patients. Lymphocytes from 3 of 6 WAS patients had a markedly reduced cell volume (approximately 50% that of normal peripheral blood lymphocytes (PBL)). The lymphocyte volume of 2 patients normalized following splenectomy, suggesting that the reduced lymphocyte volume as well as the reduced platelet size were secondary rather than primary abnormalities of WAS. Previous investigators had not proposed a common defect for both the platelets and lymphocytes in WAS; we hypothesize that a membrane glycoprotein abnormality, which increased the sensitivity of both WAS lymphocytes and platelets to splenic action, might produce platelets and lymphocytes with reduced size.

To test this hypothesis, platelets and PBL from WAS patients were radioiodolabeled, and their membrane proteins analyzed by autoradiography following SDS gel electrophoresis. Gels of WAS peripheral blood lymphocytes showed the absence of 115,000 MW glycoprotein (GPL-115) found in all normals (Fig. 1) [4]. The absence of GPL-115 was not due to the effect of the spleen since GPL-115 was absent from WAS lymphocytes both before and after splenectomy. Characterization of the lectin-binding properties of GPL-115 demonstrated that it bound to wheat germ but not lentil lectin, suggesting that it was a glycoprotein with an O-sugar linkage [5].

EBV-transformed B-cell lines were established from 3 WAS patients. These cell lines permitted us to determine the GPL-115 content of isolated B cells. Surface iodination and SDS-gel analysis demonstrated GPL-115 heterogeneity in the B-lymphoblast lines. The lymphoblasts from one patient had markedly reduced levels of GPL-115, while those from 2 other patients had relatively normal GPL-115 levels as compared to B lymphoblasts from normal individuals. These results suggest that the expression of GPL-115 is heterogeneous at the B-lymphocyte level in WAS patients, and that the GPL-115 deficiency in WAS is more severe in T lymphocytes than in B lymphocytes.

Two-dimensional electrophoresis of the surface radioiodolabeled proteins of WAS platelets revealed reduced glycoprotein 1a and 1b levels with restricted heterogeneity [6]. The platelet glycoprotein abnormalities were not secondary to the action of the spleen since equivalent abnormalities were seen in platelets from both splenectomized and nonsplenectomized WAS patients. Further, the infusion of normal platelets into a WAS patient, followed by their in vitro isolation and labeling 24 hours later, showed a normal surface labeling pattern.

These results suggest that membrane glycoprotein abnormalities may exist in both the T and B lymphocytes and the platelets of WAS patients. The GPL-115 deficiency appears to be most severe in the T lymphocytes and platelets of WAS patients, and less severe in the B lymphocytes; these findings are constant with the allelic exclusion studies of Harley et al [7] which demonstrated that T lymphocytes and platelets were invariably involved in WAS, while B lymphocytes were occasionally involved. It is possible that either GPL-115 and glycoprotein 1a-1b represent the expression of the same genetic information on different cell types or that a common enzyme is necessary for the post-

*Supported by USPHS grants RR-128, HL-24311, CA-13472, CA-29328, and CA-21225.

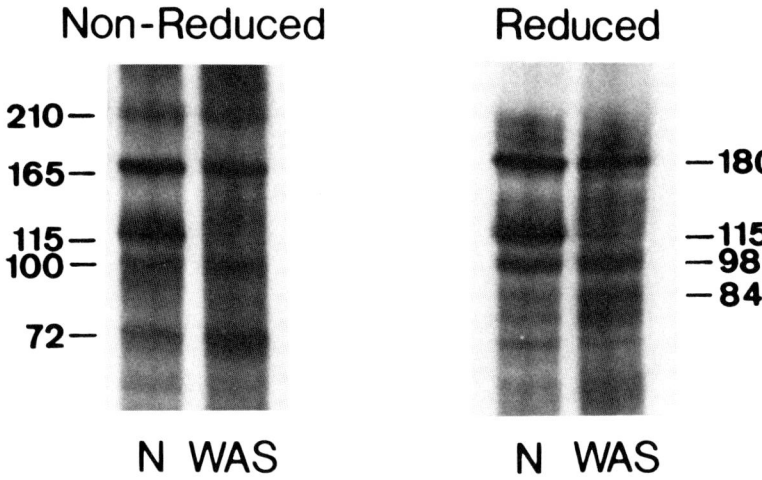

Fig. 1. Gel electrophoresis of ^{125}I labeled membranes from Normal (N) and Wiskott-Aldrich Syndrome (WAS) lymphocytes.

translational modification of both GPL-115 and glycoprotein 1a-1b.

Studies of 2 other families have suggested that GPL-115 deficiency is not invariably associated with abnormalities in platelet glycoproteins and function. In the first family, an X-linked recessive pattern of cellular ID was observed with no history of eczema or bleeding disorders. The patient was first determined to have a T-lymphocyte deficiency by Drs. Ammann and Cowan of the University of California, San Francisco. Our analysis of the patient's peripheral lymphocytes revealed no blastogenic response to mitogens or antigens, a reduced lymphocyte volume, and an absence of GPL-115. Two HLA-identical brothers had normal lymphocyte function, normal lymphocyte volume, and detectable GPL-115. The patients' platelets were normal in size, had normal glycoprotein 1a-1b content, and had normal in vitro aggregation. A second family was studied in which one child had multiple granulomas and recurrent fevers. Analysis of his PBL showed no blastogenic response to antigens, a reduced lymphocyte volume, and absence of GPL-115. His platelets had normal size, normal glycoprotein 1a-1b content, and normal in vitro aggregation. Of interest, the patient had a paternal uncle with acquired agammaglobulinemia whose peripheral lymphocytes had reduced levels of GPL-115. In these 2 families there is a clear disassociation between the lymphocyte and the platelet glycoprotein abnormalities, which suggests that the GPL-115 and glycoprotein 1a-1b abnormalities found in the WAS syndrome may be due to separate defects, or that the expression of a single primary defect is variable; those individuals with the mildest form of deficiency may have abnormalities only in their T lymphocytes, while individuals with the more severe form have abnormalities of their platelets and B lymphocytes. ADA deficiency is an example of an enzyme deficiency in which variable expression (ie variable ID) is seen.

Monoclonal and heteroantibodies to GPL-115 are presently being produced which will allow the more precise quantitation of GPL-115 and widespread patient screening. These antibodies may also allow us to determine whether GPL-115 is involved in specific T-lymphocyte functions. Since WAS patients have specific immunologic defects, including eczema, and an ability to produce antibodies to carbohydrate antigens, it may be possible to produce similar defects in vitro by incubating normal PBLs with anti-GPL-115 antibodies. The in vitro production of such abnormalities would permit the study of the relationship between lymphocyte membrane structure and function at a molecular level.

REFERENCES

1. Hirschhorn R: Defects of purine metabolism in immunodeficiency diseases. In Schwartz RS (ed): "Progress in Clinical Immunology." New York: Grune and Stratton, 1977, p 67.
2. August CS, Rosen FS, Filler RM, Janeway CA, Markowski B, Kay HEM: Implantation of a fetal thymus, restoring immunological competence in a patient

with thymic aplasia (DiGeorge's syndrome) Lancet 2:1210, 1968.
3. Lum LG, Tubergen DG, Corash L, Blaese RM: Splenectomy in the management of the thrombocytopenia of the Wiskott-Aldrich syndrome. N Engl J Med 302:892, 1980.
4. Parkman R, Remold-O'Donnell E, Kenney DM, Perrine S, Rosen FS: Surface protein abnormalities in lymphocytes and platelets from patients with Wiskott-Aldrich syndrome. Lancet 2:1387, 1981.
5. Brown WRA, Barclay AN, Sunderland CA, Williams AF: Identification of a glycophorin-like molecule at the cell surface of rat thymocytes. Nature 289:456, 1981.
6. Phillips DR: Surface labeling as a tool to determine structure-function relationships of platelet plasma membrane glycoproteins. Thromb Haemost 42:1638, 1979.
7. Harley W, Gealy WJ, Dwyer JM: Heterogeneity of allelic exclusion in Wiskott-Aldrich syndrome carriers. (Abstract) Pediatr Res 15:923, 1981.

Severe Combined Immunodeficiency (SCID) With Natural Killer (NK) Cell Predominance*

Rebecca H. Buckley, MD, Sherrie Gard, BS, Barton F. Haynes, MD, Lawrence J. Sindel, MD, Kathryn Davis, BS, Hugh A. Sampson, MD, Michael E. Ruff, MD, and Hillel S. Koren, PhD

Departments of Pediatrics, Medicine, and Microbiology and Immunology, Duke University School of Medicine, Durham, NC 27710

INTRODUCTION

Despite roughly similar clinical characteristics and functional immunologic capacities of patients with SCID, there is considerable cellular and biochemical heterogeneity within this syndrome [1,2]. Some patients have low numbers of lymphocytes bearing differentiation markers of either T- or B-cell lineage, whereas others have elevated numbers of B cells, and occasionally normal numbers of both T and B cells have been found [1]. Some, but not all, infants inheriting this syndrome in an autosomal recessive mode have been found to have a marked deficiency of the purine salvage pathway enzyme, ADA [2]. Although evidence of lymphoid cell function is generally lacking in all, including the capacities for antibody-dependent cell-mediated cytotoxicity (ADCC) and natural killing (NK) [1,3–6], Lopez et al [7] reported the detection of NK activity against herpes simplex type I (HSV-1)-infected fibroblasts in 2 infants with SCID. Prior to the studies reported here, efforts by us [4] and others [5,6] to detect NK activity against the widely used human erythromyeloid cell line, K562, have been unsuccessful. Thus, the finding of exceedingly high NK activity against this target by monocyte-depleted lymphocytes from 2 infants with SCID lacking other evidence of lymphoid cell function was unexpected. Additionally, a majority of the lymphocytes in these patients had the morphologic and phenotypic characteristics of NK cells, ie they were large granular lymphocytes (LGLs) which reacted with monoclonal antibodies to human lymphocyte membrane antigens in a pattern similar to those of NK cells [8]. These observations add yet another dimension of heterogeneity within the syndrome of SCID and offer additional information possibly relevant to NK cell lineage.

PATIENTS AND METHODS

Two female infants, one of Brazilian and the other of Iranian descent, presented to Duke University Medical Center at 3½ months and 11 days of age, respectively. The diagnosis of SCID was sought and established in the first because of an unusual oropharyngeal lesion and persistent diarrhea, and in the second because of a brother with this defect. Both infants were lymphopenic (Table 1) and had low serum Ig concentrations (*Patient #1:* IgG 185, IgA 12, IgM 3 mg/dl; *Patient #2:* IgG 690, IgA 0, IgM 10.5 mg/dl and no detectable antibodies. *Patient #1* had no detectable SIg+ B lymphocytes, whereas *Patient #2* had 33% SIg+ lymphocytes. The percentage of sheep erythrocyte-rosetting cells (E-RFC) was low in both (Table 1), and there was no response by either patient's lymphocytes to stimulation with a range of concentrations of the mitogens phytohemagglutinin (PHA), concanavalin A (Con A), pokeweed mitogen (PWM) and allogeneic cells. Erythrocytes from both infants contained normal amounts of adenosine deaminase (ADA) and nucleoside phosphorylase (NP) activity. *Patient #1* underwent bone marrow cell transplantation from her HLA-identical brother at 3½ months of age and is now fully engrafted, with normal T- and B-lymphocyte function and an XY lymphocyte karyotype. *Patient #2* underwent lectin-separated bone marrow cell transplantation [9] from her haplo-identical father at 3 weeks of age and is slowly manifesting evidence of both T- and B-cell function, with Y-body positive cells detected by quinacrine staining one month following transplantation.

Lymphocyte subpopulation enumeration and stimulation studies were carried out as previously described [1,10]. Cytofluorographic analysis of lymphoid cell populations was done on an Ortho Cytofluorograf System 50-H, using mouse monoclonal antibodies to human cell surface antigens [11] and affinity-purified, fluoresceinated goat anti-mouse IgG (Tago, Inc, Burlingame, CA). NK activity was assayed on blood mononuclear cells isolated by Ficoll-Hypaque separation and used as effectors against ^{51}Cr-labeled K562 cells [12]. In some experiments, effector cells adjusted to 1×10^6/ml in minimum essential medium (MEM) supplemented with 10% fetal calf serum (MEM-FCS 10)

*Supported by Grant #1 R01 AI18613 from NIAID and by a grant from the General Clinical Research Centers Program (RR-30).

TABLE 1. Comparison of Lymphocyte Phenotypes and Function of Two SCID Patients With Those of Normal LGLs

	Patient #1	Patient #2	Normal LGLs*
Abs. Lymph. Ct/mm^3	1005	1224	—
% LGL	71	52	85–95
Response to:			
Mitogens	0	0	?
Allogeneic cells	0	0	?
NK activity**	78.4	71.6	40–70
% of Total Lymphocytes Positive for:			
SIg	0	33	0
E-RFC	30	30	50–60
OKT3	7.9	10.4	0–17
3A1	35.6	20.4	40–47
OKT4	5.0	13.4	2–9
OKT8	19.4	21.9	19–23
OKT10	94.0	—	85–95
VEP10	93.4	78.4	85–95
OKI1	6.0	—	5–10
5E9	0	0	0

*Highly enriched by gradient isolation.
**% specific lysis of K562 in 2-hour assay @ 20:1 E:T.

were depleted of monocytes by allowing them to adhere for 1 hour at 37°C to plastic and of B cells by incubation on anti-F(ab)'2 plates before the assay. The B-cell depleted, plastic-nonadherent cells, which contained 1–2% latex-positive cells, were used as effectors. The assay was carried out in triplicate with a total volume of 0.2 ml/well in MEM-FCS 10 at effector to target cell ratios ranging from 2.5:1 to 40:1 with 1 × 10^4 targets/well, in round-bottomed microtiter plates (1S-MRC-96, Linbro Chemical Co, Inc) for 120 minutes in a 37°C humidified incubator with 7% Co_2.

RESULTS

Table 1 presents the results of lymphocyte phenotyping by AET-E-RFC, membrane immunofluorescence for surface Ig (SIg), and cytofluorography with monoclonal antibodies in the 2 SCID patients. The findings are compared with those from studies of normal LGL(s) highly enriched by density gradient isolation [8]. It can be seen that both patients had lymphocytes which formed rosettes with SE(s), though the percentages (30 for each) were lower than in normals (75.9 ± 5.4). In contrast, the percentages of lymphocytes reacting with the pan-T reagent (OKT3) were much lower, only one-third or less of the values for the E-RFC percentages. A second puzzling observation was the finding of percentages of cells reacting with the OKT8 reagent which were double the values for the OKT-3-positive cells. Since LGL(s) are known to rosette with SE(s) and bear T8 antigen (approximately 19–23%) yet have much lower reactivity with OKT3 (0–17%), this raised the possibility that the E-rosette-positive, T3-negative cells detected in these patients might be NK cells. Subsequent cytofluorographic studies of these infants' B-cell and monocyte-depleted lymphocytes with the monoclonal antibodies OKT10 and VEP10 [13] demonstrated a high degree of reactivity with both reagents (Table 1), substantiating the notion that these cells were NK-like. To explore the possibility that the high percentages of T10-positive cells were not due to activated lymphoid cells in these patients, we tested aliquots of the same cell suspensions with a monoclonal antibody recognizing the transferrin receptor (5E9), known to be an activation antigen [11], and with OKI1, which reacts with Ia-positive cells. As shown in Table 1, there were no 5E9 positive cells in either patient, and Patient #1's cells showed low reactivity (6%) with OKI1. Moreover, the level of NK reactivity of lymphoid cells from both patients was exceedingly high, causing 78.4 and 71.6% specific lysis of K562, respectively, in a 2-hour assay at an E:T ratio of 20:1 (enriched normal LGL(s) give only 40–70% specific lysis). As seen in Table 2, the pretransplant NK activities of both Patients #1 and 2 were higher at all E:T ratios than for the corresponding means for normal unfractionated lymphocytes. This activity has declined in Patient #1 following BMT and correlates with a decline in the number of T10 reactive cells (Fig. 1). In keeping with all of these observations was the finding that a majority of lymphocytes in both patients (71 and 52%, respectively) had the morphologic appearance of LGL(s), by the criteria of azurophilic granules, cell size, monocytoid nucleus, ratio of cytoplasm to nucleus, and myeloperoxidase negativity. ADCC activity was normal in both infants but only approximately half as great as the NK activity for both.

DISCUSSION

The finding of a majority of lymphocytes with NK phenotype and function in these 2 infants with SCID was novel and surprising, since our previous studies of NK activity against the K562 target in a variety of forms of primary ID had revealed SCID to be the only defect studied in which NK activity was totally lacking. This finding was confirmed by others [5,6], although NK activity against a different type of target (HSV-1 infected fibroblasts) had been observed in 2 patients with SCID by Lopez and his colleagues [7]. Indeed, of the many types of ID studied for NK activity by several groups of investigators [4–7, 14–16], this func-

TABLE 2. NK Cell Activity in 2 Patients With SCID

	% Specific Lysis (SEM) of K562				
	Patient #1			Patient #2	
E/T Ratio	(Pre-BMT)	(1 month Post-BMT)	(6 weeks Post-BMT)	(Pre-BMT)	Normal Mean ± SD
40:1	79.3 ± 4.2	—	—	—	—
20:1	78.4 ± 6.3	—	57.4 ± 2.0	71.6 ± 2.5	41.4 ± 6.4
10:1	57.3 ± 3.7	60.6 ± 1.8	44.7 ± 3.0	63.5 ± 2.5	20.7 ± 3.2
5:1	49.8 ± 4.8	53.0 ± 1.8	38.3 ± 2.0	53.7 ± 2.5	10.4 ± 1.6
2.5:1	33.0 ± 2.3	37.6 ± 2.5	—	—	—
1.2:1	26.7 ± 3.0	—	—	—	—

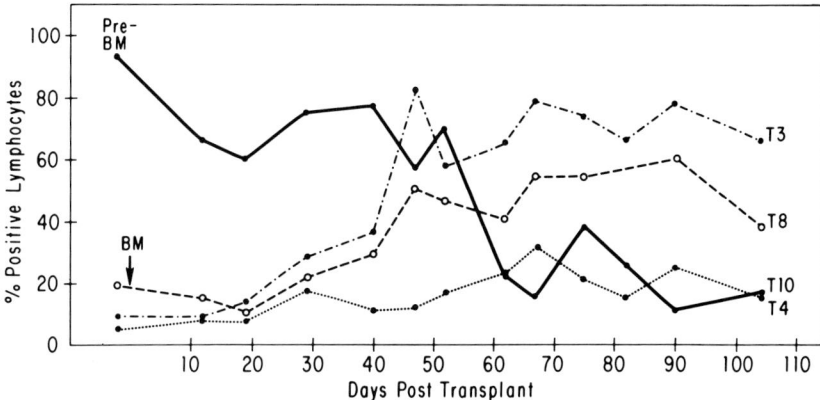

Fig. 1. Results of cytofluorographic analyses of lymphoid cells from *Patient #1* prior to and at various times subsequent to matched sib BMT. As donor cells engrafted, the very abnormally high percentage of T10 positive cells declined markedly and at present is only slightly above the normal range of 8–10%.

tion has usually been found normal in all but SCID [4–6], the Chédiak-Higashi syndrome [5,15], and X-linked lymphoproliferative disease [16]. The fact that NK function is preserved in many patients with profound T- and B-cell dysfunction suggests that NK may represent a more primitive form of host defense. The development of this function is clearly not a late event in normal human ontogeny, as it has been shown to be present in cord blood lymphocytes of full-term neonates, although at a slightly lower level than in adults [17].

The phenotype of SCID represented by these 2 infants should be suspected in patients who have much higher percentages of lymphocytes rosetting with AET or neuraminidase-treated SRBC(s) than reacting with the pan-T cell monoclonal antibody T3. This is particularly true when the percentage of cells reacting with the T8 monoclonal antibody exceeds the percentages of T3 and T4 positive cells. Highly enriched LGL(s) have been shown to have membrane receptors for SRBC, as detected by monoclonal antibodies to the E-R receptor [8]; since they are of low affinity, they are more likely to bind to modified SRBC. Similarly, higher percentages of LGL(s) have been shown to react with the T8 than with the T3 or T4 monoclonals (Table 1). Finally, the finding of a very high percentage of cells reacting with the monoclonal antibodies T10 and VEP10, and very low percentages reacting with monoclonal antibodies to the transferrin receptor (5E9, T9) and Ia (I1) is in agreement with the phenotypic characteristics of LGL(s). Low reactivity with the latter reagents is particularly important, since antigens recognized by 5E9, T9, T10, and Ia are found on rapidly dividing or activated cells of a variety of lineages [11], whereas NK cells are VEP10+ and T10+, but 5E9, T9 and Ia are negative [8]. T10 positivity alone is not sufficient to indicate that NK activity is present, as recently demonstrated by another SCID patient evaluated at this institution whose lymphocytes lacked NK activity but were both 88% T10 positive and 91% Ia positive. The finding of an increased percentage of T10 reactive lymphocytes in SCID patients had been noted previously by Vossen et al [6] and by Reinherz et al [18], who found 30% and 30–60% T10 positive lymphocytes in 1 and 4 SCID patients, respectively (normal 8–10%). However, NK activity was profoundly depressed in Vossen et al's [6] patient (T9 and Ia were not tested), and NK was not evaluated in the 4 patients of Reinherz et al [18], 2 of whose lymphocytes were also T9 positive.

Studies of NK activity in patients with primary IDs were undertaken initially to 1) clarify the role of NK in immunologic surveillance against microorganisms and neoplastic growth, and 2) gain information that might be relevant to NK cell lineage. Since SCID patients with high numbers of B cells and low numbers of T cells have had low or absent NK function [4–6], and boys with SLA who lack circulating SIg+ B cells have had normal NK function [4–6], it is generally accepted that NK cells are not of B-lymphocyte lineage. The absence or depression of NK activity in SCID, the most severely T-cell deficient of all IDs, was taken as evidence supporting a T-cell lineage for NK. However, the finding of NK function in DiGeorge syndrome [6], and in both of the present SCID cases, and in those of Lopez et al [7], argues in favor of either a separate lineage of NK from that of T cells or that NK cells may represent a very immature form of T cells. From our own observations, we have noted that NK function was lacking in 4 SCID patients who had very few E-RFC but was present in 3 SCID patients who had 30-40% E-RFC, despite complete lack of proliferative responses to T-cell mitogens in all patients. It will be of great interest to determine whether cells from SCID patients with NK cell predominance, such as the 2 in this report, can be induced by thymic hormones, lymphokines, or monokines to acquire surface markers or functions characteristic of mature T cells. Finally, the fact that lymphoid cells from both of the patients reported here evidenced both vigorous ADCC and NK gives added support to the view that both functions are mediated by the same cell [19].

REFERENCES

1. Buckley RH, Gilbertsen RB, Schiff RI, Ferreira E, Sanal SO, Waldmann TA: Heterogeneity of lymphocyte subpopulations in severe combined immunodeficiency: Evidence against a stem cell defect. J Clin Invest 58:130–136, 1976.
2. Hirschhorn R: Defects of purine metabolism in immunodeficiency diseases. Prog Clin Immunol 3:67–83, 1977.
3. Sanal SO, Buckley RH: Antibody-dependent cellular cytotoxicity in primary immunodeficiency diseases and with different normal leukocyte subpopulations: Importance of the type of target. J Clin Invest 61:1–10, 1978.
4. Koren HS, Amos DB, Buckley RH: Natural killing in immunodeficient patients. J Immunol 120:796–799, 1978.
5. Lipinski M, Virelizier J-L, Tursz T, Griscelli C: Natural killer and killer cell activities in patients with primary immunodeficiencies or defects in immune interferon production. Eur J Immunol 10:246–249, 1980.
6. Vossen JM, Astaldi A, van de Griend RJ, Dooren LJ: T cell subsets identified by monoclonal antibodies during immune reconstitution of a patient with severe combined immunodeficiency and a patient with DiGeorge's syndrome. In Touraine JL, Gluckman E, Griscelli C (eds): "Bone Marrow Transplantation in Europe. II." Amsterdam-Oxford-Princeton: Excerpta Medica, 1981, pp 218–226.
7. Lopez C, Kirkpatrick D, Sorell M, O'Reilly RJ: Association between pretransplant natural kill and graft-versus-host disease after stem-cell transplantation. Lancet 2:1103–1106, 1979.
8. Timonen T, Ortaldo JR, Herberman RB: Characteristics of human large granular lymphocytes and relationship to natural killer cells. J Exp Med 153:569, 1981.
9. Reisner Y, Kapoor N, O'Reilly RJ, Good RA: Allogeneic bone marrow transplantation using stem cells fractionated by lectins: VI. In vitro analysis of human and monkey bone marrow cells fractionated by sheep red blood cells and soybean agglutinin. Lancet 2:1320–1324, 1980.
10. Schiff RI, Buckley RH, Gilbertsen RB, Metzgar RS: Membrane receptors and *in vitro* lymphocyte responsiveness in immunodeficiency. J Immunol 112:376–386, 1974.
11. Haynes BF: Human T lymphocyte antigens as defined by monoclonal antibodies. Immunol Res 57:127–161, 1981.
12. Klein E, Ben-Bassat H, Newmann H: Properties of the K562 cell line, derived from a patient with chronic myeloid leukemia. Int J Cancer 18:421, 1976.
13. Rumpold H, Obexer G, Kraft D: Analysis of human NK cells by monoclonal antibodies against myelomonocytic and lymphocytic antigens. In Herberman RB (ed): "Natural Cell-Mediated Immunity." New York: Academic Press, 1982, vol II.
14. Pross HF, Gupta S, Good RA, Baines MG: Spontaneous human lymphocyte-mediated cytotoxicity against tumor target cells. VII. The effect of immunodeficiency disease. Cell Immunol 43:160–175, 1979.
15. Haliotis T, Roder J, Klein M, Ortaldo J, Fauci AS, Herberman RB: Chédiak-Higashi gene in humans. I. Impairment of natural killer function. J Exp Med 151:1039–1048, 1980.
16. Sullivan JL, Byron KS, Brewster FE, Purtilo DT: Deficient natural killer cell activity in X-linked lymphoproliferative syndrome. Science 210:543–545, 1980.
17. Uksila J, Lassila O, Hirvonen T: Natural killer cell function of human neonatal lymphocytes. Clin Exp Immunol 48:649–654, 1982.
18. Reinherz EL, Cooper MD, Schlossman SF, Rosen FS: Abnormalities of T cell maturation and regulation in human beings with immunodeficiency disorders. J Clin Invest 68:699–705, 1981.
19. Jensen PJ, Koren HS: Heterogeneity with the population of NK and K cells. J Immunol 124:395, 1980.

Selective Deficiency of OKT4+ Lymphocytes in a Child With Combined Immunodeficiency

Marzia Duse, MD, Rita Maccario, PhD, Luigi Nespoli, MD,
Alessandro Plebani, PhD, and Alberto G. Ugazio, MD

Department of Pediatrics, University of Pavia, 27100 Pavia, Italy

T lymphocytes expressing the OKT4 antigen (OKT4+) have been shown to provide helper function both for effector T lymphocytes and for antibody-producing B cells [1-3]. Lack of the OKT4+ subset has been described in some patients with acquired agammaglobulinemia [4]. Recently, Reinherz et al [5] reported a child with CID and loss of OKT4+ T-cell function. We report here a child with recurrent sinopulmonary and gastrointestinal infections and defective antibody- and T-cell mediated immunity associated with a low number of OKT4+ cells.

CASE REPORT

The child was born in May 1971; he has one healthy older brother. In April 1972, the first of many episodes of pneumonia and diarrhea occurred. In July 1975, he was hospitalized for pneumonia complicating measles. Mediastinal lymphadenopathy was seen by chest x ray and sarcoidosis was suspected; the patient was treated with corticosteroids and anti-tubercular therapy for a year. Despite therapy, the lymph node enlargement showed no improvement and hepatosplenomegaly became evident. In February 1977, the child was admitted to our department for the first time for pneumonia and persistent diffuse lymphoadenopathy and hepatosplenomegaly. The patient was in the 10th% for height and weight. On physical examination all superficial lymph nodes were enlarged: the liver was palpable 3 cm below the right costal margin, and the spleen 4 cm below the left costal margin. Chest x ray showed enlargement of the superior mediastinal nodes; the upper right lobe was hypotransparent. Routine hematochemical tests were normal, including RBC, WBC, and ESR. Open liver and spleen biopsies showed nonspecific inflammatory changes, and lung biopsy revealed bronchiectasis. Bone marrow smear was normal. Lymph node biopsy performed 7 days after stimulation with tetanus toxoid (TT) showed marked hypoplasia of the paracortical areas. Red cell adenosine deaminase (ADA) and nucleoside phosphorylase (NP) activity was normal, as were all tests of PMN and complement function. ANF were negative. The immunologic data are summarized in Table 1.

The patient was started on gamma globulin replacement (0.8 ml/kg/month), intermittent antibiotic treatment and postural drainage; he was discharged with a diagnosis of CID. From May 1977 to December 1979, the patient presented chronic diarrhea and several episodes of otitis and conjunctivitis, while the respiratory tract infections diminished in frequency and severity. In September 1979, the child recovered uneventfully from surgery for a kidney stone. In May 1980, therapy with thymosin fraction 5 (2 mg/kg/daily for one week and then 2 mg/kg/weekly) was started because the patient had very low serum levels of thymus dependent serum factor SF (4.7 units of activity; normal values: > 25 units of activity). As shown in Figure 1, the percentage of E+ as well as OKT3+ cells rapidly normalized, while the percentage of OKT4+ cells, as well as the other immunologic data, remained unchanged. Clinical status gradually improved. Since then he has had several minor infections of the upper respiratory tract.

DISCUSSION

Analysis of T-cell subsets with monoclonal antibodies in this child with combined deficiency of humoral and cellular immunity revealed a severe numerical defect of inducer OKT4+ cells. OKT8+ suppressor cells were present in a normal percentage and accounted for virtually all the circulating lymphocytes forming rosettes with sheep erythrocytes (E+) and recognized by OKT3 antibody.

The number of circulating lymphocytes displaying an intense focal staining for alpha-naphthyl acetate esterase (ANAE) was also severely depressed. There is evidence that ANAE+ lymphocytes [6] carry the OKT4 antigen and express helper-inducer function in vitro (C. Grossi, personal communication). The present finding of an associated deficiency of OKT4+ and ANAE+ lymphocytes further strengthens the hypothesis that both markers identify the same, or at least largely overlapping, subsets.

The severe deficiency of inducer T cells may explain the depressed antibody response to repeated antigenic challenges as well as the negative DTH skin tests and the low proliferative response of lymphocytes in vi-

TABLE 1. Immunologic Evaluation Before Thymosin Treatment

	Patient	Age normal-values[a]
T-cell subpopulations		
E+	20–30%	55–75%
OKT3+	18–27%	75± 5%
OKT4+	8–10%	44±10%
OKT8	20–25%	22± 7%
OKT6+	0– 2%	3± 2%
ANAE[b]	8–11%	57± 6%
In vitro lymphocyte response to (cpm × 10^{-3}):		
PHA	1–2.5	70–150
Con A	0.1–0.5	50–70
Candidin	0.5–1.4	16–27
TT	0.1–0.2	20–30
PWM	0.2–0.4	40–60
DTH (skin tests)		
PPD	neg.	Positive or negative according to previous antigenic exposure
SK-SD	neg.	
TT	neg.	
Candidin	neg.	
B-lymphocytes (Ig+s)	5%	5±3 %
Serum Igs (IU/ml)		
IgG	90–123	79–238
IgA	25–36	29–222
IgM	510–1350	67–310
IgE	15–20	10–90
Serum antibodies		
anti-*E coli* (U/ml)	0.7	> 50
anti-rabbit erythrocytes (titer)	1:16	>1:64
anti-tetanus toxoid (mU/ml)	3.6[c]	>100
Secretory IgA in saliva (mg/dl)	4	>0.5

[a]Data from our laboratory
[b]Staining for ANAE
[c]After antigenic stimulation

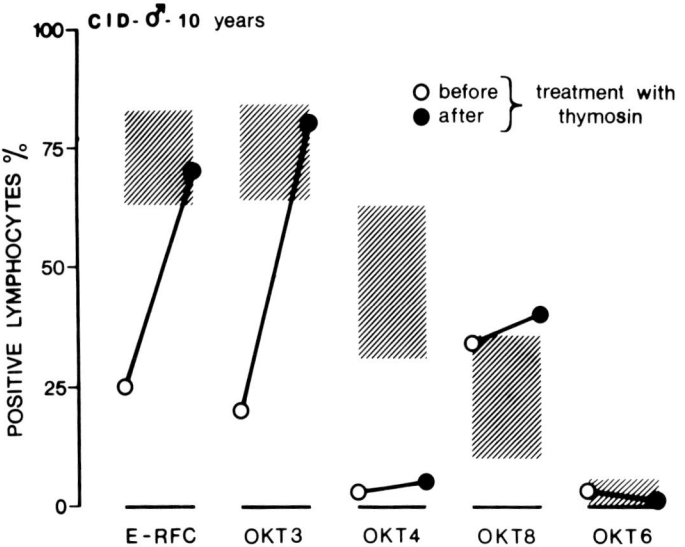

Fig. 1. Circulating T-lymphocyte subsets before and after thymosin treatment. Shaded areas represent the normal range.

tro to antigens and mitogens. A therapeutic trial with thymosin fraction 5 resulted in a significant clinical improvement, dramatic increase of the percentage of E-rosettes as well as of OKT3+ lymphocytes; however, the numbers of OKT4+ and ANAE+ cells remained low and the antibody responses, lymphocyte proliferation in vitro, and skin reactivity did not improve.

The striking increase in OKT3+ and E+ cells, but not in OKT4+ cells, which followed thymosin treatment suggests the presence of inducible precursors unable to differentiate appropriately under the influence of thymic hormones alone. This may support the hypothesis that the generation of inducer T cells in our patient is hampered by a faulty interaction between precursor T cells and thymic epithelial cells. The apparent discrepancy between the clinical and immunologic responses to thymosin treatment remains obscure.

REFERENCES

1. Reinherz EL, Kung P, Goldstein G, Schlossman SF: Separation of functional subsets of human T cells by a monoclonal antibody. Proc Natl Acad Sci USA 76:4061–4065, 1979.
2. Reinherz EL, Morimoto C, Penta AC, Schlossman SF: Regulation of B cell immunoglobulin secretion by functional subsets of T lymphocytes in man. Eur J Immunol 10:570–572, 1980.
3. Reinherz EL, Kung PC, Breard JM, Goldstein G, Schlossman SF: T cell requirements for generation of helper factor(s) in man: Analysis of the subsets involved. J Immunol 124:1883–1887, 1980.
4. Reinherz EL, Schlossman SF: The differentiation and function of human T lymphocytes. Cell 19:821–827, 1980.
5. Reinherz EL, Geha R, Wohl ME, Morimoto C, Rosen FS, Schlossman SF: Immunodeficiency associated with loss of T4+ inducer T-cell function. N Engl J Med 304:811–816, 1981.
6. Ferrari FA, Maccario R, Marconi M, Vitiello MA, Ugazio AG, Burgio V, Siccardi AG: Reliability of alpha-naphthyl acetate esterase staining of blood smears for the enumeration of circulating human T lymphocytes. Clin Exp Immunol 41:358–362, 1980.

T-Cell Subsets and Natural Killer Cells in DiGeorge and SCID Patients[*]

M.C. Sirianni, MD, L. Businco, MD, L. Fiore, MD, R. Seminara, MD, and F. Aiuti, MD

Department of Clinical Immunology, Institute of Internal Medicine III (M.C.S., R.S., F.A.), and Institute of Pediatrics (L.B., L.F.), University of Rome, 00185 Rome, Italy

The pathogenesis of most primary immunodeficiency diseases may be attributed to defects of certain stages in stem cell differentiation, along the T- and B-cellular lines [1]. The use of surface markers and monoclonal antibodies [2] for the identification of T-cell subsets has proved especially valuable for the diagnosis and pathogenesis of these diseases. Recently, a new monoclonal antibody (HNK-1 or Leu 7) [3] has been shown to identify cells featured as natural killer (NK) cells. The aim of this study was to analyze T-cell subsets, NK cells and NK activity in these patients, in order to better define the preeminent defects in some primary immunodeficiency diseases (ID).

MATERIALS AND METHODS
Patients

Three children with severe combined immunodeficiency (SCID), 2 with DiGeorge syndrome, and 3 with T-cell defect or SCID with B cells were studied. Clinical and immunologic diagnosis was made according to the criteria reported elsewhere [4]. In particular, other criteria for the differential diagnosis between SCID and T-cell defects were the presence of plasma cells and synthesis of immunoglobulins (Ig) in the latter syndrome. Normal controls were represented by a group of age/sex-matched healthy children.

[*]Supported by a grant from the Istituto Pasteur, Fondazione Cenci Bolognetti.

Analysis of Monoclonal Antibodies

Peripheral blood lymphocytes (PBL) were isolated through a Ficoll-Isopaque gradient and resuspended at 1×10^6/ml in RPMI 1640; viability was always more than 95%. T-cell subsets were determined by a panel of monoclonal antibodies (Ortho, Raritan, N.J.), already known to recognize antigens selectively expressed on cells of the T-cell lineage [3]. NK cells were enumerated by the use of HNK-1. Cells were labeled with an appropriate amount of the monoclonal antibodies and then counterlabeled with fluorescent goat anti-mouse Ig, as previously described [5]. Cells were examined for indirect immunofluorescence with a Leitz microscope.

NK activity was assayed by pelleting effector PBL and target cells (K562 and MOLT 4 cell lines) in a 4h ^{51}Cr release assay, as already described [4]. ^{51}Cr release was detected in a LKB spectrophotometer and percentage of specific lysis calculated as reported elsewhere [4].

RESULTS AND DISCUSSION

The percentage of positive cells with surface markers and monoclonal antibodies, compared to normal controls, are reported in Table 1. Functional activity of NK cells is also listed in the same Table.

The constant characteristic in all patients was the increase in percentage of cells positive for phagocytosis and stained by the antibody OKM1. All patients also showed a decrease in number of peripheral blood lymphocytes and in the proportion of SRBC positive lymphocytes, with the exception of *Case E.C.*, affected by DiGeorge syndrome. We have divided the infants with primary ID into 3 distinct groups according to their clinical criteria (from severe to relatively mild) and immunologic data, which are reported in Table 2. The first group is represented by forms of SCID with severe lymphopenia, absence of plasma cells and Ig. In all these cases, the absolute number of mature and immature T cells as well as NK cells and their activity were extremely reduced. An early block of T- and B-cell differentiation may be hypothesized.

In the second group, a decrease of lymphocytes with mature phenotypes was also present; however, in some cases, the immature thymocytes may circulate in the peripheral blood. In one of these patients, NK activity was present as well as NK cells identified by HNK-1 monoclonal antibody. The third group of children with DiGeorge syndrome was characterized by decrease of mature thymocytes and an increase of immature T-cell precursors, while NK cells were normally represented.

These findings are in agreement with the concept that NK cells originate from an early stage of cell differentiation [4,6,7] but do not definitely prove to which cell lineage they really belong. We can exclude that NK function is associated with monocytes, since all patients with

TABLE 1. Percentage of Positive Cells With Surface Markers, Monoclonal Antibodies and NK Activity in Peripheral Blood of Infants With SCID, and T-Cell Defects

Cases	Age (months)	Sex	Diag-nosis*	Lympho-cytes/mm³	SRBC	SIg	OKT10	OKT9	OKT6	OKT3	OKT4	OKT8	OKM1	HNK-1	NK Activity*		
															K-562	MOLT-4	PH
E.M.	5	M	1	250	22	0	2	10	0	3	0	1	55	0	12.7	ND	52
M.R.	6	M	1	150	16	2	6	0	2	2	1	2	83	0	8.22	10.05	85
D.F.	3	M	1	300	12	0	2	8	0	0	0	0	58	0	12.65	11.08	ND
M.S.	18	M	2	280	30	15	ND	ND	ND	28	16	10	28	0	13.74	13.20	30
P.A.	6	M	2	384	37	3	ND	ND	6	23	13	21	ND	ND	47.37	42.11	35
L.C.	13	F	2	3000	20	5	60	69	43	37	25	18	12	18	ND	ND	22
G.F.	2	M	3	300	20	35	8	1	2	22	22	8	54	6	32.98	30.47	ND
E.C.	2	F	3	4500	36	11	31	9	11	25	18	7	48	4	ND	ND	45
Normal values (mean±SD)					67 ±7.5	4.2 ±1.9	7.2 ±2.0	<1	<1	63.9 ±7.8	40.6 ±5.8	26.9 ±6.1	13.4 ±4.0	6.3 ±5.6	63.4 ±10.2	54.2 ±10.4	15.8 ±7.6

*1: SCID ADA⁺ and ADA⁻
2: SCID with B lymphocytes (?) or primary T-cell defect (?)
3: DiGeorge syndrome
SRBC: sheep red blood cells forming rosettes with T lymphocytes
SIg: surface membrane immunoglobulins
PH: phagocytosis
ND: not done
*: calculated as % of lysis (effector/target cell ratio 100:1)

TABLE 2. Monoclonal Antibodies in Peripheral Blood of Infants With SCID and T-Cell Defects

	SCID ADA⁺ and ADA⁻	Primary T-Cell Defect (?) SCID With B Lymphocytes (?)	DiGeorge Syndrome
OKT10	A	Variable	↑
OKT9	A	Variable	↑
OKT6	A	Variable	↑
OKT3	A	↓	↓
OKT4	A	↓	↓
OKT8	A	↓	↓
HNK-1	A	N	N

↑: Increased
↓: Decreased
N: Normal
A: Absent

SCID have mature functioning monocytes, revealed by the OKM1, peroxidase staining (data not shown) and phagocytosis. Since prothymocytes and thymocytes were lacking in cases of SCID, we suggest either a common precursor defect of both NK and thymic cells or the possibilty of two distinct defective progenitor cells. The presence of HNK-1⁺ cells in DiGeorge and T-cell defects is contrary to a thymic origin. However, lymphocytes with T-cell markers and without T-cell function were not completely absent in these children, and in some cases a rudimental thymus was observed. Our data do not prove whether the cell lineage of NK cells belongs to the T cell or to a separate cell line, distinct from lymphocytes or monocytes, even if data tend to support the latter hypothesis. In addition, we have demonstrated a good correlation between cells positive with HNK-1 and NK activity ($p < 0.001$). We believe that the use of monoclonal antibodies together with functional studies will permit a more precise diagnosis of SCID and related syndromes, in order to better define the therapeutic approach to these disorders.

REFERENCES

1. WHO Technical Report series: "Primary Immunodeficiencies." 630:entire volume, 1978.
2. Reinherz EL, Kung PC, Goldstein G, Schlossman SF: Discrete stages of human intrathymic differentiation: Analysis of normal thymocytes and leukemic lymphoblasts of T lineage. Proc Natl Acad Sci USA 76:4061-4065, 1979.
3. Abo T, Balch CM: A differentiation antigen of human NK and K cells identified by a monoclonal antibody (HNK-1). J Immunol 127:1024-1029, 1981.
4. Sirianni MC, Fiorilli M, Pandolfi F, Quinti I, Aiuti F: Natural killer activity and lymphocyte subpopulations in patients with primary humoral and cellular immunodeficiencies. Clin Immunol Immunopathol 21:12-19, 1981.
5. Pandolfi F, Quinti I, Frielingsdorf A, Goldstein G, Businco L, Aiuti F: Abnormalities of regulatory T-cell subpopulations in patients with primary immunoglobulin deficiencies. Clin Immunol Immunopathol 22:323-330, 1982.
6. Koren HS, Amos DB, Buckley RH: Natural killing in immunodeficient patients. J Immunol 120:796-799, 1978.
7. Abo T, Cooper MD, Balch CM: Postnatal expansion of the natural killer and killer cell population in humans identified by the monoclonal HNK-1 antibody. J Exp Med 144:321-326, 1982.

Does an Interferonopathy Underlie a Severe Combined Immunodeficiency Disease (SCID) Syndrome?

James F. Jones, MD, Linda M. Minnich, MS, David O. Lucas, PhD, Marlyn P. Langford, PhD, and G. John Stanton, PhD

Departments of Pediatrics (J.F.J.), Pathology (L.M.M.), and of Molecular and Medical Microbiology (D.O.L.), University of Arizona School of Medicine, Tucson, AZ 85724, and Department of Microbiology, University of Texas Medical Branch, Galveston, TX 77550 (M.P.L., G.J.S.)

The primary deficit in SCID is known in only the adenosine deaminase (ADA) deficiency syndrome [1]. Other patients appear to have abnormalities in stem cell development or thymic epithelial cell function suggesting additional intrinsic or extrinsic abnormalities in lymphoid cell maturation as a basis for other SCID syndromes [2,3].

The opportunity to test this concept availed itself when 2 Navajo Indian children with SCID lost T- and B-cell function which had been reconstituted after cultured thymus explant therapy. In both instances, immune function declined after a viral infection, illnesses which are often accompanied by inhibition of normal immune function [4]. An inhibitor of lymphoblastogenesis was found in 6 Navajo children and to a lesser extent in 4 Caucasian children with SCID. The inhibitor in the Navajo children was identified as interferon (IFN). The production of IFN by these patients and its possible role in the syndrome is discussed.

METHODS

Clinical and immune profiles of *Patients N1, 2, 4, 5, 6* and *C1-4* have been previously published [5-11]. *Patient N3* was diagnosed in October 1979 after a history of recurrent pneumonia, meningitis, a generalized skin rash, and failure to thrive. Laboratory values typical of SCID were found. Since no bone marrow donor was available, cultured thymus fragment therapy was given in December 1979. Within 3 weeks, lymph nodes were palpable and diarrhea had decreased. Repeat laboratory studies showed normal number of T and B lymphocytes, as well as the production of IgA, IgM and IgG. Pneumonia ensued 2 months after therapy; the initial episode resolved spontaneously but recurred one month later, at which time respiratory syncytial virus (RSV) was isolated from his pharynx. In vitro immune function declined after the initial episode and did not respond to subsequent therapy. He expired suddenly after recovery from a subsequent lower respiratory tract episode.

Serum specimens were obtained from the SCID patients at varying times during their illness. Caucasian patient sera were provided by Dr. Armond Goldman. Acute and convalescent sera from children less than one year of age with RSV which had been stored for equivalent periods at $-70°C$ (as were all of the sera) were examined for IFN activity as were age-matched controls for the IFN assay.

Reference interferons (IFNα and IFNβ) and their respective antibodies were obtained from the NIAID Antiviral Substances Program, NIH. IFNγ and anti-IFNγ were prepared as described [12].

Immune function tests were performed as previously described [5]. A standard lymphocyte stimulation assay was used to detect serum inhibitory activity. Normal lymphoid responses to mitogen were performed in cultures where patient sera replaced AB plasma or were mixed 1:1 with AB plasma. Sera from normal Navajo and Caucasian adults and children did not affect these results.

Patient serum samples were 1) dialysed against 20 volumes of pH 7.4 phosphate buffered saline for 24 hrs, 2) heated to $56°C$ for 30 min, and 3) adjusted to pH 2.0 for 24 hrs, and returned to pH 7.4 in attempts to preliminarily characterize the inhibitor. The time required for serum to inhibit lymphocyte stimulation and the viability of cells as determined by trypan blue dye exclusion was determined.

IFN activity was assayed using previously described vesicular-stomatitis virus (VSV) - HeLa cell and Sindbis virus or VSV - WISH cell systems [13]. The endpoint of the assay was 50% plaque reduction; values were compared to standards and reported in U/ml serum.

Identification of IFN types was performed by 1) incubation of sera with sodium dodecyl sulfate (SDS) (0.05% w/v) and trypsin (2.5 mg/ml w/v); 2) assay on mouse L cells; and 3) antibody neutralization using a previously published method [12]. Excess amounts of anti-IFNs were preincubated with sera prior to assay for activity. Anti-IFNs were also added to sera prior to performance of the inhibition assay. Controls included cultures with normal rabbit sera (the source of anti-IFNs). The inhibitory properties of standard

IFNs were performed by adding 1, 10, or 100 U of the standards to cultures containing 1:5000, 1:1000, or 1:300 dilutions of PHA, and 9.5, 1.0, and 5.0 μg/ml of Con A.

RESULTS

Navajo and Caucasian SCID patient sera inhibition of lymphoblastogenesis is depicted in Table 1. A 66% mean reduction was seen with the Navajo sera, versus a group mean inhibitor of 38% with the Caucasian sera. Both of the ADA-Caucasian patient sera actually caused a 5–34% increase in mitogen responses; such an increase was never seen with Navajo patients. Only minimal inhibitor was seen with *Patient N6*, the only Navajo studied after bone marrow transplantation (BMT).

Six hours of incubation were required to see an inhibitory effect; no loss of cell viability was seen with patient sera. Lowering the pH to 2.0 decreased the inhibition in *Patients N2* and *N3*, but not in *Patient N1* serum. These characteristics led to assay of the sera for IFN activity. Mean circulating levels of IFN are seen in Table 2. Mean levels for *Patients N1, N2,* and *N3* were 93, 92, and 73 U/ml; these patients had 8, 5, and 5 samples, respectively, examined. Other Navajo patients had only one specimen studied with values of 30, 33, and 100 U/ml. Caucasian *Patients C2, C3,* and *C4* had levels of 12, 4, and 4 U/ml, respectively. The virus-infected controls had decreasing levels of IFN activity as expected with resolution of infection.

IFN activity in 4 samples was decreased by treatment at pH 2.0 (Table 3) indicating the presence of IFNγ. SDS and trypsin treatment decreased IFN activity, a characteristic of IFNα. Low activity on mouse L cells also suggested IFNα activity. Incubation with anti-IFNs identified 3 types of IFN in various patient specimens (Table 4). IFNα appeared to be the dominant species. IFNγ was present only after cultured thymus explant therapy, except in *Patient N1* on 4/22/76.

Known IFNα and IFNβ inhibited Con A and PHA stimulation of normal lymphocytes; the effect of IFNα (purified to remove its inducer, staphylococcal enterotoxin A) was bimodal (Table 5). Control cultures with each IFN type showed no nonspecific stimulation of lymphocytes.

The results of incubation of patient sera with anti-IFN prior to lymphocyte stimulation are shown in Figure 1. Readily apparent abrogation of inhibitor effect was seen in 3 of 4 PHA-stimulated cultures, and a less marked removal of inhibition seen in each of the 3 Con A-stimulated cultures. IFNα appears to have been the dominant species in these samples because preincubation with anti-IFNα restored lymphocyte stimulation to expected levels in 4 of 7 cultures. IFNβ and IFNγ were likewise apparently responsible for inhibition in one culture each.

Patients N1, N2, and *N3* had IFN-inhibitor activity in their serum throughout their hospital courses irrespective of infection. For instance, *N1* was maintained in laminar flow isolation and had no viruses isolated from several cultures, but had high (>100 U/ml) levels of IFN on sev-

TABLE 1. Mean Percent Inhibition of Lymphocyte Blastogenesis by Navajo and Caucasian SCID Sera

Serum Source	PHA	Con A	PWM	Patient Mean
Navajo				
Patient N1	65(7)[a]	85(6)	76(3)	75
Patient N2	68(4)	79(4)	80(4)	76
Patient N3	62(15)	59(15)	66(12)	62
Patient N4	81(2)	89(2)	—	85
Patient N5	96(2)	95(2)	—	96
Patient N6	6(2)	23(2)	35(2)	21
Caucasian				
Patient C1	—	36(1)	28(1)	32[c]
Patient C2	34(2)[b]	21(2)	55(2)	25
Patient C3	29(2)[b]	15(2)[b]	9(2)	3
Patient C4	58(2)	51(2)	45(2)	51

[a]( )Number of sera studied.
[b]% Increase in stimulation. (These values = 0 inhibition in the patient mean computation)
[c]P = .033 by the Mann-Whitney U test. (n for Navajo = 6; n for Caucasian = 4)

TABLE 2. IFN Levels In Patient and Control Sera

IFN Level (U/ml)	Sample Source			
	SCID		Virus Infection	
	Navajo	Caucasian	Acute	Convalescent
Mean	78	7	25	7
Range	10–300	4–12	0–111	0–32
N	25	3	76	7

TABLE 3. Effect of pH 2.0 Treatment of Inhibition of Lymphoblastogenesis and IFN Activity

Source of Serum	Date	Pretreatment		Posttreatment	
		% Inhibition*	U/ml	% Inhibition	U/ml
Patient N1	2/9/77	33	20	27	<10
Patient N1	4/4/77	44	30	48	10
Patient N2	4/14/76	55	10	29	<10
Patient N3	10/26/79	56	40	30	20

*Inhibition of PHA-stimulated lymphoblastogenesis.

TABLE 4. Effect of Anti-IFN Antibody on IFN Activity (U/ml)

	Serum IFN	IFN remaining after treatment with:*						IFN type identified
		Anti-IFNα	Anti-IFNβ	Anti-IFNγ	Anti-IFNα/IFNγ	Anti-IFNα/IFNβ	Anti-IFNβ/IFNγ	
Patient N1								
4/22/76	54	0(100)**	18(66)	6(89)	6(89)	6(89)	6(89)	α,γ
7/27/76	162	18(89)	54(66)	6(96)	54(66)	54(66)	54(66)	α,γ
9/30/76	54	54(0)	6(89)	0(100)	0(100)	18(66)	6(89)	β,γ
10/14/76	18	0(100)	6(66)	18(0)	6(66)	6(66)	6(66)	α,β
Patient N2								
1/17/77	54	0(100)	18(66)	6(89)	9(100)	6(96)	0(100)	α,β,γ
2/25/74	18	0(100)	6(66)	18(0)	6(66)	6(66)	6(66)	α
Patient N3								
1/21/80	162	0(100)	0(100)	54(66)	0(100)	6(96)	0(100)	α,β,γ

*Serum samples were preincubated with 300 U of individual anti-IFN antisera or with 150 U each of 2 anti-IFN antisera prior to assay in the WISH-Sindbis assay.
**( )Percent decrease in IFN activity.

TABLE 5. Effect of IFN Standards on Mitogen Response of Normal Lymphocytes

	Concentration or Dilution of Mitogen and IFN		
	1/3000(v/v)	1/1000	1/500
PHA			
α	100,100,100*	35,28,14	106,56,44
β	400,192,100	101,86,29	42,46,24
γ	350,275,275	150,140,800	25,36,380
	0.5 μg/ml	1.0 μg/ml	5.0 μg/ml
Con A			
α	100,100,100	47,35,41	92,99,100
β	129,28,50	50,40,30	125,83,90
γ	24,33,600	79,57,20	92,67,25

*Percent of expected response in the presence of 1, 10, 100 IU, respectively, of IFN standards.

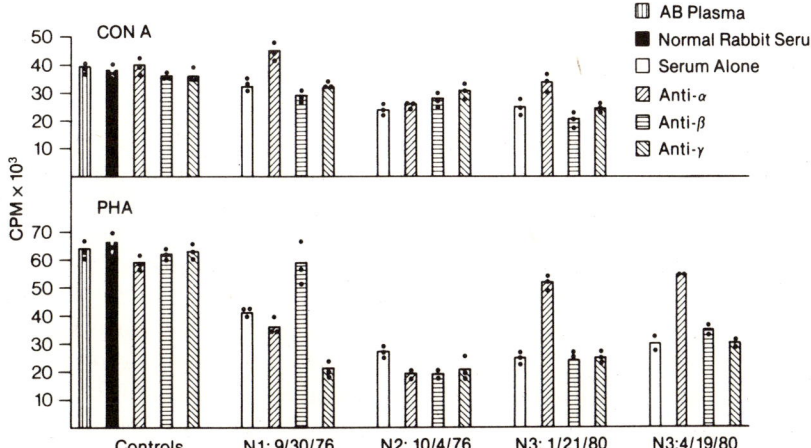

Fig. 1. Effect of anti-IFN antisera on inhibition of lymphoblastogenesis. Lymphoid cells were mixed with AB plasma, and PHA or Con A in standard lymphoblastogenesis cultures to yield the control or expected value. Normal rabbit serum and 3 rabbit anti-human IFNs were mixed with AB plasma in the other control experiments. Patient sera were then used in the cultures with and without anti-IFN antibodies. The top of the bar equals the mean of 3 replicates, and dots are the values of individual replicates.

eral occasions during that time. On the other hand, N2 had no viral infections, but did have multiple skin and blood stream bacterial infections. N3 had multiple virus infections throughout his course. Likewise, no reciprocal relationship between immune function, graft status, and inhibitor/IFN presence or levels could be demonstrated; appropriately timed samples, however, were not always available.

DISCUSSION

An inhibitor of mitogen-induced lymphoblastogenesis was identified in the sera of patients with SCID. Lymphocyte stimulation may be inhibited by a variety of substances including: macrophages and their products [14], activated T-suppressor cells and their products [15], low density lipoproteins [16], immunoglobulins in EBV infections [17], nonspecific inhibitors produced during infections [18,19], drugs [20], hormones [21], naturally occurring mediators of inflammation [22], and IFNs [23].

Physical and biologic characteristics of the inhibitor suggested that it was an IFN. Treatment of sera at pH 2.0 altered both inhibitor and IFN activity, but not to the same extent. This discrepancy could be explained by pH 2.0 stability of the major inhibitory effect or that the amount of

IFN required for inhibition of mitogenesis is less than the amount required for inhibition of virus replication.

Further evidence that the inhibitor was IFN was provided by the abrogation of inhibitor activity by anti-IFN antibodies. The one serum in which inhibition of PHA stimulation could not be removed may have contained more IFN activity than was removed under these experimental conditions. Alternatively, the inhibitor may be another substance.

The lack of volume and number of patient samples precluded clarification of specific IFN types in most instances. Although IFNα appeared to be the predominant type in most sera, it is quite likely that more than one type was present in any given sample. An equally plausible explanation for these differences is that the antisera were not sufficiently specific and thus were effective against multiple types of IFN [24].

The identification of IFN in these patients' sera and its apparent inhibitory activity support previously described inhibitory effects upon lymphocyte function for this group of glycoproteins. Blomgren et al [25] described inhibition of lymphocyte stimulation by the addition of IFNα to their assay system. Such inhibition has been observed repeatedly [23]. Exogenously administered and endogenously produced IFNs also have been shown to alter lymphocyte numbers [26] and to inhibit stimulation responses [27,28], respectively. Other workers have not observed functional changes during therapy with IFN [29].

The usual investigations of IFNs in primary immunodeficiencies have supported normal in vitro production. No comment has been made of its potential adverse effects. Miller and Hummeler [30], and Ray and Davis [31] reported normal in vitro IFNα production by cells from a patient with SCID, and patients with antibody deficiency and ataxia telangiectasia, respectively. Epstein and Ammann [32] found normal IFNγ production in culture of cells from patients with hypogammaglobulinemia and thymic hypoplasia (after fetal thymus transplantation), but diminished IFN production was seen in patients with selective IgA deficiency. Strannegard et al [33] found that cells from hypogammaglobulinemic patients produced more IFN than cells from patients with systemic lupus erythematosus or with atopic diseases.

The production of IFNs by SCID patients raises the question of their origin. Which cells produce IFN? Does the degree of maturation of the infants' cells influence both the type and quantity of IFN manufactured?

It is known that IFNα is produced by non-T leukocytes, including B, null and NK cells, as well as by macrophages [34–36]. Each patient sample but one had evidence of IFNα and this IFN appeared to be responsible for inhibitor activity in the majority of samples as well. Although the type of IFN in Patient N1's serum at 4 days of age could not be identified due to the sample volume, IFNα is the primary IFN produced at this age [37]. Of the 4 possible producer cell types, only B cells were known to be absent at this time, but we are not certain of the cell of origin of the IFN.

IFNγ is thought to be produced by B and T lymphocytes upon exposure to specific antigens or upon primary exposure to mitogens, thus implying some form of immune maturation [38]. IFNγ was also produced by each patient studied, but at times which were not related to the presence of normal immune function (Table 6). *Patient N1*, for instance, had circulating IFNγ activity at 4 months of age when circulating lymphocytes were comprised of 10% T cells, no SIg-bearing cells, and 65% EAC-positive cells; their only identifiable function was a positive mixed lymphocyte reaction (MLR). In 2 subsequent samples taken from this patient after immune reconstitution, IFNγ was the major component. No IFNγ was observed after immune function failed late in her course. Samples from *Patients N2* and *N3* were studied only after thymus fragment therapy. IFNγ was present in Patient N2 at a time when no immune responses were evident, while N3 had IFNγ after immune reconstitution. Each of these children were past the first few months of life when IFNγ is at a minimum [39]. Perhaps IFNγ production by NK cells may have been responsible for these seemingly contradictory observations in our patients [40].

Is the putative IFN-inhibitor unique to the Navajo SCID syndrome? We do not know. The inclusion of 2 Caucasian children with ADA-negative SCID may have contributed bias to the distribution of IFN observed. However, 3 of the Navajo SCID group (*N1, N2, N4*) had high percentages of circulating parallel tubular arrays (PTAs) [6]. These organelles have been recognized as a

TABLE 6. Relationship of Peripheral Blood Lymphoid Cell Types and IFN Production

Patient (age)	IFN	Lymphoid Cell Marker (%)				Function (+/−)	
		SIgM	EAC	E	PTA*(NK?)	PHA	MLC
N1 (4 day)	α	0	65	40	ND	−	+
(11 mo)	β	2	50	20	20	−	+
(4 mo)	γ	0	65	10	41	−	+
N2 (13 mo)	α,γ	0	20	7	53	−	−
N3 (5 mo)	α,γ	0	ND	56	0	+	ND

*Parallel tubular arrays

marker of Fc (EA-Hu) cells [41], which in turn have been shown to function as NK cells [42]. Recent evidence has attributed the production of at least one form of IFNα to NK cells [36]. In addition, IFNα enhances the maturation of NK cells in a positive feedback system to produce more IFNα [43].

Two final interrelated questions must be posed. Why does IFN persist in the circulation of these patients? Does circulating IFN contribute to the pathogenesis of SCID?

The primary recognized in vivo stimulus for IFN production is infection. Circulating IFN is usually seen early in the course along with other nonspecific responses, and then decreases as specific immunity develops and resolution occurs. Even though our patients had circulating IFN during periods of apparent freedom from overt infection, the lack of normal immune responses would suggest incomplete resolution of the infection resulting in persistent triggering of IFN production.

Circulating IFN is not found in normal adults or children [44–46], but has been identified in the serum of adults with autoimmune disease [45], children with Down syndrome, and Ig deficiency states [46]. Neither the specific infection status nor sequelae of circulating IFN were reported in these studies. Nude mice, animals with impaired T-lymphocyte function, are known to have higher serum IFN levels than normal animals after infection with lymphocytic choriomeningitis virus; however, IFN levels prior to infection in those animals were not reported [47].

Another explanation for the continued presence of circulating IFN is an innate abnormality in control of IFN production; this remains an untested possibility.

Since IFN affects both cell regulatory and cell growth functions, such effects could account for observed suppression of B- and T-lymphocyte numbers and responses in these patients and may have contributed to the graft failures in *Patients N1, N2, and N3*. The possible effect of IFN on cell growth may not be limited to the lymphoid system. Runting has always been an enigma in these patients; it is usually attributed to chronic infection and secondary malnutrition [48]. If IFNα is administered to suckling mice, the animals fail to grow properly, die early, and are found to have pathologic changes in their thymuses, kidneys, livers, and, in some instances, germinal centers of their spleens [49,50].

The etiology of all SCID syndromes is not known. The observations reported here suggest that development defects in the control of IFN, a group of cell regulatory glycoproteins, may play a role in the pathophysiology of these syndromes.

REFERENCES

1. Carson DA, Kay J, Seegmiller JE: Differential sensitivity of human leukemic T-cell lines and B-cell lines to growth inhibition by deoxyadenosine. J Immunol 121:1726–1731, 1978.
2. Cooper MD, Perey DY, Peterson RDA, Gabrielson AE, Good RA: The two-component concept of the lymphoid system. In Bergsma D (ed): "Immunologic Deficiency Diseases in Man." New York: The National Foundation-March of Dimes, BD:OAS IV(1):7–16, 1968.
3. Pyke KW, Dosch HM, Ipp MM, Gelfand EW: Demonstration of an intrathymic defect in a case of severe combined immunodeficiency disease. N Engl J Med 293:424–428, 1975.
4. Merigan T: Host defenses against viral disease. N Engl J Med 290:323–329, 1974.
5. Jones JF, Sieber OF Jr, Fulginiti VA, Ochs H, Schulte-Wisserman H, Hong R: Predominance of B-lymphocyte function after cultured thymus fragment therapy in severe combined immunodeficiency disease. Clin Immunol Immunopathol 17:439–450, 1980.
6. Payne C, Jones JF, Sieber OF Jr, Fulginiti VA: Parallel tubular arrays in severe combined immunodeficiency disease: An ultrastructural study of peripheral blood lymphocytes. Blood 50:55–64, 1977.
7. Sieber O, Fulginiti VA, Durie B, Salmon S: Successful immunological reconstitution in severe combined immunodeficiency disease with transplantation from a non-compatible donor. Clin Res 22:230A, 1974.
8. Murphy S, Hayward A, Troup G, Devor EF, Coons T: Gene enrichment in an American Indian population: An examination of severe combined immunodeficiency disease. Lancet 2:502–505, 1980.
9. Smith JH, Nichols MM, Goldman AS, Schmalstieg FC, Goldblum RM: Disseminated cryptococcosis in an infant with severe combined immunodeficiency disease. Hum Pathol 13:500–503,1982.
10. Mills GC, Schmalstieg FC, Trimmer KB, Goldman AS, Goldblum RM: Purine metabolism in adenosine deaminase deficiency. Proc Natl Acad Sci USA 73:2867–2871, 1976.
11. Schmalstieg FC, Tsuda H, Mills GC, Goldman AS: Immunodeficiency in a child with a healthy adenosine deaminase deficient mother. Pediatr Res 15:603, 1981.
12. Langford MP, Weigent DA, Georgiades JA, Johnson HM, Stanton GJ: Antibody to staphylococcal enterotoxin A-induced human interferon (IFNγ). J Immunol 126:1620–1623, 1981.
13. Langford MP, Stanton GJ, Johnson HM: Biological effects of staphylococcal enterotoxin A on human peripheral blood lymphocytes. Infect Immun 22:62–68, 1978.
14. Allison AC: Mechanisms by which activated macrophages inhibit lymphocyte responses. Immunol Rev 40:3–27, 1978.
15. Wolf RL, Whitsed H, Rosen FS, Merler E: A soluble inhibitor of B and T cell proliferation and antibody synthesis produced by dividing human T cells. Cell Immunol 36:231–241, 1978.
16. Chiasari FV: Immunoregulatory properties of human plasma in very low density lipoproteins. J Immunol 119:2129–2136, 1977.
17. Wainwright WH, Veltri RW, Sprinkle PM: Abrogation of cell-mediated immunity by a serum blocking factor isolated from patients with infectious mononucleosis. J Infect Dis 140:22–32, 1979.
18. Barclay GR, Keller AJ, Van Somerin V, Urbaniak SJ: Serum inhibition of lymphocyte transformation in a case of pulmonary tuberculosis. Clin Immunol Immunopathol 14:449–455, 1979.
19. Starr SE, Tolpin MD, Friedman HM, Paucker K, Plotkin SA: Impaired cellular immunity to cytomegalovirus in congenitally infected children and their mothers. J Infect Dis 140:500–505, 1979.
20. Barasoain I, Rojo JM, Portoles A: "In vivo" effects of acetylsalicylic acid and two ether-derived compounds on primary immune response and lymphoblastic transformation. Immunopharmacology 2:293–300, 1980.
21. Wang SR, Zweiman B: In vivo and in vitro effects of methylprednisolone on

human lymphocyte proliferation. Immunopharmacology 2:95-101, 1980.
22. Goodwin JS, Bankhurst AD, Messner RP: Suppression of human T-cell mitogenesis by prostaglandin existence of a prostaglandin-producing suppressor cell. J Exp Med 146:1719-1734, 1977.
23. Wallen W, Dean J, Gauntt C, Lucas D: Suppression of lymphocyte stimulation in mouse spleen cells by interferon preparations. In Geraldes A (ed): "Effects of Interferon on Cells, Viruses and the Immune System." New York: Academic Press, 1975, pp 355-365.
24. Wiranowska-Stewart M: Heterogeneity of human gamma interferon preparations: Evidence for presence of alpha interferon. J Interferon Res 1:315-321, 1981.
25. Blomgren H, Strander H, Cantell K: Effect of human leukocyte interferon on the response of leukocytes to mitogenic stimuli in vitro. Scand J Immunol 3:697-705, 1974.
26. Einhorn S, Blomgren H, Strander H: Effect of an intramuscular injection of human leukocyte interferon on blood leukocyte counts and proportions of lymphocytes forming E, EA, and EAC rosettes. Int Arch Allergy Appl Immunol 63:139-144, 1980.
27. Taylor-Papadimitriou J: Effects of interferons on cell growth and function. In Gresser I (ed): "Interferon 2." London: Academic Press, 1980, pp 13-46.
28. DeMaeyer E, Maeyer-Guignard JD: Immunoregulatory action of type I interferon in the mouse. Ann NY Acad Sci 350:1-11, 1980.
29. Rasmussen L, Merigan TC: Effect of interferon therapy on circulating lymphocytes in humans. J Interferon Res 1:101-110, 1980.
30. Miller ME, Hummeler K: Thymic dysplasia ("Swiss agammaglobulinemia") II. Morphologic and functional observations. J Pediatr 70:737-744, 1967.
31. Ray CG, Davis S: Leukocyte interferon production in immunodeficiency diseases. Lancet 1:312, 1970.
32. Epstein LB, Ammann AJ: Evaluation of T-lymphocyte effector function in immunodeficiency disease: Abnormality in mitogen-stimulated interferon in patients with selective IgA deficiency. J Immunol 112:617-626, 1974.
33. Strannegard Ö, Björkander J, Hermodsson S, Lundgren E, Strannegard IL, Westberg G: Interferon in immunodeficient patients. Ann NY Acad Sci 350:589-590, 1980.
34. Wiranowska-Stewart M, Stewart WE II: Determination of human leukocyte populations involved in production of interferons alpha and gamma. J Interferon Res 1:233-244, 1981.
35. Kirchner H, Peter HH, Hirt HM, Zawatsky R, Dalugge H, Bradstreet P: Studies of the producer cell of interferon in human lymphocyte cultures. Immunobiology 156:65-75, 1979.
36. Herberman RB, Ortaldo JR: Natural killer cells: Their role in defense against disease. Science 214:24-30, 1981.
37. Ray CG: The ontogeny of interferon production by human leukocytes. J Pediatr 76:94-98, 1970.
38. Epstein LB: The comparative biology of immune and classical interferons. In Cohen S, Pick E, Oppenheim JJ (eds): "Biology of the Lymphokines." New York: Academic Press, 1979, pp 443-514.
39. Bryson YJ, Winter HS, Gard SE, Fischer TJ, Stiehm ER: Deficiency of immune interferon production by leukocytes of normal newborns. Cell Immunol 55:191-200, 1980.
40. Herberman RB, Ortaldo JR, Timonen T et al: Interferon and natural killer (NK) cells. Tex Rep Biol Med 41:590-595, 1982.
41. Payne CM, Glasser L: Evaluation of surface markers on normal human lymphocytes containing parallel tubular assays: A quantitative ultrastructural study. Blood 57:567-573, 1981.
42. Kay HD, Bonnard GD, West WH, Herberman RB: A functional comparison of human Fc-receptor-bearing lymphocytes in natural cytotoxicity and antibody-dependent cellular cytotoxicity. J Immunol 118:2058-2066, 1977.
43. Saksela E, Timonen T, Cantell K: Cellular interactions in the augmentation of human NK activity by interferon. Ann NY Acad Sci 350:102-111, 1980.
44. Parry RP, Parry JV: Interferon assay as a diagnostic test. Lancet 1:506-507, 1981.
45. Hooks JJ, Moutsopoulos HM, Geis SA et al: Immune interferon in the circulation of patients with autoimmune disease. N Engl J Med 301:5-8, 1979.
46. Hahn T, Levin S: Interferon system assay in children. In Khan A, Hill NO, Dorn GL (eds): "Interferon: Properties and Clinical Uses." Dallas: Leland Fikes, 1980, pp 579-588.
47. Merigan TC, Oldstone MBA, Welsh RM: Interferon production during lymphocytic choriomeningitis virus infection of nude and normal mice. Nature 268:67-68, 1977.
48. Cottier H, Bürki K, Hess MW, Hassig A: Pathological considerations of immunologic deficiency diseases in man. Supra #2, pp 152-168.
49. Gresser I, Morel-Maroger L, Rivière Y et al: Interferon-induced disease in mice and rats. Ann NY Acad Sci 350:12-20, 1980.
50. Bekesi JG, Roboz JP, Zimmerman E, Holland JF: Treatment of spontaneous leukemia in AKR mice with chemotherapy, immunotherapy or interferon. Cancer Res 36:631-636, 1976.

Impaired Production of Interleukins in Patients With Cellular Immunodeficiency*

R.J. Levinsky, R. Paganelli, F. Aiuti, and P.C.L. Beverley

Department of Immunology, Institute of Child Health, London, England (R.J.L.); Cattedra di Immunologia Clinica, Rome, Italy (R.P., F.A.), ICRF Human Tumour Immunology Group, University College Hospital Medical School, London, England (P.C.L.B.)

The poor PHA response of lymphocytes from 3 patients with defects of cell-mediated immunity was restored to normal when supernatants containing Interleukin 2 (IL-2) were added to the cultures. One of 3 children with SCID also showed a partial response. There was no improvement in the normal mitogenic response of lymphocytes from patients with either the X-linked or common variable forms of hypogammaglobulinemia. All 3 patients with cell-mediated immunodeficiencies showed gross imbalance in the ratio of OKT4$^+$ to OKT8$^+$ T lymphocytes. In addition, their PHA-stimulated supernatants failed to induce proliferation of a continuous cytolytic T-cell line which was dependent upon IL-2 for growth. Our data suggest that the defect in these patients may be a failure of production of ILs but not in the acquisition of IL-2 receptors.

*This is an abstract of Dr. Levinsky's presentation. A complete and detailed report can be found in Clin Exp Immunol 51:338–344, 1983.

Dipyridamole and Intravenous Deoxycytidine Therapy in a Patient With Adenosine Deaminase Deficiency

Arthur J. Ammann, MD, Morton J. Cowan, MD, David W. Martin, MD, and Diane W. Wara, MD

Departments of Pediatrics, Biochemistry, and Medicine, University of California, San Francisco, San Francisco, CA 94143

INTRODUCTION

The treatment of choice for patients with combined immunodeficiency disease (CID) is a histocompatible, sib, bone marrow transplant (BMT). Unfortunately, relatively few patients with adenosine deaminase (ADA) deficiency have potential donors. As a result, alternative means of immunotherapy are required. In ADA deficiency, an alternative therapy which has been evaluated is that of red blood cell (RBC) transfusion, which is felt to be effective in improving the immunodeficiency by means of enzyme replacement [1,2]. The high ADA activity of RBCs provides a means of metabolizing accumulated toxic metabolites, reducing the adverse effect on immunocompetent cells, and permitting temporary recovery of the immune system. Unfortunately, only a few of the patients with ADA deficiency have responded to regular RBC infusions. In addition, the significant risk of repeated RBC transfusion, including transfusion reactions, transmittal of viral infections, and iron overload, raises serious questions about the long-term use of this approach.

Biochemical studies of patients with ADA deficiency indicate that a mechanism of immunodeficiency may be the inhibition of ribonucleotide reductase by elevated levels of deoxyATP (dATP) which accumulate within the cells secondary to elevated plasma deoxyadenosine levels [3]. In cell culture models of ADA deficiency, it has been demonstrated that deoxycytidine is capable of reversing the toxic inhibition of ribonucleotide reductase by deoxyadenosine [4]. Although this mechanism has been clearly demonstrated in an in vitro model, a reversal of toxicity in vivo with complete recovery of immunologic function has not been accomplished in patients with ADA deficiency.

We describe here an 8-year-old girl with ADA deficiency and CID who was treated with intravenous (IV) deoxycytidine and oral dipyridamole in an attempt to improve her immunologic and biochemical abnormalities.

CASE REPORT

The patient is an 8-year-old female who was well until 3 years of age, when she became ill with fever and cough, and was hospitalized for pneumonia. Previously she had been entirely well and had received all of her childhood immunizations. Following the pneumonia, she developed a picture of recurrent upper respiratory illnesses (URI) and bronchitis, and was diagnosed as having asthma. The family moved from Michigan to California because of the father's job opportunity. When evaluated by a new allergist, it was felt that the patient had pulmonary disease disproportionate to her clinical history. Severe lymphopenia was observed, and the patient was suspected of having a primary immunodeficiency disease. There was no significant family history of immunodeficiency disease. A male sib was clinically normal.

On immunologic evaluation the patient was found to have severe lymphopenia, a marked reduction in the lymphocyte response to phytohemagglutinin (PHA) and alloantigen (MLC) (Table 1). Quantitative IGs were normal. Following immunization with pneumococcal polysaccharide and keyhole limpet hemocyanin (KLH), the patient had a positive antibody response, although at a reduced level.

METHODS

ADA activity was determined using a modification of the spectrophotometric method of uric acid production, as previously described [5]. Purine and pyrimidine metabolites were measured by high-pressure liquid chromatography (HPLC) in acid soluble extracts (trioctyl-amine Freon method) which were frozen at $-70°C$ until measurements were performed [6]. Tetrahydrouridine (THU) was added to blood collection tubes in which deoxycytidine determinations were made. Purine and pyrimidine metabolites were measured using HPLC [7]. Antibody measurements for response to pneumococcal polysaccharide and KLH were performed, as previously described [8]. Peripheral blood mononuclear cells (PBMC) were obtained from heparinized peripheral blood samples, uti-

TABLE 1. Response to Deoxycytidine (50 mg/kg/24 hr)

	Pre	Post 1 week (Course #1)	Post 3 months	Post 5 months	Post 2 weeks (Course #2)	Post 1 month	Post 2 months
ATC	232 ± 27	437	—	235	256	101	159
PHA	423 ± 199	521	1,881	634	2,441	253	200
MLC	1,602 ± 456	2,124	7,261	1,403	6,498	877	3,210

ATC: Absolute T-cell count
PHA: Phytohemagglutinin
MLC: Mixed lymphocyte culture

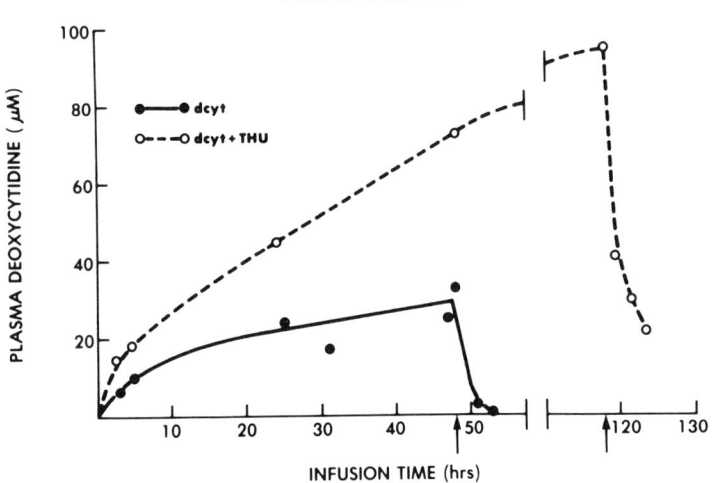

Fig. 1. Plasma deoxycytidine levels following intravenous infusion of deoxycytidine.

lizing Ficoll-Hypaque sedimentation techniques. T-cell studies included T-cell numbers and the response of PBMC to PHA and alloantigen [9].

THERAPY

The patient received 2 courses of IV deoxycytidine therapy in a dose of 50 mg/kg/24 hr for a total of 14 days for the first course and 12 days for the second course (Table 1). The first course was accompanied by an IV infusion of THU (an inhibitor of deoxycytidine deaminase) in a dose of 150 mg/kg/24 hr. The interval between the first and second course of IV deoxycytidine was 11 months. During the interval between the 2 deoxycytidine treatment courses, the patient received dipyridamole in a dose of 75 mg orally 3 times a day for a total period of 14 weeks. Dipyridamole is an inhibitor of purine and pyrimidine membrane transport.

RESULTS

ADA activity in the patient's RBCs was undetectable, while PBMC activity was 1.9% of normal controls. Levels in both parents were compatible with the heterozygote state, while the brother had normal activity. Prior to treatment, the patient's dATP level in RBCs was 200 µM (normal < 5 µM). Deoxyadenosine was elevated in her urine samples. Deoxyadenosine was not detected in plasma samples.

During IV deoxycytidine infusion an initial rapid rise in deoxycytidine levels was observed, with a subsequent more gradual increase approaching steady-state levels after 24–36 hours of therapy (Fig. 1).

When THU was added to the therapy, a steady-state level was not observed until after 72 hours of infusion. The deoxycytidine levels with THU were significantly greater than without THU (72 µM vs 30 µM, respectively). Following discontinuation of the deoxycytidine infusion, the plasma deoxycytidine levels fell rapidly, with a half-life of < 1 hr.

Biochemical measurements monitored during dipyridamole therapy included ATP/dATP ratios and concentrations. As deoxyadenosine levels were not elevated in the plasma, these could not be quantitated. Prior to dipyridamole therapy, the ATP/dATP ratios on 2 separate occasions were 9.9 and 12.9 (average 11.4). During dipyridamole therapy, ATP/dATP ratios increased gradually (16.8 to 17.8 and then to 30.6). Following discontinuation of dipyridamole therapy, values reverted to the range observed prior to therapy (10.0, 10.7). Determinations were performed on samples obtained with at least a month interval between samples (Table 2).

During the second IV infusion of deoxycytidine, THU was not administered. However, levels of plasma deoxycytidine were comparable to that observed in the first infusion without THU. A single blood sample containing a sufficient number of lymphocytes for HPLC analysis was obtained during this infusion. The dCTP levels were elevated and dATP was not detected.

IMMUNOLOGIC STUDIES

Following each course of deoxycytidine therapy, functional studies increased and subsequently returned to previous abnormal values. After the first course of deoxycytidine which was administered concomitantly with THU, the PHA response of PBMC rose to 1,881 cpm (normal > 11,750), while the MLC rose to 7,261 cpm (normal > 5,800) (Table 1).

Five months following therapy, the PHA response was 634 cpm, while the MLC response was 1,403 cpm. After the second course of deoxycytidine (11 months following the first course), the PHA rose to 2,441 cpm and the MLC rose to 6,498 cpm. One month following completion of therapy, the results were again depressed to pretreatment levels. No significant changes were observed in the absolute T-cell numbers before or after therapy following either treatment course.

In the interval between the 2 courses of IV deoxycytidine, the patient received a 3.5-month course of oral dipyridamole. After 3 months of therapy no significant changes were observed in the absolute numbers of T cells or the PHA response of PBMC (Table 2). The MLC response rose to 2,367 cpm, but this degree of response had been observed previously without any attempts at treatment. After 3.5 months of therapy the MLC became normal (7,351 cpm), while changes in the absolute number of T cells and the PHA response of PBMC were not observed. Prior to treatment, the ATP/dATP ratio averaged 11.4 in the patient's RBC extracts. During dipyridamole therapy the ATP/dATP ratio increased gradually to 16.8 and eventually reached 30.6. After cessation of therapy, immunologic studies returned to previously abnormal values and the ATP/dATP ratio fell to an average of 10.4.

DISCUSSION

In the absence of a histocompatible BMT donor, the majority of children with severe T-cell immunodeficiency lack effective alternative therapy. In patients with a defined biochemical abnormality, it may be possible to devise effective pharmacologic approaches with the potential of correcting the underlying immunodeficiency. In ADA deficiency, there are several possible mechanisms whereby immunocompetent T cells may succumb to the toxic effects which are a consequence of the ADA deficiency [10]. In vitro cell studies suggest that deoxycytidine is capable of overcoming the cell toxicity produced by deoxyadenosine [3]. Although other mechanisms such as inhibition of methylation reactions are also possible, experimental approaches to treatment are more easily approached by means of the administration of IV deoxycytidine.

The patient presented is similar to the 10–15% of patients with ADA deficiency who have CID and who present later in life [11]. She is somewhat unusual in that the diagnosis was not established until 8 years of age. The delayed diagnosis and mild clinical course may be explained on the basis of low levels of ADA activity found in the patient's PBMC, which was 1.9% of control values, while ADA activity in RBC was absent. It is of interest that there have been 2 cases reported with absent RBC ADA activity and 5% of normal ADA activity in lymphocytes with normal immunologic function [12, 13]. The data in this patient suggest that the threshold of ADA activity in lymphocytes required for normal immunologic function is somewhere between 2 and 5%.

Because the patient had a less severe form of CID and ADA deficiency, she represented an ideal candidate for attempts at biochemical therapy. The patient had normal Igs with definite antibody responses to pneumococcal polysaccharide (PPS) and KLH, although the level of response was reduced from normal. The patient also had a normal percent of T cells with a reduced absolute number. The PHA response of PBMC was absent on repeated occasions and occasionally the patient exhibited a 10–15% of normal response in MLC. Following 2 separate courses of IV deoxycytidine given 11 months apart, the patient developed an increased response of PBMC to PHA and MLC. Each time, following completion of therapy, the response returned to previously abnormal levels. Only the MLC response achieved normal values. The absolute number of T cells remained abnormal. On the first treatment course the patient also received THU, an inhibitor of deoxycytidine deaminase, in an attempt to increase the plasma levels of deoxycytidine and intracellular levels of dCTP. This was accomplished, and suggests that THU may be an effective adjunct therapy to IV deoxycytidine.

Dipyridamole is an effective inhibitor of purine and pyrimidine transport across cell membranes. An attempt was made to treat the patient with dipyrimadole to determine if deoxyadenosine could be prevented from entering the cells. Dipyridamole was administered separately from deoxycytidine so as not to prevent deoxycytidine from entering the cells. As an index of the effectiveness of this form of treatment, ATP/dATP ratios were performed before,

TABLE 2. Response to Dipyridamole (75 mg po tid)

	Pre	3 months on Dipyridamole	3.5 months on Dipyridamole	Post 3 weeks
ATC	235	137	175	—
PHA	634*	249	150	119
MLC	853*	2,367	7,351	3,200
ATP/dATP	11.4**	16.8 to 30.6 over 1 month		10.4*

ATC: Absolute T-cell count
PHA: Phytohemagglutinin
MLC: Mixed lymphocyte culture
*Average of 2
**Average of 3

during, and after treatment. Significant alterations in ratios were observed. The ATP/dATP ratio prior to therapy averaged 11.4, with a gradual increase observed during therapy to 16.8 and then to 30.6. Following cessation of a 3.5-month treatment course, the ratio returned to a value of 10.4. Following dipyridamole treatment, the patient achieved a normal MLC response (7,351 cpm), while the PHA response and the absolute numbers of T cells remained unchanged.

On 3 separate occasions and with 2 different forms of therapy, an improved immunologic response was observed in the patient. However, significant immunologic abnormalities remained. The present approach to treatment cannot therefore be considered as providing complete immunologic reconstitution. The results of these studies are nevertheless encouraging, and future trials in therapy would appear warranted. We do not feel that we have achieved an ideal treatment program utilizing a biochemical approach. Treatment with IV deoxycytidine could be provided on a regular basis, rather than for a 2-week course. In addition, more potent inhibitors of purine transport, which do not interfere with pyrimidine transport, are available. The combined therapy of IV deoxycytidine, THU, and a potent inhibitor of purine transport, given over a prolonged period of time, might lead to a synergistic effect and result in significant degrees of immunologic reconstitution.

REFERENCES

1. Polmar SJ et al: Enzyme replacement therapy for adenosine deaminase deficiency and severe combined immunodeficiency. N Engl J Med 295:1337–1343, 1976.
2. Donofrio J, Coleman MS, Hutton JJ: Overproduction of adenine deoxynucleosides and deoxynucleotides in adenosine deaminase deficiency with severe combined immunodeficiency disease. J Clin Invest 62:884–887, 1978.
3. Cohen A et al: Deoxyadenosine triphosphate as a potentially toxic metabolite in adenosine deaminase deficiency. Proc Natl Acad Sci USA 75(1):472–476, 1978.
4. Ullman B, Gudas LJ, Cohen A, Martin DW Jr: Deoxyadenosine metabolism and cytotoxicity in cultured mouse T-lymphoma cells. A model for immunodeficiency disease. Cell 14:365, 1978.
5. Cowan M, Fraga M, Andrew J et al: Purine salvage pathway enzyme activities in human T, B and null lymphocyte populations. Cell Immunol 67:121, 1982.
6. Khym JX: An analytical system for rapid separation of tissue nucleotides at low pressure on conventional anion exchanges. Clin Chem 21:1245, 1975.
7. Cohen A, Doyle D, Martin DW Jr, Ammann AJ: Abnormal purine metabolism and purine overproduction in a patient deficient in purine nucleoside phosphorylase. N Engl J Med 295:1449–1454, 1976.
8. Ammann AJ, Pelger RJ: Determination of antibody to pneumococcal polysaccharides following immunization using chromic chloride treated human red blood cells and indirect hemagglutination. Appl Microbiol 24:679–683, 1972.
9. Cowan M, Fujiwara P, Ammann AJ: Cellular immune defect in selective IgA deficiency using a microculture technique. Clin Immunol Immunopathol 17:595, 1980.
10. Hirschhorn R, Martin DW Jr: Enzyme defects in immunodeficiency diseases. Springer Seminars in Immunopathol 1:299–321, 1978.
11. Cowan M, Ammann AJ: Immunodeficiency syndromes associated with inherited metabolic disorders. In Mentzner WC (ed): "Clinics in Haematology." Philadelphia: WB Saunders, 1981, p 139.
12. Hirschhorn R, Vawter GF, Kirkpatrick JA Jr, Rosen FS: Adenosine deaminase deficiency: Frequency and comparative pathology in autosomally recessive severe combined immunodeficiency. Clin Immunol Immunopathol 14:107–120, 1979.
13. Jenkins T et al: Deficiency of adenosine deaminase not associated with severe combined immunodeficiency. J Pediatr 89:732–736, 1976.

Prenatal Diagnosis for Severe Combined Immunodeficiency

D.C. Linch, MRCP, C.H. Rodeck, MRCOG, H.A. Simmonds, PhD, and R.J. Levinsky, BSc, MD, FRCP

Institute of Child Health (R.J.L.), University College Hospital (D.C.L.), Kings College Hospital (C.H.R.), and Guy's Hospital (H.A.S.), London, England

INTRODUCTION

Severe combined immunodeficiency (SCID) is a heterogeneous syndrome inherited either as an X-linked or autosomal recessive disorder [1]. Affected children lack both CMI and humoral immunity. Most patients have an absolute deficiency of T-cell numbers, with numbers of B cells being absent, very low or very high. Within families, a similar pattern of T- and B-cell numbers is observed in affected individuals (personal experience of 6 families with more than one affected child). In 20% of the autosomal recessive type, the disease is due to a deficiency of ADA, and in these families prenatal diagnosis has been performed previously by demonstrating lack of the enzyme in amniotic cells [2]. For the remainder of cases, prenatal diagnosis has hitherto not yet been available. However, the development of monoclonal antibodies which distinguish leukocyte populations, and in particular T-cell subsets, has enabled normal ranges to be established in healthy children and adults (our unpublished data). Similarly, the diagnosis of various forms of immunodeficiency can be made by analyzing lymphocyte phenotypes. We have recently developed a method for analyzing the phenotype of leukocytes from very small samples of blood, using monoclonal antibodies and a fluorescent activated cell sorter (FACS). Using this technique, normal ranges for leukocyte populations have been established in the 2nd trimester of pregnancy on fetal blood samples (100–500 μl) obtained at fetoscopy for diagnosis of thalassemia and hemophilia [3]. It was therefore possible, knowing the phenotype of a previously affected sib, to offer prenatal advice to at-risk families during their second pregnancy. toscopy for diagnosis of thalassemia and hemophilia [3]. It was therefore possible, knowing the phenotype of a previously affected sib, to offer prenatal advice to at-risk families during their second pregnancy.

METHODS

Because < 500 μl of blood could be obtained from the midtrimester fetus at fetoscopy, it was not possible to fractionate mononuclear cells by Ficoll-Triosil centrifugation. A leukocyte-rich fraction was obtained by allowing red cells to sediment with hydroxyethyl starch (Plasmasteril) for 20 min (equal volumes added to heparanized blood sample). The nucleated cells remained in the supernatant and these were washed in the wells of a microtiter plate. The cells were stained at a concentration of 2.5–5 × 10^4 nucleated cells/ml in microtiter plates, the residual red cells acting as carrier cells for the washing steps. The following monoclonal antisera were used:

1. UCH1 which recognizes all mature T cells [4].
2. Leu 3a which recognizes helper/inducer T cells [5].
3. Leu 2a which recognizes suppressor/cytotoxic T cells [5].
4. DA2 which recognizes a nonpolymorphic determinant of HLA Dr antigen [6].
5. OKM1 which recognizes cells of the monocytic series, some granulocytes and cells with natural killer activity [7].
6. Anti-Hle-1 which reacts with all peripheral blood leukocytes [4].
7. B cells were recognized by staining surface Ig-bearing cells with fluorescent labeled rabbit or sheep antihuman Ig (Wellcome Laboratories).

The cells stained with monoclonal antisera were washed 3 times and then a second layer of fluorescent labeled sheep anti-mouse Ig. After tensive washing, the percentages of cells stained with fluorescent labeled antibodies were enumerated in a FACS. Just prior to analysis in the FACS, the residual red cells were lysed using dilute Zapoglobin (Coulter Electronics Ltd) (2 drops in 10 ml Isoton buffer—150 μl of this to 200 μl cell suspension). Fetal blood samples were obtained at fetoscopy for diagnosis of thalassemia and hemophilia and a normal range of leukocyte populations between 14–20 weeks' gestation derived [3].

The results of the whole blood analysis are expressed as a percentage of total leukocytes (Hle−1 +ve cells). On the same fetal blood specimens, control ranges were obtained for the purine salvage pathway enzymes, ADA and PNP.

PATIENTS

Three at-risk families for SCID have been screened during the 2nd trimester of pregnancy. In *Cases 1* and *2*, the index-affected children had SCID with high B-cell numbers, while the 3rd had SCID due to ADA deficiency.

Case 1

The results of the 18-week gestation fetal blood sample analysis was shown to be normal (Table 1 in

TABLE 1. % Whole Blood Leukocytes Hle-1 +ve

	UCH1 (pan T)	Leu 3a (helper T)	Leu 2a (supp/cyto-tox. T)	SIg (B)	Ba1 (B)	DA2 (HLA Dr)
CASE 1.						
Affected index* SCID sib	10	0	7	29	NT	54
Normal fetus 18/52 gest	57	40	18	7	NT	5
Baby retested* at birth	38	35	10	4	NT	20
CASE 2.						
Affected index* SCID sib	1	1	0	68	76	NT
Affected fetus 19/52 gest	0	0	5	38	36	NT
Fetal control range (n = 11; gest 14–20 weeks)	33–51	21–44	6–18	4–34	5–35	6–37

*Results expressed as % mononuclear cells after Ficoll-Triosil separation.
NT = not tested.

TABLE 2.

CASE 3 (ADA deficient)	Enzymes (nmol/mg Hb/h)	ADA	PNP
Fetal controls (n = 8)		range 31–41	range 3524–5524
Fetal SCID 18/52 gest.		<0.2	4562

dATP		
	μmol/1 packed cells	
Fetal controls (n = 8)	<40	
Fetal SCID	343	

Lymphocyte Subpopulations						
	UCH1 (pan T)	Leu 3a (helper T)	Leu 2a (supp/cytox T)	SIg (B)	DA2 (HLA Dr)	OKM1 (monocytes)
Index ADA** deficient SCID sib	1	0	0	0	21	22
Fetal SCID*	0	2	4	4	10	NT
Fetal controls* (n = 11) range	33–41	21–44	6–18	4–34	6–37	4–34

*Expressed as % of hetastarch separated whole blood leukocytes (Hle−1 +ve).
**Expressed as % of Ficoll-Triosil separated mononuclear cells.

comparison to the affected sib), and the pregnancy was continued. The normality was confirmed at birth and the child is thriving at age 10 months.

Case 2

The fetal blood analysis at 19-weeks' gestation showed absence of T cells (by E rosettes and T-cell monoclonal antisera) and very high B-cell numbers (Table 1). The fetus was aborted and the diagnosis of SCID was confirmed by absence of lymphocyte response to PHA, and histologically. At postmortem, no lymph nodes could be found; the thymus was rudimentary with fetal lobulation but there was a complete absence of any lymphocytes or thymocytes (by peroxidase staining using monoclonal antisera). The spleen showed an absence of lymphocytes in the T-cell areas around the penicillary arteries.

Case 3

The diagnosis of SCID due to ADA deficiency was confirmed in this 18-week fetus by absence of ADA activity, and accumulation of deoxyATP in the red cells. Contrary to expectations, fetal blood analysis here too showed complete absence of T-cell subpopulations (Table 2). The fetus was aborted and the diagnosis confirmed histologically.

DISCUSSION

We have previously shown that SCID can be diagnosed soon after birth by phenotype analysis of lymphocyte populations using monoclonal antisera [8]. Similarly, using these antisera and the FACS we have developed a technique of staining small numbers of cells, thereby being able to provide a leukocyte profile on very small blood samples. We have established a normal range of these leukocyte subpopulations for fetal blood from 14–20 weeks' gestation and have used this information to provide prenatal advice for 3 families at risk of having further children affected with SCID. Our results to date (one normal and 2 affected fetuses) confirm the reliability of the technique. Recently, prenatal diagnosis of SCID was established in France [9], although by using only 2 monoclonal markers. Our technique allows a greater range of antibodies to be used for a similar sized blood sample and should increase confidence in making such a diagnosis, especially when the phenotype of a previously affected sib is known. The risks of a miscarriage occurring after fetal blood sampling are < 3%, and most families would find that acceptable.

Prenatal diagnosis for SCID due to ADA has previously been performed by amniocentesis, culturing amniotic cells and measuring their enzyme activity 2–3 weeks later [2]. We have shown (*Case 3*) that it is possible to measure these purine enzymes on very small fetal blood samples and thereby rapidly establish the diagnosis. Contrary to expectations, where it was thought that the maternal circulation would deal with the accumulation of toxic deoxynucleotides and that lymphoid attrition was a late event in gestation, we found high levels of red cell dATP and a complete absence of T-cell subpopulations. Red cells actively take up adenosine type compounds [10], and this would explain the apparent inability of the maternal clearance system to dispose of these toxic metabolites, since little is left in the plasma. The combined results of raised dATP and absent T cells add further support to current thinking that the toxicity in ADA deficiency may occur at an earlier phase in the cell cycle than the ribonucleotide reductase step [11]. Whatever the mechanism, our findings indicate that in severe ADA deficiency, enzyme replacement or competitive substrate (ie deoxycytidine) therapy postnatally is never likely to succeed and the only conceivable form of treatment is bone marrow transplantation.

Our study illustrates that rapid prenatal diagnosis for the majority of cases of SCID is now available. The only variety not amenable to diagnosis is that where the child has normal percentages of T and B cells, but the cells do not function properly. Fortunately, this is the rarest variety of SCID.

ACKNOWLEDGMENTS

We thank the Leukaemia Research Fund, the Medical Research Council, and the National Fund for Research into Crippling Disease for generous grant support.

REFERENCES

1. Ammann AJ, Hong R: Disorders of the T cell system. In Stiehm ER, Fulginiti VA (eds): "Immunological Disorders in Infants and Children." Philadelphia: WB Saunders Co, 1980, pp 286–348.
2. Hirschhorn R: Clinical delineation of adenosine deaminase deficiency in enzyme defects and immune dysfunction. Ciba Found Symp 68 (New Series): 35–49, 1979.
3. Linch DC, Beverley PCL, Levinsky RJ, Rodeck CH: Phenotypic analysis of foetal blood leucocytes: Potential for antenatal diagnosis of immunodeficiency disorders. Prenatal Diagnosis 2:211–218, 1982.
4. Beverley PCL: Production and use of monoclonal antibodies in transplant immunology. Proc XI International Course on Transplant and Clinical Immunology. Amsterdam: Excerpta Medica, 1980, pp 87–94.
5. Evans RL, Wall DW, Peatsoncas GD: Thymus dependent membrane antigens in man: Inhibition of cell-mediated lympholysis by monoclonal antibodies to TH_2 antigen. Proc Natl Acad Sci USA 78:544–548, 1981.
6. Brodsky FM, Parham P, Barnstaple CJ, Crumpton MJ, Bodmer WF: Monoclonal antibodies for analysis of the HLA system. Immunol Rev 47:3–24, 1979.
7. Breard J, Reinherz EL, Kung PC, Goldstein G, Schlossman SF: A monoclonal antibody reactive with human peripheral blood monocytes. J Immunol 124:1943, 1980.
8. Levinsky RJ, Linch DC, Beverley PCL, Rodeck CH: Prenatal exclusion of severe combined immunodeficiency. Arch Dis Child 57:958, 1982.
9. Durandy A, Griscelli C, Dumez Y, Oury JF, Henrion R, Briard ML, Frezal J: Antenatal diagnosis of severe combined immunodeficiency from foetal cord blood. Lancet 1:852–853, 1982.
10. Simmonds HA, Webster DR, Perrett D, Reiter S, Levinsky RJ: Formation and degradation of deoxyadenosine nucleotides in inherited adenosine deaminase deficiency. Biosci Reports 2:303–314, 1982.
11. Fox RM, Kefford RF, Tripp EH, Taylor IW: G1 phase arrest of cultured human leukaemic T cells induced by deoxyadenosine. Cancer Res (In press)

Prenatal Diagnosis of Severe Combined Immunodeficiency and X-Linked Agammaglobulinemia

Anne Durandy, MD, and Claude Griscelli, MD

Unité d'Immunologie et d'Hématologie Pédiatriques, Département de Pédiatrie, INSERM U 132, Hôpital des Enfants Malades, 75730 Paris, France

Antenatal diagnosis of severe combined immunodeficiency (SCID) associated with a defect of adenosine deaminase (ADA) was achieved 7 years ago by assay of enzymatic activity in cultured amniotic cells [1]. The development of fetoscopy has led to the availability of pure fetal blood, allowing the antenatal diagnosis of hemoglobinopathies [2], hemophilia [3], and chronic granulomatous disease (CGD) [4]. We report here the prenatal diagnosis of SCID with alymphocytosis in a fetus at risk based on T- and B-lymphocyte marker analysis. The immunologic abnormality has been confirmed by studies performed after termination of pregnancy. We also studied other fetuses that had normal immunologic parameters permitting the continuation of pregnancy.

METHODS

Blood from 30 nonimmunodeficient fetuses and from the 7 propositi was obtained at fetoscopy according to a method described by Rodeck and Campbell [5]. Punctures were performed between 18 and 22 weeks' gestation in the vessels of the umbilical cord insertion, permitting an aspiration of 100–700 µl of fetal blood into preservative-free heparin. We investigated the immunologic status of the presumably nonimmunodeficient fetuses by taking advantage of fetal blood sampling justified for diagnosis of hemoglobinopathies. Since only an aliquot (100–150 µl) of fetal blood was available for immunologic tests, only limited investigations were performed for each fetus.

Purity of fetal blood was estimated by red blood cell size analysis with a Coulter channel analyzer and was later corroborated by the Kleihauer test. Mononuclear cells were isolated on a Ficoll-Hypaque gradient, washed, and analyzed for the markers of T and B lymphocytes. Monoclonal antibodies specific for T lymphocytes or T-cell subsets (OKT3, OKT4, and OKT8 antibodies, Ortho Pharmaceutical Corp., Raritan, NJ) were used in an indirect fluorescence test. B lymphocytes were revealed by rhodamine-labeled [F(ab)'2 fragments of anti-µ heavy chains or of anti-F(ab) IgG] antisera or rhodamine-labeled antiserum anti-δ heavy chains (Nordic Laboratory, Tilburg, The Netherlands). Monoclonal antibodies specific for β_2-microglobulin (Sera Lab, Crawley Down, Sussex, England) borne by all leukocytes or for common HLA-DR antigen (OKIa, Ortho Pharmaceutical Corp.) expressed by B lymphocytes and most monocytes, were also used in an indirect immunofluorescence test. Each fluorescence study was performed on cell suspension in a micromethod using $4-30 \times 10^3$ leukocytes; at least 250 cells were examined. Proliferative response of 40×10^3 leukocytes from fetuses or adults to PHA (10 µg/ml) (Difco Laboratories, Detroit, MI) was evaluated by incorporation of tritiated thymidine during the last 18 hours of a 3-day culture [6].

Histologic examination of fetal tissues was performed after fixation in Carnoy, Bouin, or Zenker solutions. Slides were stained with methyl green-pyronine, May-Grünwald Giemsa, or alcian blue.

CASE REPORTS

Prenatal diagnosis was attempted for 6 fetuses at risk for inherited immune deficiency: 4 for SCID due to a selective absence of precursor T cells [7], 1 for a SCID associated with a defective expression of HLA antigens [8], and 1 fetus at risk for X-linked agammaglobulinemia (SLA).

Prenatal diagnosis was also attempted in a woman who had previously given birth to a boy affected with SCID. This child died at 4 months of age with interstitial pneumonia, protracted diarrhea, and a maternofetal GVHD. Immunologic investigations performed immediately before death showed agammaglobulinemia (IgG 0.2 gm/liter, IgA and IgM not detectable), a subnormal number of lymphocytes (1.300/µl), and an absence of PHA-induced proliferation. ADA and nucleoside phosphorylase (NP) activities were found to be within normal range in both child and parents. Postmortem examination revealed a severe lymphoid depletion of spleen, lymph nodes, and thymus which did not contain Hassall corpuscles. In the absence of

TABLE 1. Immunologic Studies of 18–22 Week Fetuses

	Control fetuses (n = 30)		Fetuses at risk for immune deficiency						
			1	2	3	4	5	6	7
Lymphocytes/μl	4,200	± 1,200	3,000	3,200	1,300	NT	200	3,600	2,500
Lymphocyte markers									
OKT3	53.7 ±	8.4	65	80	62	74	1	NT	82
SIg	13.7 ±	2.5	NT	NT	34	NT	NT	NT	16
SIgM	16.6 ±	5.0	11	19	44	6.5	0	8	8
SIgD	14.2 ±	2.9	NT	NT	38	NT	NT	NT	18
Common DR	18.2 ±	10.1	NT	NT	NT	NT	NT	17	NT
β_2-microglobulin	94.7 ±	5.6	NT	NT	NT	NT	NT	88	NT
PHA-induced proliferation									
NS	0.5 ±	0.5	0.8	—	NT	0.3	NT	NT	NT
PHA	43 ±	27	36	N	NT	38	NT	NT	NT

1, 2, 3, 4 = fetuses at risk for SCID with selective absence of T cells
5 = fetus at risk for alymphocytosis and agammaglobulinemia
6 = fetus at risk for SCID with defective expression of HLA
7 = fetus at risk for SLA
N = normal, large percentage of PHA-induced blast-cells.
NS = not stimulated
NT = not tested

RESULTS

In the 37 fetuses investigated for diagnosis of hemoglobinopathies or diagnosis of SCID, contamination with maternal blood, as judged by red blood cell size and the Kleihauer test, was nil or below 3% in 31 samples and below 10% in 6 others. In the 30 presumably nonimmunodeficient fetuses, T- and B-lymphocyte membrane markers, including common HLA-DR and β_2-microglobulin, were easily detectable by immunofluorescence (Table 1). These percentages, as well as proportions of OKT4 (helper subset) and OKT8 (suppressive-cytotoxic subset) among total T-cell populations (OKT3), were comparable to those found in adults; β_2-microglobulin and HLA-DR antigens were normally found on fetal leukocyte membranes. PHA-induced proliferative responses were identical in fetuses and control adults. In 6 fetuses at risk for SCID, and in the fetus at risk for SLA, immunologic studies showed the absence of a detectable immunologic defect which was completely confirmed after birth for 3 of them (Table 1). The others are not yet born.

Pure fetal blood (500 μl) was obtained at the 22nd week of gestation from another fetus at risk for SCID (Table 1, n 5). We observed a profound lymphopenia (200/μl) characterized by a complete absence of mature T and B lymphocytes (Table 1). Termination of the pregnancy was performed by local injection of prostaglandin E_2. The fetus (a male) measured 18 cm from crown to rump and weighed 550 gm, corresponding to the presumed term. The alymphocytosis was confirmed in blood (300/μl). No T and B lymphocyte markers were detected and, as expected, PHA-induced proliferation was nil.

The macroscopic study showed no anomaly except for the weight of the thymus (0.107 gm). At the histologic examination, the lobulation of the thymus was normal, but it contained no lymphocytes and only a few Hassall corpuscles. The spleen was deprived of white pulp; the lymph nodes, normally located, were devoid of lymphocytes. No lymphocytes were observed in the gut mucosa and appendix.

DISCUSSION

The diagnosis of SCID associated with enzyme abnormality has been accomplished during intrauterine life by amniotic cell enzymatic study. In SCID without detectable enzyme deficiency, diagnosis remains possible in the prenatal period by analysis of T- and B-lymphocyte markers of pure fetal blood obtained at fetoscopy. We report the prenatal diagnosis of a SCID characterized by a profound lymphopenia and an absence of T- and B-lymphocyte surface markers. These results, compared to normal values observed in nonimmunodeficient fetuses, justified the termination of pregnancy. The diagnosis was confirmed by histologic examination, which showed a complete lymphocyte depletion of lymphoid organs. The lymphoid organs of 22-week fetuses contain easily detectable lymphocytes already organized in the spleen (white pulp) and lymph nodes [9]. In the propositus, thymus weight was one-tenth the norm for the age of gestation [10].

Other documented cases in the family, the mode of inheritance could not be defined.

The detection of lymphocyte membrane markers may permit antenatal diagnosis of several types of SCID, characterized by either absence of both T and B cells (alymphocytosis with agammaglobulinemia) or a defect of precursor T lymphocytes [7]. Furthermore, it may allow the prenatal diagnosis of SLA characterized by a complete absence of surface Ig-bearing cells. We used the same method to detect other membrane-associated antigens, such as histocompatibility antigens A-B and DR, and β2-microglobulin, known to be poorly expressed on leukocytes of some patients with SCID [8].

We must stress that prenatal diagnosis of immune deficiency can be performed only when a previously affected child in the family has been investigated. The precise abnormality of lymphocyte markers must be known to allow a prenatal diagnosis in a further pregnancy.

The mode of inheritance of an immune deficiency must also be taken into consideration because, in an X-linked inherited disease, fetoscopy would be proposed only in male fetuses of pregnant women at risk.

Other immune deficiencies are not yet detectable in the prenatal period using detection of surface antigen markers of T and B lymphocytes or proliferative response of T lymphocytes induced by mitogens. For example, prenatal diagnosis of ataxia telangiectasia or Wiskott-Aldrich syndrome cannot be performed because they are not characterized by an absence of a defined lymphocyte population or by a constant immunologic abnormality.

REFERENCES

1. Hirschhorn R, Beratis N, Rosen FS: Adenosine deaminase deficiency in a child diagnosed prenatally. Lancet 1:73, 1975.
2. Dubart A, Gooseens M, Beuzard Y, Monplaisir N, Testa U, Basset P, Rosa J: Prenatal diagnosis of hemoglobinopathies. Comparison of the results obtained by isoelectric focusing of hemoglobins and by chromatography of radioactive globin chains. Blood 56:1092, 1980.
3. Firshein S, Hoyer I, Lazarchick J, Forget B, Hobbins J, Clyne L, Pitlick F, Muir A, Markatz I, Mahoney M: Prenatal diagnosis of classic hemophilia. N Engl J Med 300:937, 1979.
4. Newburger PE, Cohen HJ, Rothschild SB, Hobbins C, Malawista SE, Mahoney M: Prenatal diagnosis of chronic granulomatous disease. N Engl J Med 300:178, 1979.
5. Rodeck CH, Campbell CH: Umbilical cord insertion as source of pure fetal blood for prenatal diagnosis. Lancet 1:1244, 1979.
6. Durandy A, Dumez Y, Oury C, Griscelli C: Prenatal testing for inherited immune deficiencies by fetal blood sampling. Prenatal Diag 2:109–113, 1982.
7. Griscelli C, Durandy A, Virelizier JL, Ballet JJ, Daguillard F: Selective defect of precursor T cells in SCID with B lymphocytes. J Pediatr 93:404, 1978.
8. Griscelli C, Durandy A, Virelizier JL, Hors J, Lepage V, Colombani J: Impaired cell to cell interaction in partial combined immunodeficiency with variable expression of HLA antigens. In Seligmann M, Hitzig WH (eds): "Primary Immunodeficiencies." INSERM Symposium No. 16. Amsterdam: Elsevier/North Holland Biomedical Press, 1980, p 499.
9. Stites P, Caldwell J, Carr M, Fudenberg H: Ontogeny of immunity in humans. Clin Immunol Immunopathol 4:519, 1975.
10. Bellanti J: General immunobiology: Concepts of immunobiology. In "Immunobiology." Philadelphia: WB Saunders, 1971, p 13.

Transplantation of Hematopoietic Cells for Lethal Congenital Immunodeficiencies*

Richard J. O'Reilly, MD, Neena Kapoor, MD, Dahlia Kirkpatrick, MD, Neal Flomenberg, MD, Marilyn S. Pollack, PhD, Bo Dupont, MD, Robert A. Good, MD, PhD, and Yair Reisner, PhD

Memorial Sloan-Kettering Cancer Center, New York, NY 10021 (R.J.O'R., D.K., N.F., M.S.P., B.D.), Oklahoma Medical Research Foundation, Oklahoma City, OK 73104 (R.A.G., N.K.), Weizmann Institute of Science, Rehovot, Israel (Y.R.)

INTRODUCTION

In 1968, HLA-histocompatible transplants of allogeneic human marrow were first applied successfully to the treatment of severe combined immunodeficiency (SCID) [1] and Wiskott-Aldrich syndrome (WAS) [2]. Since that time, marrow transplantation has rapidly emerged as a curative approach to a series of lethal congenital diseases of the lymphoid and hematopoietic systems, and as the treatment of choice for aplastic anemia [3] and for acute and chronic forms of leukemia refractory to conventional chemotherapy [4–6]. Since that time, also, patients chronically ill with lethal immunodeficiencies have continuously provided both the disease models and clinical imperatives which have led to the development of new transplantation approaches for patients lacking an HLA-identical sib donor.

In this brief review, we will summarize current results of HLA-matched marrow transplants for lethal congenital immunodeficiencies.

*This investigation was supported by PHS Grant Numbers: CA23766, CA33050, CA22507, NIH Ag03592, NF-18851, AI 19495 awarded by the National Institute of Health DHEW; and the Robert J. Kleberg and Helen C. Kleberg Foundation, the Charles A. Dana Foundation, the Lila Acheson and DeWitt Wallace Fund, the Zelda Radow Weintraub Cancer Fund, the International Paper Foundation, the March of Dimes Birth Defects Foundation #1-789.

We will also assess the experience with new transplant approaches for patients lacking HLA-identical sib donors which have been developed over the last 5 years, and describe some of the obstacles to success of unmodified or T-cell-depleted hematopoietic grafts from partially histocompatible or fully allogeneic donors which are already evident. In this analysis, we will attempt to construct testable hypotheses to explain the biology of these transplant problems, using as reference, information drawn from our own experience with such transplants in patients with SCID (24 patients), WAS (5 patients), and other lethal congenital immune disorders (7 patients).

HLA-IDENTICAL SIB MARROW GRAFTS

Transplants of HLA-identical sib marrow have long been the treatment of choice for all forms of SCID. In an updated survey of 59 patients transplanted with HLA genotypically identical marrow representing the cumulative experience of major centers treating SCID (Table 1), 34 were reported surviving with full immunologic reconstitution. Significant GVHD (grades 2–4) was observed in only 10% of cases. Failures were principally ascribed to interstitial pneumonia developing early in the course of immune reconstitution.

Both the lymphoid and platelet abnormalities of the lethal sex-linked disorder, WAS, can be corrected by a marrow transplant, provided a myeloablative agent, such as total body irradiation [7], or busulfan [8] is administered in conjunction with standard high-dose cyclophosphamide. The combination of busulfan and cyclophosphamide has been particularly tolerable, with successful grafts and long-term survival documented in each of 9 cases in which it has been used.

Transplants of HLA-identical marrow after myeloablation and immunosuppression have also been documented to correct a series of other lethal congenital diseases of host resistance, including reticular dysgenesis (R. Levinsky, personal communication), congenital agranulocytosis [9], the cartilage-hair hypoplasia syndrome [10], and chronic granulomatous disease (R. Parkman, personal communication).

TRANSPLANTS OF UNMODIFIED MARROW FROM HLA GENOTYPICALLY NONIDENTICAL BUT COMPATIBLE DONORS

Until recently, marrow transplants have been almost exclusively reserved for the patient possessing an HLA-identical sib donor. The consistent observation of lethal GVHD in SCID patients engrafted following infusions of marrow or blood from HLA haplotype mismatched parental donors [11] indicated the relatively

TABLE 1. Marrow Transplantation for SCID (International Experience)

Donor	Patients	Reconstitution T	Reconstitution B	Survival With Reconstitution	Grades 2–4 GVHD
HLA genotypically identical relative	59	41	41	34 (57%)	
HLA phenotypically identical relative	10	6	4	3 (30%)	4
HLA-D-compatible relative	11	8	6	4 (36%)	8
Unrelated HLA-D-compatible donor	4	2	1	1 (25%)	2

rigid requirement for HLA identity for marrow grafts.

From 1968 on, 21 transplants from related donors HLA genotypically identical for one haplotype, and either HLA-A,B,D phenotypically identical (10 patients), or at least HLA-D identical for the other haplotype (11 patients) have been attempted to correct SCID (Table 1). Of these patients, 10 have achieved full immunologic reconstitution, and 7 are long-term survivors. Moderate-to-severe GVHD has been observed in over half of these cases, and contributed to death in 3 cases. For a significant proportion of these cases, multiple transplants were required to achieve full engraftment and functional reconstitution, or to reverse GVH-induced aplasia [1,12,13]. More recently, this approach to donor selection has also been applied with increasing success to transplants for leukemia and aplastic anemia [14,15]. Cumulative results suggest that engraftment of HLA disparate marrow will require different or more intensive immunosuppression. At least 50% of aplastic patients transplanted from HLA partially mismatched donors, after cyclophosphamide preparation, have either failed to engraft or suffered graft rejection; up to 15% of leukemia patients have also failed to engraft despite preparation with at least 10 GRAY (Gy) total body irradiation and cyclophosphamide. The incidence and severity of GVHD has been somewhat increased [15]. Surprisingly, however, in transplants for aplasia and leukemia, this increased severity has not been correlated with genetic disparity for any one determinant within the HLA complex. Contrary to expectations, isolated disparity for HLA-D has been tolerated as well as other isolated incompatibilities (eg for HLA-A) [15]. In the end, comparative review of cumulative results suggests that transplants of HLA-nonidentical but compatible marrow are only slightly less effective than transplants from HLA-identical sibs. Improvements in these results can be expected if more intensive, yet tolerable immunosuppressive regimens are developed to insure engraftment.

Recognition of common HLA-A,B,D haplotypes also permits identification of HLA phenotypically identical unrelated donors, but only for those rare individuals who inherit 2 such haplotypes. To date, only 9 individuals have been reported to have been transplanted with marrow from an unrelated, histocompatible donor [16–23]. Of these patients, 4 (1 transplanted for SCID between 1973 and 1975 [17], 3 transplanted for aplasia in 1981 [21–23]) are alive, chimeric, with full hematopoietic and lymphoid function but with chronic GVHD. One patient transplanted for leukemia [20] experienced no GVHD, but ultimately died with leukemic relapse. A sixth patient, transplanted for chronic granulomatous disease (CGD) survives with clinical improvement, but was never convincingly engrafted [19]. This limited experience indicates the feasibility of such transplants, but underscores the possibility that graft rejection and severe GVHD may be more common, enhancing morbidity and mortality. Results of experimental marrow transplants between unrelated, DLA compatible dogs are in accord with such predictions [24].

TRANSPLANTS OF FETAL LIVER OR MARROW-DERIVED HEMATOPOIETIC CELLS FROM HLA-NONIDENTICAL DONOR

Recently, significant progress has been made in developing techniques to allow transplants of histoincompatible marrow without risk of lethal GVHD. Early studies in murine models established that GVHD is initiated by thymus-derived T lymphocytes [25]. Subsequent work in rodent systems has demonstrated that depletion of T lymphocytes from the hematopoietic grafts, or manipulation of the host environment in which alloreactive T lymphocytes develop, can permit engraftment and hematopoietic reconstitution in lethally irradiated histoincompatible marrow graft recipients without GVHD. Techniques for T-cell depletion which have been found to be effective in preventing GVHD in inbred rodent models include: transplants of fetal liver [26], treatment of allogeneic marrow or spleen cell grafts with cytotoxic antibodies specific for T lymphocytes [27–29], differential separation of hematopoietic precursors by agglutination with lectins [30] or by extended cell cultures [31], and selective elimination or "suicide" of host-specific alloreactive donor T cells by treating host-sensitized cultures of donor marrow with ^{3}H-thymidine, BUDR, viruses lytic for activated T cells, such as vesicular stomatitis virus, or idiotype specific antibodies [32–35]. In certain rodent models, GVHD may also be abrogated by pretreatment of the recipient with total lymphoid irradiation [36] or treatment with cyclosporine during the posttransplant period [37].

Experience with fully allogeneic or HLA-haplotype mismatched hematopoietic grafts in man is extremely limited, and largely derived from attempts to reconstitute lymphoid function in patients with SCID. Early transplants incorporating in vitro "suicide" techniques either did not engraft or failed to prevent GVHD [38,39]. The initial successful use of an allogeneic fetal liver transplant to provide normal lymphoid progenitors to a patient with SCID, reported by Keightley et al [40] in 1975, stimulated trials of this approach by a number of centers, including our own. In 1980, I reviewed the cumulative international experience with this approach [41]. Of 52 evaluable patients, only 19 had achieved durable engraftment; 15 achieved full or partial reconstitution of cell-mediated immunity (CMI), but only 8 formed antibody in response to immunization. Only 6 of the 52 patients (11%) achieved long-term survival. Touraine has reviewed the recent experience with this approach in Europe [42]. Of 21 patients transplanted with fetal liver, of whom 17 also received prelymphoid thymus from the same fetus, 13 achieved engraftment after one or more transplant attempts. Partial or full reconstitution of CMI was achieved in 10 patients; humoral immunity in 5. Of the 21 patients, 7 now survive 1–5 years postgrafting. Both of these reports underscore nonengraftment of fully allogeneic T-cell-depleted fetal hematopoietic cells, and the partial reconstitution achieved as the major obstacles to success. GVHD was observed in 50% of engrafted patients, but was severe only in recipients of liver and thymus from fetuses of more than 13 weeks' gestation.

From 1975 to 1981, we explored the use of fetal tissue grafts for SCID and for aplastic anemia, attempting to define the characteristics of graft and host which might influence ultimate engraftment and functional reconstitution. A total of 23 transplants of liver with or without thymus from fetuses of less than 12 weeks' gestation were administered to 8 patients with SCID. Engraftment of lymphoid precursors was documented by HLA phenotype or karyotype following 9 of the 23 transplants. Sustained engraftment of lymphoid cells from a single fetal liver source was achieved in 6 cases. We compared the fetal liver transplants which did and did not engraft. All fetal tissues were transplanted within 2 hours of elective prostaglandin or hysterotomy-induced abortion. No differences in fetal gestation age, cell viability, transplant cell dose, dose/kg/bw, or degree of HLA homology between donor and host were detected to account for the low incidence of sustained engraftment observed [41]. Clinical findings suggested that patients with SCID exhibit a variable degree of resistance to engraftment of allogeneic hematopoietic cells. Of the 6 patients who achieved durable engraftment, 4 were engrafted without preparative immunosuppression by liver cells derived from their initial fetal transplant. The other 2 patients, like the 2 fetal liver recipients in our series who were never chimeric, received multiple fetal liver and thymus transplants in sequence without engraftment, and ultimately achieved engraftment only when transplanted after preparation with either antithymocyte globulin or cyclophosphamide. A similar form of resistance was also seen in our patient transplanted from an unrelated donor, who failed to achieve sustained chimerism despite 4 marrow grafts. This patient was ultimately reconstituted only after treatment with cyclophosphamide and another transplant from the same donor [18].

Of the 6 patients engrafted with fully allogeneic fetal liver-derived T cells, 3 developed strong transformation responses to mitogens. Four patients developed normal or near normal responses to allogeneic cells, and significant responses to *Candida albicans*, to which all were heavily exposed. These results are summarized in Table 2, with responses expressed as a percent of the response of normal adult controls. Three of these patients developed antigen-specific delayed type hypersensitivity. Of the 6 engrafted patients, including the 3 who developed full or partial reconstitution of what are considered genetically unrestricted T-cell functions, only 2 were able to form specific antibody. One of these patients, whose B lymphocytes were of host type, shared HLA specificities with the engrafted fetal-derived T cells.

The other patient, who remains chimeric and reconstituted 7 years posttransplant, initially developed an effective in vivo granulomatous re-

TABLE 2. Cell-Mediated Immune Function in SCID Patients Engrafted With Allogeneic Fetal Liver and Thymus

Patient	Lymphocyte transformation*					LMIF production	DTH DNCB	Granuloma
	PHA	Con A	PWM	MLC	Candida			
K.M.	105	194	129	75	43	+	+	+
M.W.	128	138	79	94	49	+	+	NT
P.A.	34	49	27	90	30	+	+	NT
J.J.	14	7	13	57	52	−	−	−
D.V.	5	9	23	9	3	−	−	−
M.V.	7	2	10	4	1	−	−	−

*Results presented as a percent of the response of positive normal controls.
Key: LMIF = leukocyte migration inhibition factor; DTH = delayed type hypersensitivity; DNCB = dinitrochlorobenzene.

sponse, thereby clearing a disseminated *Mycobacterium avium* infection. This patient has subsequently sustained chickenpox and occasional minor upper respiratory infections. The clinical course of these infections has been mild and not different from that observed in normal children. This is the only recipient of fully allogeneic fetal liver and thymus to develop antibody responses in our series. Interestingly, this patient was unable to generate antibody either in vitro or in vivo for over one year after engraftment and reconstitution of transformation responses and delayed type hypersensitivity. During this period, T lymphocytes were found to be of donor type, while non-T populations were exclusively of host type. Thereafter, and concurrently with lymphoid infiltration and maturation of the fetal donor's thymus which had been implanted in the rectus abdominis at the time of the original infusion of fetal liver cells, E-rosette negative cells of donor origin were detected transiently. Since that time, the patient has been able to form antibody in vivo and in vitro in response to immunization. Circulating B lymphocytes have reverted to host type. Unfortunately, we have not been able to define the antibody produced as host or donor in origin. However, we have recently tested this patient and found him to be able to mount influenza virus-specific, T-cell mediated cytotoxic responses. Interestingly, the engrafted virus-sensitized fetal-type T cells, which are HLA-A,B mismatched with the host, exhibit selective toxicity against virus-infected lymphoblasts sharing the HLA specificities of the host, but *not* of the fetus. This preliminary evidence would suggest that in man, as in murine models [43,44], developing lymphoid precursors may acquire the capacity for effective T-cell-mediated interactions with cells bearing host-type histocompatibility determinants.

We initially questioned whether the persistent humoral immune deficiencies seen in most of our reconstituted fetal liver transplant recipients were merely the sequelae of partial engraftment, which was limited in all but one case to the fetal T-cell precursors. However, Kapoor, Chaganti, and Pollack (unpublished observations) evaluated these and other patients in our series. Using HLA typing and karyotypic analysis of separated macrophages, B and T lymphocytes, they demonstrated that the majority of patients transplanted with HLA-matched or partially matched marrow also failed to develop donor B lymphocytes, yet residual host B lymphocytes were able to make antibody normally both in vivo and in vitro following immunization.

Given this finding, we have hypothesized that persisting humoral immune deficiencies observed in most of our fetal liver transplant recipients reflect genetic restrictions, ie failures of T-B cooperation due to the total HLA disparity existing between donor T and host B lymphocytes. Our recent observations of virus-specific cytotoxic responses in a long-term fetal liver chimera, and Touraine's observation of virus-specific antibody formation in a fetal liver chimera whose donor T cells are fully allogeneic to the host [46] do suggest, however, that effective cooperation can develop in certain circumstances.

In murine systems it is increasingly clear that genetic restrictions are imposed on developing lymphoid cells by antigen-presenting cells, particularly in the thymus [44]. If such cells are of host-type, effective T-cell learning with host-specific restriction would be expected to occur [44]. If, however, cells of donor origin constitute the initial antigen-presenting cells migrating to the thymus, subsequent cooperative interactions between donor T cells and host cells would not be anticipated [47]. Assuming the observed humoral immune deficiencies in fully allogeneic fetal liver chimeras do reflect restrictions imposed by the genetic background of antigen-presenting cells, the high incidence of such deficiencies following fetal liver grafts suggests the latter chain of events to be the more common sequela of fetal liver transplants in man.

The problems of engraftment and restricted immunologic function might be significantly circumvented were it possible to transplant in man partially matched marrow cells containing lymphoid precursors but, like fetal liver, depleted of the T lymphocytes capable of inducing GVHD. Recently, this has been accomplished by Reisner et al [48–50] with the development of a lectin-based technique for T-cell depletion of human marrow, and more recently, with a technique by Reinherz et al [51] using a T-cell-specific monoclonal antibody for cell depletion by immune, complement-dependent cytolysis.

We have now developed an experience with soybean lectin-separated, E-rosette depleted histoincompatible marrow grafts in the treatment of SCID which we would like to review. We believe this preliminary experience already provides some insights about their potential and their limitations. The technique itself is relatively simple, and has recently been modified for separation of large volumes of human marrow [49]. As currently used, it involves Hetastarch sedimentation of red cells followed by differential agglutination and sedimentation of T cells and other mature blood elements in the marrow with soybean agglutinin, followed by removal of residual, exclusively Leu2+ T lymphocytes by E- and E_N-rosette formation and subsequent rosette depletion by differential density gradient centrifugation [49]. The $SBA^-E^-E_N^-$ marrow cells fractionated by this procedure represent

TABLE 3. SBA⁻E⁻E$_N$⁻ Marrow Cell Grafts for SCID

Patient/ UPN	Date of transplant		Preparation	Donor	Cell dose per kg	Engraftment	Chimeric state	Lymphoid reconst.	GVHD	Months surv.	Cause of failure
M.V./75	1.	12/18/80	none MTX post	father	3.4×10^7	−	−	−	0	3	graft failure
	2.	3/27/81	none	"	4.1×10^7	+	T,B part	full T,B	0	>21	−
J.S./30	1.	1/28/81	ATG,CTX	father	3.2×10^7	−	−	−	−	3	graft failure
	2.	5/07/81	none	mother	7.8×10^7	+	T,B	full T,B	0	>19	−
J.R./226	1.	12/24/81	none	father	4.3×10^7	+ trans.	T	part. T/trans	0	5	graft failure
	2.	5/20/82	none	mother	9.4×10^7	0	0	0	0	2	graft failure
	3.	7/16/82	ATG,CTX	mother	6.6×10^7	+	T	full T, early B	0	>5	−
S.H./240	1.	12/30/81	none	mother	15.8×10^7	+	T	± T	1	3	−
	2.	4/14/82	none	mother	6.7×10^7	+	T,B	full T,B	0	>8	−
A.W./266	1.	4/16/82	none	father	6.2×10^7	+	T	0	0	3	−
	2.	7/10/82	ATG,CTX	mother	7.0×10^7	+	paternal T bichimeric B	full T early B	0	>5	−
S.G./267	1.	4/30/82	none	father	9.0×10^7	+	+	none	−	3	−
	2.	7/29/82	none	father	7.1×10^7	+	+	partial T	0	>5	−

Key: UPN = unit patient number; ATG = antithoracic duct lymphocyte globulin; MTX = methotrexate; CTX = cyclophosphamide.

4–6% of the nucleated cells present in the unfractionated marrow. They contain 80–100% of the available CFU$_c$ and 70–90% of the available BFU$_e$ in the mixed marrow pool, but are depleted of T cells detectable by E-rosette formation or reactivity with T-cell-specific monoclonal antibodies, even after expansion in the presence of IL-2 or incubation with thymic supernatants. SBA⁻E⁻E$_N$⁻ marrow cells fail to respond to mitogens or to allogeneic cells by in vitro transformation. Furthermore, alloreactive cytotoxic cells cannot be generated from these cell fractions.

Initially, we tested the potential of marrow grafts depleted of T cells by this technique for restoring hematopoietic function in lethally irradiated, cyclophosphamide-treated Cynomolgus monkeys. In this model, female monkeys pretreated with 1,000–1,320r TBI and cyclophosphamide, regularly engraft following transplantation of treated marrow from unrelated MLC mismatched male donors. Animals receiving untreated marrow develop GVHD. In contrast, lectin marrow graft recipients develop neither clinical nor histologic evidence of GVHD.

In December 1980, we used our initial technique, which reversed the order of T-cell depletion steps [48] to provide a transplant for a child with SCID who was also suffering from a partially resected neuroblastoma and severe pulmonary disease due to a documented parvovirus infection. The transplant was derived from the patient's HLA-A,B,D haplotype mismatched mother. Engraftment was detected by 10 days, at which time the patient developed a generalized rash and hepatitis, suggesting mild GVHD. Skin biopsies failed to demonstrate histologic evidence of GVHD. Abnormalities cleared with a short course of prednisone. Thereafter, the patient developed partial reconstitution of T-cell function, as documented by development of E rosettes, and transformation responses to mitogens and to antigens to which the patient was exposed, specifically *Candida albicans*. Responding cells were of female karyotype and carried the maternal HLA phenotype. The preexisting parvovirus infection of the lung then became more severe, leading to death 12 weeks' posttransplant. At autopsy, lymph nodes and spleen were found to have normal architecture and were well populated with maternal lymphocytes. GVHD was not detected in any organ, including skin, liver, gastrointestinal tract, or bronchopulmonary tree. The liver was studded with micrometastases of neuroblastoma. The lung parenchyma was heavily infiltrated with lymphocytes, monocytes, and plasma cells, suggesting a strong immune response to the offending pathogen.

Encouraged by this initial experience, and having modified the procedure to the sequence of separation steps described above [49], we have since transplanted 7 more patients, 6 of whom are evaluable. These cases are detailed elsewhere [50,52]. For each of the 6 patients, an HLA-A,B,D haplotype disparate parent served as donor. The mean dose of SBA⁻E⁻E$_N$⁻ marrow cells was 6.9×10^7 cells/kg/bw. Each of the 6 patients, for reasons of engraftment or functional reconstitution, has required more than one transplant. The transplants are summarized in Table 3.

Five patients were transplanted primarily from HLA-A,B,D haplotype mismatched paternal donors. The first of these patients (*UPN/75*) was given methotrexate for GVHD prophylaxis following his initial transplant and failed to engraft, but after a secondary transplant from the father, administered without subsequent methotrexate, engrafted promptly and is now fully reconstituted 21 months' posttransplant. Another patient (*UPN/226*) was engrafted, and developed responses to mitogens and to allogeneic cells approaching 15–20% of normal within 2 months of transplant, but lost the graft in the third month. A secondary transplant from the mother also failed to take. On 7/16/82, the patient received another maternal graft after preparation with cyclophosphamide and ATG. Engraftment was first detected 15 weeks' postgrafting, but was followed by a rapid functional reconstitution. Now more than 6 months' posttransplant, he is at home and well. T-cell numbers and responses to mitogens, antigens, and allogeneic cells are normal. Immunoglobulin levels are rising; antibody responses are being evaluated. A third patient (*UPN/267*) was engrafted primarily, but it was not until 2 months after a secondary graft and 5 months after the initial transplant, that development of T cells responsive to mitogens and allogeneic cells was appreciated. Six months after the second graft, this patient remains chimeric, but with only a limited T-cell reconstitution. The other 2 patients primarily transplanted from paternal donors were already chimeric with immunologically nonreactive maternal lymphocytes presumably derived from an intrauterine transplacental infusion [53]. *Patient UPN/30* failed to engraft with paternal cells despite preparation with cyclophosphamide (50 mg/kg/day × 4). The other patient (*UPN/266*) was engrafted, but paternal cells could only be detected after in vitro culture of peripheral blood mononuclear cells with mitogen and IL-2. Functional reconstitution was not observed. Both patients received secondary transplants from their HLA haplotype mismatched mothers. The first patient (*UPN/30*) promptly engrafted with maternal cells now detected in both T- and non-T-cell fractions. He is fully reconstituted 20 months' posttransplant. The second patient (*UPN/266*) was pretreated with cyclophosphamide and ATG prior to the maternal graft. Surprisingly, the initial paternal transplant rapidly expanded after this pretreatment. After a brief period in which both maternal and paternal cells were detected in the circulation, the secondary maternal graft was lost. All circulating and mitogen-responsive T cells are of paternal origin. Six months' posttransplant, he has developed near normal reactivity to mitogens and allogeneic cells, and is generating antibody in response to immunization.

The sixth patient (*UPN/240*) to be transplanted with marrow fractionated by the current technique had also been found to be without clinical evidence of GVHD, yet chimeric with nonreactive maternal T lymphocytes prior to transplantation. This patient was primarily transplanted from his histoincompatible mother, and received a booster graft from the same donor 3 months later. This patient is now 9 months' post secondary transplant and chimeric with maternal cells in both T- and non-T-lymphocyte populations. T-cell numbers and phenotype have normalized. Responses to mitogens, antigens, and allogeneic cells are at 50% of normal values and increasing rapidly. Immunoglobulin levels are also increasing.

To summarize this experience, 7 evaluable patients with SCID have received transplants of SBA$^-$E$^-$E$_N^-$ marrow cells from HLA haplotype mismatched parental donors, each of whom has achieved durable engraftment. All 7 patients have achieved some measure of T-cell function. For 5 of these patients, cell-mediated immune function is normal as measured by in vitro lymphocyte transformation responses to mitogens, antigens, and allogeneic cells, and by their capacity to generate lymphokines in vitro and delayed typed hypersensitivity in vivo. Reconstitution of humoral immunity, with normalization of Ig levels and development of the capacity for appropriate antibody responses to diphtheria, tetanus, polio, or typhoid vaccines is complete in 3 patients, and developing in 2 other cases. Most important, only 1 of the 6 engrafted patients has shown any evidence of GVHD, and this was limited to a grade 1, biopsy-confirmed skin rash which resolved without therapy. In the 3 fully reconstituted patients who are now 9–21 months' posttransplant, engrafted parental T lymphocytes are specifically unresponsive to host HLA determinants in primary or secondary MLC, yet are fully responsive to third-party determinants. Studies to date have failed to demonstrate any specific suppressor-cell activity to explain this expression of tolerance.

The above experience clearly demonstrates that GVHD may be abrogated without compromising immunologic reconstitution if HLA incompatible marrow grafts are effectively depleted of T lymphocytes. As with fetal liver transplants, engraftment of T-cell depleted, HLA disparate marrow is more difficult to achieve. Furthermore, expansion and functional differentiation of engrafted lymphoid progenitors may be inhibited or delayed.

Histoincompatible marrow grafts treated with the T-cell specific monoclonal antibody OKT3 and complement have been used also for transplantation of a small number of patients with SCID. These patients have not survived because of either early infections or severe GVHD [54, and R. Parkman, personal communication]. Recently, however, Reinherz et al [51] have reported a patient with SCID successfully transplanted with HLA haplotype mismatched parental marrow treated with a different T-cell specific monoclonal antibody, T12, and complement. This antibody recognizes a distinct surface antigen on T cells which is much less subject to modulation than that recognized by OKT3. The patient required 3 transplants with intensive immunosuppression prior to the last 2 grafts, before engraftment and function was achieved. A severe acute GVH reaction was reversed by T12 monoclonal antibody infusions [50]. This experience reiterates the problem of engraftment. Further improvements in the methods whereby T-cell specific monoclonal antibodies such as T12 are applied to large-scale cell separations are forthcoming, which may improve the efficiency of T-cell depletions and obviate the current limitations of antibody systems employing complement to achieve selective lysis.

At least 3 features of patients with SCID may contribute to the graft resistance observed. First, a significant proportion of patients with SCID may be silently engrafted with maternal T lymphocytes which, though phenotypically dysmature and void of activity, as assessed by conventional tests of T-cell function, may actively inhibit engraftment of allogeneic cells. We have recently demonstrated 4 of 16 prospectively evaluated SCID patients to be chimeric with E+, Ia+ functionally unresponsive maternal T lymphocytes [53]. Despite clear incompatibilities between mother and child, only one of these patients exhibited clinical evidence of GVHD. Furthermore, the engrafted maternal E+ cells, unlike the mother's own cells, failed to exhibit alloreactivity against E^- lymphocytes from either the patient or his father. Yet, of the 2 patients chimeric with maternal cells who were transplanted with SBA^-E^- E_N^- paternal marrow cells, one (*UPN/60*) failed to engraft, and the other (*UPN/226*) achieved only restricted engraftment. In this patient, functional development of the paternal transplant was observed only after the patient was treated with cyclophosphamide and ATG.

Alternatively, patients with SCID may possess immunologically non-specific cell systems capable of restricting engraftment of allogeneic hematopoietic cells, such as have been described in murine models of transplantation [55]. Over half of our patients with SCID have been found to have near normal levels of "natural killer" (NK) activity [56]. Certain types of NK cells are known to be capable of suppressing the development of allogeneic hematopoietic cells [57], and have been implicated as effectors of marrow graft suppression and allogeneic resistance [58]. Interestingly, IL-2-responsive cells repeatedly cultured from the patient in our series (*UPN/226*), who rejected his paternal graft, are host-derived E+leu 1^-, 4^-, 3^-, $2\pm$, large granular lymphocytes with strong NK activity.

It is also possible that certain patients with SCID lack cells or tissues capable of producing mediators essential to the differentiation and proliferation of donor lymphoid progenitors. Certain critical accessory cells might be removed in the fractionation procedure. Alternatively, thymic defects might restrict graft development. In our patients, the thymic secretory defects seen in the majority of patients with SCID are not intrinsic to the thymus but due rather to a deficiency of inducer cells of hematopoietic origin [59]. However, a primary thymic defect might be present in rare cases [60] or, alternatively, migration of necessary inducer cells, or T-cell progenitor cells themselves might be inhibited in the allogeneic host, thereby limiting reconstitution [61]. Ongoing prospective studies are in progress to evaluate the possible contribution of each or all of these 3 factors to the graft resistance observed.

In conclusion, transplants of histocompatible marrow are being applied with continuing success to the treatment of lethal congenital disorders of the immune system. New applications of marrow transplantation and extension of modified marrow grafts to patients lacking histocompatible donors are now being explored, which should radically improve and extend the applications of marrow transplantation in the treatment of these lethal disorders.

REFERENCES

1. Gatti RA, Meuwissen HJ, Allen HD, Hong R, Good RA: Immunological reconstitution of sex-linked lymphopenic immunological deficiency. Lancet 2:1366–1369, 1968.
2. Bach FH, Albertini RJ, Joo P, Anderson JL, Bortin MM: Bone marrow transplantation in a patient with the Wiskott-Aldrich syndrome. Lancet 2:1364–1366, 1968.
3. Camitta BM, Thomas ED, Nathan DG, Gale RP, Kopecky J, Rappeport JM: A prospective study of androgens and bone marrow for treatment of severe aplastic anemia. Blood 53:504–513, 1979.
4. Thomas ED, Buckner CD, Clift RA, Fefer A, Johnson FL, Neiman PE, Sale GE, Sanders JE, Singer JW, Shulman H, Storb R, Weiden PL: Marrow transplantation for acute nonlymphoblastic leukemia in first remission. N Engl J Med 301:597–599, 1979.
5. UCLA Bone Marrow Transplantation Team: Bone marrow transplantation with intensive combination chemotherapy-radiation therapy (SCARI) in acute leukemia. Ann Intern Med 86:155–161, 1977.
6. Clift RA, Buckner CD, Thomas ED, Doney K, Fefer A, Neiman PE, Singer J, Sanders S, Stevens P, Sullivan KM, Deeg J, Storb R: Treatment of chronic granulocytic leukaemia in chronic phase by allogeneic marrow transplantation. Lancet 2:621–623, 1982.
7. Parkman R, Rappeport J, Geha R, Belli J, Cassady R, Levy R, Nathan DG, Rosen FS: Complete correction of the Wiskott-Aldrich syndrome by allogeneic bone marrow transplantation. N Engl J Med 298:921–927, 1978.
8. Kapoor N, Kirkpatrick D, Blaese RM, Oleske J, Hilgartner MH, Chaganti RSK, Good RA, O'Reilly RJ: Reconstitution of normal megakaryocytopoiesis and immunologic function in Wiskott-Aldrich syndrome by marrow transplantation following myeloablation and immunosuppression with busulfan and cyclophosphamide. Blood 57:692–696, 1981.
9. Rappeport JM, Parkman R, Newburger P, Camitta BM, Chusid MJ: Correction of

10. Sorell M, Kapoor N, Pahwa R, Halac E, Cooper D, Kirkpatrick D, Chaganti RSK, Dupont B, Good RA, O'Reilly RJ: Correction of combined immunodeficiency and agranulocytosis in a patient with cartilage-hair hypoplasia by marrow transplantation. Clin Immunol Immunopathol (In press)
11. Buckley RH: Reconstitution: Grafting of bone marrow and thymus. In Amos B (ed): "Progress in Immunology." New York: Academic Press, 1971, p 1061.
12. O'Reilly RJ, Kapoor N, Pollack M, Sorell M, Chaganti RSK, Blaese RM, Wank R, Good RA, Dupont B: Reconstitution of immunologic function in a patient with severe combined immunodeficiency following transplantation of marrow from an HLA-A,B,C nonidentical but MLC-compatible paternal donor. Transplant Proc 11:1934–1937, 1979.
13. Koch C, Henriksen K, Juhl F, Wiik A, Faber V, Anderson V, Dupont B, Hansen G, Svejgaard A, Thomsen M, Ernst P, Killman SA, Good RA, Jensen K, Muller-Berat N: Bone marrow transplantation from an HL-A non-identical but mixed-lymphocyte culture identical donor. Lancet 1:1146–1150, 1973.
14. Dupont B, O'Reilly RJ, Pollack MS, Good RA: Use of HLA genotypically different donors in bone marrow transplantation. Transplant Proc 11:219–224, 1979.
15. Clift RA, Hansen JA, Thomas ED, Buckner CD, Sanders JE, Mickelson EM, Storb R, Johnson FL, Singer JL, Goodell BW: Marrow transplantation from donors other than HLA-identical siblings. Transplantation 28:235–242, 1979.
16. Horowitz SD, Groshong T, Bach FH, Hong R, Yunis EJ: Treatment of severe combined immunodeficiency with bone marrow from an unrelated, mixed-culture non-reactive donor. Lancet 2:431–433, 1975.
17. Speck B, Zwaan FE, von Rood JJ, Eernisse JG: Allogeneic bone marrow transplantation in a patient with aplastic anemia using a phenotypically HLA identical unrelated donor. Transplantation 16:24–28, 1973.
18. O'Reilly RJ, Dupont B, Pahwa S, Grimes E, Smithwick EM, Pahwa R, Schwartz S, Hansen HA, Siegal FP, Sorell M, Svejgaard A, Jersild C, Thomsen M, Platz T, L'Esperance P, Good RA: Reconstitution in severe combined immunodeficiency by transplantation of marrow from an unrelated donor. N Engl J Med 297:1311–1318, 1977.
19. Foroozonfar N, Hobbs JR, Hugh-Jones K, Humble JG, James DCO, Selwyn S, Watson JG, Yamamuca M: Bone marrow transplantation from an unrelated donor for chronic granulomatous disease. Lancet 1:210–215, 1977.
20. Hansen JA, Clift RA, Thomas ED, Buckner CD, Storb R, Giblett ER: Transplantation of marrow from an unrelated donor to a patient with acute leukemia. N Engl J Med 303:565–566, 1980.
21. Lohrmann HP, Dietrich M, Goldman SF, Kristen T, Fliedner TM, Abt C, Pflieger H, Flad HB, Kubanek B, Heimpel H: Bone marrow transplantation for aplastic anemia from an HLA-A and MLC identical unrelated donor. Blut 31:347–354, 1975.
22. Duquesnoy RJ, Zeevi A, Marrari M, Hackbarth S, Camitta B: Bone marrow transplantation for severe aplastic anemia using a phenotypically HLA-identical, SB compatible unrelated donor. Transplantation (In press)
23. Gordon-Smith EC, Fairhead SM, Chipping PM, Hows J, James DCO, Dodi A, Batchelor JR: Bone marrow transplantation for severe aplastic anemia using histocompatible unrelated volunteer donors. Br Med J 285:835–837, 1982.
24. Storb R, Weiden PL, Graham TC, Lerner KG, Thomas ED: Marrow grafts between DLA-identical and homozygous unrelated dogs: Evidence for an additional locus involved in graft-versus-host disease. Transplantation 24:165–174, 1977.
25. Yunis EJ, Good RA, Smith J, Stutman O: Protection of lethally irradiated mice by spleen cells from neonatally thymectomized mice. Proc Natl Acad Sci USA 71:2544–2548, 1974.
26. Uphoff D: Preclusion of secondary phase of irradiation syndrome by inoculation of fetal hematopoietic tissue following lethal total body x-irradiation. J Natl Cancer Inst 20:625, 1958.
27. von Boehmer H, Sprent J, Nabholz M: Tolerance to histocompatibility determinants in tetraparental bone marrow chimeras. J Exp Med 141:322–334, 1975.
28. Onoe K, Fernandez G, Good RA: Humoral and cell-mediated immune responses in fully allogeneic bone marrow chimera in mice. J Exp Med 151:115–132, 1980.
29. Vallera DA, Youle RJ, Neville DM, Kersey JH: Bone marrow transplantation across major histocompatibility barriers. V. Protection of mice from lethal graft vs. host disease by pretreatment of donor cells with monoclonal Anti-Thy-1,2 coupled to the toxin ricin. J Exp Med 155:949–954, 1982.
30. Reisner Y, Itsicovitch L, Meshorer A, Sharon N: Hematopoietic stem cell transplantation using mouse bone marrow and spleen cells fractionated by lectins. Proc Natl Acad Sci USA 75:2933–2936, 1978.
31. Dexter TM, Spooner E: Loss of immunoreactivity in long term bone marrow culture. Nature 275:135–136, 1978.
32. Rich RR, Kilpatrick CH, Smith TK: Simultaneous suppression of responses to allogeneic tissues in vitro and in vivo. Cell Immunol 5:190–200, 1972.
33. Zoschke DC, Bach FH: Specificity of allogeneic cell recognition by human lymphocytes in vitro. Science 172:1350–1352, 1971.
34. Romano TJ, Nowakowski M, Bloom BR, Thorbecke GJ: Selective viral immunosuppression of the graft versus host reaction. J Exp Med 145:666–675, 1977.
35. Aguet M, Andersson LC, Andersson R, Wight E, Binz H, Wigzell H: Induction of specific immune unresponsiveness with purified mixed leukocyte culture-activated T lymphoblasts as autoimmunogen. II. An analysis of the effects measured at the cellular and serological levels. J Exp Med 147:50–61, 1978.
36. Slavin S, Fuks Z, Kaplan HA, Strober S: Transplantation of allogeneic bone marrow without graft-versus-host disease using total lymphoid irradiation. J Exp Med 147:963–972, 1978.
37. Powles RI, Clink HM, Spence D, Morgenstern G, Watson JG, Selby PJ, Woods M, Barrett A, Janeson B, Sloane J, Lawlor SD, Kay HEM, Lawson D, McElwain TJ, Alexander P: Cyclosporin-A to prevent graft versus host disease in man after allogeneic bone marrow transplantation. Lancet 1:327–329, 1980.
38. Parkman R, Gelfand EW, Rosen FS: Attempted immunologic reconstitution of patients with combined immune deficiency syndrome with bone marrow transplantation from histoincompatible donors. In Bergsma D (ed): "Immunodeficiency in Man and Animals." Sunderland, MA: Sinauer Associates for The National Foundation-March of Dimes, BD:OAS XI(1):417–420, 1974.
39. Salmon SE, Smith BA, Lehrer RI, Mogerman SN, Shinefield HP, Perkins HA: Modification of donor lymphocytes for transplantation in lymphopenic immunological deficiency. Lancet 2:149–150, 1970.
40. Keightley RG, Lawton AA, Cooper M: Successful fetal liver transplantation in a child with severe combined immunodeficiency. Lancet 2:850–853, 1975.
41. O'Reilly RJ, Kapoor N, Kirkpatrick D: Fetal tissue transplants for severe combined immunodeficiency—Their limitations and functional potential. In Seligmann M, Hitzig WH (eds): "Primary Immunodeficiencies." Amsterdam: Elsevier/North Holland 1980, pp 419–433.
42. Touraine JL, Griscelli C, Vossen J, Hitzig WH, Hobbs JR, Hugh-Jones K, Stoop JW, Zegers BJM, Fasth A: Foetal tissue trans-

plantation for severe combined immunodeficiency (SCID): European experience. Transplant Proc 15:1427–1430, 1983.
43. Singer A, Hathcock KS, Hodes RJ: Self recognition in allogeneic radiation bone marrow chimeras. A radiation-resistant host element dictates the self specificity and immune response gene phenotype of T-helper cells. J Exp Med 153:1286–1301, 1981.
44. Zinkernagel RM, Althage A, Callahan G, Welsh RM: On the immunocompetence of H-2 incompatible irradiation bone marrow chimeras. J Immunol 124:6, 1980.
45. O'Reilly RJ, Kapoor N, Pollack MS, Chaganti RSK, Dupont B, Kirkpatrick D, Reisner Y: Immunologic function in patients transplanted for severe combined immunodeficiency selectively engrafted with donor T lymphocytes. Behring Institute Mitteilungen 70:182–187, 1982.
46. Touraine JL: Transplantation of both fetal liver and thymus in severe combined immunodeficiency: Interaction between donor's and recipient's cells in fetal liver transplantation. In Lucarelli G, Fliedner TM, Gale RP (eds). Excerpta Medica 514:277, 1980.
47. Zinkernagel RM, Doherty PC: MHC-restricted cytotoxic T cell studies on the biological role of polymorphic major transplantation antigens determining T-cell restriction-specificity, function and responsiveness. Adv Immunol 27:51, 1979.
48. Reisner Y, Kapoor N, Kirkpatrick D, Pollack MS, Dupont B, Good RA, O'Reilly RJ: Transplantation for acute leukaemia with HLA-A and B nonidentical parental marrow cells fractionated with soybean agglutinin and sheep red blood cells. Lancet 2:327–331, 1981.
49. Kapoor N, O'Reilly RJ, Kirkpatrick D, Pollack MS, Dupont B, Good RA, Reisner Y: Restoration of immunological function by a histoincompatible T cell depleted marrow transplant in a child with severe combined immunodeficiency. (Abstract) Pediatr Res 16:224A, 1982.
50. Reisner Y, Kapoor N, Kirkpatrick D, Pollack MS, Cunningham-Rundles S, Dupont B, Hodes MZ, Good RA, O'Reilly RJ: Transplantation for severe combined immunodeficiency with HLA-A,B,D,DR incompatible parental marrow cells fractionated by soybean agglutinin and sheep red cells. Blood 61:341–348, 1983.
51. Rheinherz EL, Geha R, Rappeport JM, Wilson M, Schlossman ST, Rosen FS: Immune reconstitution in severe combined immunodeficiency following transplantation with T lymphocyte depleted HLA haplotype mismatched bone marrow. (Abstract) Clin Res 30:515A, 1982.
52. O'Reilly RJ, Kapoor N, Kirkpatrick D, Cunningham-Rundles S, Pollack MS, Dupont B, Hodes MZ, Good RA, Reisner Y: Transplantation for severe combined immunodeficiency using histoincompatible parental marrow fractionated by soybean agglutinin and sheep red blood cells: Experience in six consecutive cases. Transplant Proc 15:1431–1435, 1983.
53. Pollack MS, Kirkpatrick D, Kapoor N, Dupont B, O'Reilly RJ: Identification by HLA typing of intrauterine-derived maternal T cells in four patients with severe combined immunodeficiency. N Engl J Med 307:662–666, 1982.
54. Hayward AR, Murphy J, Githen J, Troup G, Ambroso D: Failure of a panreactive anti-T cell antibody, OKT3, to prevent graft versus host disease in severe combined immunodeficiency. J Pediatr 100:665–668, 1982.
55. Cudkowicz G, Bennett M: Peculiar immunobiology of bone marrow allografts. II. Rejection of parental grafts by resistant F_1 hybrid mice. J Exp Med 134:1513–1528, 1971.
56. Kirkpatrick D, Lopez C, Kapoor N, O'Reilly RJ, Ching C: Natural killer cell activity in marrow deficiency states. Exp Hematol 9 (Suppl 9):15A, 1981.
57. Beran M, Andersson B, Hansson M, Kiessling R: Regulation of the growth and differentiation of human committed stem cells in vitro: The role of autologous blood derived natural killer (NK) cells and macrophages. Exp Hematol 9 (Suppl 9): 144A, 1981.
58. Kiessling R, Hochman PS, Haller O, Shearer GM, Wigzell H, Cudkowicz G: Evidence for a similar or common mechanism for natural killer cell activity and resistance to hemopoietic grafts. Eur J Immunol 7:655–663, 1977.
59. Iwata T, Incefy G, Good RA, Cunningham-Rundles S, Dardenne M, Kapoor N, Kirkpatrick D, O'Reilly RJ: Circulating thymic hormone levels in severe combined immunodeficiency. Clin Exp Immunol (In press)
60. Pyke KW, Dosch HM, Ipp MM, Gelfand EW: Demonstration of an intrathymic defect in a case of severe combined immunodeficiency disease. N Engl J Med 293:424–428, 1975.
61. Stutman O, Good RA: Traffic of hemopoietic cells to the thymus: Influence of histocompatibility differences. Exp Hematol 19:12–15, 1969.

European Experience With Fetal Tissue Transplantation in Severe Combined Immunodeficiency (SCID)

Jean-Louis Touraine, MD

Transplantation and Immunobiology Unit, Hôpital Edouard Herriot, 69374 Lyon Cedex 2, France

Severe combined immunodeficiency disease (SCID) can be completely cured by bone marrow transplantation (BMT), especially from a genotypically identical donor [1]. When no compatible bone marrow donor is available, fetal liver transplantation (FLT), possibly associated with fetal thymus transplantation (FTT), has established itself as a valid alternative [2]. Because of extreme susceptibility of infants with SCID to infections, and because of the slow maturation of lymphocytes from the transplanted fetal liver cells, prolonged and complete isolation of patients treated by FLT is mandatory.

This paper reports the 62 fetal tissue transplants performed in Europe to treat 29 patients with SCID. Data have been gathered by an inquiry among the European Centers which receive infants with SCID. The results analyzed herein are representative of all fetal tissue transplants performed in Europe since 1962 for the treatment of SCID, and it is estimated that no more than 35 European patients with this condition have received FLT or FTT over the last 20 years. In this report, no mention will be made of FTT for DiGeorge syndrome or other non-SCID immunodeficiencies, of FLT for enzyme deficiencies without immunodeficiency, or of treatment of SCID patients with cultured thymic epithelial cells from postnatal thymuses.

The 29 reported patients received the 62 FTTs in the following cities: Göteborg (1 transplant in 1 patient), Leiden (8 transplants in 6 patients), London (4 transplants in 3 patients), Lyon (15 transplants in 6 patients), Paris (17 transplants in 9 patients), Utrecht (3 transplants in 1 patient), and Zürich (14 transplants in 3 patients). The mean number of sequential transplants per patient has been 2.1, with a range of 1–11 (Fig. 1).

Six patients have been treated by FTT alone, 5 patients by FLT, and 18 patients by FLT and FTT combined.

FETAL THYMUS TRANSPLANTS

The 6 patients who received FTT were 3 patients with "classic" SCID, 1 patient with the bare lymphocyte syndrome, ie combined immunodeficiency with lack of cellular expression of HLA antigens [3], 1 patient with nucleoside phosphorylase deficiency [4] (and personal communication from Dr. B.J.M. Zegers), and 1 patient with late-onset T-cell deficiency [5]. The latter 2 patients have been included in this analysis because they presented as combined immunodeficiency, although they were later considered to have a predominant T-cell deficiency. Only one patient [5] is still alive, while 2 patients died of pneumocystosis, 1 of pneumonia, 1 of lymphosarcoma and 1 of graft-versus-host disease (GVHD) following a fresh "plasma" transfusion. The first of these FTT in SCID patients was performed in 1962 [6].

FETAL LIVER TRANSPLANTS (Isolated or Associated With FTT)

Patients treated by FLT alone or in association with FTT from the same donor are described in more detail.

Characteristics of Recipients

The SCID patients were 4 infants with an adenosine deaminase (ADA) deficiency, 18 infants with normal ADA activity, and 1 infant with undetermined ADA activity. Ten of these 23 patients had a significantly reduced number of B cells, 12 had normal or high numbers of B cells, and 1 had an unknown number of B cells. Fifteen were male and 8 were female. No correlation was observed between sex of the patient or type of SCID and success rate.

Age of recipients ranged between 1 and 13 months (age at the time of the first transplant in patients who received sequential transplants). If two groups of patients are consid-

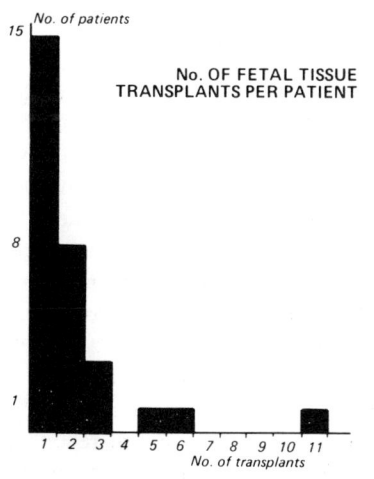

Fig. 1. Number of patients with 1 to 11 fetal tissue transplants.

ered, those with a successful outcome of FLT and those with a failure, the mean age in the former group (4.6 months) is lower than in the latter (6.0 months). If this difference is still observed in a larger series, several possible explanations should be examined: lower incidence of pre-existing infections in the youngest patients, higher percentage of take when the transplant is performed soon after birth, etc.

Characteristics of Donors and Transplanted Cells

Gestational ages of the fetal donors ranged from 7 to 20 weeks. Immunologic reconstitution was obtained independently of the donor age within this range. GVHD was observed even when the fetus was 7 or 8 weeks old but appeared to be more frequent when the age was over 13 weeks. The difference is not statistically significant, however, and some of the "oldest transplants" were not followed by GVHD. The sex of the donor was indicated in only 23 of the transplants (12 males and 11 females). A slightly lower incidence of GVHD was observed after male transplants but the difference is not significant. Relatively better results after transplants of male cells than female cells have also been recorded in BMT [7]. Because the fetal ages varied between 7 and 20 weeks, the number of nucleated cells transplanted varied from one case to another. The mean number was 6.2×10^8 but the range was very wide $(0.7-24 \times 10^8)$. The success rate was slightly better when the number of cells exceeded 1×10^8/kg of bw of the recipient or when transplants were repeated. All transplants but one were done with fresh tissues. Air transportation from one city to another within Europe, and in vitro preservation of the fetal tissues for less than 10 hours before the transplant did not appear to hinder transplant take and success.

Five patients received isolated FLT: 3 died and 2 are presently alive. Eighteen patients received both FLT and FTT: 14 died and 4 are alive. However, the latter 4 patients have an immunoreconstitution, and they are those with the longest follow-up (23-69 months) while the 2 patients alive after FLT have been followed for only 8 and 21 months, and one of them is not yet immunologically reconstituted. It is, therefore, not yet determined whether FLT can induce a degree of immunologic reconstitution as complete as FLT+FTT, both organs being provided by the same donor.

Overall Results

Table 1 summarizes the results in the 23 SCID patients treated by FLT (±FTT). Seven of the patients developed GVHD. A chimerism has been documented in 14 cases, either transiently or permanently. This chimerism was easy to demonstrate using HLA markers or chromosomal markers, in particular. T-cell reconstitution developed as a result of the transplant in 11 patients, but only 7 of them also had a B-cell reconstitution from the donor cells. In the other cases, either no B-cell development was seen, in SCID patients lacking B cells, or the host B cells became capable of differentiation into immunoglobulin-secreting plasma cells as a result of T-cell engraftment. Although the number of patients is still limited, these results show that, in many SCID patients, B cells are virtually normal and lack only the presence of normal T lymphocytes; in addition, the engraftment of completely mismatched T lymphocytes does not preclude some cooperation between host B cells and donor T cells, resulting in antibody formation [8]. It may, however, be noted that this cooperation and the production of antibodies develop relatively slowly after the evidence of T-cell reconstitution.

Patient survival after FLT is shown in Figure 2. Seventeen patients died. Factors contributing to death (one main factor in 10 patients, 2 associated factors in 7 patients) were the following: 8 septicemias, 6 GVHDs, 3 pneumonias (pneumocystis, Candida, measles virus), 2 BCG infections, 1 generalized vaccinia, 1 meningitis, 1 hemorrhage (associated with bone marrow aplasia), 1 autoimmune anemia, and 1 sudden death (aspiration). The date of death was 0.2-38 months following transplantation. Six of the 23 patients, ie

TABLE 1. Results of Fetal Liver Transplantation in Patients With SCID

No. patients treated by FLT	23
No. nucleated cells transplanted per patient	$0.7-24 \times 10^8$ (mean: 6.2×10^8)
No. patients with additional FTT	18 of the 23
GVHD	7
Documented chimerism	14
T-cell reconstitution	11
B-cell reconstitution	7
Deaths	17*
Time of death (no. months after transplantation)	0.2-38 mos
Alive	6** (26%)
Follow-up of living patients (no. months after transplantation)	8-59 mos

*The main causes of death were septicemia, GVHD, and pneumonia.
**Except for the most recently transplanted patient, all 6 infants have a total or partial immunoreconstitution. All but one, who has numerous lymphoblasts in peripheral blood, are in very good condition.
(From Touraine JL: Transplant Proc, in press, with permission.)

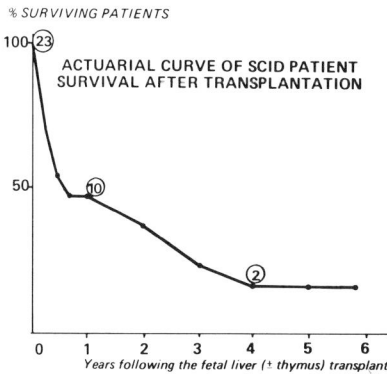

Fig. 2. Patient survival after FLT in the European series. (Figs. 2 and 3 from Touraine JL: Transplant Proc, in press, with permission.)

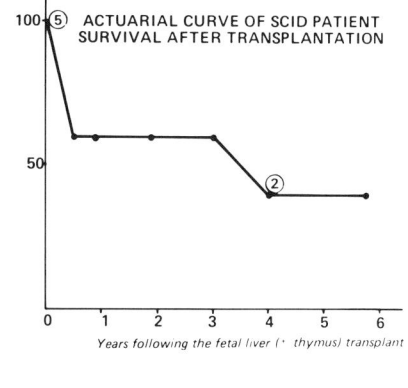

Fig. 3. Patient survival after FLT in one individual series.

TABLE 2. Favorable Factors in FLT

Patient
  Early diagnosis, isolation and treatment
  Lack of infection
  Prolonged isolation in sterile environment

Transplant
  Fresh fetal tissue
  Fetal donor 7–12 weeks of age
  Repeated transplants (2–6)
  Number of nucleated cells $> 10^8$/kg of bw of recipient
  IP or IV route
  Male donor?
  Thymus transplant syngeneic with donor liver?

Role of Compatibility?

26%, are presently alive. The follow-ups of these patients are 8, 21, 23, 34, 50, and 69 months after FLT. Five of these 6 patients have a total or subtotal reconstitution of the T-cell compartment. Except for one patient with lymphoblastosis, all living patients are in very good clinical condition.

The 2 patients with a follow-up over 4 years have been previously described [8,9]. They are very healthy and both have a full reconstitution. The grafted T cells exert normal functions, without demonstrable restriction, although donor and host cells are completely mismatched at the HLA, A, B, C, and DR loci [9,10]. Among several possible explanations, we have postulated that, in addition to the general mechanisms of "self+X" recognition, there are "allo+X" recognition structures on some T lymphocytes, the number of which would expand under the appropriate solicitations in vivo [11,12]. In both cases, immunologic reconstitution has been slow, and isolation has been a crucial factor in preventing lethal infections during the many months before immune competence was sufficient for defense against organisms. These 2 patients belong to an individual series of 5 patients homogeneously treated by FLT and syngeneic FTT from fetuses of 8–13 weeks of age. The actuarial survival curve in this series of patients treated in Lyon is shown in Figure 3. This admittedly small series demonstrates that, from 1976 to 1982, SCID patients have been offered a reasonable chance of survival and, apparently, of stable and virtually complete recovery by FLT, although the incidence of success obviously does not reach that of BMT from an HLA-identical sib.

The presently reported results are in accordance with those of a previous international survey on FLT [13] which included some of the European patients described herein. Greater heterogeneity was present in that series, with fetal ages ranging from 4 to 22 weeks. The number of patients alive at the time of the report was 12 out of 52, ie 23%, with a follow-up ranging from 1 to 72 months. Eleven of these 12 patients had been followed more than 1 year after FLT.

Detailed analysis of each factor, and of its effect on the outcome, in the European series suggests that some conditions have been more favorable (Table 2). Some conditions are associated with the patient, others with the transplant. These favorable factors are not all definitively established and deserve further studies, especially experimental work in animals. For instance, the influence of donor sex and of an associated transplant of syngeneic thymus needs a more thorough investigation.

The role of compatibility is still uncertain. HLA mismatch may delay the progression of immunologic reconstitution but certainly does not prevent it, as might have been feared from animal experiments [14].

Continuation of multicenter analyses of FLT will give more and more precise answers on such practical questions as optimal age of the fetus, optimal number of cells, the role of NK cell activity of the host, obtainment and preservation, and route of administration of fetal cells, prevention of GVHD, and optimal conditions for decontamination and isolation. The development of FTT in SCID will also lead the way to possible application in other congenital diseases, as well as in aplastic anemia and acute leukemia [15], especially if methods to accelerate the maturation and proliferation of precursor cells become available.

ACKNOWLEDGMENTS

The author thanks Doctors C. Griscelli, J. Vossen, W.H. Hitzig, J.R. Hobbs, K. Hugh-Jones, J.W. Stoop, B.J.M. Zegers, and A. Fasth for their collaboration on this article.

ADDENDUM

The patient with "lymphoblastosis" has been conclusively demonstrated to have acute lymphoblastic leukemia on transplanted cells; she now is undergoing chemotherapy (personal communication from Drs. Hugh-Jones and Hobbs).

REFERENCES

1. Bortin MM, Rimm AA: Severe combined immunodeficiency disease. Characterization of the disease and results of transplantation. JAMA 238:591–600, 1977.
2. Touraine JL, Bétuel H, Bétend B, Souillet G, Hermier M, Evrard A, Francois R: Fetal liver transplantation as an alternative to bone marrow transplantation in severe combined immunodeficiencies. Blut 41:194–197, 1980.
3. Touraine JL: the Bare Lymphocyte syndrome: Report on the Registry. Lancet 1:319–321, 1981.
4. Stoop JW, Eijsvoogel VP, Zegers BJM, Blok-Shut B, Van Bekkum DW, Ballieux RE: Selective severe cellular immunodeficiency. Effect of thymus transplantation and transfer factor administration. Clin Immunol Immunopathol 6:289–298, 1976.
5. Foroozanfar N, Yamamura M, Watson G, Weaver P, Belton EM, Lawler S, Hobbs JR: Successful thymus graft for T-cell deficiency in a 6-year-old boy. Br Med J 1:314–315, 1975.
6. Hitzig WH, Kay HEM, Cottier H: Familial lymphopenia with agammaglobulinaemia. An attempt at treatment by implantation of foetal thymus. Lancet 2:151–154, 1965.
7. Bortin MM, Gale RP, Rimm AA: Allogeneic bone marrow transplantation for 144 patients with severe aplastic anemia. JAMA 245:1132–1139, 1981.
8. Touraine JL: Transplantation of both fetal liver and thymus in severe combined immunodeficiencies. Interaction between donor and recipient cells. In Lucarelli G, Fliedner Th M, Gale RP (eds): "Fetal Liver Transplantation." Amsterdam: Excerpta Medica, 1980, pp 276–283.
9. Touraine JL: Bone marrow and fetal liver transplantation in immunodeficiencies and inborn errors. In Touraine JL et al (eds): "Transplantation and Clinical Immunology." Amsterdam: Excerpta Medica, vol 14, 1982, pp 64–71.
10. Touraine JL, Bétuel H, Bétend B, Souillet G, Touraine F: Chimerism following fetal liver and thymus transplantation: Normal lymphocyte functions despite complete HLA mismatch between cell populations. Exp Hematol 10:125–126, 1982.
11. Touraine JL: Results of fetal tissue transplantation in 25 SCID patients from the European group. In Touraine JL, Gluckman E, Griscelli C (eds): "Bone Marrow Transplantation in Europe." Amsterdam: Excerpta Medica, 1981, vol 2, pp 238–243.
12. Touraine JL, Bétuel H: Immunodeficiency diseases and expression of HLA antigens. Hum Immunol 2:147–153, 1981.
13. Gale RP: Fetal liver transplantation in man. Supra #8, pp 268–275.
14. Zinkernagel RM: The thymus: Its influence on recognition of "self major histocompatibility antigens" by T cells and consequences for reconstitution of immunodeficiency. Springer Semin Immunopathol 1:405–428, 1978.
15. Lucarelli G, Fliedner Th M, Gale RP: Supra #8.

Chimerism Following Fetal Liver Transplantation: Cell Cooperation Despite HLA Mismatch

Jean-Louis Touraine, MD, Claude Griscelli, MD, Hervé Bétuel, MD, Anne Durandy, MD, Bruno Bétend, MD, and Gérard Souillet, MD

Transplantation and Immunobiology Unit, (J.L.T.), Centre de Transfusion (H.B.), Service de Pédiatrie (B.B.), Hôpital E. Herriot, Lyon, France, Unité d'Hémato-Immunologie Infantile, Hôpital Necker-Enfants Malades, Paris, France (C.G., A.D.), Service de Pédiatrie, Hôpital Debrousse, Lyon, France (G.S.)

When no compatible donor is available for a bone marrow transplant, patients with severe combined immunodeficiency (SCID) can be treated by fetal liver transplantation (FLT) [1]. In such circumstances, no attempt is made to match donor and host for HLA antigens. It is thought that stem cells of the fetal liver become tolerant to the antigens of the host, and that GVHD only develops when some more or less differentiated T cells are present in the injected cell suspension.

We report herein 4 SCID patients in whom sustained reconstitution of the T-cell compartment resulted from transplantation of fetal liver (and of associated syngeneic fetal thymus in 3 of the patients). These children provide us with a unique opportunity to study the effects of HLA mismatch on cell cooperation in humans with long-term chimerism.

Patient 1

Sergio S. has received 2 fetal liver and thymus transplants. He progressively developed a full immunologic reconstitution (Tables 1 and 2). After a sterile isolation of 534 days, the infant went back to his family. He is presently in perfect condition, 69 months after the transplant, and he lives a normal life. His defense against viral infections is normal.

The HLA phenotypes of host and donor were:
Host:
A3 A33 B14 B47 DR4 DR5

Fetal donor:
A1 A2 B18 B27 DR1 DR7

No HLA A, B, or DR specificity was therefore shared by donor and recipient.

By separation of T- and B-lymphocyte populations, followed by HLA typing, it was demonstrated that all T lymphocytes were of donor origin, while B lymphocytes were of host origin. The monocyte population included two varieties of cells: some monocytes derived from donor cells, others from host cells.

Despite complete HLA mismatch at the A, B, and DR loci, T lympho-

TABLE 1. Reconstitution of CMI in *Patient 1*

S . . . (fetal liver + thymus transplants)
Results 3½ years later
HTLA$^+$ lymphocytes	:71%
E-RFC	:58%
Igs$^+$ lymphocytes	:12%
Proliferative responses to mitogens:	
O	: 867 dpm ± 83
Con A	: 385,259 dpm ± 22,871
PHA	: 458,136 dpm ± 9,321
PWM	: 22,495 dpm ± 2,563
(idem 5½ years later)	

T-cell cytotoxic responses normal toward a large variety of target cells. No important restriction of T-cell cytotoxic functions imposed by either the donor MHC or the host MHC.

TABLE 2. Reconstitution of Humoral Immunity in *Patient 1*

● **Immunoglobulins**

	Before the transplant	Day 500	Day 2000
IgM	Low	Normal	Normal
IgG	Low	Normal (restricted heterogeneity)	Normal (normal heterogeneity)
IgA	Low	Normal	Normal
IgD	Low	Low	Normal
IgE	Low	Low	Normal

● **Allohemagglutinins**

	Before the transplant	Day 1000
Anti-A	0	1/8
Anti-B	0	1/16

● **Antibodies following vaccination on day 1000**

	Before vaccination	After vaccination
Antipolio I (titer)	⩽8	64
II (titer)	⩽8	64
III (titer)	⩽8	128
Anti-diphtheria toxoid (U/ml)	⩽0.01	1
Anti-tetanus toxoid (U/ml)	0.5	1

cytes did cooperate with B lymphocytes and exerted effector functions on various other host cells.

Patient 2

Aurélie C. has received 5 fetal liver and thymus transplants. She developed a progressive, and slow, immunologic reconstitution up to complete level in 3 years. She was in sterile isolation for 3½ years, after which she went back to her family. This child is now in perfect condition, 50 months after the transplant. Her defense against viral infections is normal. The number of T lymphocytes, their proliferative responses to mitogens and the immunoglobulin levels are virtually normal. Cytotoxic function of T lymphocytes and antibody production are present.

The HLA phenotypes of host and donor were:
Host:
A2 A11 B15 B35 DR5 DR6
Fetal donor:
A1 A33 B5 B16 — —

No HLA A or B specificity was shared by donor and recipient. The DR phenotype of fetal cells has not yet been determined.

By separation of T- and B-lymphocyte populations, followed by HLA typing, it was demonstrated that a) most T lymphocytes were of donor origin and the others were of host origin, b) approximately 50% of B lymphocytes were of donor origin and 50% were of host origin.

In this child, cell cooperation is present but it is difficult to determine which type of B cells cooperate with donor type T cells.

Patient 3

Nicholas R. had a rapid T-cell reconstitution, in two months, following a fetal liver and thymus transplant but he remained profoundly hypogammaglobulinemic. He then developed a very severe autoimmune hemolytic anemia with panagglutinating IgG and complement on his own erythrocytes and in serum. This hemolytic anemia led to rapid deterioration of his general condition which, in association with septicemia, resulted in death after 12 months (3 months after a splenectomy).

The HLA phenotypes of host and donor were:
Host:
A2 A24 B5 — DR4 DR6
Fetal donor:
A2 — B40 — — —

At least one HLA antigen (A2) was shared by donor and recipient.

All T lymphocytes were of donor origin; some B lymphocytes were of donor origin, others were of host origin.

The degree of cell cooperation has been difficult to ascertain with precision in this child. Many speculations can be put forward to explain the autoimmune hemolytic anemia. It

TABLE 3. Immunologic Reconstitution in *Patient 4*

The T-cell reconstitution initiated at 5 months and was complete at 9 months.
Ig levels still low:
  IgM 0.3 (but present prior to transplantation)
  IgG 4.6 (injected γglobulins)
  IgA 0.08
Antibody production low and dissociated:
  Polio +
  Diphtheria + weak
  Tetanus + weak
  Candida 0
  Anti-B ½

may, for instance, be hypothesized that the chimerism itself is responsible for this complication in certain circumstances. It might also indicate that some fetal cells have not acquired the self tolerance in the environment of the recipient's thymus.

Patient 4

Albert B. had progressive T-cell reconstitution after one FLT (Table 3). He presently is in perfect clinical condition, 21 months after transplantation. The T-cell reconstitution is complete but antibody production is still very weak and dissociated.

The HLA phenotypes of host and donor were:
Host:
A32 A33 B14 B27 DR2 DR3
Fetal donor:
A2 A33 B14 — — —

At least 2 HLA antigens (A33 and B14) were shared by donor and recipient.

All T lymphocytes were of donor origin; some B lymphocytes were of donor origin, others were of host origin.

In this child, cell cooperation is still very incomplete. As far as antibody production is concerned, antibody titers are low, even after vaccination, and dissociated.

DISCUSSION

From the study of these 4 patients, the development of cell populations

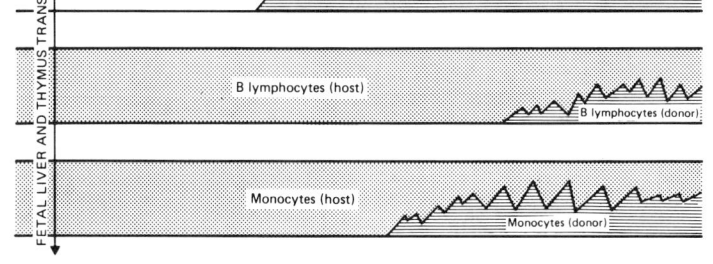

Fig. 1. Development of T lymphocytes, monocytes, and B lymphocytes from transplanted fetal liver cells, and establishment of chimerism with both donor and host mononucleated cells. From J.L. Touraine et al: Exp Hematol 10, (Suppl 10):125–126, 1982, with permission.

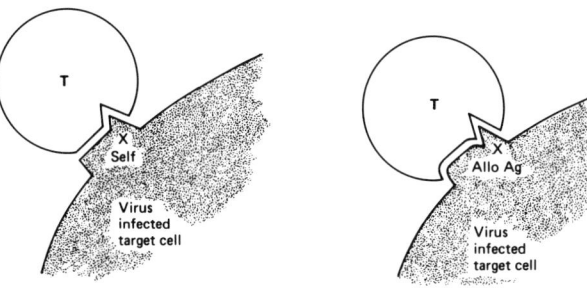

Fig. 2. Hypothesis of 2 types of T lymphocytes differentiating in the thymus, one with "Self + X" recognition structures (left), the other with "Allo + X" recognition structures (right).

following FLT can be envisioned as schematically represented in Figure 1.

Cooperation of donor cells with host cells has been a matter of much debate in different conditions and models both in humans [2,3] and in experimental animals [4]. In brief, animal studies predicted a low or absent interaction of donor T lymphocytes with the various cells of an HLA mismatched host [5]. In some patients, however, T lymphocytes of donor origin have been shown to cooperate with host cells despite an HLA mismatch. Several explanations can account for this lack of major allogeneic restriction [3]. In particular, it is possible that "Allo + X" recognition structures exist on some T cells, the number of which would expand under the appropriate solicitations in vivo (Fig. 2) [3,6].

REFERENCES

1. Touraine JL: European experience with fetal tissue transplantation in severe combined immunodeficiency (SCID). This volume.
2. Griscelli C, Durandy A, Ballet JJ, Prieur AM, Hors J: T- and B-cell chimerism in two patients with severe combined immunodeficiency (SCID) after transplantation. Transplant Proc 9:171–175, 1977.
3. Touraine JL: Cooperation between thymus and transplanted precursor cells during reconstitution of immunodeficiencies with bone marrow or fetal liver cells. In Thierfelder S, Rodt H, Kolb HJ (eds): "Immunobiology of Bone Marrow Transplantation." Berlin: Springer Verlag, 1980, pp 141–148.
4. Katz DH, Hamaoka T, Benacerraf B: Cell interactions between histo-incompatible T and B lymphocytes. II. Failure of physiologic cooperative interactions between T and B lymphocytes from allogeneic donor strains in humoral response to hapten-protein conjugates. J Exp Med 137:1405–1418, 1973.
5. Zinkernagel RM: The thymus: Its influence on recognition of "Self Major Histocompatibility Antigens" by T cells and consequences for reconstitution of immunodeficiency. Springer Semin Immunopathol 1:405–428, 1978.
6. Touraine JL, Bétuel H: Immunodeficiency diseases and expression of HLA antigens. Hum Immunol 2:147–153, 1981.

Problems of Mismatched Bone Marrow Transplantation for Severe Combined Immunodeficiency After Soybean Lectin Fractionation

Roland J. Levinsky, BSc, MD, FRCP, E.G. Davies, MRCP, M. Butler, FIMLS, A. Abai, BSc, D.C. Linch, MRCP, and A.H. Goldstone, MRCP

Institute of Child Health, London WC1N 1EH (R.J.L., E.G.D., M.B., A.A.), and University College Hospital, London (D.C.L., A.H.G.), England

INTRODUCTION

In mice and rats, transplantation across major histocompatibility barriers is possible without fatal GVHD developing, only when all alloreactive theta (θ)-positive cells are removed prior to infusion of bone marrow [1,2]. The mortality increases dramatically when splenocytes containing immunocompetent T cells are added back to the bone marrow infusion [3]. In man, there is so far no antibody which recognizes the theta equivalent; therefore, other measures to remove these cells are necessary. The galactose-binding lectins, soybean agglutinin (SBA) and peanut agglutinin (PNA) selectively bind to hemopoietic precursors in the marrow of the mouse; the stem cells isolated in this way fully reconstitute hemopoietic function in lethally irradiated H2 incompatible mice without GVHD [3]. In man, SBA binds to mature cells; thus, the stem cell-enriched fraction is obtained by negative selection. Applying this technique, Reisner et al [4] obtained full engraftment in a leukemic patient mismatched with the parental donor at the A, B, and C, but not DR loci.

Accordingly, we have applied the same technique of bone marrow fractionation to the transplantation of 5 babies with SCID using one of the parents as donors. In 4 of the cases there was a haplotype mismatch, but one child was phenotypically A, B, C, and DR identical with her mother, although with a very strong MLR.

METHODS

One liter of bone marrow (fraction 1) was harvested from the donor; it was concentrated to 250 ml on a cell separator and the red cells separated by sedimentation with hydroxyethyl starch (fraction 2). The white cells were incubated with SBA (2 mg/ml) for 5 minutes and the agglutinated (fraction 3) and unagglutinated (fraction 4) separated on a 5% BSA gradient. Residual T cells were then removed by 2 rosetting steps with neuraminidase-treated SRBC followed by Ficoll-Triosil centrifugation. Fraction 5 consisted of the E +ve cells from the first rosetting step, fraction 6: the cells from the first Ficoll-Triosil interface, while fraction 7 were the E −ve cells from the second rosetting step used for the transplant. All fractions were evaluated morphologically and by monoclonal antisera for colony-forming activity and for MLR.

RESULTS

Bone Marrow Separation

A representative separation (Case 2) is shown in Table 1. The number of nucleated cells in fraction 7 was approximately 5% of those found in the original marrow (fraction 1). Fraction 7 retained 47% of the original erythroid burst-forming activity (BFUe), and 66% of the granulocyte colony-forming activity (CFU$_{GM}$). It was considerably enriched for myelocytes and for cells bearing the immature OKT10$^+$ antigen. Of 5 separations used for the transplants, the final fraction consistently contained <0.5% mature T cells (defined by E-rosetting and by monoclonal antiserum UCH1) and had no reactivity in MLR against a third unrelated party.

In a natural killer cell (NK) assay against MOLT 4 cell line, fraction 7 showed approximately one-third of the activity of fraction 1. All children received approximately 1×10^8 nucleated fraction 7 cells/kg/bw.

Patients Posttransplant

Case 1

This 9-month-old male SCID with high B-cell numbers received a haplotype mismatch graft from his father. He showed engraftment by day 28 with 26% T cells (UCH1 +ve) which responded to PHA (stimulation index 4). However, he developed adenovirus hepatitis and died of this on day 37. At postmortem, there was no evidence of GVH.

Case 2

This 8-month-old male SCID with ADA deficiency received a haplotype mismatch graft from his mother. The final fraction (No. 7) had 0.2% T-cell contamination. He showed engraftment by day 25. Normal numbers of mature T cells (65% UCH1 +ve) were rapidly established but with a very abnormal helper/suppressor (OKT4$^+$/OKT8$^+$) ratio of 1:6. All the T cells were maternal by HLA typing. PHA-stimulation index was normal (>10). B-cell en-

TABLE 1. Representative Bone Marrow Fractionation *Case 2*

Fraction No.	Cells %	T cells (UCH1) %	OKT10 %	MLR SI	BFUe %	CFU$_{GM}$ %	NK %	Erythroid precursors %	Myeloid precursors %
1	100	19	4	2.4	100	100	32	13	13
2	52	8	4	1.65	81	81	10	9	17
3	22	11	4	2.85	5	4	1	15	7
4	8	11	12	<1.0	52	78	35	0.5	41
5	2	31	8	1.7	—	—	23	0	23
6	6	1	20	<1.0	—	—	13	0	56
7	4.8	0.2	34	<1.0	47	66	9	0	57

Cells % = percentage nucleated cells; 100% is that of starting marrow
UCH1 = monoclonal antibody recognizing all T cells
OKT10 = monoclonal antibody recognizing lymphoid and myeloid precursors
MLR = mixed lymphocyte reaction expressed as a stimulation index (SI)
BFUe = erythroid burst-forming units; 100% is that of starting marrow
CFU$_{GM}$ = monocyte/granulocyte colony-forming units; 100% is that of starting marrow
NK = natural killer cell activity against MOLT 4 cell line expressed as % chromium release
Erythroid and myeloid precursors expressed as percentage of nucleated cell count.

TABLE 2. *Case 3* **(ADA Deficiency)**

	E. rosettes	UCH1 (pan T)	OKT4 (helper T)	OKT8 (suppressor T)	OKT6 (cortical thymocytes)	OKT10 (lymphoid precursors)	WT1 (pan T, thymocytes undifferentiated leukemia)
At diagnosis	<1	1	3	1	1	7	NT
After regular transfusions	<1	1	1	0	0	8	NT
10/52 after transplant	32	13	14	7	2	40	63
18/52 after transplant	52	50	21	13	1	12	NT

NT = not tested

graftment was slow, appearing first at 3 months. Initially, at 28 days posttransplant, there was mild skin GVH which responded to steroids, but by 60 days this had become worse with gut and liver involvement. By days 90–120, GVH was at stage III–IV and could not be controlled with high dose steroids plus azathioprine. His bone marrow became hypocellular with no megakaryocytes. Throughout this time the T-cell numbers and helper/suppressor ratio of 1:6 remained constant. Intermittently very high numbers of cells bearing DR$^+$ antigens were seen. The child died at 6-months postgraft of severe GVH. Following this experience, we decided to add cyclosporin A from day −2 to day +100 as a precaution against the T-cell contamination. The drug was given either orally or intravenously twice daily attempting to maintain trough levels at 100–300 ng/ml.

Case 3

This 6-month-old female SCID with ADA deficiency received a phenotypically identical, but MLR incompatible, bone marrow from her mother. Engraftment was severely delayed, but at 6-weeks postgraft she developed immature T cells in her blood. These were E-rosette positive, OKT10 positive, and WT1 positive (this latter monoclonal antisera recognizes mature T cells, thymocytes, and undifferentiated leukemias [5]), but were OKT3, OKT4, OKT8, and OKT6 negative (Table 2). This cell type remained constant until 12-weeks postgraft despite treatment with crude fraction V (TP1) and synthetic (TP5) thymic hormone. Cyclosporin A was stopped at 10 weeks. At 14-weeks postgraft, the cells matured with full graft take and strong PHA stimulation index (SI) (>10) (Fig. 1). She began producing antibody, but recently, shortly after discharge, has developed an aggressive Coombs-positive autoimmune hemolytic anemia (IgG antibody) which is requiring high dose steroids to suppress hemolysis. There have never been any other signs or symptoms of GVH.

Case 4

This 8-month-old male SCID with ADA deficiency received a haplotype mismatch graft from his father. Graft

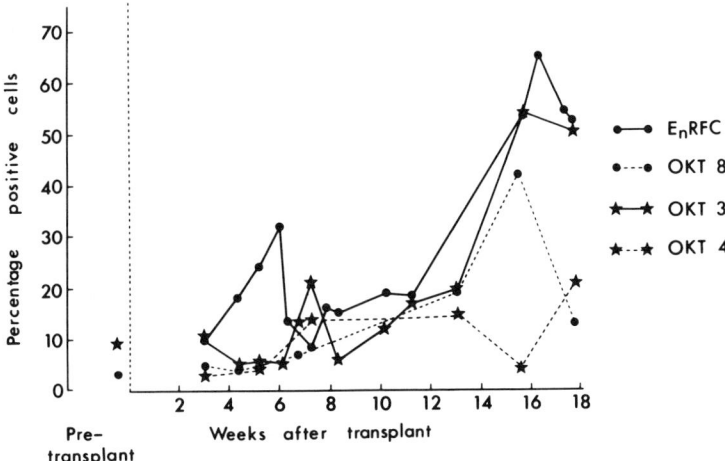

Fig. 1. Posttransplant course of *Case 3* illustrated by rising percentage of T-cell subpopulations. E_nRFC = E rosettes; OKT3 = pan T cell; OKT4 = helper/inducer T cell; OKT8 = suppressor cytotoxic T cell.

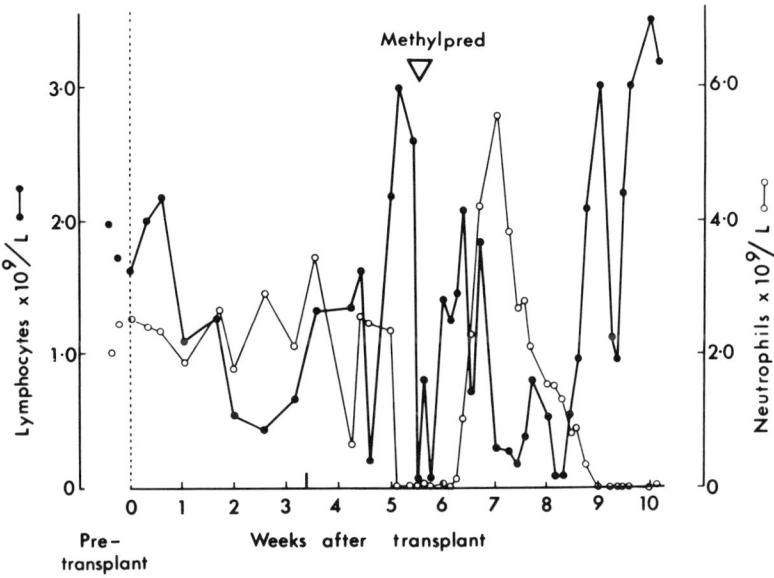

Fig. 2. Reciprocal relationship between lymphocyte and neutrophil count as T-cell engraftment occurred in *Case 5*. Neutrophil count only returned following steroid suppression. Methylpred=methylprednisolone pulse therapy 30 mg/kg/iv for 4 days.

take has been very slow and 18-weeks postgraft he has 30% E-rosetting cells but only 15–18% of these show mature $OKT3^+$, $OKT4^+$, and $OKT8^+$ antigens; his cells still do not respond to PHA or MLR. Cyclosporin A was stopped at 10 weeks. At present he is very well and is thriving. At no time has he shown any signs of GVH.

Case 5

This 5-month-old male SCID with high B-cell numbers received a haplotype mismatch graft from his father. There was evidence of full graft take by day 35, but soon after this he developed mild liver GVH. As his T-cell numbers became normal, he dropped his neutrophil count and his bone marrow showed an excess of monocytoid cells with almost complete absence of myeloid precursors. Neutrophils reappeared after methyl-prednisolone pulse therapy (Fig. 2) but disappeared again 4 weeks later as the T-cell graft returned. Following further methylprednisolone pulse therapy he was treated with daily prednisolone which is being tapered gradually. At 14-weeks posttransplant he is thriving with a normal neutrophil count, full T-cell take, but is still on cyclosporin A and low-dose prednisolone. He has no signs of GVH.

DISCUSSION

Our mixed experience of mismatched bone marrow transplantation indicates that it is possible to cross histocompatibility barriers in man but that it is not without problems. The technique of fractionation using SBA and 2 E-rosetting steps is cumbersome and time-consuming (the procedure takes approximately 15 hours). The technique is efficient if performed carefully, and reliably leaves a homogeneous precursor cell type which is 99% viable and with <0.5% T-cell contamination. To date, we have not been able to achieve anything approaching that efficiency using monoclonal antibodies.

We have achieved engraftment of T cells (and B cells in some cases) in all the children, but graft take has been very slow. Since using cyclosporin A in addition, we have not had any aggressive acute GVH and the drug appears to prevent skin GVH. We do not believe that graft take is further delayed *(Case 5)*. The excessively prolonged take with immature T cells was confined to the 2 children with ADA deficiency. Both were more severely affected than *Case 2* in that they did not respond at all to repeated red cell transfusions. It is possible that damage to thymic epithelium by the toxic deoxynucleotides is a factor in their slow thymic/T-cell maturation. We can surmise from these 2 children that the early prethymic T cell expresses E-rosette receptors, OKT10 and WT1 antigens, but not OKT6, OKT3, 4, or 8 antigens.

To date, none of the children can be considered cured, since *Case 3* has an autoimmune hemolytic anemia requiring steroid suppression, *Case 4* still shows immature T-cell engraftment, and *Case 5* is still on cyclosporin A and low-dose steroids. However, the experience of these latter 3 SCID children is very encouraging. The combination of T-cell removal from bone marrow plus cyclosporin A may allow haplotype mismatched bone marrow grafting without severe GVHD to be performed for any condition, when techniques have been further refined.

ACKNOWLEDGMENTS

We thank Dr. Y. Reisner for teaching us the technique, the Leukaemia Research Fund for generous support, and Sandoz Ltd for supplies of cyclosporin A.

REFERENCES

1. Once K, Fernandez G, Good RA: Humoral and cell-mediated immune responses in fully allogeneic bone marrow chimera in mice. J Exp Med 151:115, 1980.
2. Muller-Ruckholtz W, Wotlge WU, Muller-Hermelink HK: Bone marrow transplantation in rats across strong histocompatibility barriers by selective elimination of lymphoid cells in donor marrow. Transplant Proc 8:537, 1976.
3. Reisner Y, Itzicovitch L, Meshorer A, Sharon N: Haemopoietic stem cell transplantation using mouse bone marrow and spleen cells fractionated by lectins. Proc Natl Acad Sci USA 75:2933, 1978.
4. Reisner Y, Kapoor N, Pollack MS, Dupont B, Chagant RSK, Good RA, O'Reilly RJ: Transplantation for acute leukaemia using HLA A, B, C non-identical parental marrow cells fractionated with soy bean agglutinin and sheep red blood cells. Lancet 2:327, 1981.
5. Tax WJM, Willems HW, Kibbcluar MDA, De Groot J, Capel PJA, De Waal RMW, Reekers P, Koene RAP: Monoclonal antibodies against human thymocytes and T lymphocytes. In Peeters H (ed): "Protides of the Biological Fluids." New York: Pergamon Press, 1981, vol 29, p 701.

SECTION 3
DISORDERS AFFECTING B LYMPHOCYTES

Diagnosis Criteria and Classification of Human Primary Defects of Humoral Immunity

Maxime Seligmann, MD, and Jean-Jacques Ballet, MD

Laboratory of Immunochemistry and Immunopathology, INSERM U 108, Research Institute on Blood Diseases of University Paris VII and Laboratory of Oncology and Immunohematology of CNRS, Hôpital Saint-Louis, 75475 Paris Cedex 10, France

Interactions and cooperation between B cells, T cells and macrophages in the regulation of immune responses render the usual distinction of immunodeficiencies (ID) into deficiencies in cell-mediated immunity (CMI), deficiencies in antibody production, and combined deficiencies of both functions somehow arbitrary and difficult. However, a predominant and primary defect of humoral immunity (ie diminished or absent antibody response to infections or injected antigens, with preserved, or largely preserved, immune responses of the T cells) characterizes the deficiencies of humoral immunity (HID) which will be considered here.

Any attempt to classify primary ID must be based on current information about: 1) phenotypic expression of abnormalities, 2) mode of inheritance, 3) association with certain characteristic clinical abnormalities, 4) presumed level of faulty cellular differentiation, 5) possible pathogenetic mechanisms, and 6) presumed nature of the basic defect. However, we wish to underline that, in spite of increasing knowledge, the nature of the basic defect remains unknown in most HID syndromes and that all our own attempts to classify primary ID [1,2], as well as those of the successive WHO expert committees, remain unsatisfactory, most patients still belonging to a "waste basket" under the heading of "common variable ID" which encompasses a heterogeneous group of poorly classified patients.

DIAGNOSIS CRITERIA

The main clinical feature leading to diagnosis of HID is the recurrence of invasive pyogenic infections. It should be remembered, however, that, in some conditions, such as selective IgA deficiency, an appreciable number of individuals remain healthy throughout life, and diagnosis may be by a laboratory finding. In certain cases, clinical manifestations may be delayed in life (ie agammaglobulinemia with thymoma, common variable ID (CVID), or transient (transient hypogammaglobulinemia of childhood).

Although humoral ID are defined by impaired *antibody* production, the deficiency in serum immunoglobulins (Ig) usually represents the main biologic feature. No major difficulty arises in defining cases with marked depression of all or most Ig classes.

The theoretic rationale for delineating entities in which only one Ig class is deeply depressed may be questioned. For instance, in selective IgA deficiency which was considered to be the best example of such a single Ig class defect, it was shown that IgG_2 and sometimes IgG_4 subclasses may be greatly reduced [3]. Moreover, selective IgA deficiency is a rather frequent finding in family members of patients with CVID.

Selective deficiency of some IgG subclasses, although of clinical significance, may be underestimated when the IgG_1 subclass is unaffected, since total IgG levels may remain within normal limits. The availability of monoclonal antibodies specific for each IgG subclass will probably make possible the recognition of an increasing number of IgG subclass deficiencies. The evaluation of in vivo antibody responses to various antigens (including polysaccharide antigens) is crucial in such patients, and also in the rare group of patients with ID who appear to manifest only a failure to produce normal specific antibody titers while maintaining normal (or elevated) serum levels of all Ig classes (and subclasses?) [4].

It is of note that important spontaneous fluctuations of Ig levels are not uncommon during the course of some HID (mainly CVID), suggesting abnormalities in regulatory mechanisms. Imbalances in Ig-light chain and γ-heavy chain isotypes are not uncommon in patients with primary hypogammaglobulinemia [5].

The mode of inheritance is of major interest in the classification of those ID which are clearly familial. It is of note that several ID syndromes appear inherited as an X-linked condition, suggesting an important and yet undefined role of the X chromosome in the expression of immunologic functions. We wish to emphasize that important variations in the phenotypic expression of ID may occur within members of a given family, showing that a same genetic defect may lead to different immunologic patterns [6]. It should be recalled that many of the adult-onset variable Ig deficiencies are genetically determined, even though the exact mode of inheritance cannot be ascertained in most cases.

ASSOCIATED CLINICAL ABNORMALITIES

Whereas several primary ID (such as ataxia telangiectasia (AT) or the Wiskott-Aldrich syndrome (WAS)) are mainly defined and classified according to associated characteristic clinical features, the only meaningful association within HID is the coexistence of thymoma and agammaglobulinemia. In this respect, the recently described cases of X-linked hypogammaglobulinemia associated with an isolated growth hormone deficiency [7] appear of interest.

The incidence of autoimmune disorders and malignancies is high among patients with ID. Although predominant in certain categories, these associated conditions are not helpful for the classification of ID. Moreover, they may even be misleading in reaching a diagnosis. For instance, the respective priority of ID or lymphoid malignancy may be difficult to establish in some patients, and family history is of particular help.

POTENTIAL PATHOGENIC MECHANISMS

The ontogeny and continual differentiation of the human B-cell lineage is now known in some detail [8]. Current knowledge of this framework has allowed us to elucidate the level of faulty B-cell differentiation in several primary defects of humoral immunity. The enumeration of pre-B cells in the bone marrow, and of circulating B lymphocytes with characterization of the isotypes of their membrane-bound Ig are of utmost importance.

The mechanisms responsible for the failure to produce antibodies cannot be deduced from the mere phenotype of circulating B (or T) cells, and remain unknown for many patients although progress has been made in recent years. It should be stressed that, whatever the level in the B-cell differentiation pathway where the apparent defect lies, the faulty B-cell development and failure of Ig production may be due a) to an intrinsic abnormality of B cells, and/ or b) to the deficiency of any factor required for their differentiation and produced by other cell types, such as helper factors of T cells, and/or c) to the presence of suppressor factors or inhibitory substances. It should also be remembered that the study of circulating cells does not take into account possible microenvironmental influences.

To explore these potential mechanisms, which are not mutually exclusive, a variety of in vitro procedures have been developed. Defects in the maturation of the patients' B cells into Ig-producing plasma cells are studied after stimulation by polyclonal activators of B cells, such as T-cell factors, or pokeweed mitogen (PWM) which is the best established T-cell dependent activator, *Nocardia opaca* and other mitogens. Transformation by Epstein-Barr virus (EBV), a T-helper (Th) cell independent activator, has also been used successfully. The latter procedure has allowed cell lines derived from patients with HID to develop as well as somatic cell hybrids enabling biochemical and genetic investigations to be performed [9]. The in vitro stimulation of specific antibody production, without the use of a polyclonal activator, has been successfully studied using SRBC, influenza, tetanus-toxoid (TT) and ΦX 174 antigens. On the other hand, immunoregulatory T-cell functions are evaluated by co-culture experiments and functional studies of T-cell subsets which are usually correlated with a given phenotype of their membrane-bound antigens.

Levels of Arrested B-Cell Differentiation and Functional B-Cell Defects

In this section we wish to review briefly the main data available on developmental arrests of the B-cell lineage in some HID syndromes and on functional in vitro studies of B cells, aiming to establish or to rule out the existence of an intrinsic B-cell defect.

In most patients with X-linked agammaglobulinemia (SLA), circulating B lymphocytes are absent and pre-B cells are present in the bone marrow. No lymphoblastoid cell lines could be established from the peripheral blood of such patients. However, a group of unique EBV-containing cell lines were derived from bone marrow [10]. Some of these lines resembled pre-B cells and other possible precursors of pre-B cells without detectable Ig molecules. The possibility that some of these cell lines reflect abnormal Ig synthesis characteristic of SLA has not been ruled out. In contrast, in those very rare cases of SLA where circulating B cells are present, these cells could be hybridized with mouse myeloma cells. These hybrids were found to synthesize and secrete human Ig [11].

In patients with selective IgA deficiency, IgA-bearing lymphocytes are always present in the blood [12], and PWM is able to induce differentiation into IgA-plasma cells [13]. The majority of these circulating IgA-bearing lymphocytes express surface IgM and IgD as well as IgA and are therefore not mature activated lymphocytes [14]. This finding is in agreement with the relatively low percentage of IgA-plasma cells obtained after in vitro stimulation.

In ID with hyper-IgM (which are often but not always transmitted as an X-linked trait), circulating B cells bearing IgG or IgA are absent, although all 3 IgD-IgM-bearing B-cell subsets are present [15]. Circulating plasmacytoid IgM-secreting cells are found. Circulating B cells from these patients could not be triggered in vitro by EBV or mitogens to produce IgG; they secrete only IgM [16]. Therefore, this syndrome appears to be characterized by an intrinsic defect in B-cell isotype switch.

Some ID patients fail completely to produce Ig molecules with κ chains. In these patients with κ-chain deficiency, the precise level of faulty cellular differentiation may be equivocal. In one patient [17], a normal κ/λ ratio was found among circulating B lymphocytes and also for cytoplasmic Ig in in vitro PWM-induced plasma cells. In another patient [18], circulating B lymphocytes bore Ig molecules with λ-light chains exclusively; however, in such a patient, κ-chain-containing plasma cells could be obtained after stimulation by PWM. Thus, the deficiency in κ-chain production may result from either an abnormality of in vivo terminal differentiation of B_K lymphocytes or to an intrinsic abnormality of the κ-polypeptide chain.

In agammaglobulinemia with thymoma there is usually a lack or considerable decrease in circulating B cells and bone marrow pre-B cells.

Transient hypogammaglobulinemia of infancy is characterized by normal numbers of circulating B lymphocytes with normal isotypic diversification of their membrane-bound Ig. There is a block of in vivo terminal differentiation into plasma cells, contrasting with normal Ig in vitro production after EBV transformation. These findings strongly suggest an immunoregulatory defect.

Since CVID represents a heterogeneous group of disorders, it could be expected that the findings in these patients would display a great degree of heterogeneity. The patients are clearly heterogeneous in terms of the site of the block in B-cell differentiation and in the pathogenetic mechanism that leads to the defect in Ig synthesis [15, 19, 20]. The study of circulating B lymphocytes, including the determination of isotypes of their surface Ig molecules, and of in vitro Ig production, allows delineation of some categories with CVID.

Many patients have near normal or moderately low numbers of circulating B cells, with absence of B lymphocytes bearing IgM without IgD, and of SIgG-positive cells; thus the circulating lymphocytes are "immature." Another subset of patients has very low numbers of circulating B cells and normal numbers of bone marrow pre-B cells. A third subgroup of patients, including the majority of those presenting with considerable follicular hyperplasia of lymph nodes, has near normal or increased number of circulating B lymphocytes, without major abnormalities in isotypic diversification of their surface Ig suggesting a block in terminal differentiation. Some patients may show considerable variations in the numbers of circulating B cells, depending mainly upon intercurrent infections [21].

In some patients, mainly within the second category, B cells do not produce Ig for export in response to mitogenic stimulation or following EBV transformation. In other patients, B cells are found which are not triggered to Ig secretion by T-dependent activators such as PWM, but which do produce Ig when transformed by EBV. Finally, B cells from some patients do synthesize and secrete Ig in vitro after T-dependent or T-independent polyclonal activation.

Two other minor but well-defined categories are delineated from such studies within patients with CVID. One of these subgroups is characterized by near normal numbers of circulating B cells with increased numbers of IgG-bearing lymphocytes. These patients have bone marrow plasma cells and fail to secrete IgG, secondary to the production of an altered heavy chain [22, 23]. The last category is featured by low or very low numbers of circulating B lymphocytes, with preserved normal isotypic diversification of their membrane-bound Ig molecules and without evidence of faulty differentiation. These patients have autoantibodies to B cells [24].

Defective T-Cell Control of B-Cell Differentiation

Since the original observation of Waldmann et al [25] that suppressor cells may play an important role in the pathogenesis of hypogammaglobulinemia, a large body of evidence supports the occurrence of imbalanced immunoregulatory T-cell functions in some patients with HID.

All data in this field of investigation should be interpreted with great caution. It may be somewhat hazardous to elaborate pathogenetic mechanisms on the sole basis of imbalances in T-cell subsets identified by their antigenic markers which do not always correlate with the results of functional studies. For instance, some patients with ID were found to have nonfunctional T4+ cells, ie a lack of Th-cell function contrasting with normal numbers of circulating cells belonging to the T4+ inducer subset [26].

A number of issues have been raised concerning the observations made in co-culture experiments [27]. The results obtained in these experiments should take into account several parameters such as the critical T/B-cell ratio, the number of monocytes, the possible occurrence of mixed lymphocyte reactions, the nature of the polyclonal B-cell activator, and the administration of previous gamma globulin therapy. Suppressive activity may affect the synthesis of all Ig classes or of only one Ig class, may lead to κ/λ imbalances, or even affect Ig secretion [28]. Furthermore, the target of excessive suppressor activity should be studied whenever possible.

The demonstration of unequivocal defective T-cell control does not necessarily mean that it represents a primary pathogenetic mechanism causing hypogammaglobulinemia and that an intrinsic B-cell defect should be ruled out. The co-existence of a dual B-and T-cell primary dysfunction due to the same basic defect is a theoretic possibility. Excessive T-cell suppressor activity may constitute a secondary phenomenon. The secondary development of circulating suppressor T cells does indeed occur in patients with hypogammaglobulinemia and a primary B-cell defect, such as SLA [29]. In this respect, one

TABLE 1.

Designation	Usual Phenotypic Expression			Presumed Level of Faulty B-Cell Differentiation
	Serum Ig	Serum Antibodies	Circulating B Cells	
SLA	↓↓(All)	↓↓	Usually absent	Pre-B cell
Ig deficiency with increased IgM	↓↓ IgG and IgA ↑ IgM and ± IgD	↓ IgG and IgA Ab	• Normal IgM-and IgD-bearing cells • No IgG-or IgA-bearing cells • Plasmacytoid IgM-secreting cells	Failure of IgM B cell switch to IgG
"Selective" IgA deficiency	1) ↓↓ IgA 2) ↓ IgA with IgG2 (and IgG4)	↓↓ IgA Ab ↓ IgA and IgG$_2$ Ab	Presence of IgA-bearing cells expressing simultaneously IgM and/or IgD	"Immature" Bα lymphocytes
Selective deficiency in other Ig class or subclass	↓ IgM ↓ IgG subclass	↓ Ab of the deficient class/ subclass	? Normal ?	? Terminal differentiation Unknown
Secretory piece deficiency	↓↓ Secretory IgA	↓↓ Secretory IgA Ab		
Kappa-chain deficiency	↓↓ κ	↓	↓Bκ in some	Unknown
Antibody deficiency with normal or hypergammaglobulinemia	Normal or elevated	↓ To most antigens	Near normal	Unknown
Transient hypogammaglobulinemia of infancy	↓ IgG	↓	Normal	Terminal differentiation
Transcobalamin II deficiency	↓ IgG	↓	Normal	Terminal differentiation
ID with thymoma	↓ (All)	↓	Absent or very low	Pre-B cell precursor ? HSC
X-linked hypogammaglobulinemia with growth hormone deficiency	↓↓ (All)	↓	Absent or very low	? Pre-B cell
CVID with predominant Ig deficiency	↓	↓	1) Near normal (with absence of SIgM +/SIgD- and of SIgG+ cells) 2) Very low 3) Near normal or increased 4) Near normal with increased numbers of SIgG cells 5) Low with normal subsets	1) Immature lymphocytes 2) Pre-B cell or early lymphocyte 3) Terminal differentiation 4) Defect in Ig secretion 5) No evidence of faulty differentiation

Continued

TABLE 1. (continued)

Designation	Possible Pathogenetic Mechanism(s)			Nature of Basic Defect	Inheritance	Characteristic Associated Features
	Intrinsic B-Cell Defect	Abnormal T-Cell Control	Others			
SLA	+	0	—	Unknown	X-linked	—
Ig deficiency with increased IgM	+	?0	—	Unknown	X-linked > AR > unknown	—
"Selective" IgA deficiency	?+	?+ (IgA-specific suppressor activity or inadequate help)	—	Unknown	Unknown > AR > AD (frequent in families with variable ID)	—
Selective deficiency in other Ig class or subclass	?+	?+ (Specific T-suppressor activity)	—	Unknown	Unknown > AR	—
Secretory piece deficiency			Mucosal epithelial cell	Unknown	Unknown	—
Kappa-chain deficiency	?+	0	—	Unknown	Unknown	—
Antibody deficiency with normal or hypergammaglobulinemia	?0	?+ (Defective help)	?	Unknown	Unknown > AR	—
Transient hypogammaglobulinemia of infancy	?0	+ Lack of T-helper activity	—	Unknown	Unknown (frequent in heterozygous individuals in families with SCID)	—
Transcobalamin II deficiency	?+	?0	—	Metabolic effects of vitamin B_{12} deficiency	AR	1) Pancytopenia with megaloblastic anemia 2) Intestinal villous atrophy 3) Defect in granulocyte bactericidal activity
ID with thymoma	?+	+ (Excessive T suppressor activity)	—	Unknown	Unknown	1) Thymoma 2) Eosinopenia 3) Erythroblastopenia 4) Aplastic anemia
X-linked hypogammaglobulinemia with growth hormone deficiency	+	0	—	Unknown	X-linked	Short stature
CVID with predominant Ig deficiency	+ (0 in some cases)	+ In some cases: a) Excessive T-suppressor activity b) Absent or defective helper T cells c) Autoantibodies to helper T cells	Autoantibodies to B cells	Unknown (except for abnormal H chain in subgroup 4)	Unknown > AR > AD	—

should recall the elegant experiments of Blaese et al [30] demonstrating at the same time that suppressor T cells develop in bursectomized and irradiated chicken, and that these suppressor T cells do cause agammaglobulinemia when transferred to syngeneic normal birds.

Defective T-cell help. Of particular interest is the numeric and functional deficiency in T4+ helper cells found, in the absence of excessive suppression and of an intrinsic B-cell defect, in infants with transient hypogammaglobulinemia [31].

A small subset of patients with CVID has a profound deficiency of Th-cell function [20], in the presence or absence of T4+ cells [26,32]. Defective help has also been demonstrated by Ochs et al (this volume) in patients with HID and elevated gamma globulins. The possible role of autoantibodies to Th cells should also be mentioned [33].

Excessive suppressor T-cell activity. Excessive suppressor cell activity consistently has been found in patients with hypogammaglobulinemia associated with thymoma [25]. In such immunodeficient patients with red cell aplasia, an effect of suppressor T cells on both Ig production and erythroid differentiation has been demonstrated [34].

Some patients with CVID possess an increased number of T5/T8 suppressor cells that were activated in vivo, as judged by the expression of Ia antigens on their cell surface [32]. Carefully controlled co-culture experiments demonstrate that excessive suppressor T-cell activity appears to be the primary pathogenetic mechanism in a subgroup of patients with CVID who have no demonstrable B-cell defect [27]. In contrast, the occurrence of excessive suppression appears to be a secondary phenomenon in some other patients, and the absence of any T-cell immunoregulatory abnormality in many others should be outlined [20]. Little information is currently available concerning the suppressor role of monocytes, which may be of importance in some patients [35,36].

A T-cell mediated specific suppression of IgA synthesis has been observed in some [37], but not all [38], persons with selective IgA deficiency. The primary pathogenesis of this syndrome remains speculative since inadequate T-cell help has also been advocated [39] and since there is much evidence in favor of an intrinsic B-cell defect [38].

Antibody-mediated elimination of B-lymphocytes. Elimination of B-lymphocytes by autoantibodies specific for B cells has been documented in a patient of Tursz et al [24]. The autoantibody nature of the anti-B-cell antibodies and their pathogenetic role leading to HID was demonstrated by removal of the antibodies by massive plasmaphereses which were followed by a dramatic and transitory increase in B-cell numbers.

PRESUMED NATURE OF THE BASIC DEFECT

There is still a considerable lack of knowledge in this field.

Whereas the nature of the basic enzymatic defect has been elucidated in some SCIDs and T-cell immunodeficiencies (reviewed by Rochelle Hirschhorn in this volume), the low enzymatic activities described in patients with HID, such as 5′nucleotidase or cytosol enzymes, presumably reflect B-cell immaturity rather than a basic underlying metabolic defect [40]. The occurrence of depressed humoral and cellular immunity in some children with biotin-dependent carboxylase deficiencies should be mentioned [41].

The nature of the basic defect is unknown in most HID syndromes. Exceptions to this rule are the few patients with CVID who fail to secrete Ig molecules where the production of an abnormal γ-chain has been demonstrated, and the ID syndrome associated with transcobalamin II deficiency [42] where vitamin B_{12} deficiency results in a defective DNA methylation.

The search for Ig-gene abnormalities in patients with HID has been disappointing up to now, even in instances such as ID with hyper-IgM or κ-chain deficiency where such abnormalities could be expected.

The complexity of the relationship between humoral ID and viral infections should be recalled. The secondary nature of ID following in utero rubella infection is well established. Immunodeficiencies, presumably secondary to cytomegalovirus infections, are reported with increasing frequency. Epstein-Barr virus infection activates the suppressor/cytotoxic T-cell subset which becomes Ia+ during acute infectious mononucleosis [43]. In this regard, the X-linked susceptibility to EBV leading to transient or permanent hypogammaglobulinemia, as well as fatal mononucleosis, aplastic anemia, and B-cell lymphoproliferative disorders [44] is of particular interest. This syndrome may be considered as primary ID. The immune defect in these patients and family members at risk is possibly not selective but generalized, since abnormal antibody responses to bacteriophage ΦX 174 have been demonstrated by Ochs et al (this volume).

In Table 1 we have attempted to classify the various primary humoral immunodeficiencies according to the above-mentioned parameters.

REFERENCES

1. Seligmann M, Fudenberg HH, Good RA: A proposed classification of primary immunologic deficiencies. Am J Med 45:817–825, 1968.
2. Cooper MD, Lawton AR, Preud'homme JL, Seligmann M: Primary antibody deficiencies. Springer Sem Immunopathol 1:265–281, 1978.
3. Oxelius V-A, Laurell AB, Lindquist B, Golebiowska H, Axelsson U, Bjorkander J: IgG subclasses in selective IgA deficiency: Importance of IgG_2-IgA deficiency. N Engl J Med 304:1476–1477, 1981.

1981.
4. Blecher TE, Soothill JF, Voyce MA, Walker WHC: Antibody deficiency syndrome. A case with normal immunoglobulin levels. Clin Exp Immunol 3:47–51, 1968.
5. Yount WJ, Hong R, Seligmann M, Good R, Kunkel HG: Imbalances of gamma globulin subgroups and gene defects in patients with primary hypogammaglobulinemia. J Clin Invest 49:1957–1966, 1970.
6. Wedgwood RJ, Ochs HD: Variability in the expression of X-linked agammaglobulinemia: The coexistence of classic X-LA (Bruton type) and "common variable immunodeficiency" in the same families. In Seligmann M, Hitzig WH (eds): "Primary Immunodeficiencies." INSERM Symposium No 16. New York: Elsevier, 1980, pp 69–78.
7. Fleisher TA, White RM, Broder S, Nissley PS, Blaese RM, Mulvihill JJ, Olive G, Waldmann TA: X-linked hypogammaglobulinemia and isolated growth hormone deficiency. N Engl J Med 302:1429–1434, 1980.
8. Cooper MD: Pre B cells: Normal and abnormal development. J Clin Immunol 1:81–89, 1981.
9. Schwaber J: Agammaglobulinemia in vitro: Lymphoid cell lines and somatic cell hybrids. Supra #6, pp 49–57.
10. Fu SM, Hurley JN, McCune JM, Kunkel HG, Good RA: Pre-B cells and other possible precursor lymphoid cell lines derived from patients with X-linked agammaglobulinemia. J Exp Med 152:1519–1526, 1980.
11. Schwaber JF, Rosen FS: Induction of human immunoglobulin synthesis and secretion in somatic cell hybrids of mouse myeloma and human B lymphocytes from patients with agammaglobulinemia. J Exp Med 148:974–979, 1978.
12. Preud'homme JL, Griscelli C, Seligmann M: Immunoglobulin on the surface of lymphocytes in fifty patients with primary immunodeficiency diseases. Clin Immunol Immunopathol 1:241–256, 1973.
13. Wu LYF, Lawton AR, Cooper MD: Differentiation capacity of cultured B lymphocytes from immunodeficient patients. J Clin Invest 52:3180–3189, 1973.
14. Conley ME, Cooper MD: Immature IgA B cells in IgA deficient patients. N Engl J Med 305:495–497, 1981.
15. Schwaber JF, Rosen FS: Isotypes of surface immunoglobulin on B lymphocytes from patients with immune deficiency. J Clin Immunol 2:30–34, 1982.
16. Schwaber JF, Lazarus H, Rosen FS: IgM-restricted production of immunoglobulin by lymphoid cell lines from patients with immunodeficiency with hyper IgM (dysgammaglobulinemia). Clin Immunol Immunopathol (19:91–97, 1981.
17. Barandun S, Morell A, Skvaril F, Oberdorfer A: Deficiency of kappa- or lambda-type immunoglobulins. Blood 47:79–89, 1976.
18. Zegers BJM, Maertzdorf WJ, Van Loghem E, Mul NAJ, Stoop JW, Van der Laag J, Vossen JJ, Ballieux RE: Kappa chain deficiency. An immunoglobulin disorder. N Engl J Med 294:1026–1030, 1976.
19. De Gast GC, Wilkins SR, Webster ADB, Rickinson A, Platts-Mills TAE: Functional "immaturity" of isolated B cells from patients with hypogammaglobulinemia. Clin Exp Immunol 42:535–544, 1980.
20. Platts-Mills TAE, De Gast GC, Webster ADB, Asherson GL, Wilkins SR: Two immunologically distinct forms of late onset hypogammaglobulinemia. Clin Exp Immunol 44:383–388, 1981.
21. Seligmann M, Preud'homme JL, Brouet JC: B and T cell markers in human proliferative blood diseases and primary blood diseases and primary immunodeficiencies, with special reference to membrane bound immunoglobulins. Transplant Rev 16:85–113, 1973.
22. Ciccimara F, Rosen F, Schneeberger E, Merler E: Failure of heavy chain glycosylation of IgG in some patients with common variable agammaglobulinemia. J Clin Invest 57:1386–1390, 1976.
23. Schwaber J, Rosen F: Somatic cell hybrids of mouse myeloma cells and B lymphocytes from a patient with agammaglobulinemia: Failure to secrete human Ig. J Immunol 122:1849–1854, 1979.
24. Tursz T, Preud'homme JL, Labaume S, Matuchansky C, Seligmann M: Autoantibodies to B lymphocytes in a patient with hypoimmunoglobulinemia: Characterization and pathogenic role. J Clin Invest 60:405–410, 1977.
25. Waldmann TA, Broder S, Blaese RM, Durm M, Blackman M, Strober W: Role of suppressor T-cells in pathogenesis of common variable hypogammaglobulinemia. Lancet 2:609–613, 1974.
26. Reinherz EL, Geha RS, Wohl ME, Mordioto C, Rosen RS, Schlossman SF: Immunodeficiency associated with loss of T4+ inducer T-cell function. N Engl J Med 304:811–816, 1981.
27. Waldmann TA, Broder S, Goldman CK, Marshall S, Muul L: Suppressor cells in common variable immunodeficiency. Supra #6, pp 119–128.
28. Seligmann M: Classification of human primary B cell immunodeficiencies. In Doria G, Eshkol A (eds): "The Immune System: Functions and Therapy of Dysfunction." New York: Academic Press, 1980, pp 129–137.
29. Siegal FP, Siegal M, Good RA: Suppression of B cell differentiation by leukocytes from hypogammaglobulinemic patients. J Clin Invest 58:109–112, 1976.
30. Blaese RM, Weiden PL, Koski I, Dooley N: Infectious agammaglobulinemia: Transmission of immunodeficiency with grafts of agammaglobulinemic cells. J Exp Med 140:1097–1101, 1974.
31. Siegel RL, Issekuts T, Schwaber J, Rosen FS, Geha RS: Deficiency of T-helper cells in transient hypogammaglobulinemia of infancy. N Engl J Med 305:1307–1313, 1981.
32. Reinherz EL, Cooper MD, Schlossman SF, Rosen FS: Abnormalities of T cell maturation and regulation in human beings with immunodeficiency disorders. J Clin Invest 68:699–705, 1981.
33. Rubinstein A, Sicklick M, Mehra V: Antihelper T cell autoantibody in acquired agammaglobulinemia. J Clin Invest 67:42–50, 1981.
34. Litwin SD, Zanjani ED: Lymphocytes suppressing both immunoglobulin production and erythroid differentiation in hypogammaglobulinemia. Nature 266:57–58, 1977.
35. Eibl MM, Mannhalter JW, Zielinski CC, Ahmad R: Defective macrophage-T-cell interaction in common varied immunodeficiency. Clin Immunol Immunopathol 22:316–322, 1982.
36. Krantman HJ, Saxon A, Stevens RH, Stiehm ER: Phenotypic heterogeneity in X-linked infantile agammaglobulinemia with in vitro monocyte suppression of immunoglobulin synthesis. Clin Immunol Immunopathol 20:170–178, 1981.
37. Waldmann TA, Broder S, Durm M, Meade B, Krakauer R, Blackman M, Goldman C: Defect in IgA secretion and in IgA specific suppressor cells in patients with selective IgA deficiency. Trans Assoc Am Physicians 89:215–224, 1976.
38. Cassidy JT, Oldham G, Platts-Mills TAE: Functional assessment of B-cell defect in patients with selective IgA deficiency. Clin Exp Immunol 35:296–305, 1979.
39. King MA, Wells JV, Nelson DS: IgA synthesis by peripheral blood mononuclear cells from normal and selectively IgA deficient subjects. Clin Exp Immunol 38:306–315, 1979.
40. Webster ADB: Metabolic defects in immunodeficiency diseases. Clin Exp Immunol 49:1–10, 1982.
41. Cowan MJ, Wara D, Packman S, Ammann AJ, Yoshino M, Sweetman L, Nyhan W: Multiple biotin-dependent carboxylase deficiencies associated with

defects in T-cell and B-cell immunity. Lancet 2:115–118, 1979.
42. Seger R, Galle J, Wildfeuer A, Frater-Schroeder M, Linnel J, Hitzig WA: Impaired functions of lymphocytes and granulocytes in transcobalamin II deficiency, and their response to treatment. Supra #6, pp 353–362.
43. Reinherz EL, O'Brien C, Rosenthal P, Schlossman SF: The cellular basis for viral induced immunodeficiency: Analysis by monoclonal antibodies. J Immunol 125:1269–1274, 1980.
44. Purtilo DT: Pathogenesis and phenotypes of X-linked lymphoproliferative syndrome. Lancet 1:882–884, 1976.

A National Registry for Primary Immunodeficiency Syndromes in Italy: A Report for the Period 1972–1982

G. Luzi, MD, L. Businco, MD, and F. Aiuti, MD

Department of Clinical Immunology (G.L., F.A.), Department of Pediatrics I (L.B.), University of Rome, 00185 Rome, Italy

In Italy, cooperation among various Departments permitted the formation of a National Registry for Immunodeficiencies (Registro Italiano per le Immunodeficienze Primitive: R.I.I.P.) in 1977 [1].

We report here a summary of the results obtained up to April, 1982.

MATERIALS AND METHODS

An immunologic schedule was prepared, and various Italian Research Groups made specific diagnoses for their patients under observation. Data were periodically sent to the Department of Clinical Immunology or Department of Pediatrics, University of Rome, where the schedules were examined.

Primary immunodeficiencies were diagnosed according to the WHO report on immunodeficiencies [2]. The general scheme used was as follows: 1) humoral defects, 2) cellular defects, 3) T and B CIDs, 4) nonspecific immunity defects.

RESULTS AND DISCUSSION

Table 1 reports the results on primary immunodeficiencies in Italy up to April, 1982, and the incidence of neoplastic and autoimmune diseases.

Table 2 shows the number and the percentage of immunodeficient patients according to the WHO criteria.

Tables 3 and 4 report the incidence of neoplastic and autoimmune diseases in the various forms of primary immunodeficiencies observed.

The role of immunologic registries for immunodeficiencies is very impor-

TABLE 1. Immunodeficiencies Registered in the Italian Registry for Immunodeficiencies: 1982

Total number of registered patients	884
Immunodeficiencies with a specific diagnosis	797
Other immunodeficiencies	87
Associated tumors	19 (2.38% of 797 patients)
Associated autoimmune diseases	47 (5.89% of 797 patients)

TABLE 2. Primary Immunodeficiencies in the Italian Registry for Immunodeficiencies: 1982

Diagnosis	Patients	(%)
SCID	45	5.64
lymphoreticular dysgenesis	2	0.25
Swiss type	27	3.38
ADA defect	4	0.50
with B lymphocytes	12	1.50
PNP	2	0.25
DiGeorge	8	1.00
T-lymphocyte defects	58	7.27
Bruton	33	4.14
CVH	117	14.68
IgA defect	354	44.40
Selective IgG and/or IgM defect	22	2.76
Hypogammaglobulinemia with hyper IgM	5	0.62
ID and short-limbed dwarfism	6	0.75
ID and ataxia telangiectasia	50	6.27
Wiskott-Aldrich	14	1.75
Nonspecific immunity	64	8.02
ID with hyper IgE	12	1.50
chronic granulomatous disease	12	1.50
C' fraction defect	13	1.63
others	27	3.38
CMCC	19	2.38

TABLE 3. Tumors Associated With Primary Immunodeficiencies Registered in I.R.I.D.

Diagnosis	Cases	Tumors	Percentage
SCID	45	2	4.44
Primary T-cell defects	58	2 (2 lymphomas)	3.44
Bruton	33	2	6.06
CVH	117	1	0.85
IgA defects	354	5 (1 neuroblastoma; 1 carnioph.)	1.41
Ataxia telangiectasia and immunodeficiency	50	6 (1 lymphoma; 3 ALL; 1 mesothelioma)	12.00
Wiskott-Aldrich	14	1	7.14

cranioph. = craniopharyngioma
ALL = acute lymphatic leukemia

TABLE 4. Autoimmune Diseases Associated With Primary Immunodeficiencies Registered in I.R.I.D.

Diagnosis	Cases	Autoimmune Diseases	Percentage
SCID	45	3	6.66
Primary T-cell defects	58	4[a]	6.89
Bruton	33	2[b]	6.00
Hypogammaglobulinemia and hyper IgM	5	2	40.00
IgA defects	354	29[c]	8.19
Wiskott-Aldrich	14	1	7.14
Ataxia Telangiectasia and immunodeficiencies	50	1[d]	2.00
CVH	117	5[e]	4.27

[a]3 cases of hemolytic anemia
[b]1 case of rheumatoid arthritis and 1 case of hemolytic anemia
[c]1 case of systemic lupus, 1 case of rheumatoid arthritis, 1 case of hemolytic anemia, and 1 case of thrombocytopenic purpura
[d]1 case of hemolytic anemia
[e]3 cases of hemolytic anemia.

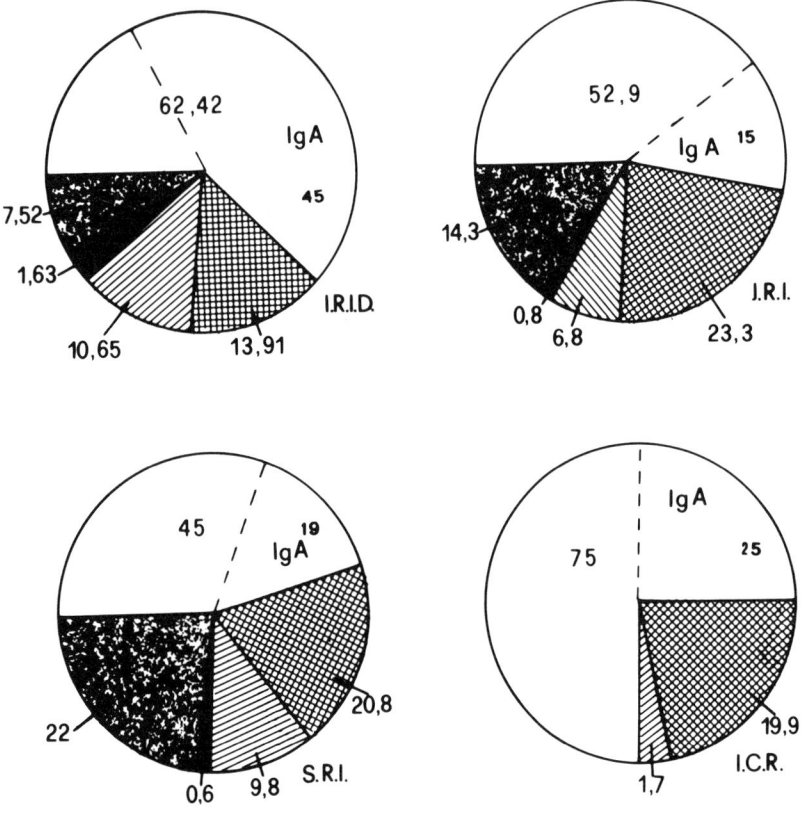

I.R.I.D.: italian registry for immunodeficiencies
J.R.I.: japanese registry for immunodeficiencies
S.R.I.: swedish registry for immunodeficiencies
I.C.R.: immunodeficiency and cancer registry (U.S.A.)

Percentage of distribution as follow:
- humoral defects
- combined immunodeficiencies
- T cell defects
- non specific immunodeficiencies
- C' defects

Figure 1.

tant for identifying new pathologic forms, and for enabling the evolution of correlated or secondary diseases to be pursued. From the Italian Registry for Immunodeficiencies and from the data of other reports such as the American Registry for Immunodeficiencies and Cancer [3], the Japanese National Survey for Primary Immunodeficiencies [4], and the Swedish Registry for Imunodeficiencies [5], a prevalence of humoral defects and specifically IgA defects have been observed (Fig. 1) [6]. Patients with IgA defects suffer from a high incidence of autoimmune diseases (8.19% Table 4), and arthritis, and although most of them do not have severe symptoms, many show frequent infections of the respiratory tract and intestinal giardiasis.

Common variable hypogammaglobulinemia (CVH) and selective immune globulin defects have been diagnosed in people of different ages. We want to underline the familial incidence of IgA in male sons of CVH mothers (personal data not reported).

In Table 2, the group of T-cell deficiencies has been separated from patients with pure DiGeorge syndrome and chronic mucocutaneous candidiasis (CMCC).

From the general evaluation of the data of R.I.I.P., Japanese, American, and Swedish reports, we can make some observations: 1) a prevalence of humoral defects with respect to other primary immunodeficiencies; in particular a high incidence of IgA defects in all reports; 2) the same range of T-cell defects in Italian and Swedish reports; 3) small different percentages of SCID were found in all the Registries.

In the Italian Registry, a high incidence of viral forms is described in T-cell defects, a prevalence of bacterial diseases in humoral defects, and an association of both viral and bacterial forms in SCIDs.

In primary immunodeficiencies, it is important to evaluate tumors and autoimmune diseases. Particularly ataxia telangiectasia, Wiskott-Aldrich syndrome, and SCIDs show the highest incidence of neoplastic diseases.

Our data both as absolute values and distributions are in agreement with those of other registries.

We stress that the highest incidence of autoimmune disorders was found in patients with humoral immune defects (CVH, IgA, hypogammaglobulinemia).

REFERENCES

1. Aiuti F, Giunchi et al: Le immunodeficienze primitive in Italia. Folia Allergol Immunol Clin 25:7–15, 1977.
2. W.H.O.: Classification of primary immunodeficiencies. N Engl J Med 288:966–975, 1973.
3. Spector BD, Perry GS III, Kersey JH: Genetically determined immunodeficiency diseases and malignancy. Report from the Immunodeficiency Cancer Registry. Clin Immunol Immunopathol 11:12–29, 1978.
4. Haykawa H, Iwata T, Yata J, Kobayashi N: Primary immunodeficiency syndrome in Japan. I. Overview of nationwide survey on primary immunodeficiency syndromes. J Clin Immunol 1:31–39, 1981.
5. Fasth A: Primary immunodeficiency disorders in Sweden: Cases among children 1974–1979. J Clin Immunol 2:86–92, 1982.
6. Luzi G, Bonomo R: Le immunodeficienze primitive in Italia: 1972–1981. In Aiuti F, Fiorilli M (eds): "Le Immunodeficienze Primitive in Italia." Rome: Field Educational Italy, 1982, pp 4–9.

Failure of Isotype Progression in Hypogammaglobulinemia and During Normal B-Cell Ontogeny

R. Scott Pereira, MRC Path, Susan R. Wilkins, BSc, A. David Webster, FRCP, Geoffrey L. Asherson, FRCP, FRCPath, and Thomas A.E. Platts-Mills, FRCP

Divison of Allergy and Clinical Immunology, Department of Medicine, University of Virginia, Charlottesville, VA 22908 (T.A.E.P.-M.), Division of Immunological Medicine (S.R.W., G.L.A., A.D.W.), and Division of Rheumatology (R.S.P.), Clinical Research Centre, Harrow HA1 3UJ, England

Patients with late-onset or common variable hypogammaglobulinemia (CVID) have at least two different patterns of immunologic abnormalities [1]. In some cases, the T cells show increased suppressor activity in vitro [1,2]; in these cases an increased proportion of T cells have phenotypic markers associated with suppression [3]. This group of patients often has very low numbers of circulating B cells (<1%) [4], and it is these cases which may be associated with thymoma [5]. However, the majority of patients with CVID do not have abnormal T cells as judged either by phenotypic markers [3,6] or by in vitro function [1,7,8]. These patients also have normal or near normal numbers of circulating cells which bear surface IgM [4,9]. Using pokeweed mitogen (PWM) and normal T-cell help, the quantities of IgM produced by these cells vary from near normal to very low, while IgG production is very low or absent [2,4,10]. Using Epstein-Barr virus (EBV) [11], and measuring Ig production by RIA [4,12,13], these cells produce normal quantities of IgM and IgD but still fail to produce IgA and IgG. When T-depleted (or cyclosporin A-treated) mononuclear cell cultures are stimulated with EBV, the response is very consistent both in timing, maximum quantity of IgM produced, and particularly the ratio of IgM:IgG (normal mean 2.8; normal range 1.0–8.5), so that it is possible to compare different groups of patients or controls on a statistical basis [12] (Fig. 1).

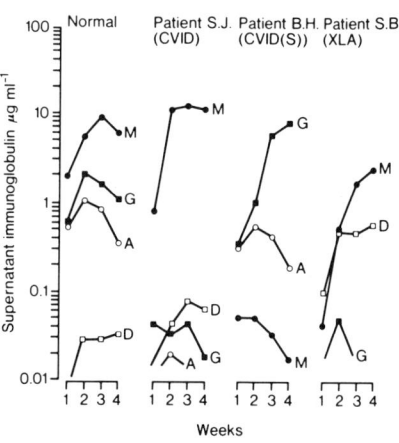

Fig. 1. Ig production following EBV stimulation of non-T cells in vitro. Typical results are shown for a normal donor; Patient S.J. with CVID and normal T cells; Patient B.H. with CVID and abnormal increased in vitro suppressor activity (CVID(S)); and Patient S.B. with X-linked agammaglobulinemia (XLA) (see ref. 12 for details).

B cells which bear surface IgM and IgD but not IgG or IgA appear early in human fetal development and are dominant in cord blood [14]. When stimulated with EBV in vitro these cells consistently produce normal quantities of IgM with a mean IgM:IgG ratio of 62 (range 10–1000) [12]. This pattern persists in the peripheral blood of most infants up to the age of 9 months. In the fetus, these B cells can be regarded either as immature or virgin, since they have not yet reacted with specific antigen; the B cells may be controlled by T cells since cord blood T cells show profound suppressor activity [15]. However, a population of similar immature B cells appears to be present in normal adult bone marrow [16] and normal adult peripheral blood [17,18]. When B cells from patients with CVID are stimulated with EBV in vitro the Ig production (IgM:IgG ratio, 34; range 12–714) is very similar to that seen with cord blood B cells [12]. These similarities lead to the conclusion that the patient's B cells are normal immature B cells. It seems likely that the production of immature B cells by the fetal liver or bone marrow is continuous from the early fetus onward, and may well be under physiologic rather than immunologic control. In most patients with CVID this production of SmIgM and SmIgD+ve cells appears to be fully normal, as is their production of pre-B cells [19]. Using either PWM or EBV in vitro, it is not possible to shift these patients' B cells to produce IgG or IgA; however, this is equally true for fetal B cells.

In considering the causes of antibody deficiency in patients with CVID, it is worth considering what the defect is. These patients have low serum IgG, IgA, and IgE with low or normal levels of serum IgM. When exposed to antigens in vivo either naturally or by immunization they fail to produce antibody responses [20]. These antigens include: diphtheria toxoid (normally an IgG_1 and IgG_3 response in man), inhalant allergens (normally an IgG_4, IgA and IgE response) [21,22], and also pneumococcal polysaccharide (normally an IgG_2 and IgM response) [23]. The failure to produce IgM antibody to pneumococcal polysaccharide is particularly interesting since these patients can produce normal quantities of IgM in vitro, so that the failure is not due to a failure of isotype progression in the simple sense of the ability to express a particular DNA heavy chain code. The patterns of isotype expression in human antibody responses imply that the normal controls, which may be genetic or dependent on dosage or route of immunization [24], direct progression toward a group of isotypes rather than toward a particular isotype. There is now convincing evidence that the ability to respond to inhalant allergens, ie atopy, represents a control over IgG and IgE antibody production equally [21]. Studies on Ig heavy chain DNA codes in mice suggested that the isotypes were arranged linearly and that progression was orderly with deletion of earlier codes [25]. It is now clear that genes are not automatically deleted [25]. More important, recent human results suggest that there may be considerable duplication on chromosome number 14 with isotype codes arranged in groups, ie α_2 with epsilon, α_1 with a pseudogene for epsilon, and γ_2 with γ_4 [25,26]. The exciting possibility is that the pattern of isotype responses seen in man has a direct relationship to the arrangement of heavy chain codes in groups (Fig. 2). The implication is that T cells control the direction of expression rather than controlling the switch to a particular isotype.

There are several reasons why apparently normal immature or virgin B cells in patients with CVID might fail to produce antibody responses in vivo. It is possible that these cells have a subtle defect which prevents their progression, or that the patients' T cells have a defect which prevents help in vivo. However, it seems more likely that the defect is a failure of antigen presentation either because T cells fail to recognize the antigen, or because macrophages fail to present, or because the normal microenvironment is absent. The positive evidence from the patients is that they have abnormal lymphoid architecture, and follicles are very rare [20]. However, whatever the underlying cause, it appears likely that the absence of isotype progression beyond IgM in circulating B cells is secondary to a failure of specific antibody responses. If isotype progression normally only occurs as part of specific immune responses then the lack of isotype progression seen in the patients' circulating B cells may simply reflect the fact that these patients fail to make specific immune responses. At present, we are unable to detect any difference between the patients' B cells and normal fetal B cells, and it seems unlikely that these B cells have any intrinsic abnormality.

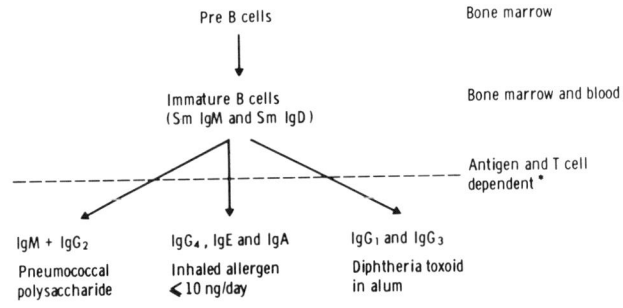

Fig. 2. Isotype 'progression' in human antibody responses.

REFERENCES

1. Platts-Mills TAE, de Gast GC, Webster ADB, Asherson GL, Wilkins SR: Two immunologically distinct forms of late-onset hypogammaglobulinaemia. Clin Exp Immunol 44:383–388, 1981.
2. Waldmann TA, Broder S, Blaese RM, Durm M, Blackman M, Strober W: Role of suppressor T-cells in pathogenesis of common variable hypogammaglobulinaemia. Lancet 2:609–613, 1974.
3. Pereira RS, Platts-Mills TAE: Lymphocyte subsets in hypogammaglobulinaemia. In Janossy G (ed): "The Lymphocytes." "Clinics in Haematology." Philadelphia: WB Saunders, 1982, vol II, no 3, pp 589–605.
4. de Gast GC, Wilkins SR, Webster ADB, Rickinson A, Platts-Mills TAE: Functional "immaturity" of isolated B cells from patients with hypogammaglobulinaemia. Clin Exp Immunol 42:535–544, 1980.
5. Waldmann TA, Broder S, Durm M, Blackman M, Krackauer R, Meade B: Suppressor T cells in the pathogenesis of hypogammaglobulinaemia associated with thymoma. Trans Assoc Am Physicians 88:120, 1975.
6. Siegel RL, Issekutz T, Schwaber J, Rosen FS, Geha RS: Deficiency of T helper cells in transient hypogammaglobulinaemia of infancy. N Engl J Med 305:1307–1313, 1981.
7. Geha RS, Schneeberger E, Merler E, Rosen FS: Heterogeneity of "acquired" or common variable agammaglobulinaemia. N Engl J Med 291:1–6, 1974.
8. Moretta L, Mingari MC, Webb SR, Pearl ER, Lydyard PM, Grossi CE, Lawton AR, Cooper MD: Imbalances in T cell subpopulations associated with immunodeficiency and autoimmune syndromes. Eur J Immunol 7:696–700, 1977.
9. Wu LYF, Lawton AR, Cooper MD: Differentiation capacity of cultured B lymphocytes from immunodeficient patients. J Clin Invest 52:3180, 1973.
10. de la Concha EG, Oldham G, Webster ADB, Asherson GL, Platts-Mills TAE: Quantitative measurements of T- and B-cell function in "variable" primary hypogammaglobulinaemia: Evidence for a consistent B-cell defect. Clin Exp Immunol 27:208–215, 1977.
11. Bird AG, Britton S, Ernberg J, Nilsson

12. K: Characteristics of Epstein-Barr virus activation of human B lymphocytes. J Exp Med 154:832–839, 1981.
12. Pereira RS, Webster ADB, Platts-Mills TAE: Immature B cells in fetal development and immunodeficiency; studies of IgM, IgG, IgA and IgD production *in vitro* using Epstein-Barr virus activation. Eur J Immunol 12:540–546, 1982.
13. Tosato G, Magrath IT, Koski IR, Dooley NJ, Blaese RM: B cell differentiation and immunoregulatory T cell function in human cord blood lymphocytes. J Clin Invest 66:383–388, 1980.
14. Gathings WE, Lawton AR, Cooper MD: Immunofluorescent studies of the development of pre B cells, B lymphocytes and immunoglobulin isotype diversity in humans. Eur J Immunol 7:804, 1977.
15. Hayward AR, Lydyard PM: Suppression of B lymphocyte differentiation by newborn T lymphocytes with an Fc receptor for IgM. Clin Exp Immunol 34:374–378, 1978.
16. de Gast GC, Platts-Mills TAE: Functional studies on lymphocytes in adult human bone marrow. II. Isolated surface IgM positive cells. J Immunol 122:285–290, 1979.
17. Ault KA, Unanue ER: Failure of B lymphocytes in human blood to regenerate surface immunoglobulin after its removal by antibody. J Immunol 119:327–329, 1977.
18. Ault KA, Towle M: Human B lymphocyte subsets: I. IgG bearing B cell responses to pokeweed mitogen. J Exp Med 153:339–351, 1981.
19. Pearl E, Vogler LB, Okos AJ, Crist WM, Lawton AR, Cooper MD: B lymphocyte precursors in human bone marrow: An analysis of normal individuals and patients with antibody-deficiency states. J Immunol 120:1169–1175, 1978.
20. Asherson GL, Webster ADB: "Diagnosis and Treatment of Immune Deficiency Diseases." Oxford: Blackwell, 1980, pp 37–60.
21. Platts-Mills TAE: Immediate hypersensitivity. In Lachmann PJ, Peters DK (eds): "Clinical Aspects of Immunology," 4th Ed. Oxford: Blackwell, 1982, pp 615–620.
22. Van der Giessen M, Homan WL, Van Kernebeek G, Aalberse RC, Dieges PH: Subclass typing of IgG antibodies formed by grass pollen allergic patients during immunotherapy. Int Arch Allergy Appl Immunol 50:625, 1976.
23. Latiff AAA: Antibody response to pneumococcal polysaccharide vaccine in humans. Clinical study on the use of such vaccine to test for immunodeficiency. Ph.D. thesis, Brunel University, London.
24. Gearhart PJ, Cebra JJ: Differentiated B lymphocytes potential to express particular antibody variable and constant regions depends on site of lymphoid tissue and antigen load. J Exp Med 149:216–227, 1979.
25. Marcu KB: Immunoglobulin heavy-chain constant-region genes. Cell 29:719–721, 1982.
26. Max EE, Battey J, Ney R, Kirsch IR, Leder P: Duplication and deletion in the human immunoglobulin E genes. Cell 29:691–699, 1982.

Recurrent Infections in Children With "Selective" IgA Deficiency: Association With IgG2 and IgG4 Deficiency

Alberto G. Ugazio, MD, Theo A. Out, PhD, Alessandro Plebani, PhD, Marzia Duse, MD, Virginia Monafo, MD, Luigi Nespoli, MD, and G. Roberto Burgio, MD

Department of Pediatrics, University of Pavia, 27100 Pavia, Italy (A.G.U., A.P., M.D., V.M., L.N., G.R.B.), Central Laboratory of the Netherlands Red Cross Blood Transfusion Service and Laboratory for Experimental and Clinical Immunology, University of Amsterdam, The Netherlands (T.A.O.)

Selective IgA deficiency, the most frequent primary immunodeficiency [1], is associated with a wide variety of clinical manifestations, ranging from recurrent infections to atopy, autoimmune disorders, and malabsorption [1,2]; many subjects with IgA deficiency are apparently healthy [3]. The mechanisms underlying the variability of the clinical expression of selective IgA deficiency are still obscure. Various studies of humoral and cell-mediated immunity (CMI) [1,2,4] have so far failed to provide better insight into the problem.

Oxelius et al [5] have provided evidence recently that selective IgA deficiency is frequently associated with deficiency of serum IgG2 and that the combined deficiency of IgA and IgG2 is associated with greater susceptibility to infections. In the present study of 36 children with selective IgA deficiency, problems with recurrent infections were found to be associated with IgG4 as well as IgG2 deficiency.

METHODS

Thirty-six children with selective IgA deficiency, 21 males and 15 females ranging from 2–12 years of age, were included in the study. Twenty-one matched healthy children with comparable geographic and socioeconomic environments served as controls.

Samples of serum and saliva were stored at $-20°C$ until they were assayed. Levels of IgG, IgA and IgM were assessed by single radial diffusion; low levels of serum IgA and secretory IgA were measured by electroimmunoassay [6]. Serum IgE was measured by PRIST (Pharmacia). Levels of IgG1, IgG2, IgG3, and IgG4 were measured by single radial diffusion and compared to age-normal values as previously described [7].

RESULTS

The associated diseases in the 36 IgA-deficient patients are indicated in Table 1, and the sites of infection seen in the 13 infection-prone children are reported in Table 2.

Serum levels of IgA were <0.5 mg/dl in 15 subjects, between 0.5 and 5 mg/dl in 9, and >5 mg/dl but <-2 SD of the age-normal mean in 12. No significant association was found between serum IgA levels and recurrent infections. Secretory IgA was undetectable (<0.5 mg/dl) in the 15 children with serum IgA <0.5 mg/dl, and low but detectable in all the other subjects.

Serum IgE levels in patients with (50 ± 91 U/ml) and without recurrent infections (150 ± 260 U/ml) were not significantly different ($p>0.5$).

In the 21 age-matched healthy controls, IgG1, IgG2, IgG3, and IgG4 levels were always within age-normal values [7].

IgG1 levels were low for age in 3 patients, 2 with upper respiratory tract infections (URTI) and one apparently healthy.

IgG3 levels were low in 1 child with URTI.

Serum IgG2 was low for age or undetectable in 9 children, 8 of them had recurrent infections (Table 2) and the remaining patient had Silver-Russell dwarfism. As shown in Table 3, the correlation between IgG2 deficiency and recurrent infections was highly significant.

Serum IgG4 levels were low for age or undetectable in 8 children; in 4 of them IgG4 and IgG2 deficiency were associated. As reported in Table 4, IgG4 deficiency and recurrent infections were significantly associated.

DISCUSSION

In the present study of 36 children with selective IgA deficiency, a combined deficiency of IgG2 and IgG4 was found in 4, of IgG2 in 5, and of

TABLE 1. Associated Diseases in the 36 IgA-Deficient Patients

Associated Disease	Number of Affected Patients
Recurrent infections	13
Atopic disease	10
Malabsorption	4
Endocrine diseases	3
Autoimmune disorders	2
Seizures	2
Silver-Russell syndrome	1
None	1

TABLE 2. Serum Levels of IgG Subclasses in 13 Children With Selective IgA Deficiency and Recurrent Infections

Patient	Age (years)	Sex	Site of infections[a]	Serum IgA level[b]	Serum levels of IgG subclasses expressed as percentage of a standard serum			
					IgG1	IgG2	IgG3	IgG4
Combined IgA-IgG2 deficiency								
C.A.	6	F	LRTI	<0.5	130	*10*[c]	20	<10
B.V.	5	F	LRTI	0.5–5	90	*40*	50	*<10*
C.G.	4	M	LRTI	<0.5	70	*20*	330	*<10*
S.V.	3	M	LRTI	0.5–5	90	*40*	60	60
C.V.	5	F	URTI	>5	70	*20*	40	*<10*
L.R.	5	F	URTI	>5	*30*	*<10*	*<10*	*<10*
P.S.	9	M	LRTI	>5	90	*40*	50	*<10*
N.R.	2	M	URTI	>5	*50*	*10*	30	30
Isolated IgA deficiency								
L.F.	5	M	URTI	<0.5	220	80	160	*30*
R.R.	12	F	URTI	<0.5	180	280	160	120
V.M.	9	F	URTI	<0.5	270	140	90	*<10*
V.A.	5	M	LRTI	<0.5	170	90	30	160
S.V.	4	M	URTI	0.5–5	220	100	80	320

[a]LRTI = Lower respiratory tract infections; URTI = Upper respiratory tract infections including pharyngo-tonsillitis, otitis, and sinusitis.
[b]<0.5 = <0.5 mg/dl; 0.5–5 = between 0.5 and 5 mg/dl; >5 = >5 mg/dl but <−2SD of the age-normal mean.
[c]Italicized values are below the lower limit of the age-normal range.

TABLE 3. Association of IgG2 Deficiency and Recurrent Infections

	Serum IgG2 Levels	
	Low	Normal
IgA deficiency		
With recurrent infections	8	5
Without recurrent infections	1	22

$X^2 = 11.6$
$p < 0.001$

TABLE 4. Association of IgG4 Deficiency and Recurrent Infections

	Serum IgG4 Levels	
	Low	Normal
IgA deficiency		
With recurrent infections	6	7
Without recurrent infections	2	21

$X^2 = 4.7$
$p < 0.05$

IgG4 in 4. Thirteen children had severe recurrent infections, and 10 of these had a deficiency of either IgG2 or IgG4. Statistical analysis showed that susceptibility to infection among the children with selective IgA deficiency was significantly associated with IgG2 deficiency ($p < 0.001$) and also with IgG4 deficiency ($p < 0.05$); the combined deficiency of both subclasses did not appear to increase susceptibility to infection.

IgG2 deficiency has been found in association with IgA deficiency in patients with ataxia telangiectasia [8] who are known to suffer from recurrent severe sinopulmonary infections. Furthermore, most antibodies directed against the bacterial polysaccharide capsular antigens which are important virulence factors for bacteria, such as type b *Haemophilus influenzae* and pneumococci, belong to the IgG2 subclass; in fact, patients with IgG2 deficiency have been shown to improve on Ig therapy [9,10].

The possible pathogenetic significance of the IgG4 deficiency is quite obscure, especially in view of the observation that IgG4 is undetectable in the serum of 1 of 4 normal subjects [5].

When patients were divided into 3 groups according to their serum IgA levels (ie <0.5 mg/dl; between 0.5 and 5 mg/dl; >5 mg/dl but <−2 SD of the age-normal mean), no correlation was found with susceptibility to infections. Similarly, presence or absence of secretory IgA, as well as serum IgE levels, was not correlated with susceptibility to infections.

In agreement with the previous data of Oxelius and co-workers the results of the present study indicate that IgG2 deficiency plays an important role in determining the susceptibility to infections in some children with IgA deficiency. However, 5 of the 13 children with selective IgA deficiency and recurrent infections did not present an associated IgG2 deficiency, thus suggesting that IgG2 deficiency is certainly not the only factor causing infection-proneness in selective IgA deficiency. Children with combined IgA-IgG2 deficiency should theoretically benefit from Ig therapy, but the potential benefits of this approach should be carefully weighed against the possible risks of anaphylactic reactions with Ig administration to IgA-deficient subjects.

REFERENCES

1. Buckley RH: Clinical and immunologic features of selective IgA deficiency. In Bergsma D (ed): "Immunodeficiency in

1. Man and Animals." Sunderland, MA: Sinauer Associates for the National Foundation-March of Dimes, BD:OAS XI(1):134–141, 1975.
2. Burgio GR, Duse M, Monafo V, Ascione A, Nespoli L: Selective IgA deficiency: Clinical and immunological evaluation of 50 pediatric patients. Eur J Pediatr 133:101–106, 1980.
3. Koistinen J: Selective IgA deficiency in blood donors. Vox Sang 29:192–205, 1975.
4. Ammann AJ, Hong R: Disorders of the IgA system. In Stiehm RE, Fulginiti VA (eds): "Immunologic Disorders in Infants and Children." Philadelphia: WB Saunders, 1980, pp 260–273.
5. Oxelius V-A, Laurell AB, Lindquist B, Golebiowska H, Axelson U, Björkander J, Hanson LA: IgG subclasses in selective IgA deficiency. N Engl J Med 304:1476–1477, 1981.
6. Burgio GR, Lanzavecchia A, Plebani A, Jayakar S, Ugazio AG: Ontogeny of secretory immunity: Levels of secretory IgA and natural antibodies in saliva. Pediatr Res 14:1111–1114, 1980.
7. van der Giessen M, Rossouw E, van Teen TA, van Loghem E, Zegers BJM, Sander PC: Quantification of IgG subclasses in sera of normal adults and healthy children between 4 and 12 years of age. Clin Exp Immunol 21:501–509, 1975.
8. Oxelius V-A, Berkel AI, Hanson LA: IgG2 deficiency in ataxia-telangiectasia. N Engl J Med 306:515–517, 1982.
9. Oxelius V-A: Chronic infections in a family with hereditary deficiency of IgG2 and IgG4. Clin Exp Immunol 17:19–27, 1974.
10. Hanson, LA, Björkander J, Oxelius V-A, Wadsworth C: Indications and limitations of parenteral immunoglobulin treatment: Prophylactic intramuscular gammaglobulin treatment. In Nydegger UE (ed): "Immunochemotherapy." London: Academic Press, 1982, pp 423–430.

IgG_2 and IgG_3 Subclass Deficiencies in Selective IgA Deficiency in the United States

Charlotte Cunningham-Rundles, MD, PhD, Vivi-Anne Oxelius, MD, PhD, and Robert A. Good, MD, PhD

Memorial Sloan-Kettering Cancer Center, New York, NY 10021 (C.C.-R.), Institute of Medical Microbiology, University of Lund, Lund, Sweden (V.-A.O.), Oklahoma Medical Research Foundation, Oklahoma City, OK 73104 (R.A.G.)

Human IgG is composed of 4 subclasses based on antigenic differences in the polypeptide chain [1,2]. The approximate percentages of the IgG subclasses of normal adult IgG are IgG_1, 66%, IgG_2, 23%, IgG_3, 7%, and IgG_4, 4% [3]. Structural or regulator gene abnormalities of IgG subclasses could result in a lack of the capacity to synthesize specific types of heavy chains which would produce disproportionate levels of IgG subclasses, since heavy chains are synthesized at separate, although closely linked, loci [4]. In addition to their genetic implications, IgG subclass imbalances are of importance because of the variable distribution of biologic properties of antibodies among such subclasses and because certain antibody populations may be markedly restricted to a single IgG subclass [3]. An example of such antibody restriction is the IgG_2 antibody subclass, which appears to contain the majority of antibody directed against bacterial polysaccharides [5]. Imbalances of IgG subclasses have previously been reported [5–10]. Recently, Oxelius reported that 7 of 37 IgA-deficient individuals in Sweden who had repeated infections were IgG_2 subclass deficient [11]. Interestingly, of the 11 healthy IgA-deficient subjects (located through population screening), none had IgG_2 deficiency. IgG_2 levels should be determined for all symptomatic IgA-deficient individuals since such patients may benefit from gamma globulin prophylaxis (if anti-IgA antibodies are absent) [12].

METHODS

Patients were referred to the Immunodeficiency Clinic of the Memorial Sloan-Kettering Cancer Center and were diagnosed as having selective IgA deficiency if their serum IgA were less than 5 mg/dl and other immunoglobulins were in the normal range. Six IgA-deficient patients, previously described [13], were found through screening of the patients referred to this medical center for evaluation and treatment of various cancers.

Quantitative studies of IgG subclasses were performed by electroimmunoassay described by Oxelius and Laurell [14–16]. In this method, the differences in electrophoretic mobility between the IgG subclasses are used: IgG_4 is located anodally, IgG_3 cathodally, and IgG_2 and IgG_1 both anodally and cathodally. With this method the results are obtained more quickly than with other immunoprecipitation techniques.

Qualitative studies of IgG subclasses were performed by crossed immunoelectrophoresis [17]. This method reveals more details about the distribution of IgG subclasses in the electrophoretic field than immunoelectrophoresis.

Purification of IgG subclass myeloma proteins was done by preparative electrophoresis [14], Sephadex G200 gel filtration, and DEAE chromatography.

Specific anti-IgG_1, anti-IgG_2, anti-IgG_3, and anti-IgG_4 antisera were raised in rabbits. A modification of the method by Spiegelberg and Weigle [18] has been described.

RESULTS

Thirty-nine IgA-deficient subjects were studied (Table 1). Of these, 3 adults had IgG_2 levels which were at least 2 standard deviations (SD) depressed from the mean, and 1 child (*Case 10*) had a level which was depressed by 1 SD from the normal mean. In addition, 2 patients had IgG_3 levels falling below 2 SD from the mean, and one other had a level falling 1 SD below the mean. One patient with IgG_2 deficiency (*Case 4*) was also IgG_3 deficient.

Table 2 indicates the clinical problems of these 6 patients with subclass deficiencies. Two had lymphoproliferative malignancies, one is healthy, 2 have recurrent upper respiratory infections (one of which also has celiac disease; and one cancer) and one other patient has spastic colitis.

DISCUSSION

Previously, Oxelius et al have shown that 7 of 37 (19%) IgA-deficient patients had IgG_2 deficiency, while none of the 11 healthy IgA-deficient individuals had this defect. In this study we show that 3 of 39 (7.7%) IgA-deficient patients were IgG_2-deficient (2 SD below the mean). Of this IgA group, since all but *Case 8* (who is a laboratory technician) had been referred for significant medical problems, these data indicate that combined IgA and IgG_2

TABLE 1. IgG Subclasses in Selective IgA Deficiency

Patient number	Age/Sex		IgG$_1$* gm/liter	IgG$_2$ gm/liter	IgG$_3$ gm/liter	IgG$_4$ gm/liter
1	14	M	8.84	3.83	0.39	0.29
2	5	F	8.50	1.93	0.11	0.75
3	60	M	9.18	2.40	0.99	<0.01
4	62	F	3.54	0.77↓	0.18↓	<0.01
5	4	M	8.84	3.66	0.26	<0.01
6	52	M	4.69	2.80	0.60	0.85
7	50	M	0.54	0.33↓	0.47	<0.01
8	32	F	6.26	3.13	0.26↓	0.15
9	19	F	10.20↑	3.66	0.95	0.12
10	7	F	4.49	0.83↓	0.60	0.15
11	11	M	6.53	3.03	0.55	0.17
12	15	F	9.18	2.20	0.42	0.21
13	32	F	7.14	4.00	0.51	0.15
14	10	F	8.84	3.66	0.69	0.17
15	12	M	9.52	2.20	0.38	0.22
16	10	F	10.20↑	3.33	0.84	<0.01
17	5	M	9.52	3.66	0.31	0.43
18	10	M	12.58↑	2.13	0.95	0.16
19	20	F	5.85	1.53	0.45	<0.01
20	32	F	3.26	4.66	0.51	0.35
21	7	F	9.52	3.83	0.42	0.14
22	35	M	5.85	3.50	0.15↓	0.22
23	20	F	9.52	3.23	0.71	<0.01
24	5	F	9.86	1.20	0.64	<0.01
25	26	M	6.80	3.23	0.12	<0.01
26	10	M	9.52	3.33	0.58	<0.01
27	50	M	7.14	5.00	1.39	<0.01
28	2	M	7.14	1.67	0.18	<0.01
29	13	F	7.14	3.00	0.57	<0.01
30	10	M	6.80	1.80	0.45	<0.01
31	23	F	25.84↑	4.33	2.56↑	0.22
32	8	F	11.56↑	1.00	0.35	0.24
33	19	F	7.48	0.77↓	0.41	<0.01
34	10	F	13.60↑	2.33	0.61	1.28↑
35	61	F	6.80	3.33	1.06	0.01
36	10	F	9.52	4.00	0.47	0.94
37	38	F	11.56↑	3.26	0.91	0.24
38	13	F	14.28↑	2.13	0.61	<0.01
39	59	F	6.19	1.20	1.13	<0.01

*Normal ranges for adults: IgG$_1$ = 7.55, SD = 2.45; IgG$_2$ = 3.80, SD = 1.50; IgG$_3$ = 0.73, SD = 0.26; IgG$_4$ = 0.55, SD = 0.63. For Case 10, the IgG$_2$ mean normal for age = 2.57, SD = 1.10.

TABLE 2.

Case Number	Deficiency	Clinical Diagnosis
4	IgG$_2$,IgG$_3$	Lymphoma (poorly differentiated)
7	IgG$_2$	Lymphoma (well-differentiated lymphocytic)
8	IgG$_3$	Healthy
10	IgG$_2$	Celiac disease, recurrent upper respiratory tract infections
22	IgG$_3$	Intermittent spastic colitis
33	IgG$_2$	Recurrent upper respiratory tract infections, cancer

deficiency is not as frequently found in the United States as it is in Sweden [11]. Two of our IgG$_2$ subclass deficient patients have a history of repeated bacterial infections; this association was reported in the previous study and may be due to a lack of specific antibody to bacterial polysaccharides [11].

IgG$_3$ deficiency was not observed in the Swedish IgA-deficient patients, but in the current study, 3 patients (one of whom was also IgG$_2$-deficient) were IgG$_3$-deficient. One of these individuals was healthy, one had lymphoma, and one had spastic colitis.

As in the Swedish report, IgG subclass elevations were also noticed in this population; an IgG$_1$ increase was found in 8 of 39 (21%), and increases of IgG$_3$ and IgG$_4$ in one individual each. The meaning of this is unknown, although a specific chronic antigenic stimulation is possible.

It is interesting that 2 of the 4 IgG$_2$-deficient subjects in this study have a lymphoid malignancy. Although this IgG subclass immunoglobulin defect could be produced by suppressive influences of the malignancy, IgG subclass studies in non-IgA-deficient patients with similar lymphoid malignancies would have to be performed to clarify this possibility. One might speculate that since IgA and IgG$_2$ deficiency seem to be linked abnormalities in ataxia telangiectasia (AT) [14], an immune defect which has a very high frequency of lymphoreticular malignancies [19], the subjects in our study who have these defects could be heterozygous for the AT gene. The incidence of the carrier state of AT is believed to approach 1% in the general population [20], but as yet, no distinct methods for the identification of heterozygosity have been identified.

We conclude that in our population, IgG$_2$ deficiency is not as frequently associated with IgA deficiency as has been reported in Sweden, but that IgG$_3$ deficiency may be more commonly found in this disorder. This study suggests that patients with these linked immunologic defects may have an increased incidence in lymphoproliferative disorders.

REFERENCES

1. Grey HM, Kunkel HG: H chain subgroups of myeloma proteins and normal 7S γ-globulin. J Exp Med 120:253, 1964.
2. Terry WD, Fahey JL: Subclasses of human γ_2-globulin based on differences in the heavy polypeptide chains. Science 146:400, 1964.
3. Yount WJ, Kunkel HG, Litwin SD: Studies of the Vi (γ_{2c}) subgroup of γ-globulin. A relationship between concentration and genetic type among normal individuals. J Exp Med 125:177, 1967.
4. Natvig JB, Kunkel HG, Gedde-Dahl T: Genetic studies of the heavy chain subgroups of G-globulin. Recombination between the closely linked cistrons. Gammaglobulins. Structure and control of biosynthesis. In Killander J (ed): "Proceedings of the Nobel Symposium." Stockholm: Almqvist and Wiskell, 1967, vol 3, p 313.
5. Yount WJ, Dorner MM, Kunkel HG, Kabat EB: Studies on human antibodies. VI. Selective variations in subgroup composition and genetic markers. J Exp Med 127:633, 1968.
6. Terry WD: Variations in the subclasses of IgG. In "Immunologic Deficiency Diseases in Man." Birth Defects* 4(1):357–363, 1968.
7. Schur PH, Borel H, Gelfand EW, Alper CA, Rosen FS: Selective gammaglobulin deficiencies in patients with recurrent pyogenic infections. N Engl J Med 293:631, 1970.
8. Yount WJ, Hong R, Seligmann M, Good RA, Kunkel HG: Imbalances of gammaglobulin subgroups and gene defects in patients with primary hypogammaglobulinemia. J Clin Invest 49:1957, 1970.
9. Morell A, Skvaril F, Radl J, Dooren LJ, Barandun S: IgG subclass abnormalities in primary immunodeficiency diseases. In "Immunodeficiency in Man and Animals." Birth Defects* 11(1): 108, 1975.
10. Oxelius V: Chronic infections in a family with hereditary deficiency of IgG_2 and IgG_4. Clin Exp Immunol 17:19, 1974.
11. Oxelius V, Laurell AB, Lindquist B, Golebiowska H, Axelsson U, Bjorander J, Hanson LA: IgG subclasses in selective IgA deficiency. N Engl J Med 304:1476–1477, 1981.
12. Seligmann M, Chairman; Cunningham-Rundles C, Hanson L, Hitzig W, Knapp T, Lambert P, Nydegger U-E, Soothill J, Rosen F, Thompson R, Wedgwood R: The appropriate uses of human immunoglobulin in clinical practice. WHO Bulletin, 1981.
13. Cunningham-Rundles C, Pudifin D, Armstrong D: Selective IgA deficiency and neoplasia. Vox Sang 38:61–67, 1980.
14. Oxelius V: Quantitative and qualitative investigations of serum IgG subclasses in immunodeficiency disease. Clin Exp Immunol 36:112–116, 1979.
15. Laurell C-B: Quantitative estimation of proteins by electrophoresis in agarose gel containing antibodies. Anal Biochem 15:45, 1966.
16. Laurell C-B: Electroimmunoassay. Scand J Clin Lab Invest 29 (Suppl) 124:21, 1972.
17. Laurell C-B: Antigen antibody crossed electrophoresis. Anal Biochem 10:358, 1965.
18. Spiegelberg HL, Weigle WO: The production of antisera to human gammaglobulin subclasses in rabbits using immunological unresponsiveness. J Immunol 101:377–380, 1968.
19. Biggar WD, Good RA: Immunodeficiency in ataxia-telangiectasia. Supra #9, p 271.
20. Bridges BA, Harnden DG: Untangling ataxia-telangiectasia. Nature 289:222–223, 1981.

*Birth Defects: Original Article Series, published for March of Dimes Birth Defects Foundation.

Pre-B Cells in X-Linked Agammaglobulinemia*

Jerrold Schwaber, PhD

Children's Hospital Medical Center, Department of Pathology, Harvard Medical School, Boston, MA 02115

INTRODUCTION

X-linked agammaglobulinemia (SLA) is a congenital antibody deficiency disease which is inherited in a sex-linked manner. In addition to profound deficiency of serum Igs, the most consistent finding in patients with this disease is the absence of circulating B lymphocytes [1, 2]. Most patients with this disease fail to develop cells of the antibody producing lineage beyond the stage of pre-B cells [3]. Only a few patients with documented family histories of X-linkage of agammaglobulinemia have been found to have peripheral blood B lymphocytes [4, and J. Schwaber, unpublished results].

Pre-B cells are the earliest recognized precursors of Ig-producing cells. They are characterized by scant cytoplasmic immune fluorescence to mu chains, in the absence of cytoplasmic fluorescence to light chains and surface Ig fluorescence to either light or heavy chains [5–7]. Surface Ig-bearing B lymphocytes arise in cultures containing pre-B cells, although direct evidence that they arise from pre-B cells is lacking [8].

In vitro analogs of mouse pre-B cells have been established by transformation with Abelson murine leukemia virus [9, 10] and by fusion with mouse myeloma cells [11, 12]. Studies of Abelson virus-transformed cell lines have shown that expression of mu H chain may occur prior to rearrangement of the L-chain genes [13]. Whether pre-B cells express the mu H chain as a membrane Ig is controversial [14,15]. Fusion of mouse pre-B cells with a light-chain-producing mouse myeloma cell line resulted in expression of surface IgM, demonstrating that the membrane form of mu H chain is produced by pre-B cells [11]. Efforts to directly demonstrate mu H chain on the cell surface without light chain, however, have failed to distinguish between membrane mu chain and secreted mu chain in transit through the membrane. Human pre-B cell lines have been established from bone marrow of patients with SLA by transformation with Epstein-Barr virus (EBV) [16, 17]. These cell lines produce mu H chain without detectable light chain, similar to Abelson virus-transformed mouse pre-B cell analogs.

Examination of the mu H chains produced by pre-B-cell analogs suggests that some pre-B cells may produce incomplete molecules. Two of the pre-B-cell lines established from an SLA patient produced mu chains which were reduced in size compared to normal mu chains [16, 17]. A mouse pre-B-cell hybrid produced mu chains which were also reduced in size [15]. The deletion resulting in these reductions in size has not been identified.

Ig-heavy-chain genes undergo a sequence of alterations during differentiation to the mature gene set coding for a complete molecule [18–20]. An intermediate stage of this process of rearrangement has been identified in Abelson virus-transformed cell lines. Alt and Baltimore [21] have shown that the J_H- and D-region genes, corresponding to the third hypervariable region of the antibody H chain, are rearranged in a cell line prior to translocation of a specific V_H-region gene, coding for the remainder of the V_H of the antibody molecule [22]. Early forms of Ig heavy-chain genes may be transcribed. Kemp et al [23] have demonstrated transcription of murine mu-H-chain gene prior to rearrangement of the J_H, D, and V_H genes, yielding spliced, polyadenylated RNA sequences coding for C_{mu} without V_H region. These C_{mu} RNA sequences have been identified in cells of presumed B, T, and myeloid lineages. However, efforts to demonstrate translation of these sequences have been unsuccessful [24, 25].

We have examined pre-B cells from a patient with SLA, as fresh bone marrow, as EBV-transformed cell lines, and as pre-B-cell hybrids, to determine whether they produce mature mu H chains. Our results indicate that the mu chain produced is an immature form, representing either constant region of mu chain alone (C_{mu}) or the intermediate product of D-J_H-C_{mu}.

V_H FLUORESCENCE

As a working hypothesis, we proposed that the pre-B cells from patients with SLA produced mu H chains without variable region. To test this hypothesis, we prepared a fluorescent antiserum specific for V_H region antigen. Anti-V_H was isolated from the IgG fraction of goat anti-

---

*Supported by grants from the March of Dimes Birth Defects Foundation, USPHS, NIH, and a Scholar Award from the Leukemia Society of America, Inc.

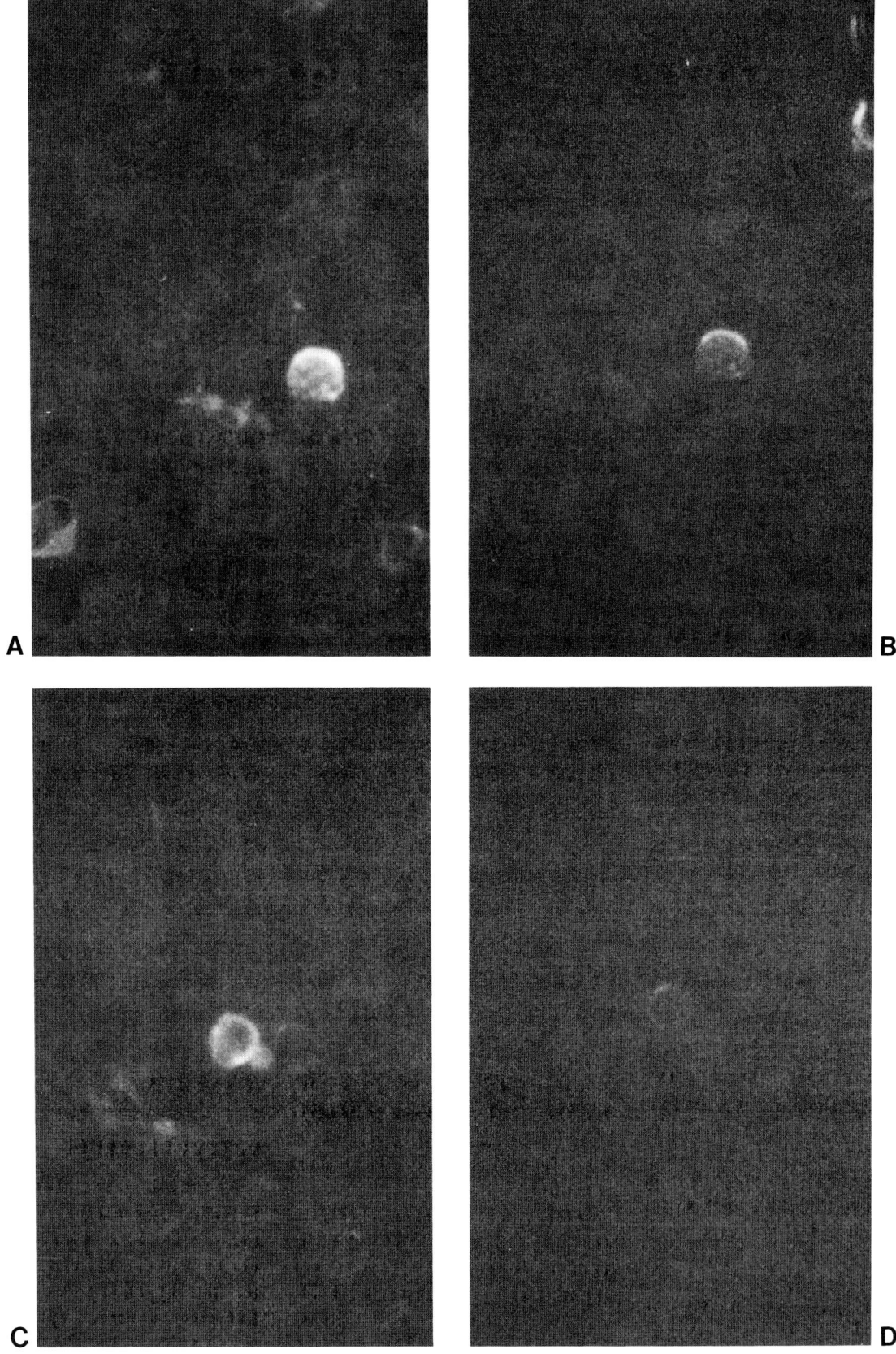

serum to the Fab' fragment of human IgG (Cappel Laboratories, Cochranville, PA). The IgG was pepsin digested, chromatographed in Sephadex G-150 to isolate the Fab$_2$' fragment, affinity purified on human IgM coupled to Sepharose 4B, and then conjugated with fluorescein isothiocyanate (FITC, Baltimore Biological Laboratories) as previously described [26]. The critical step in preparation of this antiserum is isolation of the antibodies which react with both IgG Fab' and IgM. Theoretically, this isolation relies on the conserved framework of V_H regions common to all H-chain isotypes. Reactivity of the antiserum with V_H protein independent of H-chain isotype was demonstrated on a panel of well-characterized human B-cell lines and human-human hybrid cells [27–29, and J. Schwaber, unpublished results]. Anti-V_H reacted with all 5 cell lines tested and, in double label experiments, reacted only with Ig-positive cells. One of these cell lines, LAZ 166, produced delta H chain without L chain, demonstrating the reactivity of anti-V_H with free H chains.

Fig. 1. Pre-B-cell immune fluorescence. Bone marrow cells from normal individuals were stained with peroxidase conjugated antiserum to human Ig for surface Ig, placed on microscope slides with a cytocentrifuge, fixed at −20° for 15 minutes with acetone, washed extensively in PD (phosphate buffered saline without divalent cations) over 30 minutes, and stained with FITC-conjugated anti-V_H and TMRITC-conjugated anti-mu [26]. After staining, the cells were reacted with o-phenylenediamine in 0.1 M citrate buffer, pH 4.5, to develop the peroxidase-conjugated antibody to SIg and so to discriminate B lymphocytes from pre-B cells. A) Normal bone marrow with TMRITC (anti-mu) fluorescence; B) normal bone marrow with FITC (anti-V_H) fluorescence. Bone marrow cells from a patient with SLA were placed on microscope slides with a cytocentrifuge, fixed with acetone, and stained with FITC anti-V_H and TMRITC anti-mu. C) SLA bone marrow with TMRITC (anti-mu) fluorescence; D) SLA bone marrow with FITC (anti-V_H) fluorescence.

TABLE 1. Expression of V_H Region Protein by Pre-B Cells

	% Cytoplasmic mu+ Surface mu− Cells*	% Cytoplasmic mu+ Cells which are V_H+ Cells
Normal		
1	18	94.0
2	36	95.1
3	31	94.4
SLA		
T	24	0

Bone marrow slides were stained with anti-mu and anti-V_H. From normal individuals, surface Ig was stained with peroxidase. More than 300 pre-B cells were examined for V_H region protein from each individual.
*Percent of mononuclear cells.
T is the initial of the last name of the SLA patient.

To test the specificity of anti-V_H, Fv fragments, composed of V_H and V_L, were prepared by the cold pepsin digestion method of Lin and Putnam [30]. Briefly, pooled human IgG was treated with pepsin (1 mg/25 mg) for 48 hours at 4°, with addition of more pepsin after 24 hours, followed by chromatography in Sephacryl S-300. Two peaks, corresponding to Fab' and Fv by molecular weight, were isolated. A second run of the Fv peak through Sephacryl S-300 confirmed the migration pattern. Anti-V_H staining of the cell lines was completely eliminated by preincubation of the anti-V_H with Fv at a molar ratio of 4:1 (Fv:anti-V_H). In contrast, staining was not removed by absorption of anti-V_H with free L chains, and was not blocked by preincubation of the cells with antiserum to human L chains.

Bone marrow was examined from 3 normal individuals. Cells were stained with peroxidase conjugated anti-Ig for surface Igs, rhodamine conjugated, affinity purified, Fab$_2$' fragments of antiserum for C_{mu}, and fluorescein conjugated anti-V_H. Eighteen to 35% of mu-positive cells were cytoplasmic mu+ and surface mu−, ie pre-B cells. Ninety-four to 96% of these pre-B cells reacted with anti-mu and with anti-V_H (Figs. 1A and B, and Table 1).

Bone marrow from a patient with SLA was then examined. This patient had pre-B cells but no SIg-bearing cells, eliminating the necessity for the peroxidase stain for SIg [3, and J. Schwaber, unpublished results]. More than 300 pre-B cells were identified from each patient by cytoplasmic fluorescence with antiserum to mu chain. None of these SLA pre-B cells reacted with anti-V_H (Figs. 1D and E, and Table 1).

PRE-B CELL mRNA

A human-human pre-B cell hybrid analog was established to examine RNA coding for mu chain without associated V_H region. SLA bone marrow was fused with the LSM 2.7 human myeloma cell line [31]. This myeloma cell line does not produce Ig of its own, lacks detectable mRNA for Igs and has deleted its C_{mu} gene (J. Schwaber, unpublished results). 10^7 LSM 2.7 myeloma cells were fused with 10^8 bone marrow cells with 50% polyethylene glycol 6000. Hybrid cells were isolated in HAT half selective medium as described by Littlefield [32], and modified by Davidson [33]. Hybrid colonies were not cloned in order to examine RNA from as large an initial sample of pre-B cells as possible.

The resulting hybrid cells, named LSM-T, were examined for V_H expression and found to retain the C_{mu}+ V_H− phenotype of the parental cells. In a Northern blot analysis [34]

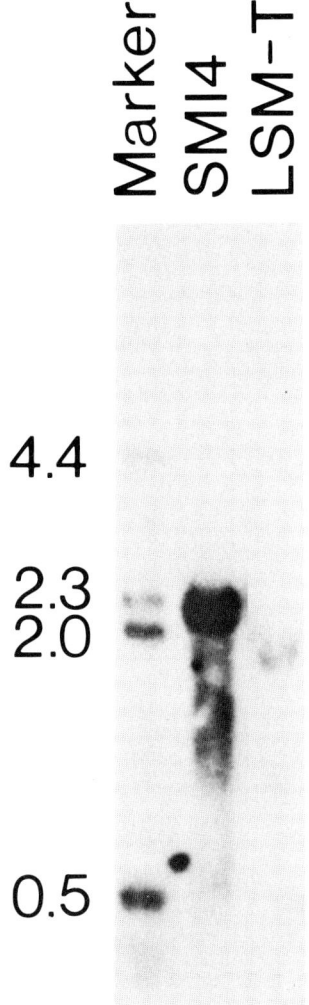

Fig. 2. Northern blot hybridization of RNA from SLA pre-B-cell hybrid. RNA was isolated from 5×10^8 cells of each hybrid by lysis in guanidine HC1, followed by differential precipitation in ethanol, and phenol:(chloroform: isoamyl alcohol) [1:(24:1)] extraction [35]. Twenty micrograms of total RNA were treated with glyoxal and electrophoresed in 1.2% agarose gels as described by Thomas [34]. RNA was transferred from the gel to nitrocellulose in 20X SSC, pH 7.5, air dried, and baked at 80° for 2 hours. Clone PmuHN2, representing cDNA coding for C_{mu} (1.6 kb starting at base 30 of the CH1 domain) cloned in PAT 153 (H. Molgaard, unpublished results) was used as probe. Total plasmid was digested with Pst1 and labeled with ^{32}P dCTP using T4 DNA polymerase [36]. Filters were hybridized in 50% formamide, 1X Denhart's, 100 µg sonicated, salmon sperm DNA, 0.1% SDS with 5X SSC, and washed to 0.1X SSC with 0.1% SDS at 60°. Filters were autoradiographed for 24–72 hours at −70° with intensifying screen. SMI4 is a normal B-cell line which produces IgM. LSM-T is a human hybrid formed with bone marrow from SLA patient N. Lambda DNA digested with Hind III was used as molecular weight marker.

of RNA from LSM-T, mu-chain mRNA migrated as a 2.0–2.1-kb band. In contrast, mu mRNA from SMI4, a normal IgM-producing B-cell line migrated as a 2.3–2.4-kb band (Fig. 2). The reduction in size of the mu mRNA from LSM-T, approximately 300 nucleotides, corresponds to the 300 nucleotide size of the V_H region [37].

PRIMED cDNA

The reduction in size of the pre-B cell mu RNA was localized by primer-extension analysis [38] to the 5' portion (V_H region) of the mRNA. A 61 nucleotide primer, composed of nucleotides 47–108 of the mu CH1 domain, was isolated from the pmuHM2 mu-cDNA clone (see legend to Fig. 3). Following hybridization with cellular RNA [42], reverse transcriptase was used to copy the RNA to its 5' terminus [40]. Normal mu mRNA from the B-cell line SMI4 yielded primed cDNA fragments corresponding to 550 nucleotides in length (Fig. 3). In contrast, mu mRNA from the SLA pre-B-cell hybrid LSM-T yielded primed cDNA fragments co-migrating with the 238/242 nucleotide marker. This result demonstrates that the reduction in size of the mRNA is due to absence of the V_H region.

DISCUSSION

Pre-B cells from a patient with SLA produced an incomplete mu H chain. None of the pre-B cells examined from this patient's bone marrow reacted with fluorescent antiserum specific for V_H region protein. A human-human pre-B-cell hybrid analog was also found to express C_{mu} without associated V_H region fluorescence. The mu-chain mRNA produced by this hybrid was 200–300 bases smaller than the normal mu mRNA produced by a B-cell line. By primer-extension analysis, this reduction in size was found to represent 300 bases at the 5' terminus of the molecule. This loss of RNA se-

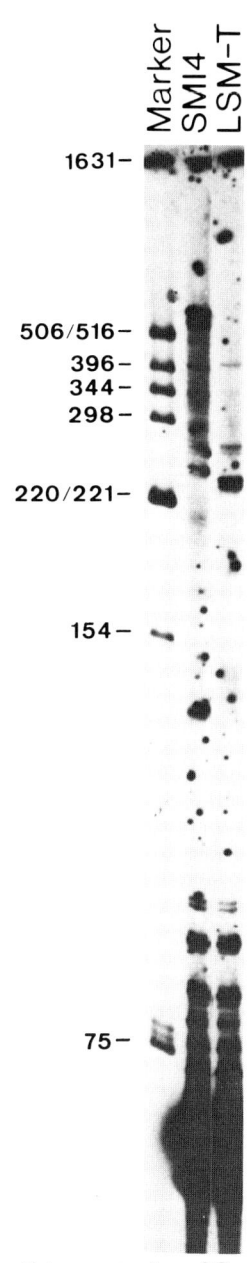

Fig. 3. Primer extension of C_{mu} CH1 fragment on pre-B-cell RNA. RNA was isolated from SLA pre-B-cell hybrid as described in the legend to Fig. 2. C_{mu} cDNA insert from clone PmuHN2 was digested with Hinf 1, 5' end labeled with 32 P gamma ATP, using polynucleotide kinase [39], and digested with EcoR1. A 61 nucleotide fragment corresponding to bases 47–108 of the CH1 domain of mu chain was isolated from a 10% acrylamide gel. Labeled primer and 25–50 µg of total cell RNA were denatured in hybridization buffer [40] and incubated for 20 hours at 51° followed by ethanol precipitation. Hybridized primer was extended with AMV reverse transcriptase according to Treisman et al [38]. Reactions were phenol extracted, ethanol precipitated, and electrophoresed for 2 hours at 2000 volts (V) in 8% acrylamide gels containing 6 M urea [41]. Size markers were plasmid PBR 322 digested with Hinf 1 and 5' end labeled. SMI4 is a normal IgM-producing B-cell line, LSM-T is an SLA pre-B-cell hybrid.

quence is sufficient to include the entire V_H region. No full size mu mRNA was found in either analysis.

We propose that pre-B cells producing mu chain without V_H region represent the earliest stage of identifiable B-lymphocyte precursor. Production of this incomplete molecule probably precedes translocation of a particular V_H region gene adjacent to the C region gene set. We have not determined whether D and J have undergone rearrangement from the embryonic configuration in these pre-B-cell hybrids. However, preliminary results with 2 pre-B cell lines from a single SLA patient suggest that their J region genes have undergone rearrangement from the embryonic configuration.

The Ig molecule produced by these early pre-B cells is composed of either C_{mu} alone, or of C_{mu} in association with rearranged J_H and D region genes, corresponding to the third hypervariable region of V_H [42]. Physiologically, a D-J_H-C_{mu} molecule may represent a primordial antibody molecule, which would have lowered antibody affinity in conjunction with broadened specificity. This primordial antibody molecule might serve as an early antigen receptor, providing a basis for selecting particular clones for expansion. Alternatively, translation of C_{mu} completely lacking the V_H region protein may serve as a regulatory molecule controlling rearrangement of a V_H gene. Resolution between these alternative shortened mu-chain products requires further experiments.

In this model of pre-B cell differentiation, SLA occurs secondary to a failure to differentiate, associated with a failure to translocate V_H region genes. Expression of V_H region protein may be required prior to expression of L-chain genes, or of switching from one H-chain isotype to another. Alt et al [13] proposed a similar regulatory role for immunoglobulin L chains in H-chain isotype expression. The X-linkage of this disease suggests that the failure to translocate V_H region genes is not due to an abnormality of the Ig H-chain structural genes which are on chromosome 14 [35]. Rather, enzymes specific for translocation of V_H genes or regulatory sites necessary for pre-B cells to differentiate to a stage utilizing these enzymes may be encoded on the human X chromosome.

REFERENCES

1. Geha R, Rosen F, Merler E: Identification and characterization of subpopulations of lymphocytes in human peripheral blood after fractionation on discontinuous gradients of albumin. J Clin Invest 52:1726–1734, 1973.
2. Siegal F, Pernis B, Kunkel H: Lymphocytes in human immunodeficiency states: A study of membrane associated immunoglobulins. Eur J Immunol 1:482–486, 1971.
3. Pearl E, Vogler L, Okos A, Christ W, Lawton A, Cooper M: B lymphocyte precursors in human bone marrow. J Immunol 120:1169–1181, 1978.
4. Schwaber J, Lazarus H, Rosen FS: Restricted classes of immunoglobulin produced by a lymphoid cell line from a patient with agammaglobulinemia, Proc Natl Acad Sci USA 75:2421–2423, 1978.
5. Osmond D, Nossal GJV: Differentiation of lymphocytes in mouse bone marrow. Cell Immunol 13:132–138, 1974.
6. Raff M, Megson M, Owen J, Cooper MD: Early production of intracellular IgM by B lymphocyte precursors in mouse. Nature 259:224–226, 1976.
7. Cooper MD: Pre-B cells: Normal and abnormal development. J Clin Immunol 1:81–89, 1981.
8. Lau C, Melchers F, Miller R, Phillips R: In vitro differentiation of B lymphocytes from pre-B cells. J Immunol 122:1273–1277, 1979.
9. Pratt D, Strominger J, Parkman R, Kaplan D, Schwaber J, Rosenberg N, Scher C: Abelson virus transformed lymphocytes: Null cells that modulate H-2. Cell 12:683–690, 1977.
10. Siden E, Baltimore D, Clark D, Rosenberg N: Immunoglobulin synthesis by lymphoid cells transformed in vitro by Abelson murine leukemia virus. Cell 16:389–396, 1979.
11. Burrows P, LeJeune M, Kearney J: Asynchrony of immunoglobulin chain synthesis during B cell ontogeny. Nature 280:838–840, 1979.
12. Kloppel T, Kubo R, Cain P, Browne C, Colon S, Kearney J, Grey H: Structural analysis of the mu chains synthesized by fetal liver hybridomas. J Immunol 126:1346–1350, 1981.
13. Alt F, Rosenberg N, Lewis S, Thomas E, Baltimore D: Organization and reorganization of immunoglobulin genes in A-MULV transformed cells: Rearrangement of heavy but not light chain genes. Cell 27:381–390, 1981.
14. Burrows P, Kearney J, Lawton A, Cooper M: Pre-B cells. J Immunol 120:1526–1531, 1978.
15. Melchers F, Abramzuk J: Murine embryonic blood between day 10 and 13 of gestation as a source of immature precursor B cells. Eur J Immunol 10:763–767, 1980.
16. Fu S, Hurley J, McCune J, Kunkel H, Good R: Unusual lymphoid cell lines derived from patients with immunodeficient states. In Seligmann M, Hitzig W (eds): "Primary Immunodeficiencies." New York: Elsevier/North Holland, 1980, pp 59–67.
17. Fu S, Hurley J, McCune J, Kunkel H, Good R: Pre-B cells and other possible precursor lymphoid cell lines derived from patients with X-linked agammaglobulinemia. J Exp Med 152:1519–1526, 1980.
18. Brack C, Hirama M, Lenhard-Schuller R, Tonegawa S: A complete immunoglobulin gene is created by somatic recombination. Cell 15:1–14, 1978.
19. Early P, Huang H, Davis M, Calame K, Hood L: An immunoglobulin heavy chain variable region gene is generated from three segments of DNA: VH, D, and JH. Cell 19:981–992, 1980.
20. Perry R, Kelley D, Coleclough C, Kearney J: Organization and expression of immunoglobulin genes in fetal liver hybridomas. Proc Natl Acad Sci USA 78:247–251, 1981.
21. Alt FW, Baltimore D: Joining of immunoglobulin heavy chain gene segments: Implications from a chromosome with evidence of three D-J_H fusions. Proc Natl Acad Sci USA 79:4118–4122, 1982.
22. Davis M, Calame K, Early P, Livant D, Joho R, Weissman I, Hood L: An immunoglobulin heavy chain gene is formed by at least two recombination events. Nature 283:733–739, 1980.
23. Kemp D, Harris A, Adams J: Transcripts of the immunoglobulin C_{mu} gene vary in structure and splicing during lymphoid development. Proc Natl Acad Sci USA 77:7400–7404, 1980.
24. Walker I, Harris A: Immunoglobulin C_{mu} RNA in T lymphoma cells is not translated. Nature 288:290–293, 1980.
25. Walker I, Harris A: Mu polypeptide phenotypes of lymphoid and myeloid cell lines containing RNA transcripts of the

immunoglobulin C_{mu} gene. J Immunol 127:561-566, 1981.
26. Schwaber J, Rosen FS: Isotypes of surface immunoglobulin on B lymphocytes from patients with agammaglobulinemia. J Clin Immunol 2:30-34, 1982.
27. Schwaber J, Lazarus H, Rosen FS: Bone marrow-derived lymphoid cell lines from patients with agammaglobulinemia. J Clin Invest 62:302-310, 1978.
28. Schwaber J, Klein G, Ernberg I, Rosen A, Lazarus H, Rosen F: Deficiency of Epstein-Barr virus (EBV) receptors on B lymphocytes from certain patients with agammaglobulinemia. J Immunol 122:2191-2199, 1979.
29. Schwaber J, Cohen EP: Human × mouse somatic cell hybrids secreting immunoglobulin of both parental types. Nature 244:444-446, 1973.
30. Lin LC, Putnam F: Cold pepsin digestion: A novel method to produce the Fv fragment from human immunoglobulin M. Proc Natl Acad Sci USA 75:2649-2653, 1978.
31. Schwaber J, Posner M, Schlossman S, Lazarus H: Human-human hybrids secreting pneumococcal antibodies. Hum Immunol (In press)
32. Littlefield JW: The use of drug resistant markers to study the hybridization of mouse fibroblasts. Exp Cell Res 41:190-196, 1966.
33. Davidson R: Regulation of melanin synthesis in mammalian cells, as studied by somatic hybridization. III. A method of increasing the frequency of cell fusion. Exp Cell Res 55:424-426, 1969.
34. Thomas P: Hybridization of denatured RNA and small DNA fragments transferred to nitrocellulose. Proc Natl Acad Sci USA 77:5201-5205, 1980.
35. Croce C, Shander M, Martinis J, Cicurel L, D'Anconna G, Dolby T, Koprowski H: Chromosomal location of the genes for human immunoglobulin heavy chains. Proc Natl Acad Sci USA 76:3416-3419, 1979.
36. Challberg M, Englund P: Specific labeling of 3' termini with T4 DNA polymerase. Methods Enzymol 65:39-42, 1980.
37. Gough N, Barnard O: Sequences of the joining region genes for immunoglobulin heavy chains and their role in generation of antibody diversity. Proc Natl Acad Sci USA 78:509-513, 1981.
38. Treisman R, Proudfoot NJ, Shander M, Maniatis T: A single-base change at a splice site in a Beta°-thalassemic gene causes abnormal RNA splicing. Cell 29:903-911, 1981.
39. Chaconas G, van de Sande J: 5' ^{32}P labeling of RNA and DNA restriction fragments. Methods Enzymol 65:75-85, 1980.
40. Favaloro J, Treisman R, Kamen R: Transcription maps of polyoma virus-specific RNA: Analysis by two-dimensional nuclease S1 gel mapping. Methods Enzymol 65:718-749, 1980.
41. Maxam A, Gilbert W: Sequencing end-labeled DNA with base-specific chemical cleavages. Methods Enzymol 65:499-559, 1980.
42. Weigert M, Gatmaitan L, Loh E, Schilling J, Hood L: Rearrangement of genetic information may produce immunoglobulin diversity. Nature 276:785-790, 1978.

Lymphoid Cell-Derived Lectin-Like Receptor Molecules as Immunoregulatory Signals in Immunodeficiency

R. Michael Blaese, MD, Andrew V. Muchmore, MD, and Giovanna Tosato, MD

Cellular Immunology Section, Metabolism Branch, National Institutes of Health, Bethesda, MD 20205

A considerable body of evidence has recently appeared to suggest that lectin-carbohydrate interactions at the cell surface may play an important role in the recognition of foreignness by nonimmune mononuclear phagocytes (MNP) [1]. Lectins capable of interacting with foreign cells can be demonstrated on invertebrate MNP, the coelomocytes, and this recognition mechanism has been preserved during evolution and can be demonstrated on murine and human monocytes/macrophages as well [2–6]. Evidence for the potential role of cellular lectins in the function of the specific immune system has also been presented. The lymphokine MIF binds to a fucosidase-sensitive receptor on the macrophage [7]. The action of lymphocyte-derived chemotactic factor (LDCF) is blocked by the sugar L-rhamnose. Antigen-induced human T-cell proliferation is blocked by certain nontoxic simple sugars [8].

Plant lectins induce lymphoid cells to perform almost all of the functions seen in specific, antigen-induced immune responses. They can induce T cells to proliferate; B cells to produce immunoglobulin (Ig); monocytes, polymorphonuclear neutrophilic leukocytes (PMNs), K cells, and T cells to kill foreign targets; T cells and monocytes to produce lymphokines and monokines which in turn affect the function of other lymphoid cells; suppressor activity in both T cells and monocytes; and T-cell helper function [9]. This broad array of immune cell activation by lectins which bind to specific saccharide structures on the membranes of lymphoid cells must be more than mere coincidence, and suggests that similar structures and molecules may be important elements in normal immunoregulatory processes.

A widely studied immunoregulatory system involves the stimulation of lymphoid cell cultures with the plant lectin, Con A. Con A-stimulated cells have been shown to suppress mitogen- and alloantigen-stimulated T-cell proliferation, as well as Ig and antibody production in mitogen- or antigen-stimulated lymphocyte cultures. Recently, we have described studies of suppressor factors found in the supernatants of Con A-stimulated cultures of human peripheral blood mononuclear cells [10–12]. Forty-eight-hour Con A-stimulated culture supernatants added to fresh lymphocyte cultures will suppress the proliferative response of T cells to mitogens and antigens and the production of Ig in response to pokeweed mitogen (PWM) or the Epstein-Barr virus (EBV). Significantly, partial purification of this supernatant activity by gel filtration showed a dissociation between the suppressor activity for T-cell proliferation and the activity which inhibited Ig production by B cells. Table 1 lists the characteristics of these soluble immune suppressor supernatant activities, SISS-T and SISS-B, respectively. SISS-T has a molecular weight of 30–45,000 and its production is very dependent on monocytes. SISS-B has a molecular weight of 60–80,000 and is a T-cell product. The table also lists the effect of adding various monosaccharides to lymphocyte cultures treated with these suppressor factors. Alpha-methyl mannoside, the sugar to which Con A binds most avidly, has no effect on the suppression induced by either supernatant factor, indicating that the suppression observed is not due to free Con A carried over in the supernatants. The action of SISS-T was essentially totally reversed by N-acetylglucosamine. L-rhamnose had no effect on the activity of SISS-T. By striking contrast, N-acetylglucosamine had no effect on the suppression of Ig production induced by SISS-B. In this case, however, L-rhamnose was found to reverse this supernatant suppressor activity. These data indicate that a plant lectin (Con A) which binds preferentially to mannose-like sugar residues on lymphoid cell membranes induces subpopulations of these cells to produce their own lectin-like biologically active factors with distinctly different sugar-binding specificities. SISS-B binds to L-rhamnose-like sugar residues on the surface of B lymphocytes and this interaction suppresses the B cells' capacity to be activated to produce Ig. SISS-T binds to an N-acetylglucosamine containing membrane components on the T cell, resulting in suppression of T-cell proliferation. Interestingly, the plant lectin, wheat-germ agglutinin, also has binding specificity for N-acetylglucosamine, and this nonmitogenic lectin also functions as a di-

TABLE 1. Characteristics of Soluble Immune Suppressor Supernatants, SISS-T and SISS-B, Produced by Con A-Stimulated Human Mononuclear Cells

	SISS-T	SISS-B
Molecular size	30–45,000	60–80,000
Producer cell	Adherent cell dependent	T cell
Site of action	T cell	B cell
Time of maximal factor appearance in culture	48 hrs	8 hrs
Functional effect of monosaccharide addition		
Alpha-methyl mannoside	None	None
N-acetylglucosamine	Reverse suppression	None
L-rhamnose	None	Reverse suppression
L-fucose	None	ND

TABLE 2. Suppression of Ig Production in Co-cultures of Normal (NL) Mononuclear Cells and T Cells From a Patient With Infectious Mononucleosis (IM)

		Culture Stimulant	
		PWM	EBV
		Ig-Secreting Cells/Culture	
NL-MNC[a]		7,800	6,300
IM-MNC		250	500
NL-MNC+	NL-T[b]	7,200	—[e]
NL-MNC+	IM-T	500	—
NL-MNC+	IM-T$_{xr}$[c]	6,700	—
NL-B[d]		50	8,000
IM-B		250	7,300
NL-B+	IM-T	200	—
IM-B+	NL-T	5,800	—
IM-B+	IM-T	300	600

[a]5×10^5 mononuclear cells.
[b]5×10^5 T cells.
[c]2,000 rads gamma irradiation.
[d]5×10^5 B cells.
[e]Not done because allogeneic cell mixtures are normally suppressed in EBV-stimulated cultures.

rect suppressor signal for T-cell proliferation [13].

SISS-T and SISS-B are lectin-like effector molecules produced by lymphoid cells stimulated with another lectin. We wondered if examples of a similar suppressor mechanism could be found in the disorders of man characterized by excessive in vivo suppressor activity. A common disease of man which is regularly associated with intense suppressor T-cell activity is infectious mononucleosis (IM) [14]. EBV, the agent which causes IM, is a unique viral pathogen in that it attacks the immune system directly and almost exclusively. B lymphocytes, the target of EBV, are induced to proliferate and differentiate to produce Ig by the virus [15]. In vitro, EBV-infected B cells transform into permanently growing cell lines; in vivo, EBV is thought to cause the B-cell tumor, African Burkitt lymphoma. In normal subjects with acute EBV infection (ie IM), the immune system responds to this infection by generating an intense suppressor T-cell response. These suppressor T cells, which account for the majority of the "atypical lymphocytes," are able to prevent further B-cell activation by this virus. Table 2 illustrates the results obtained in studies of the peripheral lymphocytes from a typical patient with IM. The cultured mononuclear cells from the IM patient failed to make significant Ig in vitro in response to either PWM or EBV. Importantly isolated patient T cells suppressed Ig production by normal mononuclear cells by over 90%. This suppressor activity was sensitive to irradiation. The patient B cells were able to respond normally when separated from their autologous T cells.

To test whether the suppression associated with IM was related to the lectin-like activity seen with SISS-T and SISS-B, we added various monosaccharides to PWM-stimulated co-cultures of patient T cells mixed with normal mononuclear responder cells. Table 3 shows the results of one such study. Again, the response of the normal cells was markedly suppressed by the patient T cells. Neither N-acetylglucosamine nor L-rhamnose, the sugars which inhibit SISS-T and SISS-B, had any effect on this suppression. Neither did gentiobiose, L-fucose, or N-acetylgalactosamine. However, the addition of either D-mannose or alpha-methyl mannoside to these co-cultures showed a striking reversal of the expected suppression [16]. In dose-response studies (not shown), progressive reversal of the suppression was seen as higher concentrations of mannose were added to the co-cultures. At 25 mM mannose, four times as many patient T cells were required to achieve an equivalent level of suppression to that seen in co-cultures not containing mannose. Since these compounds are permitting a suppressed culture to respond normally, simple toxicity as an explanation for their effects is unlikely. Thus, these studies also support the concept that

TABLE 3. Reversal of Infectious Mononucleosis T-Cell-Mediated Suppression of Ig Production by Mannose

Cells		Sugar	Ig-Secreting Cells per PWM Stimulated Culture
NL-MNC[a]	—	—	6,700
+	IM-T[b]	—	500
+	+	L-rhamnose[c]	750
+	+	N-acetylglucosamine	600
+	+	L-fucose	300
+	+	N-acetylgalactosamine	800
+	+	Gentiobiose	400
+	+	D-mannose	5,200
+	+	Alpha-methyl mannoside	5,600

[a]NL-MNC, 5×10^5 normal mononuclear cells.
[b]IM-T, 1×10^6 infectious mononucleosis T cells.
[c]Sugars present at 25 mM final concentration.

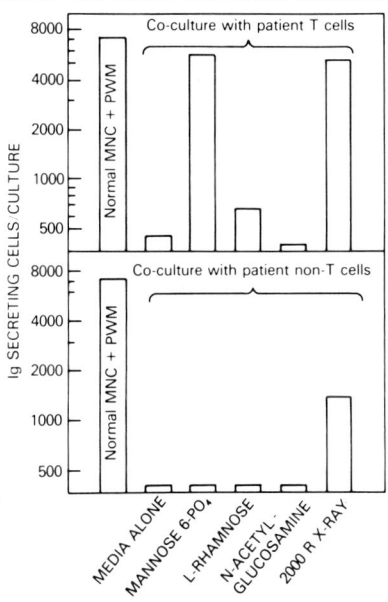

Fig. 1. The effect of irradiation and the addition of various monosaccharides on the suppressor activity of T cells and non-T cells from a patient with agammaglobulinemia.

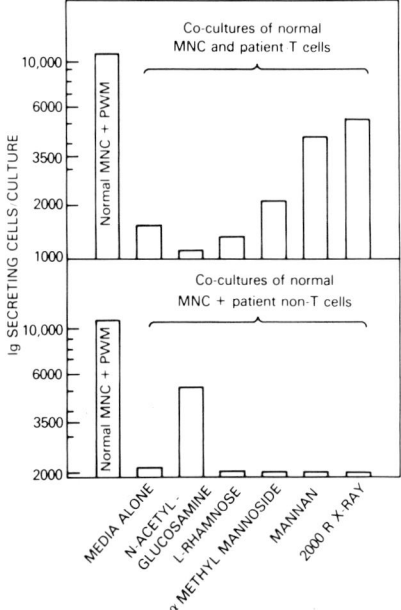

Fig. 2. Reversal of suppressor T-cell activity by a mannose polymer and reversal of suppressor monocyte activity by N-acetylglucosamine.

important immunoregulatory signals may involve the interaction of effector lectin-like receptors with cell membrane saccharide structures.

Certain patients with adult-onset hypogammaglobulinemia also have excessive suppressor activity when co-cultured with normal lymphoid cells. Figures 1 and 2 illustrate the results of co-culture studies of 2 patients who were found to have excessive suppressor activity in both their T cells and non-T cells (probably monocytes). In Figure 1, co-cultures demonstrated that both the patient's T-cell suppressor and the non-T-cell suppressor were at least partially radiosensitive, but that only the T-cell suppressor activity could be reversed by any of the monosaccharides tested. In this case, mannose 6-PO_4 almost totally restored the response of the indicator population to PWM, while L-rhamnose and N-acetylglucosamine had no effect. The T-cell suppressor shown in Figure 2 was also radiosensitive, while the non-T suppressor was not. N-acetylglucosamine had a significant effect on the non-T suppressor, and none at all on the T-cell suppressor. Conversely, a mannose polymer, yeast mannan, substantially reversed the suppression induced by the patient T cells, but not that induced by the non-T suppressor.

Our knowledge of the chemical-molecular basis of immunoregulatory processes is still in its infancy. We know something about the types of cells involved in these processes, some of their distinctive cell surface phenotypes as revealed by heteroantisera and monoclonal antibodies, and some of the characteristics of their secreted factors which have immunoregulatory activity. We believe that the present studies and others [17–24] add an additional clue to the solution of this puzzle by suggesting that some immunoregulatory processes involve the interaction of cell-bound or secreted lectin-like factors which bind to target cell receptors consisting of specific sugar polymers. The membranes of all cells are rich in saccharide molecules, primarily in the form of glycoproteins and glycolipids. It is our challenge to now determine with precision the nature of these immunoregulatory signals and their cellular receptors. In addition, each of the sugar-modulated immunoregulatory processes described is nonspecific in that they affect the proliferation of T cells in general, and the production of Ig by all B cells. Although there is an important need for such nonspecific, polyclonal immunoregulatory mechanisms in host defense (eg IM), it is also our challenge to determine whether similar regulatory mechanisms are operative at the level of the antigen-specific response. The evidence for the capacity of both plant and endogenous animal lectins to activate and regulate a wide spectrum of immune responses is compelling, and most certainly justifies continued exploration of the role of the sugar-coating on cells as a critical receptor site for the control of cell function.

REFERENCES

1. Muchmore AV, Blaese RM: Evidence that monocyte mediated cellular recognition phenomena are mediated by receptors with specificity for simple oligosaccharides. In Unanue ER, Rosenthal AS (eds): "Macrophage Regulation of Immunity." New York: Academic Press, 1980, pp 505–517.
2. Decker JM, Elmholt A, Muchmore AV: Spontaneous cytotoxicity mediated by invertebrate mononuclear cells toward normal and malignant vertebrate target: Inhibition by defined mono- and disaccharide. Cell Immunol 59:161–170, 1980.
3. Decker JM, Muchmore AV, Blaese RM: Spontaneous cytotoxicity mediated by invertebrate mononuclear cells exhibits broad target specificity and is inhibited by specific monosaccharides. In Resch K, Kirchner H (eds): "Mechanisms of Lymphocyte Activation." Amsterdam: Elsevier, 1980, pp 326–328.
4. Muchmore AV, Decker JM, Blaese RM: Spontaneous cytotoxicity by human peripheral blood monocytes: Inhibition by monosaccharides and oligosaccharides. Immunobiology 158:191–206, 1981.
5. Kolb H, Kolb-Backofen V, Schlepper-Schofer J: Cell contacts mediated by D-galactose-specific lectins on liver cells. Biol Cell 36:301–308, 1979.
6. Wier DM: Surface carbohydrates and lectins in cellular recognition. Immunol Today 1:45–51, 1980.
7. Remold HG: Requirements for α-L-fucose on the macrophage membrane receptor for MIF. J Exp Med 138:1065–1076, 1973.
8. Muchmore AV, Decker JM, Blaese RM: Evidence that specific oligosaccharides block early events necessary for the expression of antigen specific proliferation by human lymphocytes. J Immunol 125:1306–1311, 1980.
9. Oppenheim JJ, Rosenstreich DL: "Mitogens in Immunobiology." New York: Academic Press, 1976.
10. Greene WC, Fleisher TA, Waldmann TA: Soluble suppressor supernatants elaborated by concanavalin A-activated human mononuclear cells. I. Characterization of a soluble suppressor of T cell proliferation. J Immunol 126:1185–1191, 1981.
11. Fleisher TA, Greene WC, Blaese RM et al: Soluble suppressor supernatants elaborated by concanvalin A-activated human mononuclear cells. II. Characterization of a soluble suppressor of B cell immunoglobulin production. J Immunol 126:1192–1197, 1981.
12. Fleisher TA, Greene WC, Uchiyama T et al: Characterization of a soluble suppressor of human B cell immunoglobulin biosynthesis produced by a continuous human suppressor T cell line. J Exp Med 154:156–167, 1981.
13. Greene WC, Waldmann TA: Inhibition of human lymphocyte proliferation by the nonmitogenic lectin wheat germ agglutinin. J Immunol 124:2979–2987, 1980.
14. Tosato G, Magrath I, Koski I et al: Activation of suppressor T cells during Epstein-Barr-virus-induced infectious mononucleosis. N Engl J Med 301:1133–1137, 1979.
15. Kirchner H, Tosato G, Blaese RM et al: Polyclonal immunoglobulin secretion by human B lymphocytes exposed to Epstein-Barr virus in vitro. J Immunol 122:1310–1313, 1979.
16. Tosato G, Pike SE, DeSeau V et al: Reversal of infectious mononucleosis suppressor T cell activity by a monosaccharide. Clin Res 30:516, 1982.
17. Koszenowski UH, Karmer M: Selective inhibition of T suppressor-cell function by a monosaccharide. Nature 289:181–184, 1981.
18. Forbes JT, Bretthauer RK, Oeltmann TH: Mannose 6-, fructose 1-, and fructose 6-phosphates inhibit human natural cell-mediating cytotoxicity. Proc Natl Acad Sci USA 78:5797–5801, 1981.
19. Mann DL, Muchmore AV: Inhibition of DRw antisera reactivity by mono- and oligosaccharides. J Immunol 124:2218–2221, 1980.
20. Teodroescu M, Mayer EP, Dray S: Identification of fine human lymphocyte subpopulations by their differential binding of various strains of bacteria. Cell Immunol 29:352–361, 1977.
21. McKenzie IFC, Clarke A, Parish CR: Ia antigenic specifications are oligosaccharides in nature: Hapten inhibition studies. J Exp Med 145:1039–1053, 1977.
22. Tomaska LD, Parish CR: Inhibition of secondary IgG responses by N-acetyl-D-galactosamine. Eur J Immunol 11:181–186, 1981.
23. MacDermott RP, Kienker LJ, Bertovich MJ et al: Inhibition of spontaneous but not antibody-dependent cell-mediated cytotoxicity by simple sugars: Evidence that endogenous lectins may mediate spontaneous cell-mediated cytotoxicity. Immunology 44:143–152, 1981.
24. Stutman O, Dien P, Wisun RE et al: Natural cytotoxic cells against solid tumors in mice: Blocking of cytotoxicity by D-mannose. Proc Natl Acad Sci USA 77:2895–2898, 1980.

T Cells and T-Cell Subsets in a Large Population of Patients With Primary Immunodeficiency*

Rebecca H. Buckley, MD, Sherrie Gard, BS, Richard I. Schiff, MD, PhD, and Hugh A. Sampson, MD

Departments of Pediatrics and of Microbiology and Immunology, Duke University School of Medicine, Durham, NC 27710

During the past decade rapid advances have been made in technology permitting the identification and enumeration of human lymphoid cell populations and subpopulations [1,2]. This has been hastened considerably by the development of monoclonal antibodies recognizing cell-surface antigens characteristic of different developmental stages and functions of T lymphocytes [2]. It was expected that these antibodies would prove useful in the elucidation of basic abnormalities underlying primary immunodeficiency (ID) disorders. Thus, in the 2 years since their development, hybridoma antibodies to human T-cell subsets have been employed by a number of investigators in the analysis of lymphoid cell populations from a variety of patients with well-defined primary immune defects [3-8]. While abnormalities in the numbers of T cells and T-cell subsets have been reported in several of these disorders [3-8], they have not been observed consistently in some, raising the question of whether such subset abnormalities are etiologic or occur as a consequence of unknown primary biologic errors in these defects. Moreover, the resultant phenotypic findings have not necessarily correlated with lymphocyte functional abnormalities in such patients. The purposes of this study were to determine 1) the intra- and inter-subject variability of results of cytofluorographic analyses of blood lymphocytes from normal donors, and 2) how often statistically significant deviations from these results occur in patients with well-defined primary ID diseases, so as to assess the usefulness of this type of analysis in elucidating basic mechanisms underlying such disorders.

PATIENTS AND METHODS

Fifty-four patients with well-defined primary ID diseases being followed on a regular basis at the Duke University Clinical Research Center (RR-30) had heparinized venous blood samples obtained on one or more occasions for cytofluorographic analyses. The population consisted of 19 patients with common variable immunodeficiency (CVID), 11 with X-linked agammaglobulinemia (SLA), 5 with SCID, 3 with X-linked immunodeficiency with hyper IgM (HypM), 3 with the Wiskott-Aldrich syndrome (WAS), 3 with the hyper IgE syndrome (HypE), 2 with Nezelof syndrome (NEZ), 1 with antibody deficiency and normal immunoglobulins (ADNIg), 1 with DiGeorge syndrome (DiG), 5 with transient hypogammaglobulinemia of infancy (THI), and 1 with chronic mucocutaneous moniliasis (CMC). Twenty-seven healthy adults donated heparinized venous blood samples on from 1-20 occasions which served as simultaneous controls for the patient samples.

Lymphocyte subpopulation enumeration and stimulation studies were carried out as previously described [1]. Cytofluorographic analysis of lymphoid cell populations were done on an Ortho Cytofluorograf System 50-H, using mouse monoclonal antibodies to human cell surface antigens [9] and affinity-purified, fluoresceinated goat anti-mouse IgG (Tago, Inc, Burlingame, CA). Patient group means were compared with those from the normal control population by Student's t test.

RESULTS

Table 1 summarizes group means for percentages of lymphocytes reacting with the pan-T reagent (T3), the monoclonal antibody recognizing the helper/inducer T-cell subpopulation (T4), the monoclonal antibody recognizing the cytotoxic/suppressor T-cell subset (T8), and for the ratios of the percentages of T4 to T8 positive cells for the entire patient and control populations. The means ± SD for the normal group were: T3 75 ± 7, T4 52 ± 9, T8 27 ± 9, and T4/T8 2.1 ± 0.8. In data not shown, individual mean percentages ± SD for these same parameters in 10 normal controls studied on more than one occasion (2-20 times) were determined; surprisingly, SDs were found to be as high or higher than for the entire normal group's mean percentages in 7/10 cases. Thus, the intra-subject (presumably biologic) variability in the results of these cytofluorographic analyses was equal to or greater than the inter-subject variability in this group of normal subjects.

For the two large groups of agammaglobulinemic patients (SLA and CVID), means differed statistically

*Supported by Grant #1 R01 AI18613 from NIAID and by a grant from the General Clinical Research Centers Program (RR-30).

TABLE 1. Comparison of Mean Percentages of Immunodeficient Patients' T Cells and Subsets With Those of Normals

		Mean % Total Lymphocytes ± SD			
Group	No.	T3	T4	T8	T4/T8 ± SD
1. SLA	11	82† ± 12	54 ± 17	34† ± 9	1.8 ± 0.9
2. CVID	19	70 ± 12	48 ± 12	29 ± 11	1.9 ± 1.0
3. THI	5	71 ± 5	57 ± 4	21 ± 8	3.0† ± 0.7
4. HypM	3	55*** ± 15	40 ± 19	19 ± 5	2.1 ± 0.9
5. HypE	3	72 ± 19	44 ± 6	26 ± 5	1.7 ± 0.1
6. ADNIg	1	90	59	27	2.2
7. WAS	3	28*** ± 18	26*** ± 15	10** ± 4	3.1 ± 0.6
8. DiG	1	26***	19**	13	1.6
9. NEZ	2	64 ± 31	46 ± 21	17 ± 8	3.0 ± 0.5
10. CMC	1		33†	30	1.1
11. SCID	5	6*** ± 3	6*** ± 5	9*** ± 10	1.7 ± 1.6
12. Normals	27	75 ± 7	52 ± 9	27 ± 9	2.1 ± 0.8

†p value = < 0.05 by Student's *t test*.
*p value = < 0.02 by Student's *t test*.
**p value = < 0.01 by Student's *t test*.
***p value = < 0.0001 by Student's *t test*.

from those of normals only for the SLA group, where higher percentages of cells reacting with the pan-T reagent (T3: 82 ± 12 vs 75 ± 7, p = < 0.05) and with the suppressor/cytotoxic reagent (T8 34 ± 9 vs 27 ± 9) were noted. Individual patient data are not presented, but we observed an increased percentage of cells of the suppressor phenotype (ie > 2 SD of the normal mean percentage for T8+ cells, or > 44%) in only 3/19 CVID and also found a significant increase in 2/11 SLA. Similarly, a decreased percentage of cells with the helper phenotype (ie < 2 SD of the normal mean percentage for T4+ cells or < 34%) was noted in 3/19 patients with CVID and in 1/11 patients with SLA. Both types of abnormalities occurred simultaneously in only 2 patients from these groups (1 with SLA and 1 with CVID). T4/T8 ratios were significantly higher than that of the normal group (ie > 3.7) in only 1 patient with CVID and significantly lower (ie < 0.5) in only 1 patient with SLA.

Table 2 presents the individual patient data for those with miscellaneous antibody deficiency syndromes (THI, HypM, HypE, and ADNIg). The only deviations from normal were a significantly higher mean T4/T8 ratio for the THI group (3.0 ± 2.0 vs 2.1 ± 0.8, p = < 0.05) and a significantly lower mean percentage of T3+ cells in HypM (55 ± 15 vs 75 ± 7, p = < 0.0001). We did not observe T4 deficiency in a single patient with THI. The low mean percentage for T3+ cells in HypM is accounted for by low percentages (ie < 61%) in 2 of the 3 patients in this group. Of particular note is the fact that neither individual HypE patient nor group means for T4+ or T8+ cells or for T4/T8 ratios differed at all from the normal group.

In contrast to infrequent abnormal findings in cytofluorographic studies of blood lymphocytes from patients with antibody deficiency disorders, patients with T-cell dysfunctions had relatively more deviations from the norm (Tables 3 and 4). Mean percentages of T3+, T4+, and T8+ cells were significantly (p = < 0.01-< 0.0001) lower than normal for the WAS group, and T3+ and T4+ cells were also low in patients with DiG and CMC (Table 3). Mean percentages for the NEZ group did not differ significantly from normal, although T3+ and T4+ cells were below 2 SD of the normal group in 1 of the 2 patients with this diagnosis.

The most striking abnormalities were seen in patients with SCID (Table 4). Mean percentages of E-RFC, T3+, T4+, and T8+ cells were extremely low (23, 6, 6 and 9%, respectively, p = < 0.0001). In contrast, mean percentages of SIg+ and VEP 10/T10+ cells were significantly higher than in normals. It should be noted, however, that there was considerable heterogeneity within this group with respect to numbers of both B and T cells, with 2 infants lacking detectable SIg+ cells and percentages of E-RFC being considerably higher in 3 of the patients than in the other 2. Of particular interest are the high percentages of T10+ cells in all 3 infants in this group evaluated with this reagent and the normal percentages of T8+ cells in 2 of these 3. In one case *(#5)* T10 positivity occurred in association with a high percentage of Ia+ cells, whereas in the other 2 cases there was no other marker to suggest cell activation. As reported elsewhere in this volume, we observed high natural killer (NK) cell activity against the erythromyeloid line K562 by lymphocytes from the 3 patients with the highest percentages of E-RFC, whereas NK function was absent in the other 2. In *Patients 3* and *4,* who

TABLE 2. T Cells and Subsets in 12 Patients With Miscellaneous Antibody Deficiency Syndromes

Subject	% Total Lymphocytes			T4/8
	T3	T4	T8	
Transient Hypogammaglobulinemia of Infancy				
1. S.H.	67	56	10	5.6
2. F.H.	70	57	29	2.0
3. J.C.	78	62	26	2.4
4. E.C.	69	52	24	2.2
5. A.H.	69	56	18	3.1
Mean ± SD	71 ± 5	57 ± 4	21 ± 8	3.0* ± 2.0
X-Linked Immunodeficiency With Hyper IgM				
1. D.Mc.	72	60	24	2.5
2. D.L.	45	21	21	1.0
3. J.Y.	47	38	14	2.8
Mean ± SD	55** ± 15	40 ± 19	19 ± 5	2.1 ± 0.9
Hyper IgE Syndrome				
1. A.T.	88	48	32	1.5
2. J.B.	75	46	26	1.8
3. J.W.	51	38	21	1.8
Mean ± SD	72 ± 19	44 ± 6	26 ± 5	1.7 ± 0.1
Antibody Deficiency With Near Normal Igs				
1. B.L.†	90	59	27	2.2
Normals (27)				
Mean ± SD	75 ± 7	52 ± 9	27 ± 9	2.1 ± 0.8

*p value = < 0.05 when compared in Student's *t test* with appropriate normal mean.
**p value = < 0.0001 when compared in Student's *t test* with appropriate normal mean.
†analysis done on SRBC purified T cells.

TABLE 3. T Cells and Subsets in 7 Patients With Miscellaneous Cellular Immunodeficiencies

Subject	% Total Lymphocytes			T4/T8
	T3	T4	T8	
Wiskott-Aldrich Syndrome				
1. B.H.	8	9	5	2.4
2. C.C.	44	35	13	3.6
3. M.T.	32	34	12	3.4
Mean ± SD	28*** ± 18	26*** ± 15	10** ± 4	3.1 ± 0.6
DiGeorge Syndrome				
1. R.K.	26***	19**	13	1.6
Nezelof Syndrome				
1. G.W.	86	61	23	3.4
2. J.H.	42	31	11	2.7
Mean ± SD	64 ± 31	46 ± 21	17 ± 8	3.0 ± 0.5
Chronic Mucocutaneous Moniliasis				
1. S.C.	57*	33†	30	1.1
Normals (27)				
Mean ± SD	75 ± 7	52 ± 9	27 ± 9	2.1 ± 0.8

†p value = < 0.05 when compared with appropriate normal mean in Student's *t test*.
*p value = < 0.02 when compared with appropriate normal mean in Student's *t test*.
**p value = < 0.01 when compared with appropriate normal mean in Student's *t test*.
***p value = < 0.0001 when compared with appropriate normal mean in Student's *t test*.

had exceedingly high NK activity, the phenotype of their lymphoid cells was more fully characterized and found to be E-RF+, 3A1+, T8+, T10+, T3−, 5E9−, and Ia−. Finally, it should be noted that, despite these striking deviations from the norm in percentages of cells reacting with the monoclonal antibodies recognizing T-cell surface antigens in patients with T-cell dysfunction, no statistically significant abnormalities are noted for any mean T4/T8 ratios. Indeed, only one individual patient with cellular immunodeficiency (*#3* of the SCID group, Table 4) had an abnormal T4/T8 ratio (0.3).

DISCUSSION

The results of monoclonal antibody studies of T lymphocytes from the 81 subjects evaluated by our group over the past 2 years, while useful in revealing limitations and low-cost effectiveness of this type of analysis, were generally disappointing in the insight they provided in understanding basic mechanisms of primary ID. This study is the first to address the question of intra-subject variability in percentages of total T cells and T-cell subsets in a normal control population. Surprisingly, that variability (presumably biologic) was as great as the inter-subject variability among the 27 different normal controls studied. Moreover, the inter-subject variability was comparable to that reported for other groups of normal controls [3,5,8]. This suggests that cytofluorographic studies of T cells and subsets in disease 1) are not likely to be useful in revealing small differences in percentages, and 2) would necessarily have to be repeated on one or more occasions to confirm the consistency of any abnormalities (or lack of them).

The finding that T-cell phenotypes in most patients with severe humoral ID are not statistically different from those of normal controls indicates that cytofluorographic studies with monoclonal antibodies to T cells and subsets are least cost-effective in this type of patient. While imbalances in numbers of cells of the helper and suppressor phenotype have been reported in CVID [3,5,8], suggesting that either excessive suppression or defective help could be etiologic in the failure of these patients' SIg+ B

TABLE 4. Lymphocyte Membrane Markers in 5 Patients With SCID

Subject	% of Total Lymphocytes									
	SIg+	E-RFC	T3	3A1	T4	T8	T4/8	5E9	VEP10 T10	OKI1
1. J.K.	0	41	4	—	2	3	0.7	—	—	—
2. K.G.	74	14	5	—	8	2	3.9	—	—	—
3. L.C.	0	30	8	—	5	19	0.3	0	93	6
4. A.M.	33	30	10	15	13	22	0.6	0	78	—
5. D.M.	17	2	3	12	3	1	3.0	0	88	91
Mean ± SD	25* ± 31	23* ± 15	6* ± 3		6* ± 5	9* ± 10	1.7 ± 1.6	0	57* ± 50	30 ± 53
Normal Mean ± SD	8 ± 3	76 ± 5	75 ± 7		52 ± 9	27 ± 9	2.1 ± 0.8		8 ± 2	

*p value = < 0.0001 when compared in Student's *t test* with appropriate normal mean.

cells to differentiate [10], such abnormalities have also been noted in SLA patients [3,5,8] who lack SIg+ B cells. In the present study, both CVID and SLA patients evidenced abnormal percentages of T4+ and/or T8+ lymphocytes, although there were very few in either group. Moreover, previous studies of suppressor cell function in many of these same patients [11] revealed excessive suppression by T cells of both SLA and CVID patients. Indeed, in unpublished Ig synthesis studies done on most of the patients presented here, there was often evidence of excessive suppressor cell function even when phenotypes were normal (and vice versa). However, in virtually all patients with either SLA or CVID whom we have studied, their B cells did not differentiate normally in response to polyclonal activators, even when normal T help was provided, suggesting intrinsic B-cell defects.

In contrast to a report by Siegel et al [7], we did not find a deficiency of T cells of the helper phenotype in any of the 5 infants with THI. Indeed, surprisingly, the only mean T4/T8 ratio differing significantly from normal was that of the THI group, in which the high ratio of 3.0 indicated more helper than suppressor cells in the THI patients than in normals. The reason for this discrepancy is unclear, although differences in diagnostic criteria are felt to be the most likely explanation. We consider it necessary for a patient to have serum concentrations of one or more Ig(s) below the 95% confidence interval for age on 2 or more occasions, and to give evidence of normal antibody-forming capacity for establishment of this diagnosis [12]. Few clinical characteristics, only one Ig determination, and no antibody titers were given for the patients of Siegel et al [7], who had primarily selectively IgG deficiency. Other causes of IgG deficiency did not appear to have been excluded. For example, IgG concentrations can be selectively and transiently decreased in infants recovering from diarrhea, and lymphocytes as well as Ig can be lost into the gut in that circumstance.

We also failed to confirm the reported deficiency of T8+ cells [6] in the HypE syndrome [13]. Again, the reason for this discrepancy is not apparent, but differences in patient definition are again suspect. We have also been unable to confirm the reported [14] deficiency of T8+ cells in atopic eczema, another condition characterized by elevated serum IgE concentration. In unpublished studies of 30 patients with severe atopic dermatitis, we found percentages of T cells of both subsets, as well as T4/T8 ratios, to be indistinguishable from those of normal controls.

Even though there was a relatively high frequency of abnormal percentages of total T cells and of T-cell subsets in patients with various forms of cellular immunodeficiency in this as well as in other studies [3,5], this did not amplify information already obtained by E-RF cell studies except in SCID. Surprisingly, mean T4/T8 ratios did not differ significantly from normal in any of these disease states. In 2 patients in the SCID group, the results of monoclonal antibody analyses led to the suspicion that most cells were NK-like. Even though functional studies confirmed the latter, this information nevertheless did not provide a better understanding of the as yet unknown primary biologic error(s) in SCID. It is possible, however, that, as new reagents are developed which distinguish other early differentiation markers or subsets of T cells, useful information can be gained from cytofluorographic studies of blood lymphocytes from patients with cellular ID disorders. For the present, it would appear that, with the exception of SCID, monoclonal antibody analysis of T cells and subsets offers little advantage over the far more cost-effective E-RFC assay.

REFERENCES

1. Schiff RI, Buckley RH, Gilbertsen RB, Metzgar RS: Membrane receptors and in vitro responsiveness of lymphocytes in human immunodeficiency. J Immunol 112:376–386, 1974.
2. Reinherz EL, Schlossman SF: The differentiation and function of human T lymphocytes. A review. Cell 19:821–827, 1980.

3. Phan-Dinh-Tuy F, Durandy A, Griscelli C, Bach MA: T cell subset analysis by monoclonal antibodies in primary immunodeficiencies. Scand J Immunol 14:193–200, 1981.
4. Reinherz EL, Geha RS, Wohl ME, Morimoto C, Rosen FS, Schlossman SF: Immunodeficiency associated with loss of T4+ inducer T cell function. N Engl J Med 304:811–816, 1981.
5. Reinherz EL, Cooper MD, Schlossman SF, Rosen FS: Abnormalities of T cell maturation and regulation in human beings with immunodeficiency disorders. J Clin Invest 68:699–705, 1981.
6. Geha RS, Reinherz EL, Leung D, McKee KT Jr: Deficiency of suppressor T cells in the hyperimmunoglobulinemia E syndrome. J Clin Invest 68:783–791, 1981.
7. Siegel RL, Issekutz T, Schwaber J, Rosen FS, Geha RS: Deficiency of T helper cells in transient hypogammaglobulinemia of infancy. N Engl J Med 305:1307–1313, 1981.
8. Pandolfi F, Quinti I, Frielingsdorf A, Goldstein G, Businco L, Aiuti F: Abnormalities of regulatory T cell subpopulations in patients with primary immunoglobulin deficiencies. Clin Immunol Immunopathol 22:323–330, 1982.
9. Haynes BF: Human T lymphocyte antigens as defined by monoclonal antibodies. Immunol Res 57:127–161, 1981.
10. Waldmann TA, Broder S, Blaese RM, Durm M, Blackman M, Strober W: Role of suppressor T cells in pathogenesis of common variable hypogammaglobulinemia. Lancet 2:609–613, 1979.
11. Herrod HG, Buckley RH: Use of a human plaque forming cell assay to study peripheral blood B cell activiation and excessive suppressor cell activity in humoral deficiency. J Clin Invest 63:868–876, 1979.
12. Tiller TL, Buckley RH: Transient hypogammaglobulinemia of infancy: Review of the literature, clinical and immunologic features of 11 new cases, and long-term follow-up. J Pediatr 92:347–353, 1978.
13. Buckley RH, Wray BB, Belmaker EZ: Extreme hyperimmunoglobulinemia E and undue susceptibility to infection. Pediatrics 49:59–70, 1972.
14. Leung DYM, Rhodes AR, Geha RS: Enumeration of T cell subsets in atopic dermatitis using monoclonal antibodies. J Allergy Clin Immunol 67:450–455, 1981.

Treatment of Defects of Humoral Immunity

Martha Eibl, MD

Institute of Immunology, University of Vienna, Vienna, Austria

Patients with B-cell deficiency are an inhomogeneous group, both with respect to the nature of the immunologic defect and to the clinical manifestation. Clinical symptomatology does not always correlate with the extent of the immunologic defect recognized, but improving diagnostic possibilities may help to clarify some of these fictitious discrepancies [1–3].

Most patients with B-cell defects are unduly susceptible to infections with pyogenic microorganisms. Severe acute and chronic infections, like purulent meningitis and chronic lung disease, make the prognosis of these patients poor, if diagnosis and therapy are delayed [4]. Even though resistance to different viral infections often has been described as normal, severe chronic ECHO virus infections causing chronic encephalitis and dermatomyositis-like syndromes have been observed [4–7]. Inflammatory joint disease resembling juvenile rheumatoid arthritis has been described [8, 9]. In addition, an increased frequency of malignancies is known to appear. Substitution therapy with normal human gamma globulin has been shown to be effective for the prophylaxis of infections [10–12] and in the therapy of ECHO virus infection [13]. These preparations have improved prognosis of hypogammaglobulinemic patients, as well as the clinical situation in patients with other antibody deficiency syndromes suffering from recurrent infections [4, 11]. Gamma globulin is also effective in controlling symptoms of inflammatory joint diseases in agammaglobulinemic patients, while the influence on the occurrence and frequency of malignancies is still not clarified.

The continuous administration of Serum Immune Globulin (human) (SIGH) for intramuscular (im) use was the form of therapy most widely used in the treatment of patients with clinical and laboratory evidence of antibody deficiency, and its efficacy has been well documented [12, 14–17]. The im preparations used contain mainly IgG, different amounts of IgA, and traces of IgM. The recommended dose was 25 mg/kg/week.

SIGH for im use is prepared from plasma by cold ethanol fractionation. It is a 15–18% solution of mainly IgG. To guarantee consistency with regard to antibody spectrum, plasma of at least 1,000 donors has to be fractionated per pool. The different fractionation procedures of different manufacturers yield products which are similar in composition, physicochemical properties, and antibody content [18, 19]. Despite these similarities, differences have been noticed in the content of aggregates and fragments before and during storage. Antibodies are enriched 10–20-fold as compared to plasma, and both the spectrum and quality of the antibodies are comparable to that in the starting material [19]. As for the safety of these im preparations, use has proven that if the single donations of plasma are free of detectable hepatitis B_s antigen, and if appropriate fractionation methodology is used, the end product can be considered safe with regard to the transmission of viral hepatitis. On the other hand, hepatitis has been transmitted by SIGH occasionally when inadequate starting material and/or fractionation methodology was used [20–24].

SIGH for im use usually has high anticomplementary activity and contains variable amounts of aggregates [19]. The advantages of SIGH for im use must not be overlooked: different products from different manufacturers are similar in quality; IgG subclass distribution is almost equal to subclass distribution in plasma; the whole antibody spectrum and all Fc effector functions are preserved.

It has been assumed that these contaminating protein aggregates are responsible for the severe adverse reactions caused by these preparations when given intravenously [25–28]. The im application of these products has been associated with adverse reactions as well, especially in the agammaglobulinemic. In Lars Hanson's patients, 15 of 27 [29], and 15% of the patients in Thompson's series [17], showed adverse reactions. In 9 of Thompson's 123 patients, therapy had to be discontinued because of adverse reactions. These patients did well on plasma infusions, but long-term plasma treatment is always accompanied by the increased risk of hepatitis transmission.

The question that had been asked at several occasions was: Is IgG sufficient for replacement therapy in patients lacking all classes of immunoglobulin (Ig)? Experience has shown that it is. But there were also reports that periodic plasma infusions improved clinical results in congenital Ig deficiencies [30]. Still, problems in the management of patients were apparently more closely connected with difficulties in applying optimal dosage than with the class of antibody.

A preparation enriched in IgM has been available for several years, but limited experience does not allow us to answer several open questions regarding its safety and efficacy [31].

An IgA-enriched preparation is also available, but since patients with IgA deficiency can develop antibodies to IgA, the parenteral use of such a preparation has been considered of questionable advantage. A WHO expert committee advises strongly against this therapy in the IgA-deficient [32]. IgA deficiency occurs with a frequency of one in 700, and most individuals with this deficiency are asymptomatic. They do not need any therapy. Whenever the lack of IgA alone is associated with clinical symptoms, it is more likely the lack of secretory IgA than that of IgA. There is not enough evidence to prove that the IgA administered im will enter secretions.

In some IgA-deficient patients with recurrent sinusitis, bronchitis, and/or pneumonia, an additional antibody deficiency, namely IgG_2, could be identified. IgG_2 deficiency is more likely to be connected with the clinical manifestations observed than with IgA deficiency, and some of these patients respond well to therapy with IgG [32].

Intravenous (IV) Ig preparations for the treatment of B-cell deficiencies were considered desirable for the following reasons: the im injections are painful, and the amounts that can be given by this route are limited; maximum serum levels are not reached before 24 hours after injection and may take up to 3 days. In vivo recovery is hardly above 50%. Alterations in the IgG molecule may occur at the injection site [33]. Long-term exposure to mercury compounds is not devoid of toxicity [34].

SIGH had to be further treated to arrive at a product that can be given in a convenient time period in large enough quantities. Different methods of degradation and purification have been used, and a fair number of preparations are now available for clinical use [33].

Besides the obvious advantages of the IV application, there are new questions arising: different products show wide variation in quality [33], and great differences in subclass distribution [35]; part of the antibody spectrum can be missing; and Fc effector functions can be lost, preserved in part, or preserved completely [36–38]. The available intravenous Ig preparations can be divided into 3 major groups:

1. Enzymatically modified preparations. These are preparations treated with pepsin and plasmin.
2. Chemically modified preparations. Chemical modification is achieved by B-propiolactone, reduction and alkylation, or sulfonation. One preparation with both chemical and enzymatic treatment is applied successively (pH4 and traces of pepsin).
3. Different products are available in which IgG can be considered as unmodified. They include an "untreated" Scottish im gamma globulin, and IgG purified by $Si\ O_2$ sepharose, DEAE sepharose,

TABLE 1. Available Intravenous Ig Preparations: Enzymatically Treated

Procedure	Producer	Country	Product
Pepsin	Behringwerke	Germany	Gamma-venin
	Nikon Seiyaku	Japan	Glovenin
	Kaketsukeu	Japan	Immunoglobulin IV
	Fujoroki	Japan	Globulin V
Plasmin	Hyland	USA	Immunoglobulin IV
	Michigan	USA	
	Green Cross	Japan	Venoglobin
	Merieux	France	Rhodiglobin

TABLE 2. Available Intravenous Ig Preparations: Chemically Treated

Procedure	Producer	Country	Product
β-propiolactone	Biotest	Germany	Intraglobulin
pH4 + treated pepsin	SRC, Sandoz	Switzerland	Sandoglobin
Reduced, alkylated	Cutter	USA	Polyglobin
Sulfonated	Teijin	Japan	Venilon
	Behringwerke	Germany	Venimmun

TABLE 3. Available Intravenous Ig Preparations: Unmodified

Procedure	Producer	Country	Product
$Si\ O_2$ QAE sepharose	Condie	USA	
DEAE sepharose stabilized with albumin	Kabi	Switzerland	Gammonativ
DEAE sepharose	Winnipeg		
PEG/HES	Armour	USA	Immunoglobin 7s
PEG	Green Cross	Japan	Venoglobin
	Immuno	Austria	Endobulin
Cohn II + III + PEG	Continental	Canada	
Ethanol	Scottish National Blood Transfusion Service	Great Britain	

polyethyleneglycol/hydroxy ethyl starch (PEG/HES) purification, and other PEG purification methods (Tables 1, 2, 3).

A few details about the structure and functions [39, 40] of IgG are essential in the assessment of composition, properties and functional capacity of different IV globulin products [41]. IgG is a three-dimensional structure composed of 3 covalently linked regions [42]. Two of these, designated Fab, are identical and bind antigen. The third, the Fc region, has been identified as the site of antibody effector function. IgG is made of heavy (gamma) and light chains (kappa or lambda) held together by disulfide and weak covalent bonds. Both the heavy and the light chains have regions with constant amino acid sequences (C_L, C_H1, C_H2, C_H3) and with variable amino acid sequences (V_1 and V_H). The Fab fragment is composed of V_1, V_H, and C_H1, the Fc fragment of $2(C_H2$ and $C_H3)$.

Fab and Fc fragments interact through the hinge region. The interchain disulfide bridges must be intact to have an unimpaired effect on the Fc effector functions. There are indications that both Fab regions must bind to the antigen to induce complement (C') activation by the classic pathway. The antigen combining site is the most resistant against chemical treatment and enzymatic splitting [43]. Virus neutralization or binding to bacterial antigen is similar in pepsin- or plasmin-treated IgG to preparations containing the intact molecule [44–46].

In contrast, the hinge region of a molecule is the most sensitive for chemical treatment. This makes it understandable that different effector functions are highly vulnerable in the course of enzymatic chemical treatment, while the reactivity with the antigen is preserved [44, 47].

There are 4 different subclasses of IgG: IgG 1 (approx. 70%), IgG 2 (approx. 15%), IgG 3 (approx. 10%), IgG 4 (approx. 5%). Individual subclasses differ antigenically by minor changes on the heavy chains but show major differences in biologic activity, eg IgG 1 and IgG 3 activate the classic pathway of C' effectively, IgG 2 to some extent, IgG 4 not at all. Ig2 contains most of the antibodies against polysaccharides, IgG3 some of the antiviral antibodies, etc.

Functions connected with the Fc region of the molecule [48] include:
C1q binding (C_H2) near the hinge region [49]
C' activation (requires intact hinge region)
Half-life (catabolism C_H2) [49]
Passage through membranes - placenta intact Fc [50, 51]
Interaction with receptor cells:

Phagocytic cells [52–54]	Immune regulatory and effector cells
Granulocytes (C_H2, C_H3)	T cells (C_H3) [56–58]
Monocytes (C_H2, C_H3)	B cells (C_H3) [59, 60]
(Mø possibly possess receptors)	NK (C_H3) [61]
(1 for phagocytosis, 1 for cytotoxicity)	K cells [62, 63]
Cytophilic qualities [55]	Mast cells [64]

Laboratory techniques to assess the structural integrity of Fc (in the C_H2 C_H3 domain) involve adsorption on protein A of *Staphylococcus aureus* and the measurement of increased anticomplementary activity after heat treatment [65–67]. For the estimation of efficacy of an intravenous Ig preparation the following items are of importance: 1) Antibody activity with respect to combining with the antigen; 2) subclass distribution (are all subclasses present?); 3) biologic half-life of the preparation (variations in different diseases); 4) different Fc dependent effector functions [66–68]; and 5) clinical experience.

It has been known from the work of Weil et al in 1938 [69] and Kass et al in 1940 [70] that from the experience gained with equine antitoxins, antibodies can be treated with proteolytic enzymes and will not lose their activity to combine with and neutralize the respective antigen (toxins). This knowledge has been utilized in the development of the first human IV gamma globulin product, a pepsin-treated preparation of Behringwerke, which has been in clinical use for several decades. Mainly composed of Fab₂ fragments, it cannot activate C' via C1 and has no opsonizing capacity for *Staphylococcus aureus* [68], *Serratia marcescens* [47], and *E. coli* [71]. With a half-life of approximately 24 hours, it has never been considered suitable for replacement therapy [26] in patients with antibody deficiency, but because of its complete lack of anticomplementary activity it was assumed to be absolutely safe. This assumption has to be modified, since a recent controlled study demonstrated lack of efficacy in patients with severe infections, and adverse reactions in 9 of the 146 patients treated [72].

Enzyme-Treated Products

Plasmin-treated products show great variations in fragmentation [36], subclass composition [35], amount of aggregates, etc (Table 4). This can be explained by varying intensity of the enzymatic treatment applied.

The Fc fragment can be damaged to different degrees by changing conditions slightly. The IgG subclasses show dissimilar susceptibility to proteolytic cleavage; IgG 1 and IgG 3 are more sensitive; IgG 2 is especially resistant. Biologic half-life of the plasmin-treated preparations will vary depending on the percentage of fragments, and the same is true for different effector functions (Table 4).

Apparently good clinical results have been obtained with the Michigan preparation [73], the product showing the lowest fragmentation,

TABLE 4. Aggregation and Fragmentation of Enzyme-Treated Intravenous Ig

Producer	Method	Fragments (in %)	Monomers (in %)	Aggregates (in %)
Behringwerke	pepsin	80–91	11–17	2–9
Hyland	plasmin	40–65	39–55	1–5
Merieux	plasmin	65	32	3D
Green Cross	plasmin	50–60	40–50	<5
Michigan	plasmin	7–12	85–90	3

but the rate of adverse reactions was comparable to the rate seen with unmodified gamma globulin products. Most of the enzyme-treated products are highly fragmented, have short half-lives, Fc functions are lost to a great extent, and adverse reactions are still occurring and are comparable in rate and severity to the side effects of chemically treated or unmodified preparations.

Chemically Modified Products

Different kinds of chemical treatment will produce different structural and functional changes on the IgG molecule. Procedures acting on disulfide bonds will have a great influence on the functional capacity of the hinge region. Low pH treatment renders the region between C_H2 and C_H3 susceptible to cleavage by proteolytic enzymes [43].

The biologic half-lives of individual preparations range between 10 and 22 days. The adsorption on Staph protein A varies, and this could reflect differences in the interaction with receptors on phagocytic cells.

The β-propiolactone-treated, the sulfonated, and the product obtained by alkylation and reduction have lost their capacity to increase anticomplementary activity after heat treatment [66]. It is important to realize that in the chemically modified and in the unmodified group of IV gamma globulins, certain preparations have been further developed, and in reality each of these represents at least two generations of products. This might help to explain the differences found in the composition, properties, and clinical results in apparently one and the same product at different times [25, 36].

In general, the first generation of these products gave satisfactory results for potency, but had a varying and often unacceptable rate of adverse reactions. Products of the second generation have significantly less adverse reactions, but the question of potency has to be reestablished [74].

One preparation among the chemically treated modified products — treated with β-propiolactone [75] — has a shortened half-life [76], adsorbs only about 50% on Staph aur protein A. It has been considered efficacious in several clinical reports, mainly as adjunct therapy in bacterial infections [77].

The sulfonated Teijin preparation has been widely used in Japan with a great variety of indications [78]. One of the interesting aspects of this product is that it has a high anticomplementary activity, but the rate of adverse reactions reported in wide clinical application in several hundreds of patients is not higher than the rate seen with other products with negligible anticomplementary activity [79].

Among the chemically modified Ig preparations, the two products accumulating most of the clinical experience are the Swiss Red Cross (pH4 pepsin) [80–82] and the Cutter (reduced alkylated)Ig [83, 84]. Both can be looked upon as second-generation products.

Sandoglobulin has been efficacious in the substitution therapy of B-cell deficiencies and in the treatment of idiopathic thrombocytolenic purpura (ITP). The preparation still causes adverse reactions considered as severe. Three of 27 patients in the Sloan-Kettering study had to be withdrawn due to severe reactions to infusions [85]. The second generation of the alkylated reduced Ig preparation with 10% maltose added produces negligible adverse reactions (3 in 26) [74]. The effectiveness in the substitution therapy of antibody-deficient patients was at equal dose levels unexpectedly slightly below the im regime [84].

The various unmodified Ig products contain all of the Ig subclasses; their biologic half-life is unchanged and each of them will activate C' when heated. Adverse reactions have been a problem with some of these products. The injection of steroids had been advocated to diminish adverse reactions of a Scandinavian preparation [86].

The product I am using is a PEG preparation manufactured in Austria [87, 88]. It is a second- (or multi-) generation IV gamma globulin causing only negligible adverse reactions. The potency is superior to im gamma globulin at similar dose levels, and we were able to treat 4 patients who could not be treated with im preparations because of adverse reactions [89]. One of these patients was an agammaglobulinemic with recurrent severe infections and a disabling arthritis. The patient is doing very well, and arthritic symptoms disappeared completely in the course of the intravenous Ig therapy.

Safety of Intravenous Ig Preparations

Views on the pathophysiology of adverse reactions have been changing, and previous concepts must be amended in view of recent experimental work and clinical experience.

Aggregates are likely to cause adverse reactions, but complement activation can no longer be regarded as the only pathophysiologic pathway [90] (Table 5). IgG contaminants trigger the release of pharmacologically active molecules from monocytes, macrophages, and leukocytes. These substances, like prostaglandin E [91, 92] or platelet activating factor [93, 94], are known to produce fever,

TABLE 5. Factors Considered Responsible for Adverse Reactions in Ig Preparations

Products	ACA* % C1 q Binding	PKKA** % BOB Reference***	No. of Patients Treated	No. of Patients Showing Adverse Reactions	Therapy Discontinued
Sulfonated Teijin	82	0	541	14	
PEG-treated Immuno	0	112-720	143	5 minimal	0
Alkylation reduction Cutter	2	12	29	3 minimal	0
pH4 + pepsin SRC	0	0	27	3 severe	3
Pepsin-treated Behringwerke	0	11	146	9 (2 severe)	5

*anticomplementary activity.
**prekallikrein activator.
***Bureau of Biologies, reference preparation for PKKA.

changes in blood pressure, bronchospasm, leukopenia, etc, symptoms well known in the course of adverse reactions to intravenous Ig (Table 6). These substances might also be released by IV gammaglobulin reacting with circulating antigens present in certain agammaglobulinemic patients [85, 95]. The experience that pharmacologic agents like aspirin, given prior to IV gamma globulin infusions, could ameliorate side effects is in accordance with the assumption that these reactions might be caused by prostaglandin release. A further common experience, that patients suffering from an acute infection will show adverse reactions to an infusion of intravenous Ig, while tolerating the same lot and the same amount at other occasions, can also be explained on these grounds. Hyperreactivity of macrophages is known to appear during infectious episodes and the release of mediators might be facilitated. Activation of the kinin system can be followed by localized or generalized changes in vascular tonus and permeability [96]. An activator of this system, prekallikrein activator (PKKA), was detected in different amounts in blood products [96] causing adverse reactions. A clear dose relationship could not be established.

It had been assumed that PKKA could be responsible for adverse re-

TABLE 6. Adverse Reactions to IV-Administered Ig

Fever	Chest tightness
Chills	Dyspnea
Facial flush	Wheezing
Tachycardia	
Palpitation	Urticaria
Lowering of blood pressure	Rash
Shock	Anxiety
Lumbar pain	Nervousness
Abdominal pain	Headache
Nausea	
Vomiting	

actions caused by intravenous Ig as well [97]. We have clear evidence that high PKKA content of a product is not necessarily associated with the occurrence of adverse reactions.

Not a single adverse reaction has been observed with 3 individual lots having PKKA activities of 720%, 560%, and 120%, respectively, of the Bureau of Biologies (BOB) reference preparation (Table 5). A total of 308.7 gm have been used. Treated patients included agammaglobulinemics who were known to be "reactants," and patients with ITP who received 400 mg/kg on 5 consecutive days. In vitro experiments demonstrated that the kallikrein-generating potential of these preparations is neutralized by minimal amounts of plasma in a dose-dependent way (Philapitsch, personal communication, manuscript in preparation).

Experimental models would be desirable, but are not widely used to detect contaminants in IV gamma globulin preparations. Assuming that several substances may be involved or that the same substances would produce different reactions at different dose levels, it might be useful to have individual experimental systems for the individual reactions known to occur, like lowering of blood pressure, leukopenia (leukocyte activation, release of leukotrienes [slow reacting substances] and prostaglandins), platelet activation, bronchoconstriction, activation of the coagulation system. A dog model provided a reliable tool with clear and reproducible dose-related response of changes in blood pressure and leukopenia (personal communication, Dr. Raberger, Institute of Pharmacology, University of Vienna).

Allosensitization in connection with intravenous Ig application does occur [98]. Antibodies against IgA can be the cause of anaphylactic reactions [99–101]. IgE antibodies against allogeneic IgG have been detected in certain patients [102], as well as antibodies of other Ig classes [98] which are of less importance in the context of adverse reactions [103, 104].

Because intravenous Ig products can be infused in larger quantities, freedom of isoagglutinins and non-agglutinating antibodies against red cell antigen is important, otherwise hemolytic reactions might occur in the recipients.

As the transmission of ubiquitous viruses, like cytomegalo [105] and Epstein-Barr virus (EBV) [106], is of growing concern, it would be useful to include antibody determinations against these viruses.

The experience with viral hepatitis has shown that HB_s antibody, present in the final product, is a safeguard to avoid transmission of this disease.

The efficacy of any preparation will relate to the content of its protective antibodies. Large enough pools of starting material will guarantee a broad spectrum of antibodies, if all the subclasses are present in a given preparation.

Assessment of the integrity (or impairment) of the Fc fragment, like substantial increase of anticomplementary activity after heating or binding to protein A of Staph, as well as the evaluation of Fc-mediated properties like biologic half-life, or opsonizing capacity, will certainly provide more indication for potency than the antigen reactive capacity alone.

CONCLUSION

There are acceptable intravenous Ig preparations available in the treatment of patients with antibody deficiency syndromes. Recent clinical and experimental experience can help to further improve both the safety and efficacy. Since large amounts of certain products can be infused without adverse reactions, optimal dose on an individual basis can now be applied in patients previously difficult to treat. It appears likely that Ig treatment will continue to be our basic tool in the treatment of patients with antibody deficiency syndromes.

REFERENCES

1. WHO Report: Immunodeficiency. Clin Immunol Immunopathol 13:297–359, 1979.
2. Cooper MD, Lawton AR, Miescher PA, Müller-Eberhard HJ: "Immune Deficiency." Berlin, Heidelberg, New York: Springer-Verlag, 1979.
3. Wedgwood RJ: "X-linked agammaglobulinemia," Seligson D (ed): CRC Handbook Series in Clinical Laboratory Science. West Palm Beach, Fl: CRC Press, 1978, Section F, Part 1, pp 41–50.
4. Rosen FS: The immunodeficiency syndromes. Section II. Diseases with abnormal immune responses. In Samter M (ed): "Immunological Diseases," 3rd Ed. Boston: Little, Brown & Co, Inc, vol 1, 1978, pp 472–498.
5. Ziegler JB, Penny R: Fatal ECHO 30 virus infection and amyloidosis in X-linked hypogammaglobulinemia. Clin Immunol Immunopathol 3:347–352, 1975.
6. Bardelas JA, Winkelstein JA, Secto DSY, Tsai T, Rogol AD: Fatal ECHO 24 infection in a patient with hypogammaglobulinemia: Relationship to dermatomyositis-like syndrome. J Pediatr 90:396–399, 1977.
7. Lyon G, Griscelli C, Fernandes-Alvarez E, Prats-Vinas J, Lebon P: Chronic progressive encephalitis in children with X-linked hypogammaglobulinemia. Neuropaediatrie 11:57–71, 1980.
8. Good RA, Rötstein J, Mazzitello WF: The simultaneous occurrence of rheumatoid arthritis and agammaglobulinemia. J Lab Clin Med 49:343–357, 1957.
9. Janeway CA, Gitlin D, Craig JM, Grice DS: "Collagen disease" in patients with congenital agammaglobulinemia. Trans Assoc Am Physicians 69:93–97, 1956.
10. Janeway CA, Rosen FS: The gamma globulins: IV. Therapeutic uses of gamma globulin. N Engl J Med 275:826–831, 1966.
11. Barandun S, Skvaril F, Morell A: Prophylaxe und Therapie mit γ-Globulin. Allgemeine Charakterisierung und klinische Anwendung von γ-Globulin-Präparaten. Teil II: Klinische Anwendung von γ-Globulin Präparaten. Schweiz Med Wochenschr 106:580–586, 1976.
12. MRC. Medical Research Council Report SRs 310. London:HMSO, 1970.
13. Mease PJ, Ochs HD, Wedgwood RJ: Successful treatment of echovirus meningoencephalitis and myositis-fasciitis with intravenous immune globulin therapy in a patient with X-linked agammaglobulinemia. N Engl J Med 304:1278–1280, 1981.
14. Barandun S, Riva G, Spengler GA: Immunologic deficiency diagnosis, forms and current treatment. In Bergsma D (ed): "Immunologic Deficiency Diseases in Man." The National Foundation-March of Dimes, BD:OAS IV(1): 40–52, 1968.
15. Gitlin D, Janeway CA: Agammaglobulinemia. Congenital acquired and transient forms. Prog Hematol 1:318–329, 1956.
16. Domz CA, Dickson DR: The agammaglobulinemias. Relations and implications. Am J Med 23:917–927, 1957.
17. Thompson RA, Rees-Jones A: The antibody deficiency syndrome: A report on current management. J Infect 1:49–60, 1979.
18. Immunoglobulin Federal Register, vol, 45, No 74:25739–25748, April 15, 1980.
19. Finlayson JS: Immune globulins. Semin Thromb Hemostas. 6(1):44–74, 1979.
20. Tabor E, Gerety RJ: Transmission of hepatitis B by immune serum globulin. Lancet 2, 1293, 1979.
21. John TJ, Ninan GT, Rajagopalan HS, John F, Flewett TH, Francis DP, Zuckerman AJ: Epidemic hepatitis B caused by commercial human immunoglobulin. Lancet 1, 1074, 1979.
22. da Silva LC, Sette H, Antonacio F, Lopes JD: Commercial gammaglobulin (CGG) as a possible vehicle of transmission of HBsAG in familial clustering. Rev Inst Med Trop Sao Paolo 19:352–354, 1977.
23. Petrilli FL, Crovari P, De Flora S: Hepatitis B in subjects treated with a drug containing immunoglobulins. J Infect Dis 135:252–258, 1977.
24. Keusch GT, Olsson RA, Troncale FJ: Asymptomatic hepatitis in adults given γ-globulin for prophylaxis. Arch Intern Med 124:326–329, 1969.
25. Barandun S, Kistler P, Jeunet F, Isliker H: Intravenous administration of human gammaglobulin. Vox Sang 7:157–174, 1962.
26. Fudenberg H, Good RA, Goodman HC, Hitzig W, Kunkel HG, Roitt IM, Rosen FS, Rowe DS, Seligmann M, Soothill JR: Primary immunodeficiencies. Report of a World Health Organization Committee. Pediatrics 47:927–946, 1971.
27. Merler E, Rosen FS, Salmon S, Crain JD, Janeway CA: Studies with intravenous gamma globulin. Vox Sang 13: 102–103, 1967.
28. Janeway CA: The development of clinical uses of immunoglobulins: A review. In Merler E (ed): "Immunoglobulins: Biologic Aspects and Clinical Uses." Natl Acad Sci USA 1970, pp 3–14.
29. Hanson LÅ, Björkander J, Ljunggren Ch, Oxelius V-A, Wadsworth Ch: Problems with use of immunoglobulins

in treatment of immunodeficient patients. In Alving BM, Finlayson JS (eds): "Immunoglobulins: Characteristics and Uses of Intravenous Preparations." US Dept of Health and Human Services, Public Health Services, 1979, pp 151–159.
30. Buckley RH: Replacement therapy in immunodeficiency. In Thompson RA (ed): "Recent Advances in Clinical Immunology." Edinburgh and London: Churchill Livingstone, 1977, pp 219–244.
31. Tympner KD: Zur Therapie mit Immunglobulinen (IgG, IgA und IgM) im Kindesalter. Monatsschr Kinderheilkd 118:330–335, 1970.
32. Appropriate uses of human immunoglobulin in clinical practice: Memorandum from an IUIS/WHO meeting. WHO Bulletin, 60:43–47, 1982.
33. Ochs HD: Intravenous immunoglobulin therapy of patients with primary immunodeficiency syndromes: Efficacy and safety of a new modified immune globulin preparation. Supra #29, pp 9–14.
34. Haeney MR, Carter GF, Yeoman WB, Thompson RA: Long-term parenteral exposure to mercury in patients with hypogammaglobulinaemia. Br Med J 2:12–14, 1979.
35. Skvaril F, Probst M, Steinbuch A, Steinbuch M: Distribution of IgG subclasses in commercial and some experimental γ-globulin preparations. Vox Sang 32:335–338, 1977.
36. Römer J, Morgenthaler JJ, Scherz R, Skvaril F: Characterization of various immunoglobulin preparations for intravenous application. I. Protein composition and antibody content. Vox Sang 42:62–73, 1982.
37. Barandun S, Skvaril F, Morell A: Prophylaxe und Therapie mit γ-Globulin. Allgemeine Charakterisierung und klinische Anwendung von γ-Globulin-Präparaten. I. Teil: Allgemeine Charakterisierung der γ-Globulin-Präparate. Schweiz Med Wochenschr 106:533–542, 1976.
38. Morell A, Schürch B, Ryser D, Hofer F, Skvaril F, Barandun S: In vivo behaviour of gamma globulin preparations. Vox Sang 38:272–283, 1980.
39. Morell A, Skvaril F: Struktur und biologische Eigenschaften von Immunglobulinen und γ-Globulin-Präparaten. II. Eigenschaften von γ-Globulin-Präparaten. Schweiz Med Wochenschr 110:1–6, 1980.
40. Pinteric L, Painter RH, Connell GE: Ultrastructure of the Fc fragment of human immunoglobulin G. Immunochemistry 8:1041–1045, 1971.
41. Stiehm ER: Standard and special human immune serum globulins as therapeutic agents. Pediatrics 63:301–319, 1979.
42. Amzel LM, Poljak RJ: Three dimensional structure of immunoglobulins. Annu Rev Biochem 48:961–997, 1979.
43. Stanworth DR, Turner MW: Immunochemical analysis of immunoglobulins and their sub-units. In Weir DM (ed): "Handbook of Experimental Immunology". Oxford, London, Edinburgh, Melbourne: Blackwell Scientific Publications, 1979, Chapter 6.
44. Scheiermann N, Kuwert EK: Untersuchung menschlicher Gammaglobulinpräparate. I. Mitteilung: Virales Antikörper profil. Med Klin 74:820–824, 1979.
45. Wirsing CH, Finger H, Jansen P, Trobisch H: Gehalt an spezifischen Antikörpern in handelsüblichen intravenös applizierbaren Gammaglobulinpräparaten. Blut 36:211–216, 1978.
46. Kunz CH, Hofmann H, Stary A: Der Gehalt an Antikörpern gegen Viren in einigen Gammaglobulinpräparaten. Wien Klin Wochenschr 89:203–206, 1977.
47. Traub WH: Failure of a commercial, intravenously applicable IgG F(ab)$_2$ preparation (Gamma-Venin) to enhance human serum bactericidal activity against Serratia marcescens. Zbl Bakt, I, Abt Orig 249:504–511, 1981.
48. Painter RH: The Fc fragment and the effector function of human IgG. In Nydegger UE (ed): "Immunotherapy. A Guide to Immunoglobulin Prophylaxis and Therapy." London, New York, Toronto, Sydney, San Francisco: Academic Press, 1981, pp 27–35.
49. Nevin C, Gorick HG, Gorick B: C1q - an effector molecule for IgG. Ibid, pp 37–45.
50. Jenkinson EJ, Billington WD, Elson J: Detection of receptors for immunoglobulin on human placenta by EA rosette formation. Clin Exp Immunol 23:456–461, 1976.
51. Matre R, Tonder O, Endreson C: Fc receptors in human placenta. Scand J Immunol 4:741–745, 1975.
52. Unkeless JC, Eisen HN: Binding of monomeric immunoglobulins to Fc receptors of mouse macrophages. J Exp Med 142:1520–1533, 1975.
53. Heusser CH, Anderson CL, Grey HM: Receptors for IgG: Subclass specificity of receptors on different mouse cell types and the definition of two distinct receptors on a macrophage cell line. J Exp Med 145:1316–1327, 1977.
54. Foster DE, Dorrington KJ, Painter RH: An analysis of the structural requirements in human IgG1 for binding to the Fc receptor of human monocytes. J Immunol 124:2186–2190, 1980.
55. Inchley Ch, Grey HM, Uhr JW: The cytophilic activity of human immunoglobulins. J Immunol 105:362–368, 1970.
56. Morgan EL, Thoman ML, Weigle WO: Enhancement of T lymphocyte functions by Fc fragments of immunoglobulins. I. Augmentation of allogeneic mixed lymphocyte culture reactions requires I-A- or I-B-subregion differences between effector and stimulator cell populations. J Exp Med 153:1161–1172, 1981.
57. Fridman WH, Goldstein P: Immunoglobulin-binding factor present on and produced by thymus-processed lymphocytes (T cells). Cell Immunol 11:442–455, 1974.
58. Andersson B, Skoglund A CH, Rönnholm M, Lindstein T, Lamon EW, Whited Colisson E, Walia AS: Functional aspects of IgM and IgG Fc receptors on murine T lymphocytes. Immunol Rev 56:1–50, 1981.
59. Basten A, Miller JFAP, Sprent J, Pye J: A receptor for antibodies on B lymphocytes. I. Method of detection and functional significance. J Exp Med 135:610–626, 1972.
60. Dickler HB, Kunkel HG: Interaction of aggregated γ-globulin with B lymphocytes. J Exp Med 136:191–196, 1972.
61. Herbermann RB, Djeu JY, Kay DH, Ortaldo JR, Riccardi C, Bonnard GD, Holden HT, Fragnani R, Santoni A, Puccetti P: Natural killer cells: Characteristics and regulation of activity. Immunol Rev 44:43–70, 1979.
62. Perlmann P, Perlmann H, Wigzell H: Lymphocyte mediated cytotoxicity in vitro. Induction and inhibition by humoral antibody and nature of effector cells. Transplant Rev 13:91–114, 1972.
63. MacLennan ICM: Antibody in the induction and inhibition of lymphocyte cytotoxicity. Transplant Rev 13:67–90, 1972.
64. Ovary Z: Passive cutaneous anaphylactic reactions as tools in the study of the structure of the IgG molecule. Immunochemistry 15:751–754, 1978.
65. Deisenhofer J, Jones A, Huber R, Sjodahl J, Sjoquist J: Crystallization, crystal structure analysis and atomic model of the complex formed by a human Fc fragment and fragment B of protein A from Staph. aureus. Hoppe Seyler's Z Physiol Chem 359:975–985, 1978.
66. Römer J, Späth PJ, Skvaril F, Nydegger UE: Characterization of various immunoglobulin preparations for intravenous application. II. Complement ac-

tivation and binding to Staphylococcus protein A. Vox Sang 42:74–80, 1982.
67. Ceska M: Binding of protein A to some human gamma-globulins used intravenously. Vox Sang 40:395–402, 1981.
68. van Furth R, Leijh PCJ: Functional interactions of various commercial gammaglobulin preparations with Staphylococcus aureus and granulocytes. Supra #48, pp 181–190.
69. Weil AJ, Partentjew IA, Bowman KL: Antigenic qualities of antitoxins. J Immunol 35:399–412, 1938.
70. Kass EH, Scherago M, Weaver RH: J Immunol 45:87, 1942. As cited in Fortsch der Serologie, Steinkopff D (ed). Darmstadt: H Schmidt Verlag, 1955.
71. Eibl M, Friers G: Hemmung der Opsonisierung von E. coli durch enzymatisch gespaltene Gammaglobuline. Wien Klin Wochenschr 90:717–721, 1978.
72. Lindquist L, Lundbergh P, Maasing R: Pepsin-treated human gamma globulin in bacterial infections. A randomized study in patients with septicaemia and pneumonia. Vox Sang 40:329–337, 1981.
73. Magylavy DB, Cassidy JT, Tubergen DG, Petty RE, Chisholm R, McCall K: Intravenous gamma globulin in the management of patients with hypogammaglobulinemia. J Allergy Clin Immunol 61:378–383, 1978.
74. Ochs HD, Buckley RH, Pirofsky B, Fischer SH, Rousell RH, Anderson CJ, Wedgwood RJ: Safety and patient acceptability of intravenous immune globulin in 10% maltose. Lancet 2:1158–1159, 1980.
75. Stephan W: Undergraded human immunoglobulin for intravenous use. Vox Sang 28:422–437, 1975.
76. Bläker F, Hellwege HH, Mai K: Plasma-Elimination intravenös verträglicher menschlicher Immunglobuline bei Patienten mit humoralen Immundefekten. Untersuchungen zur Schutzwirkung und Schutzdauer nach passiver Immunisierung. Dtsch Med Wochenschr 97:1151–1156, 1972.
77. Neu IS, Pelka RB: Immunglobuline bei bakteriellen und viralen Meningitiden. Ergebnisse einer kontrollierten randomisierten klinischen Studie intravenöser und intrathekaler Applikation. Fortschr Med 100:802–809, 1982.
78. Masaoka T: The clinical effect of GGS on severe infections in the field of internal medicine. In Mashimo K (ed): "Proceedings of Symposium on Immunoglobulin Therapy." Tokyo: Medical Information Services, 1980, pp 81–89.
79. Matsumoto S: Side reactions to immune serum globulin administered by intravenous infusion. Ibid, pp 101–109.
80. Barandun S, Morell A, Skvaril F: Clinical use of intravenous gamma-globulin. Bibl Haematol 46:170–174, 1980.
81. Sidiropoulus D, Böhme U, v Muralt G, Morell A, Barandun S: Immunglobulin-substitution bei der Behandlung der neonatalen Sepsis. Schweiz Med Wochenschr 111:1649–1655, 1981.
82. Hansi W, Kratzsch G, Heimpel H: Klinische Erfahrungen mit einem neuen intravenös applizierbaren Immunglobulin-Präparat. Dtsch Med Wochenschr 105:1675–1680, 1980.
83. Nolte MT, Pirofsky B, Gerritz GA, Golding B: Intravenous immunoglobulin therapy for antibody deficiency. Clin Exp Immunol 36:237–243, 1979.
84. Wedgwood RJ, Ochs HD: The safety, acceptability and effectiveness of immunoglobulin modified for intravenous use. Supra #48, pp 331–356.
85. Cunningham-Rundles C, Day NK, Wahn V, Smithwick EM, Siegal FP, Gupta S, Good RA: Reactions to intravenous gammaglobulin infusions and immune complex formation. Ibid, pp 447–450.
86. Gislason D, Hanson LÅ, Kjellman H, Ljunggren C, Malmberg R. Intravenous gamma-globulin infusions in patients with hypogammaglobulinemia. Vox Sang 34:143–148, 1978.
87. Pietrogrande MC, Dellepiane RM, Varin E, Corona F, Capello M, Bardare M: La gammaglobuline e.v. a Fc intatto nella terapie dei Deficit immunitari infantili. In Aiuti, Fiorelli FM (eds): "Le Immunoglobuline Primitive in Italia." Field Education Italia, Acta Medica Rome, 1982, pp 89–96.
88. Eibl M: Intravenous immunoglobulins: Clinical and experimental studies. Supra #29, pp 23–30.
89. Tinelli M, Minoli L, Perucca F: Schema terapeutico immunosostitutivo in un caso di agammaglobulinemia ad esordio tardivo. VI Congresso Nazionale della Società Italiana di Immunologia e Immunopathologia, Abstract, 1982.
90. Rosen F: In panel discussion on indications and limitations of immunoglobulin prophylaxis and therapy. Supra #48, pp 451–460.
91. Goodwin JS, Webb DR: Review: Regulation of the immune response by prostaglandins. Clin Immunol Immunopathol 15:106–122, 1980.
92. Passwell JH, Dayer JM, Merler E: Increased prostaglandin production by human monocytes after membrane receptor activation. J Immunol 123:115–120, 1979.
93. Philp RB: Methods of testing proposed antithrombotic drugs. V. Platelet activating factor (PAF). Florida: CRC Press, 1981, pp 114–128.
94. Camussi G, Aglietta M, Coda R, Bussolino F, Piacibello W, Tetta C: Release of platelet-activating factor (PAF) and histamine. II. The cellular origin of human PAF: Monocytes, polymorphonuclear neutrophils and basophils. Immunology 41:191–199, 1981.
95. Delire M, Masson PL: The detection of circulating immune complexes in children with recurrent infections and their treatment with human immunoglobulins. Clin Exp Immunol 29:385–392, 1977.
96. Alving BM, Hojima Y, Pisano JJ, Mason BL, Buckingham RE Jr, Mozen MM, Finlayson JS: Hypotension associated with prekallikrein activator (Hageman-factor fragments) in plasma protein fraction. N Engl J Med 299:66–70, 1978.
97. Alving BM, Tankersley DL, Mason BL, Condie RM, Finlayson JS: Biologic activities of enzymic contaminants in immunoglobulin preparations. Supra #48, pp 161–170.
98. Stiehm ER, Fudenberg HH: Antibodies to gammaglobulin in infants and children exposed to isologous gamma-globulin. Pediatrics 35:229–235, 1965.
99. Schmidt AP, Taswell HF, Gleich GJ: Anaphylactic transfusion reactions associated with anti-IgA antibody. N Engl J Med 280:188–193, 1969.
100. Bjerrum OJ, Jersild C: Class-specific anti-IgA associated with severe anaphylactic transfusion reactions in a patient with pernicious anaemia. Vox Sang 21:411–424, 1971.
101. Leikola J, Koistinen J, Lehtinen M, Virolainen M: IgA-induced anaphylactic transfusion reactions: A report of four cases. Blood 42:111–119, 1973.
102. Ropars C, Geay-Chicot D, Cartron JP, Doinel C, Salmon C: Human IgE response to the administration of blood components. II. Repeated gammaglobulin injections. Vox Sang 37:149–157, 1979.
103. Henney ChS, Ellis EF: Antibody production to aggregated human gammaglobulin in acquired hypogammaglobulinemia. N Engl J Med 278:1144–1146, 1968.
104. Ropars C, Caldera LH, Griscelli C, Homberg JC, Salmon C: Anti-immunoglobulin antibodies in immunodeficiencies: Their influence on intolerance reactions to gamma-globulin administration. Vox Sang 27:294–301, 1974.
105. Gottlieb MS, Schroff R, Schanker HM, Weisman JD, Fan PT, Wolf RA, Saxon A: Pneumocystis carinii pneumonia and mucosal candidiasis in previously healthy homosexual men: Evidence of a new acquired cellular immunodeficiency. N Engl J Med 305:1425–1431, 1981.
106. Schwartz RS: Epstein-Barr virus - oncogen or mitogen? N Engl J Med 302:1307–1308, 1980.

Use of Intravenous pH 4.0 Treated Gamma Globulin in Humoral Immunodeficiency Disease*

Charlotte Cunningham-Rundles, MD, PhD, Elizabeth M. Smithwick, MD, Frederick P. Siegal, MD, Noorbibi K. Day, PhD, Alise Lion, RN, Joseph O'Malley, MD, Silvio Barandun, MD, and Robert A. Good, MD, PhD

Memorial Sloan-Kettering Cancer Center, New York, NY 10021 (C.C.-R., E.M.S., A.L.), Mt. Sinai Hospital, New York, NY 10029 (F.P.S.), Oklahoma Medical Research Foundation, Oklahoma, OK 73104 (N.K.D., R.A.G.), The American Red Cross, Washington, DC (J.O'M.), University of Berne, Berne, Switzerland (S.B.)

INTRODUCTION

Human immunoglobulin preparations have been used for the treatment of primary humoral immunodeficiency disease since the first report of a patient with agammaglobulinemia who benefited by intramuscular (im) injections of an alcohol-fractionated (Cohn Fraction II) IgG-enriched preparation [1]. Other reports confirmed the benefits of im gamma globulin in hypogammaglobulinemia [2–4]. However, the volume of Ig which can be given im is limited by muscle mass, which is unfortunate since the patients receiving 50 mg/kg/wk of IgG may have fewer infections than those receiving 25 mg/kg/wk [5]. In addition, im preparations cannot be given intravenously because they produce severe anaphylactic reactions due to the presence of aggregates [6,7]. The introduction of intravenous (IV) gamma globulin preparations promises to alleviate these problems since large doses of immunoglobulin can be easily and safely administered [8,9]. This report describes the use of pH 4.0 treated IV gamma globulin as compared to conventional therapy with im gamma globulin in a large clinic of patients with primary immunodeficiency disease.

*Supported in part by USPHS grants CA 19267, AI 19495.

MATERIALS AND METHODS

Patients

Forty-three patients with antibody deficiency have been treated in this ongoing study. Thirty-two of these patients have common varied immunodeficiency (CVID), 3 have X-linked agammaglobulinemia (SLA), 2 have IgM deficiency, 1 each have Nezelof syndrome, SCID, thymoma and agammaglobulinemia, lymphoma or leukemia and secondary hypogammaglobulinemia, and antibody deficiency with normal levels of Igs. Diagnoses were established according to criteria established by the World Health Organization [10]. Patients were considered for this study if the serum IgG level were <400/mg/dl and/or if significant responses to injected antigens (such as pneumovax or diptheria tetanus toxoid) could not be demonstrated. All patients had clinical histories of repeated bouts of bacterial infections.

At the start of the study the age range of the patients was 5–63; 24 were males, 19 were female. Twenty-nine of these patients had been previously treated for at least 2 years with im gamma globulin (Gamastan, Cutter Laboratories) 25–35 mg/kg/wk or plasma; in almost all instances they have been continually followed for 2–6 years by the same physician at either Memorial Hospital or Mt. Sinai Hospital.

Intravenous Gamma Globulin Preparation

The IV gamma globulin ("Sandoglobulin") is supplied by the Swiss Red Cross through collaboration with the American Red Cross; it is derived from a Cohn Fraction II preparation made pH 4.0 by the addition of HCl in the presence of traces of pepsin and then brought to neutrality and lyophilized [11]. Infusions are given at 300 mg/kg every 3 weeks, using 3% solutions in the initial infusion and 6% solutions thereafter.

Design of Study

The intention of the study is to test the safety and efficacy of this IV gamma globulin in treating antibody deficiency states when the mean IgG concentration was elevated to a level considered within the normal range for age. Since the majority of patients had already had 2–6 years of treatment with im gamma globulin, we elected to initiate one year of treatment with IV gamma globulin in order to compare the clinical condition of these patients during the treatment year with the calendar year immediately preceding the treatment period. Each patient (or parent or guardian) is asked to maintain a diary and to record the days in which school or work is missed or a temperature over 100.8°F is noted: specific complaints, amounts and name

TABLE 1.

21	patients finished 12 months
10	patients finished in 1982
2	patients will finish in 1983
3	patients had infusion reactions leading to cessation of treatment (#25, 28, 29)
2	dropped out
2	had treatment cancelled by their M.D.
1	died of lymphoma
1	is getting Cutter IV gamma globulin at home
1	had marrow transplant
43	Total

TABLE 2. Number of Days for Which Infections Were Recorded During Control and Treatment Years*

Acute Infection	Control	Year	Treatment	Year
Upper respiratory tract**	1020	(18)†	622	(18)
Bronchitis**	709	(16)	424	(14)
Gastrointestinal tract	225	(12)	209	(10)
Pharyngitis**	176	(16)	156	(15)
Otitis media	140	(8)	108	(6)
Conjunctivitis	112	(3)	102	(3)
Pneumonia	61	(5)	41	(3)
Dental abscess	30	(1)	0	
Urinary tract	0		13	(2)
	2473		1675	

*For the 18 patients for whom a control year of im gamma globulin could be compared to the treatment year of IV gamma globulin.
†The number of patients who had these disorders.
**Diagnostic categories were determined by the major complaint: URI—predominant symptoms of rhinitis, sinusitis; bronchitis—coughing with production of purulent sputum; pharyngitis—sore throat or tonsillitis.

of all antibiotics and all other medicines taken are recorded. These diaries are collected periodically and reviewed by the clinical research nurse. If a new infection appeared, appropriate cultures or x rays were obtained.

RESULTS

Table 1 outlines the disposition of patients in this clinical trial as of 8/1/82.

Comparisons of Treatment and Control Years

Eighteen of the 21 patients who have completed one year's treatment with IV gamma globulin had had at least one year's previous treatment with im gamma globulin and these 18 serve as the group in which the relative efficacy of IV vs im gamma globulin can be compared. For the im gamma globulin year (control year), these 18 patients had a total of 1,131 days sick, 940 days with fever, 2,980 days with antibiotic treatment, and 61 days in the hospital. For the IV gamma globulin treatment year, there was a total of 327 days sick, 145 days with fever, 1,064 days on antibiotics, and 41 days in the hospital. All patients except 2 reported improvements in the treatment year as opposed to the control year, although a few individuals reported much greater differences in these parameters than did the others.

Table 2 lists the actual number of acute and chronic illnesses recorded for the control year as opposed to the treatment year for the same 18 patients. Also given for both years are the number of patients (in parenthesis in each column) who were ill with these disorders. Most improvements from the control to the treatment year were found in upper respiratory tract infections and bronchitis; many less were noted for pharyngitis, otitis, and conjunctivitis. Since only 5 patients had pneumonia, 2 had urinary tract infections and 1 had a dental abscess, it is difficult to conclude benefit for these particular illnesses.

Adverse Reactions

The total number of infusions (to 8/1/82) given to the entire population is 638. Sixteen reactions in a total of 7 patients have occurred, resulting in a reaction incidence of 2.5%. Reactions to infusions could be divided clearly into 3 types.

Type 1–mild, occurring at the time of infusion and related to speed of infusion (2 patients);

Type 2–moderate and occurring during or within 1 to 2 hours after the infusion had been completed (2 patients);

Type 3–severe and occurring during the time of the infusion, possibly continuing after the infusion was finished (3 patients).

In the case of the severe reactions, one patient had lymphoma, an IgM paraprotein and a markedly depressed (<2 SDs) CH50, C1q, and C3, and high levels of circulating immune complexes before infusion. After infusion, complement and components C1q and C3 decreased further and higher levels of immune complexes appeared. Another patient, who also had lymphoma and an IgM paraprotein, had chest pain, hypotension, and pallor during the infusion. His already low complement levels (CH50, C1q, and C3 $<$ 2SDs of normal) were further depleted after each infusion. A third patient, who was found to have a preexisting anti-IgA antibody, had abdominal pain, nausea, and myalgias lasting from 1–16 hours without change in vital signs. Evaluation of her complement components performed pre- and postinfusion have been reported [12].

DISCUSSION

This study reports clinical and laboratory observations made for a large group of patients with humoral IDs who have been infused with pH 4.0 treated IV gamma globulin. A total of 43 patients have been treated between 3/20/80 and 8/1/82. The intention of this study is to test the safety and possible efficacy of this preparation when given at a dose of 300 mg/kg/3 wks.

Judging by parameters of number of illnesses, days sick, days with fever, hospitalizations, and antibiotic usage, 16 of 18 patients who had had at least one year's previous treatment with im gamma globulin and then completed one year of IV gamma globulin therapy, were distinctly improved by the latter therapy. Two patients with CVID were not improved; these patients are considered treatment failures. If, in addition, the 3 patients who stopped treatment due to reactions to the infusions, and the 2 patients who dropped out of the study, are considered treatment failures, there were 7 individuals in a total of 23 who did not respond favorably to IV gamma globulin. This indicates a 30% failure rate and a 70% benefit rate.

Striking differences in the number of days missed from work or school, days with fever, and days antibiotics were used were reported for the control and treatment years. Since 8 of the 18 individuals compared in this way do not go to work or school, the number of days estimated for being sick is probably the least reliable category; patients were asked to decide how many days they *would* have stayed home. In addition, since patients usually took their own temperatures, the number of days with fever could contain errors. The number of days in which antibiotics were taken is a more reliable index of improvement. Since only 5 patients were hospitalized, and 3 were hospitalized twice, it is difficult to use this category as an index of clinical improvement. However, using the verbal reports of the entire patient group and their written diaries, it is quite clear that the majority of these patients perceive a distinct benefit from this IV gamma globulin.

As noted by others, chronic illness may not be particularly altered by IV gamma globulin treatment [9,13]. We confirm this view, as chronic diarrhea associated with nodular lymphoid hyperplasia or malabsorption, and chronic lung disease were not improved in our study. Incidence of conjunctivitis, otitis media, and urinary tract infection were also not influenced by IV gamma globulin treatment.

CONCLUSIONS

In conclusion, we find that the majority of patients with humoral ID may be expected to improve when treated with this preparation of IV gamma globulin at this dosage schedule. Reactions were encountered in 2.5% of infusions; if patients with IgM paraproteins or anti-IgA antibodies are excluded, a reaction rate of 1% might be expected. Patient tolerance is excellent.

REFERENCES

1. Bruton OC: Agammaglobulinemia. Pediatrics 9:722–728, 1952.
2. Stiehm ER (ed): "Immunologic Disorders and Children." Philadelphia: WB Saunders, 1973, pp 145–147.
3. Ammann AJ, Hong R: "Cellular Immunodeficiency Disorders." Philadelphia: WB Saunders, 1973, pp 236–272.
4. Janeway CA: "The Development of Clinical Uses of Immunoglobulins," Merler E (ed). Natl Acad Sci Libr Cong, 1970, pp 3–14.
5. Hill LE, Mollison PL: Conclusions. In "Hypogammaglobulinemia." United Kingdom, MRC Spec Rep Ser No. 310, 1971.
6. Barandun S, Kistler P, Jeunet F et al: Intravenous administration of human gammaglobulin. Vox Sang 7:157–162, 1962.
7. Soothill JF: Reactions to immunoglobulin. Supra #5.
8. Barandun S, Morell A, Skvaril F: Clinical experiences with immunoglobulin for intravenous use. In Alving BM, Finlayson JS (eds): "Immunoglobulins: Characteristics and Uses of Intravenous Preparations." Bethesda: US Dept of Health and Human Services, 1980.
9. Nolte MT, Pirofsky B, Gerritz GA, Golding B: Intravenous immunoglobulin therapy of antibody deficiency. Clin Exp Immunol 36:237–243, 1979.
10. Report of a WHO scientific group. Immunodeficiency. WHO Tech Rep Ser 630:3–80, 1978.
11. Barandun S: Use of intravenous gammaglobulin in the treatment of severe bacterial infection. Vox Sang 37:117–119, 1979.
12. Wahn Y, Poleshuck L, Gupta S, Cunningham-Rundles C, Good RA, Day NK: Evidence of IgA-IgG complexes associated with C3 split products in common variable immunodeficiency. Clin Res 29:1981.
13. Ammann AJ, Ashman RF, Buckley RH, Hardie WR, Krantman HJ, Nelson J, Ochs H, Stiehm ER, Tiller T, Wara DW, Wedgwood R: Use of intravenous gammaglobulin in antibody immunodeficiency: Results of a multicenter controlled trial. Clin Immunol Immunopathol 22:60–67, 1982.

Intramuscular and Intravenous Administration of Immunoglobulin to Patients With Hypogammaglobulinemia

L.Å. Hanson, MD, J. Björkander, MD, and C. Wadsworth, PhD

Department of Clinical Immunology, Institute of Medical Microbiology (L.A.H., C.W.), and Division of Allergy, Department of Medicine I (J.B.), University of Göteborg, Göteborg, Sweden

Hypogammaglobulinemia is usually regarded as a rare disease. In two recent surveys in Sweden we have found 3/100,000 among children and 2/100,000 among adults [1] (unpublished research). In the county around our hospital a frequency twice the expected was found [1]. This could be due to our long-term interest in these patients and suggests that the real frequency of hypogammaglobulinemia may be much higher than presently known.

We were appalled to discover that patients with common variable hypogammaglobulinemia often had not been correctly diagnosed until long after the onset of clinical symptoms: the mean delay was 12 ± 12 years [2,3]. Furthermore, after diagnosis many of the patients had received inadequate Ig prophylaxis, defined as <25 mg/kg/week [4]. The presence of chronic lung damage, which is a major threat to these patients, could be related to such inadequate prophylaxis.

LUNG FUNCTION AND IMMUNOGLOBULIN PROPHYLAXIS IN HYPOGAMMAGLOBULINEMIA

Careful work-up of the lung function of hypogammaglobulinemia patients is important. Determinations of $FEV_{1.0}$ and/or vital capacity demonstrated deteriorated function in 9/26 patients, but the single breath N_2 test showed abnormal findings in 18/26 patients [3], illustrating that these patients must be discovered earlier and treated more efficiently.

The occasionally dramatic side effects of intramuscular Ig injections [5] not only alarm the patients and the physicians, but contribute to insufficient Ig prophylaxis. After such untoward effects, many patients were left without prophylaxis or with doses which were too small. Although we found a significant relationship between decreased lung function and

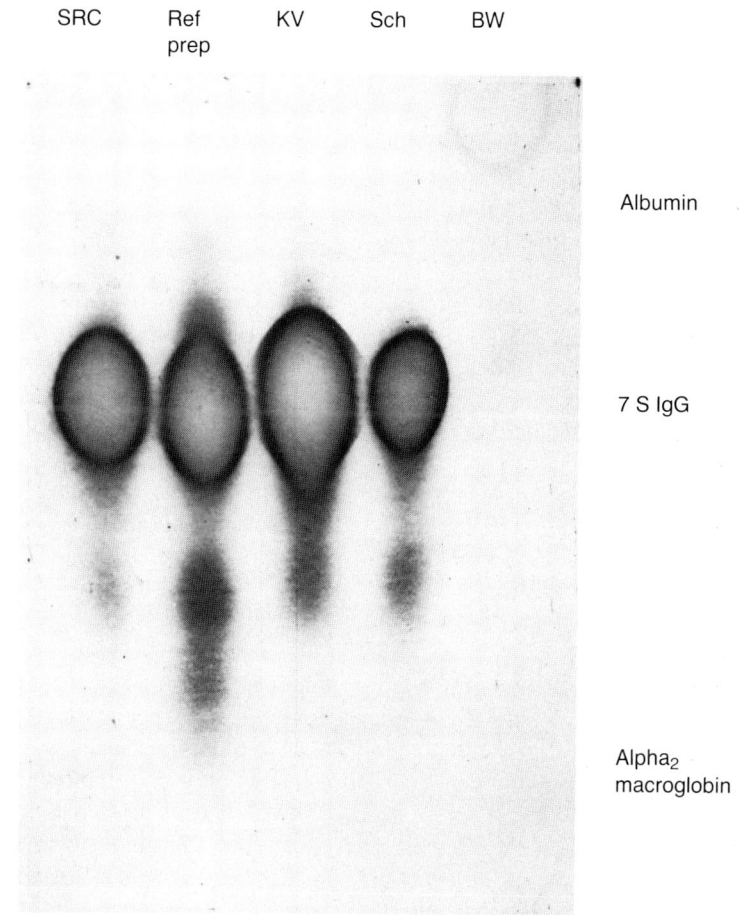

Fig. 1. Immuno-gel filtration analyses of IV immunoglobulin preparations from different manufacturers: Swiss Red Cross, a reference preparation, KabiVitrum, Schura, and Behringwerke (BW). After chromatography through a thin layer of Sephadex G 200 superfine, the IgG is precipitated by anti-IgG incorporated in the agarose slab which is superimposed on the Sephadex. Only small fragments of Fc are demonstrated in the BW preparation (Gammavenine) since the antiserum was very low in anti-Fab. For relative amounts of monomeric (7 S halos), dimeric and polymeric IgG see Table 1. Buffer flow (↓) and filtration positions of some human serum components are indicated.

TABLE 1. Immuno-Gel Filtration Analysis of IgG Components in IV Immunoglobulins (Relative amounts according to area of precipitates using the Schura preparation as reference)

IgG components	SRC	Ref prep	Kabi	Schura
7S				
halos	1.31	1.38	1.78	1.00
dimers	0.95	1.71	0.96	1.00
polymers	0	1.24*	0	0

*in relation to dimers

inadequate Ig prophylaxis among 24 patients with CVID [2,3], we have followed one patient with very low serum Ig levels and normal lung function, who has refused Ig injections for many years.

Igs FOR INTRAVENOUS USE

The possibility of administering the Ig prophylaxis intravenously has been studied by several investigators [2,5–7]. There has been variable success, but recently some new Ig preparations have been presented with favorable results. Among them is a preparation produced by KabiVitrum AB, Sweden, using basically a Cohn cold ethanol method. It is stabilized by addition of albumin and contains no IgG fragments, some dimers but no, or only traces of, larger aggregates which have been connected with side effects [2,5]. This is illustrated by immuno-gel filtration analyses (Fig. 1, Table 1). This largely nonmodified IgG preparation has a half-life ranging from 20–25 days using anti-HBs as a marker [8].

With im administration of Ig it can be difficult to reach over 2 gm/liter of IgG in the patient's circulation without repeatedly giving huge painful injections. With the presently available material for IV use we can easily reach normal serum levels of IgG in 2 days in a desperately ill patient (Fig. 2).

It is also possible to give larger doses so that the infusions can be given less often during continuous prophylaxis. It is eminently practical for the patient, as well as the hospital, to be able to give the Ig infusions only every 5th week (Fig. 3). We

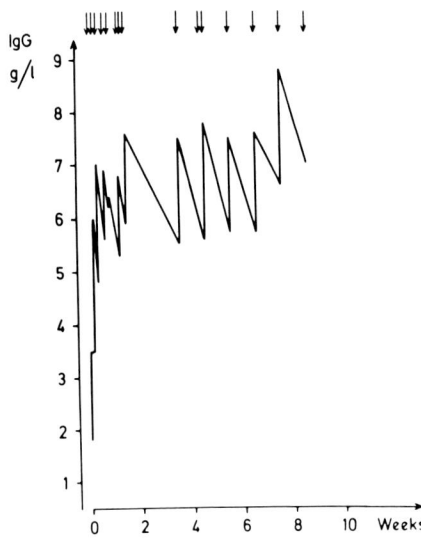

Fig. 2. Ig given intravenously in repeated infusions to a patient with hypogammaglobulinemia quickly increasing the serum IgG level.

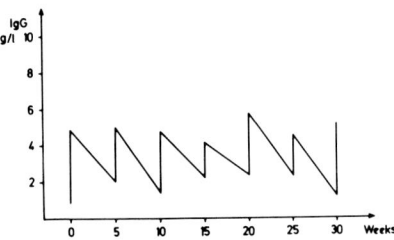

Fig. 3. IV infusions of Ig every 5 weeks (130 mg/kg) to a patient with common variable hypogammaglobulinemia.

have not completed studies, however, to exclude that IgG 3 with a shorter half-life does not get too low with these longer intervals.

Side Effects

To date, we have given 350 IV infusions with this new Ig preparation. We have encountered side effects in only 5 instances. In 3, it was a matter only of a temperature rise of 1°C (one of these patients had a cold). The fourth case was the very sick patient shown in Figure 2 who was in a respirator after pneumothorax, apnea, asystole, and subcutaneous emphysema. In connection with an IV infusion he became anuric, but he had 11 other infusions simultaneously; he has since accepted numerous regular Ig infusions without any problems. The fifth case, a patient with bronchopneumonia, reacted with dyspnea, chills, and back pain, when the infusion rate was increased rapidly from the initial 0.25 ml/min to 4 ml/min. Thereafter, she has readily accepted the infusions at a rate of 0.5 ml/min. Patients who have been given the IV infusions rarely want to return to the im mode of administration.

SUMMARY

Hypogammaglobulinemia patients, who seem to be more numerous than previously known, have an unacceptable diagnostic delay of 12 years. They often get insufficient Ig prophylaxis, frequently due to the side effects caused by the im administration.

A new Ig preparation for IV use has been utilized, which is much more acceptable to the patients, causing very few side effects. In contrast to im preparations, IV immunoglobulin can be used at high doses, quickly normalizing the patient's serum IgG level, and seems to permit longer intervals between infusions during long-term prophylaxis.

REFERENCES

1. Fasth A : Primary immunodeficiency disorders in Sweden: Cases among children, 1974-1979. J Clin Immunol 2:86-92, 1982.
2. Hanson LÅ, Björkander J, Oxelius V-A, Wadsworth C: Indications and limitations of parenteral immunoglobulin treatment: Prophylactic intramuscular immunoglobulin in therapy. In Nydegger UE (ed): "Immunohemotherapy. A Guide to Immunoglobulin Prophylaxis and Therapy." New York: Academic Press, 1981, pp 423-430.
3. Björkander J, Bake B, Hanson LÅ: Hypogammaglobulinemia, delayed diagnosis, inadequate treatment and abnormal lung function. Am J Med (Submitted for publication).
4. British Medical Research Council: "Hypogammaglobulinemia in the United Kingdom." SRS 310, Medical Research Council, Her Majesty's Stationary Office, London, 1971.
5. Hanson LÅ, Björkander J, Ljunggren C, Oxelius V-A, Wadsworth C: Problems with use of immunoglobulins in treatment of immunodeficient patients. In Alving B, Finlayson FS (eds): "Immunoglobulins: Characteristics and Uses of Intravenous Preparations." Washington DC: Department of Health and Human Services. DHHS Publication No (FDA) -80-9905, 1980, pp 151-159.
6. Pirofsky B, Anderson CJ, Bardana EJ Jr: Therapeutic and detrimental effects of intravenous immunoglobulin therapy. Supra #2, pp 15-22.
7. Cunningham-Rundles C, Day NK, Wahn V, Smithwick EM, Siegal FP, Gupta S, Good RA: Reactions to intravenous gammaglobulin infusions and immune complex formation. Supra #5, pp 447-449.
8. Iwarson SA, Wahl M, Hermodson S, Kjellman H: Influence of pharmacokinetic factors on the effect of hepatitis B immunoglobulin therapy. In "Proceedings of the Third International Symposium on Viral Hepatitis." New York City: The Franklin Institute Press, 1981, pp 754-755.

Individualization of Gamma Globulin Dosage in Patients With Humoral Immunodeficiency*

Richard I. Schiff, MD, PhD, Christine Rudd, D Phar, Ruby Johnson, and Rebecca H. Buckley, MD

Departments of Pediatrics (R.I.S., R.J., R.H.B.), Microbiology and Immunology (R.H.B.), and Pharmacy (C.R.), Duke University School of Medicine, Durham, NC 27710

For nearly 30 years, injections of exogenous gamma globulin have been used at a fixed dose of 100 mg/kg/mo in the treatment of severe humoral immunodeficiency disorders. Since neither this nor other doses have ever been subjected to a controlled study of efficacy in the treatment of such defects, it is unknown whether 100 mg/kg/mo of IgG is either an adequate or an ideal quantity for replacement therapy. When therapy was formerly restricted to unmodified Cohn Fraction II, it was difficult to increase the quantity because of the difficulty in injecting large volumes intramuscularly. With the recent development of safe and effective IV IgG preparations [1,2], however, there is no longer a restriction on the amount of IgG that can be infused. Thus, knowledge of the optimal dose for replacement therapy becomes of practical importance.

The present study was undertaken to 1) determine whether there are significant between-subject differences in the metabolism of IgG in patients with severe humoral deficiency, and 2) to evaluate the effect of increasing doses of IV gamma globulin on the serum concentrations and half-life of IgG in such subjects.

PATIENTS AND METHODS

Fourteen patients with well-defined humoral immunodeficiency [3] were treated for a 12-month period with a β-propiolactone-stabilized IV preparation of IgG, Intraglobin® (Biotest Serum Institut GmbH, Frankfurt, FRG). Thus far, 8 of the patients have had 2 IgG half-life studies completed and these comprise the basis of this report. The 8 patients who have completed the study thus far ranged in age from 3–30 years (Table 1). *Patients BD and CD are identical twins, and KW and MW are brothers.* All patients were receiving some form of gamma globulin replacement at the beginning of the study. The study was divided into 2 phases. In the first 6 months, all patients were infused every 28 days with a standard dose of 100 mg/kg of IgG. Serum IgG concentrations were determined immediately before and after each infusion by single radial diffusion in agar gel, using antisera and reference standards prepared in our laboratory [4]. All samples for a given half-life study were tested simultaneously on a single antibody agar plate, but monthly samples for peak and trough levels were assayed when obtained. After the 4th infusion of the standard dose, the IgG half-life was determined for each patient by measuring serum IgG concentrations immediately before and after the infusion and on 1, 2, 5, 7, 10, 14, 21, and 28 days later. The half-life was determined using standard equations for 1st order elimination: $T\ ½ = .693/K$ where K is calculated for the slope of the line of log IgG concentration vs time, as determined by least squares analysis. As has been shown previously [5], elimination of nondenatured, unmodified IgG follows a rapid initial redistribution or alpha phase and a slower terminal beta phase; the half-life was calculated using the slope of the beta phase. Thus,

$$K = \frac{2.3\ (\log\ conc_2 - \log\ conc_1)}{time\ interval}$$

This constant K was then used to calculate the dose necessary to maintain a minimum serum IgG concentration of 200 mg/dl:

$$C_{pss}\ min = \frac{dose\ (e^{-KT})}{v_d\ (1 - e^{-KT})}$$

where C_{pss} is the desired minimal concentration, V_d is the volume of distribution, and T is the dosing interval (in this case, 28 days). V_d is determined by extrapolating the β-slope back to 0 days to determine C_{pO}, and then calculated using the equation $V_d = dose/C_{pO}$.

In the second 6 months, patients were given an individualized dose that was calculated from the half-life study to result in a serum concentration of 200 mg/dl 28 days after the infusion. Peak and trough IgG concentrations were monitored monthly, and the IgG half-life was then redetermined for each patient after the last dose. All patients were seen monthly on the Duke University Clinical Research Unit (RR-30) and were examined at the time of their infusions. Records were kept on the

---

*Supported in part by Grant #1 R01 AI18613 from NIAID and by a grant from the General Clinical Research Centers Program (RR-30).

TABLE 1. Effects of Adjusted Dose of IgG on Trough IgG Concentrations in Patients With Primary Immunodeficiency

	Patients			Phase 1 (Standard Dose)		Phase 2 (Adjusted Dose)	
	Dx	Age	Sex	Dose (mg/kg)	Mean trough IgG conc. (mg/dl)	Dose (mg/kg)	Mean trough IgG conc. (mg/dl)
A)							
KW	CVID	20	M	100	236	100	204
MW	CVID	19	M	100	266	100	227
B)							
CB	CVID	30	F	100	198	120	152
AP	CVID	16	F	100	173	150	166
JY	HypM	19	M	100	137	150	139
C)							
BD	CVID	16	M	100	105	300	175
CD	CVID	16	M	100	145*	250	160
MtW	XAG	3	M	100	63	200	167

*Received blood and plasma during surgery.

TABLE 2. Effects of Gamma Globulin Infusions on Catabolism of IgG

Patient	Phase 1 Standard (100 mg/kg) Dose of IgG			Phase 2 Adjusted Dose of IgG			
	Conc. of IgG (mg/dl)		T½ (Days)	Dose (mg/kg)	Conc. of IgG (mg/dl)		T½ (Days)
	Pre	Post			Pre	Post	
CB	198	416	36.5	120	152	403	49.6
BD	105	262	32.0	300	175	637	35.7
CD	145	297	46.5	250	160	644	49.6
AP	173	403	31.0	150	166	478	64.0
KW	236	514	80.6	100	204	532	85.6
MW	266	520	34.0	100	241	488	86.0
MtW	56	244	26.3	200	167	500	39.6
JY	137	309	37.5	150	139	388	37.0

incidence of infections and the frequency of additional antibiotic usage.

RESULTS

The 2 patients listed in section A of Table 1 were infused with 100 mg/kg/mo in both phases of the study. Both consistently had trough serum IgG concentrations above 200 mg/dl one month postinfusion. Neither showed a significant change in their mean trough serum IgG concentration between the 2 phases. The 3 patients in section B of Table 1 received 120–150 mg/kg in the second phase of the study. Despite this increase, their mean trough serum IgG concentrations were the same or lower in the second phase of the study. The 3 patients in section C of Table 1 received 200 to 300 mg/kg/mo in phase 2 and all but CD showed a significant rise in mean trough serum IgG concentrations. Despite the rises in trough serum IgG concentrations, however, it can be seen that the desired serum IgG concentration of 200 mg/dl was not achieved. The mean serum IgG concentration for *Patient CD* was raised temporarily in the first phase by his having received blood and plasma during surgery; this could have affected his mean trough serum IgG concentration in phase 1 sufficiently to make the rise during phase 2 appear insignificant. *Patient MtW* had very low initial levels of IgG and had not yet reached a steady state by the 12th month.

As is seen in Table 2, the half-life of IgG determined in the initial phase of the study for each patient was highly variable for these 8 patients, ranging from 26.3 days *(MtW)* to 80.6 days *(KW)*. There was poor correlation between the mean trough serum IgG concentrations and the IgG half-life for an individual patient. In contrast to our suspicions, none of the patients showed a shortening of the IgG half-life (calculated from the beta phase) in the second half of the study, regardless of whether the mean trough serum IgG concentration was raised. In several patients *(CB, AP, MW,* and *MtW)*, the T ½ for IgG was considerably longer in the second 6 months. This did not appear to be due to an increased amount of IgG infused, since *MW* received 100 mg/kg in both phases of the study. Those patients infused with increased doses of IgG in the 2nd phase did show the expected increase in their serum concentrations immediately postinfusion, especially *BD, CD,* and *MtW* who received 300, 250, and 200 mg/kg, respectively.

An example of the pattern of variation in pre- and postinfusion IgG concentrations is shown in Figure 1. *Patient BD's* pattern typifies that seen in patients receiving very high doses, with very high initial IgG concentrations and a modest increase in trough IgG concentrations. *Patients CB, AP,* and *JY* had similar curves but did not increase their trough IgG concentrations in spite of receiving 120–150 mg/kg/mo.

The lack of an increase in the trough IgG concentration in patients receiving higher doses of IgG suggested to us that elimination might have become more rapid but, as noted above, this was apparently not due to a shorter half-life. This contradiction is partly explained in Figure 2 where it can be seen in *Patient*

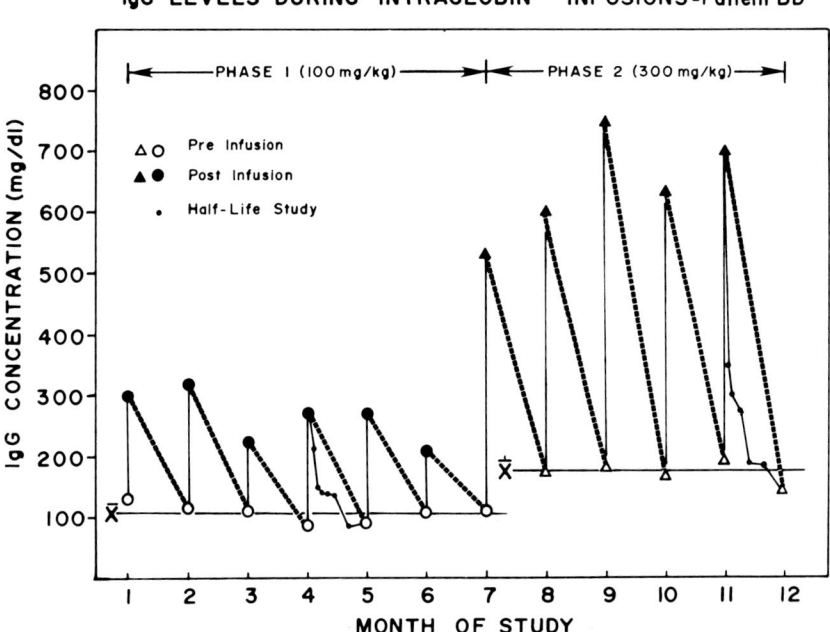

Fig. 1. Fluctuations in serum IgG concentrations during monthly infusions of β-propiolactone stabilized IgG (Intraglobin®) in *Patient BD*. The means of preinfusion serum IgG concentrations for the 2 phases of the study are indicated by the x̄ symbol and horizontal line. The dashed line represents a theoretic decline only; the actual decline in IgG concentrations can be seen in the 2 half-life studies.

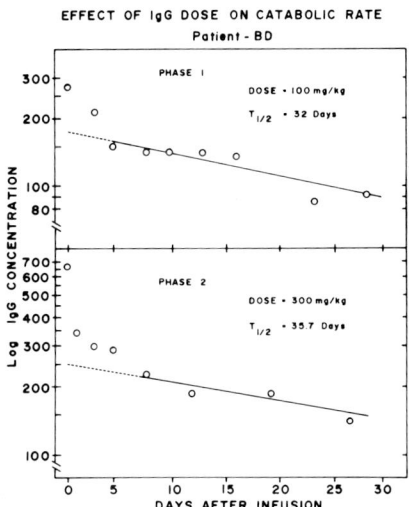

Fig. 2. IgG half-life studies for *Patient BD* infused monthly with 2 doses of IV IgG (Intraglobin®). The T ½ is proportional to the slope of the line log concentration vs time (beta phase). The dotted line depicts the extrapolation to 0 days to determine C_{pO}. The alpha phase, not drawn in, is the slope of the curve connecting the points in the first 5 days.

BD that the initial redistribution and elimination (alpha) phase is more profound when higher doses are infused. Despite greater losses in the alpha phase, the trough serum IgG concentration was increased, but not as much as had been estimated on the basis of half-life alone.

There were no significant adverse reactions in over 200 infusions of Intraglobin® during the one-year period of this study. All patients were in reasonably good health throughout; the exception was *Patient CD*, who underwent lobectomy for bronchiectasis between the 3rd and 4th months of the study. He did well subsequently. Infections in the group were limited to sinusitis, bronchitis, and pharyngitis. There was no demonstrable difference in the incidence of infections or in the requirement for additional antibiotics in the 2 phases of the study.

DISCUSSION

These studies demonstrate that there is marked variability in the serum IgG half-life in patients with severe primary humoral immunodeficiency, ranging from 26–80.6 days. These half-lives are generally much greater than the range reported for normal subjects (14–28 days), as determined by the turnover of radiolabeled normal IgG [5]. In a more recent study using IV injections of trace amounts of radiolabeled commercial Cohn Fraction II, the IgG T ½ in 14 normal volunteers ranged from 7.3–18.3 days [1]. In several studies, plasma IgG half-lives in immunodeficient patients have been found to be prolonged (range of 23–70 days) relative to those of normals [5–7], similar to the range found in the present study.

Studies by Waldmann and Strober [6] showed a correlation between the serum IgG concentration and the plasma half-life, with the shortest half-lives occurring in patients with myeloma, and the longest half-lives in patients with hypogammaglobulinemia. In our study, we did not observe a correlation between the T ½ and the trough serum IgG concentration; ie patients with the shortest half-lives did not necessarily have the lowest trough serum IgG concentrations. However, our patients all had severe hypogammaglobulinemia and the range of IgG concentrations examined was not as extensive as in Waldmann and Strober's study.

In previous studies of serum IgG T ½, only trace amounts of radiolabeled IgG were injected to determine the T ½ of the endogenous IgG; the quantities of IgG injected were insufficient to substantially alter serum IgG concentrations. There are no published data in man on the effect of the quantity of IgG infused on the IgG half-life. In the mouse, infusions of increasing quantities of either human or mouse IgG, but not of IgA or IgM, were found to shorten the half-life of IgG [8]. In the present study, there was no shortening of the IgG T ½ with increased doses of IgG in any patient, regardless of whether or not the mean trough IgG concentrations were increased.

Infusion of very large doses of IgG (200–300 mg/kg) resulted in significant increases in trough serum IgG concentrations but not to the projected concentration calculated on the basis of half-life. As discussed above, the half-life was not shortened with increased doses. The apparent contradiction between the increased peak levels of IgG in patients receiving higher doses of IgG and the failure to raise trough levels was explained by a more profound fall during the early or alpha phase rather than a change in the serum T ½. The alpha phase usually consists primarily of equilibration of undenatured IgG between the intravascular and extravascular compartments, but the fact that several days often elapsed in our studies with modified IgG before the onset of the beta phase suggests a more complex process. Damage to IgG molecules during purification and radioiodination can result in rapid elimination from the body [5].

Thus, it is possible to increase trough serum IgG concentrations in patients with severe humoral immunodeficiency without altering the IgG half-life, but complex factors causing early elimination make calculation of the required dose difficult. It is likely that it will be necessary to evaluate the early elimination phase characteristic of each of the specific IV IgG preparations to be used, since data derived from one preparation cannot necessarily be extrapolated to others.

There was no difference between the incidence of infections or in the need for additional antibiotics in the 2 phases (standard dose vs half-life dose) of our study. In view of the limited state of our knowledge regarding metabolism of various commercial IgG preparations, the current cost of administering high doses, and the uncertainty of the optimal dose of IgG for regular replacement therapy, only those patients with very low trough serum IgG concentrations and an unsatisfactory clinical course should be considered candidates for routine high-dose therapy at present.

REFERENCES

1. Morell A, Schurch B, Ryser D, Hofer F, Skvaril F, Barandun S: *In vivo* behaviour of gamma globulin preparations. Vox Sang 38:272–283, 1980.
2. Romer J, Morgenthaler J-J, Scherz R, Skvaril F: Characterization of various immunoglobulin preparations for intravenous application. Vox Sang 42:62–73, 1982.
3. Report of a World Health Organization Committee. Pediatrics 47:927–946, 1971.
4. Buckley RH, Dees SC, O'Fallon WM: Serum immunoglobulins. I. Levels in normal children and in uncomplicated childhood allergy. Pediatrics 41:600–611, 1968.
5. Wells JV, Fudenberg HH: Metabolism of radio-iodinated IgG in patients with abnormal serum IgG levels. II. Hypogamma-globulinemia. Clin Exp Immunol 9:775–783, 1971.
6. Waldmann TA, Strober W: Metabolism of immunoglobulins. Prog Allergy 13:1–110, 1969.
7. Stiehm ER, Vaerman J-P, Fudenberg HH: Plasma infusions in immunologic deficiency states: Metabolic and therapeutic studies. Blood 28:918–937, 1966.
8. Fahey JL, Robinson AG: Factors controlling serum-globulin concentration. J Exp Med 118:845–868, 1968.

Subcutaneous Infusion of Gamma Globulins in the Management of Agammaglobulinemic Patients

Alberto G. Ugazio, MD, Marzia Duse, MD, Alessandro Plebani, PhD, Luigi D. Notarangelo, MD, and G. Roberto Burgio, MD

Department of Pediatrics, University of Pavia, 27100 Pavia, Italy

Intramuscular injection of human standard globulins (HSG) is effective for the prevention of infections in patients with agammaglobulinemia or severe hypogammaglobulinemia [1,2]. However, intramuscular replacement has several disadvantages: a) because of the large volume that has to be used, local pain at the site of injection is distressing for the patient, and especially in older children may lead to noncompliance; b) because of the large volume required it is difficult to maintain serum IgG levels of at least 200 mg/dl, generally accepted as adequate [1]; and c) in most patients, maintenance of these serum IgG levels does not prevent recurrent sinopulmonary infections which might be relieved by maintaining higher serum IgG concentrations [3]. These disadvantages have prompted search for alternatives such as substitution with human plasma [4] or IV gamma globulin preparations [5]; however, both alternatives require frequent infusions in a hospital day-care unit under close supervision, and the former carries the risk of hepatitis.

Following the initial trial of Berger et al [6] we studied [7] the safety and efficacy of subcutaneous infusion of intramuscular (im) preparations of HSG in 14 patients with X-linked agammaglobulinemia (SLA); we also assessed biologic activity of the IgG absorbed.

METHODS

Patients. Fourteen children with SLA, ranging in age from 4 to 15 years were included in the study. All patients had previously been treated with weekly im injections of HSG in a maintenance dose of 0.2–0.4 ml/kg/wk. Blood was drawn one week after the last im injection (just before the first subcutaneous infusion), at weekly intervals for one month, and then monthly. Blood was allowed to clot at room temperature for 30 minutes, and the serum was stored in liquid nitrogen until used.

Infusion. The technique for slow subcutaneous infusion was adapted from Berger et al [6]. Briefly, HSG available for im use were purchased from Immuno (Wien) and administered subcutaneously by an MS16 Pye Dynamics syringe driver (Bushey, Herefordshire U.K.). A 25-gauge Butterfly needle was inserted subcutaneously in the anterior abdominal wall, and if no blood return was observed, it was connected to a disposable syringe mounted on the pump.

After a loading dose of 100 mg/kg daily for 5–10 days, 50–100 mg/kg were given once a week at a rate of 1–3 ml/hr over 6–8 hours. The first 5–10 infusions were carried out in the hospital in order to teach the patient and/or his parents to use the device at home.

Igs and antibodies. Serum Ig levels were quantitated by automated nephelometry [8]. IgG antibodies directed against tetanus toxoid (TT) were assayed in serum samples, as well as in HSG preparation, by means of an ELISA technique in microtiter plates; results were expressed in mU/dl with reference to a standard serum. The complement-fixing capacity of the anti-TT antibodies in serum samples, as well as in HSG preparations, was evaluated in microtiter plates coated with TT by a microcomplement fixation technique; complement-fixing activity was calculated as percent of the activity of a standard serum by comparing the time necessary to reach 50% hemolysis (tH50) of the sample to the tH50 of different dilutions of the standard serum.

Direct and alternative pathways of complement. Activity of the direct pathway was evaluated by means of a micromodification of the hemolytic technique described by Mayer [9]; activity of the alternative pathway was evaluated by a micromodification of the hemolytic technique with rabbit erythrocytes described by Siccardi et al [10]. For both pathways activity was expressed in hemolytic units/ml (HU/ml).

RESULTS

Clinical data. After 3–9 months of treatment with subcutaneous infusion, all 14 children are clinically well and no severe infections have been observed. No alterations of the usual hematochemical parameters including RBC, WBC, and platelet counts, clotting factors, or liver enzymes have been observed. After 480 infusions carried out so far, only 7 have resulted in transient painful reactions at the injection site. The subcutaneous (sc) infusion was preferred to im injection by all children more than 6 years old because it was less painful.

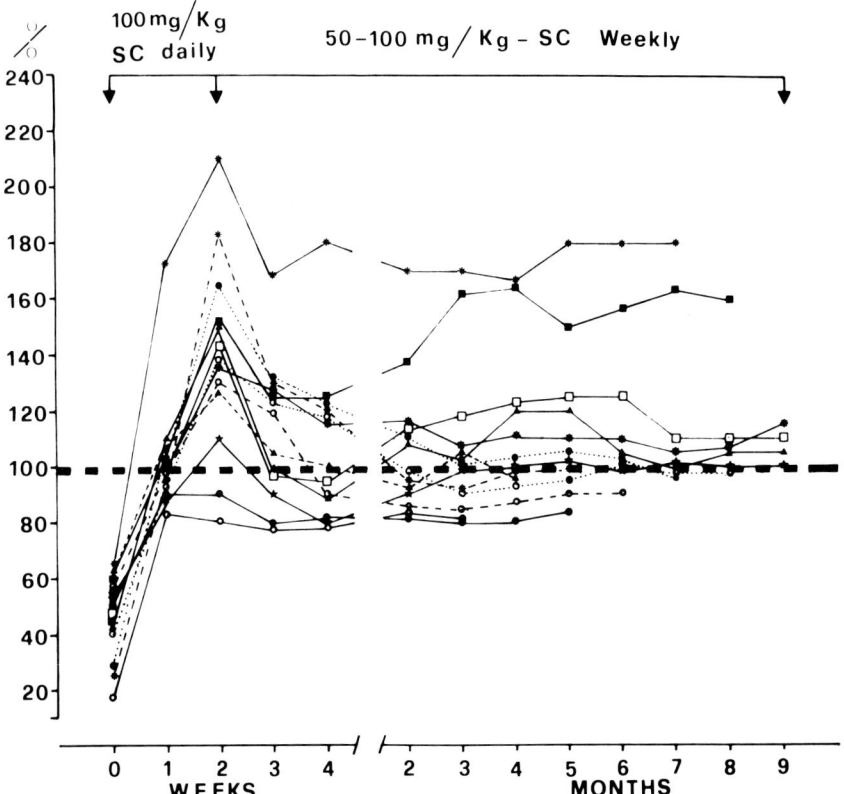

Fig. 1. Serum IgG levels in 14 children with SLA on replacement therapy with slow sc infusion of HSG. IgG values are expressed as percent of the lower limit of the age-normal range (broken horizontal line); values at 0 weeks indicate the level monitored 1 week after the last conventional im injection just before beginning sc replacement.

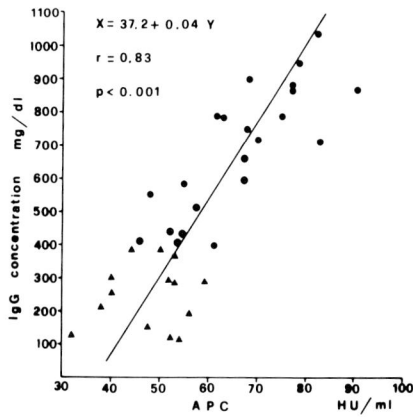

Fig. 2. Correlation between activity of the alternative pathway of complement (APC) and serum IgG levels in serum samples from the children with SLA, before (▲) and during (●) replacement therapy with slow sc infusion of HSG. Each point represents one sample.

Serum IgG levels. As shown in Figure 1, serum IgG levels expressed as percent of the lower limit of the age-normal range, ranged from 15–60% (mean 42 ± 18%) during conventional im treatment, and from 80–170% (mean 105 ± 28%) during maintenance with sc infusion.

Antibody activity of circulating IgG. In order to establish whether the IgG absorbed from the subcutaneous depot retained antibody activity, anti-TT IgG antibodies as well as their complement-fixing capacity were determined both in the HSG preparation and in serum samples. The HSG preparation used contained 550 mU/mg of IgG, while in the 5 subjects tested the IgG absorbed retained antibody activity ranging from 250 mU/mg (45%) to 450 mU/mg (82%). The complement-fixing activity of the anti-TT IgG antibodies absorbed in the serum of the 5 subjects tested ranged from 40–75% of that of the HSG preparation infused.

Direct and alternative pathway of complement. Activity of the direct pathway of complement was within normal limits in all subjects on conventional im replacement and did not vary significantly during treatment with sc infusions (data not shown).

During conventional im treatment, activity of the alternative pathway of complement was low in all 14 patients, ranging from 31–59 HU/ml with a mean of 47 ± 13 HU/ml (normal range: 63–132, mean 96 ± 13 HU/ml). When patients were switched to sc infusion, repeated assessment of alternative pathway activity showed a dramatic increase up to 67 ± 10 HU/ml (range: 47–90). As reported in Figure 2, statistical analysis showed that alternative pathway activity and serum IgG levels were highly correlated.

DISCUSSION

The present study of 14 children with SLA shows that replacement therapy can be safely carried out by weekly subcutaneous (sc) infusion of HSG. It was also reported in another study [11] that sc infusion is much better tolerated than im injection, especially in older children, and allows administration of larger amounts of HSG, thus usually permitting attainment of age-normal serum IgG levels. As a rule, the procedure is carried out at home while the child is sleeping or playing; no school days are lost because of hospitalization which is necessary when substitution is performed with plasma or IV gamma globulins. No major side effects were recorded and the rare painful reactions were rapidly alleviated by gentle massage. As no severe infections have been observed, sc replacement is likely to be at least as effective as conventional im replacement; the possible advantage of maintaining age-normal IgG levels is currently being investigated in a controlled clinical trial.

About 40–60% of the IgG injected im is destroyed locally by proteolytic enzymes [12]. In the present study we have shown that from 40–82% of the IgG absorbed from the subcutaneous site of infusion retains biologic activity as assessed by an ELISA technique as well as by a complement-fixing assay.

Low activity of the alternative pathway of complement has already been reported in agammaglobulinemic patients; the activity reportedly improved after addition of IgG in vitro [13]. In our patients treated with conventional im HSG, activity of the alternative pathway was still low and normalized only when age-normal levels of serum IgG were attained by means of sc infusions. Antibodies are certainly involved in activation of the alternative pathway possibly by protecting the C3bBb convertase from inactivation by serum inhibitors [14]; in fact, some human antivirus antibodies have been shown to enhance activation of the alternative pathway by virus-infected cells [15], and there is evidence that bacteria normally unable to activate the alternative pathway are transformed into activators by interaction with specific antibodies [16]. Thus, it is conceivable that deficiency of the alternative complement pathway contributes significantly to the high susceptibility to infections of agammaglobulinemic patients.

The results of the present study show that the relatively low levels of serum IgG maintained by conventional im replacement are not sufficient for normalization of the alternative pathway of complement which is attained only when IgG levels reach age-normal values. Therefore, attainment of high serum IgG concentrations by subcutaneous infusion of HSG may offer the advantage of providing a large amount of antibodies available not only for opsonization of microorganisms through the classic pathway, but also for normalization of the alternative pathway of complement.

REFERENCES

1. Janeway CA, Rosen FS: The gamma globulins. IV. Therapeutic uses of gammaglobulin. N Engl J Med 275:826–831, 1966.
2. Medical Research Council Working Party: Hypogammaglobulinemia in the United Kingdom. Lancet 1:163–169, 1969.
3. Wedgwood RJ, Ochs HD: The safety, acceptability and effectiveness of immunoglobulin modified for intravenous use. In Nydegger UE (ed): "Immunohemotherapy." London: Academic Press, 1981, pp 351–355.
4. Stiehm ER: Plasma therapy: An alternative to gamma globulin injections in immunodeficiency. In Bergsma D (ed): "Immunodeficiency in Man and Animals." Sunderland, MA: Sinauer Assoc for The National Foundation-March of Dimes, BD:OAS XI(1):343–346, 1975.
5. Alvin BM, Finlayson JS (eds): "Immunoglobulins: Characteristics and Uses of Intravenous Preparations." DHHS Publication No(FDA)-80-9005, U.S. Gov. Printing Office, 1980.
6. Berger M, Cupps TR, Fauci AS: Immunoglobulin replacement therapy by slow subcutaneous infusion. Ann Intern Med 93:55–56, 1980.
7. Ugazio AG, Duse M, Re R, Mangili G, Burgio GR: Subcutaneous infusion of gammaglobulins in management of agammaglobulinemia. Lancet 1:226, 1982.
8. Walker WHC, Gauldie J: Automated determination of immunoglobulins. In Ritchie RF (ed): "Automated Immunoanalysis." New York: Marcel Dekker, 1978, pp 203–225.
9. Mayer MM: Complement and complement fixation. In Kabat EA (ed): "Experimental Immunochemistry," 2nd Ed. Springfield: Charles C Thomas, 1971, pp 133–240.
10. Siccardi AG, Marconi M, Ferrari FA, Fortunato A, Giannetti A, Sacchi FT, Beretta A, Ugazio AG, Jayakar SD: High incidence and heterogeneity of functional defects of the alternative pathway of complement among atopic children. J Clin Lab Immunol 3:165–170, 1980.
11. Roord JJ, Van Der Meer JWM, Kuis W, De Windt GE, Zegers BJM, van Furth R, Stoop JW: Home treatment in patients with antibody deficiency by slow subcutaneous infusion of gammaglobulins. Lancet 1:689–690, 1982.
12. Hitzig WH: Summary of therapeutic applications of immunoglobulins. Supra #3, pp 435–440.
13. Corry JM, Polhill RB, Edmonds SR, Johnston RB: Activity of the alternative complement pathway after splenectomy: Comparison to activity in sickle cell disease and hypogammaglobulinemia. J Pediatr 95:964–969, 1979.
14. Isliker H, Nydegger UE: The complement system: Immunopathogenic mediator and regulator of immunoglobulin interactions. Supra #3, pp 47–60.
15. Perrin LH, Joseph BS, Cooper NR, Oldstone MBA: Mechanism of injury of virus-infected cells by antiviral antibody and complement. Participation of IgG F(ab')2 in alternative complement pathway. J Exp Med 143:1027–1041, 1976.
16. Edwards M, Nicholson-Weller A, Baker CJ, Kasper DL: The role of specific antibody in alternative complement pathway mediated opsonophagocytosis of type III group streptococcus. J Exp Med 151:1275–1287, 1980.

Treatment of Antibody Deficiency Syndromes With Subcutaneous Infusion of Gamma Globulin

John J. Roord, Jos W.M. van der Meer, Wietse Kuis, and Ralph van Furth, MD

Department of Immunology, University Children's Hospital "Het Wilhelmina Kinderziekenhuis," Utrecht, The Netherlands (J.J.R., W.K.); Department of Infectious Diseases, University Hospital, Leiden, The Netherlands (J.W.M.v.d.M., R.v.F.)

INTRODUCTION

Patients with one of the various forms of hypogammaglobulinemia frequently suffer from infections with encapsulated bacteria. The upper and lower respiratory tracts are most often involved in these infections. Infections of the skin, eyes and intestinal tract also are often encountered. Secondary septicemia, bacterial meningitis, osteomyelitis or arthritis may occur [1]. The most important pathogens that can be isolated in these infectious episodes are *Streptococcus pneumoniae* and *Haemophilus influenzae;* group A hemolytic streptococci, *Staphylococcus aureus* and *Neisseria meningitidis* also may cause infections.

Most viral infections usually run a benign course presumably because cell-mediated immunity is intact. However, paralytic poliomyelitis resulting from either live, attenuated vaccine or wild-type poliomyelitis virus has been reported [1,2]; persistent ECHO-virus infections of the CNS, often presenting as a dermatomyositis-like syndrome, usually have a fatal outcome [3]; infection with hepatitis B virus often leads to chronic progressive hepatitis [1]. These data underline the critical role of Igs in the eradication of some viruses. On the other hand, they may indicate that in hypogammaglobulinemia a distinct T-cell dysfunction also may be present. This hypothesis is supported by the observation that malignancies and autoimmune diseases are more often seen in patients with antibody deficiency syndromes than in the normal population [1].

INTRAMUSCULAR ADMINISTRATION OF GAMMA GLOBULINS

In the first patient, diagnosed as agammaglobulinemia, the benefit of the administration of gamma globulin was shown with respect to the many bacterial infections [4]. Since then gamma globulin administration has become the treatment of choice in patients with hypogammaglobulinemia.

Several routes for administration of the Igs have been used; they all have their advantages and disadvantages (Table 1). Over the last 30 years, Igs were usually administered by the intramuscular (im) route. The preparations are isolated from large pools of plasma obtained from healthy donors or from human placentas, and this guarantees a broad spectrum of specific antibodies. The dose of gamma globulin that provides an effective prophylaxis to bacterial infections was found empirically [1]. Invasive bacterial infections can be prevented if the serum IgG is kept above approximately 2 gm/L. Most patients achieve this level if they receive 0.6 ml of the regular 16% gamma globulin preparation/kg/bw (= 100 mg IgG/kg) every 3–4 weeks intramuscularly. This interval is acceptable because the half-life of the im immunoglobulin preparations is in the order of 3 weeks. A newly diagnosed patient is given a double or triple dose the first time. Higher substitution (200 mg IgG/kg/bw 3–4 weeks) gives better infection prevention [1], but this substitution usually can not be achieved because of discomfort to the patient. Otitis/sinusitis and bron-

TABLE 1. Advantages and Disadvantages of the Different Routes of Ig Administration

	Gamma Globulin			
	im	IV	sc	Plasma
Pain	+++	±	±	±
Resorption	incomplete	complete	?	complete
Anaphylactoid reactions	occasionally	occasionally	none	occasionally
Hepatitis B virus transmission	none	none	none	occasionally
t 1/2 IgG	± 20 days	10–20 days	20 days	20 days
IgA/IgM substitution	none	none	none	some
Other disadvantages	injection volume	Ig fragments; MPS blockade	administration during ± 7 hrs	administration 1–2 hrs

chitis/bronchopneumonia still occur in patients substituted with 100 mg IgG/kg every 3–4 weeks, and antibiotics are frequently needed; even surgical intervention may be necessary. The im administration is not only painful but can also lead to (severe) anaphylactoid reactions, probably due to the absorption of aggregated IgG to the vascular compartment; this in turn may lead to complement activation.

REPLACEMENT THERAPY BY PLASMA TRANSFUSIONS

Plasma transfusions (10–15 ml/kg at 3-week intervals), have been advocated also in the treatment of patients with antibody deficiency syndromes [5–7]. This regimen has the theoretic advantage of the administration of certain amounts of IgM and IgA, which may have some positive effect in infection prevention. However, since the half-life for IgM and IgA is only several days, substitution for these Ig classes is only accomplished by frequent infusions. Another advantage is that large doses of Igs can be given. Moreover, the administered Igs are undenatured and other serum proteins, especially complement components that may be of immunologic importance, are provided. However, the procedure is laborious: the patient must come to the hospital to receive an IV line, and the infusion must take place under medical supervision. Virus transmission (especially hepatitis B and cytomegalovirus) and transfusion reactions are a real risk. An additional disadvantage may be that the spectrum of specific antibodies of one donor is limited.

INTRAVENOUS ADMINISTRATION OF GAMMA GLOBULINS

Because of the limitations of im administration, several attempts have been made to infuse the Igs intravenously.

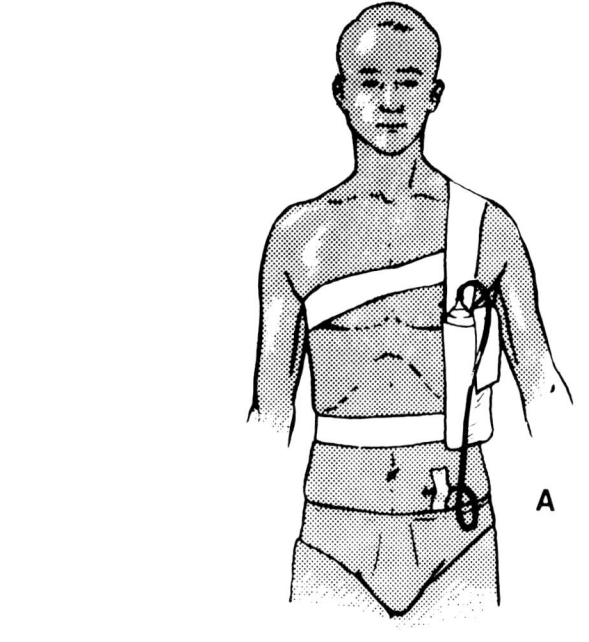

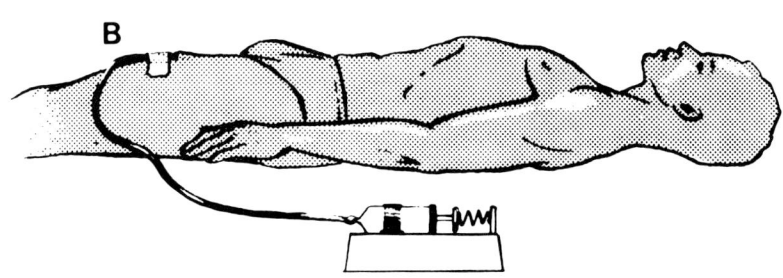

Fig. 1. Slow subcutaneous infusion of gamma globulin with a small infusion pump. 16% human IgG for im use is infused via a scalp vein needle inserted in the sc tissue of A) the abdominal wall, or B) the upper leg. By sc infusion 15–25 ml can easily be administered weekly at an infusion rate of 2–3 ml/hr, either in the daytime or during sleep.

nously. The conventional human serum Ig preparations can induce catastrophic vasomotor reactions due to complement activation by IgG aggregates [8,9]. By modification of the IgG molecule, the anti-complementary activity can be removed permitting IV administration; although acid and pepsin treatment [10] or deaggregation by the human enzyme plasmin [11] reduced vasomotor reactions, the IgG half-life was also shortened, thereby limiting clinical usefulness. More recently, chemically modified Ig preparations have been manufactured for IV use [9,12–14] that have a half-life comparable to the im preparations. However, the modification procedure of some preparations has affected the opsonic capacity of the immunoglobulin [15,16].

Another disadvantage of IV administration of Igs is that the patient becomes very dependent on the physician; he has to attend the hospital each 2–3 weeks. Furthermore, side effects occur up to approximately 5%, and the IV preparations are much more expensive than the im. Still, advantages of the IV injection are apparent: large doses may be

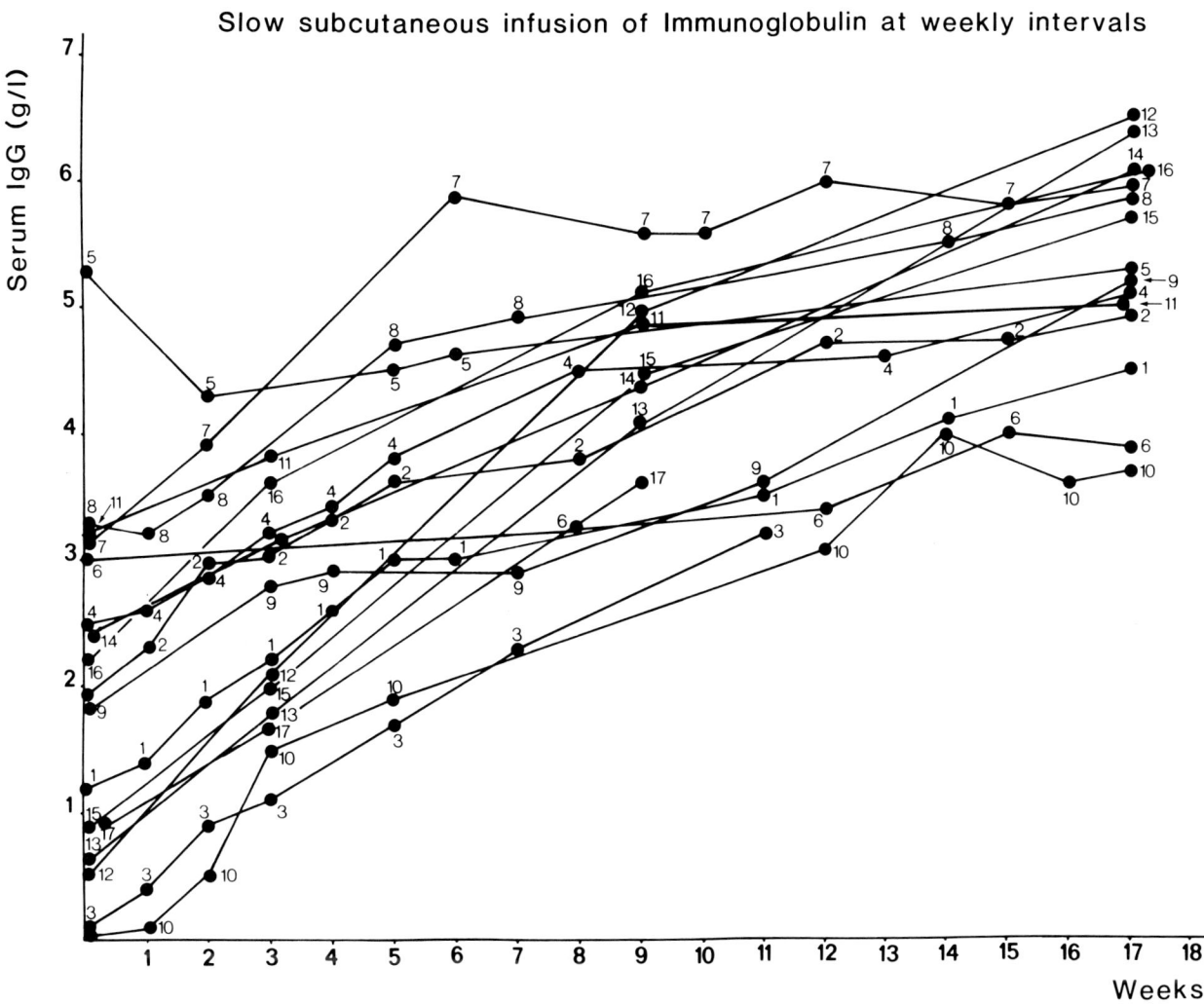

Fig. 2. Serum IgG levels following weekly sc IgG administration. All patients received approximately 50 mg IgG/kg/bw/week (16% Ig preparation provided by Central Laboratory of the Netherlands, Red Cross Blood-transfusion Service, Amsterdam). Patient 17 received 10 ml, patients 1–4, 13, 15 and 16 received 15 ml, patients 5–7, 9–12 and 14 received 20 ml, and patient 8 received 25 ml gamma globulin sc per week. The data of 3 additional patients, who started on daily sc infusions, are not given.

given by a single infusion and the Igs are directly available to fulfill their biologic function. It has been reported recently that IV administration of IgG preparations has led to a transient rise in platelet counts in a number of patients with idiopathic thrombocytopenic purpura, probably due to blockade of the Fc-receptor of the phagocytic cells [17]. This blockade might also take place in the immunocompromised, hypogammaglobulinemic patient and impair the clearance of opsonized bacteria by macrophages in the liver and spleen. Thus, it adversely affects the host defense against infections.

SUBCUTANEOUS ADMINISTRATION OF GAMMA GLOBULINS

It has been shown recently that im immunoglobulin preparation can also be given by slow subcutaneous (sc) infusion [18–20], and high serum IgG levels can be reached easily by high-dose substitution. At least 50 mg IgG (0.3 ml of the 16% preparation) per kilogram bodyweight at an infusion rate of 2–3 ml per hour can be given weekly. After a short period of instruction, the patients are able to infuse themselves at home during the day by a portable pump or at night during sleep (Fig. 1). During sc treatment there is initially a gradual increase of the serum IgG level and levels ⩾ 3 gm/L can easily be reached (Fig. 2). No side effects have been seen in over 2,000 sc transfusions, whereas several patients had severe anaphylactoid reactions from their previous treatment (im gamma globulin administration). Occasion-

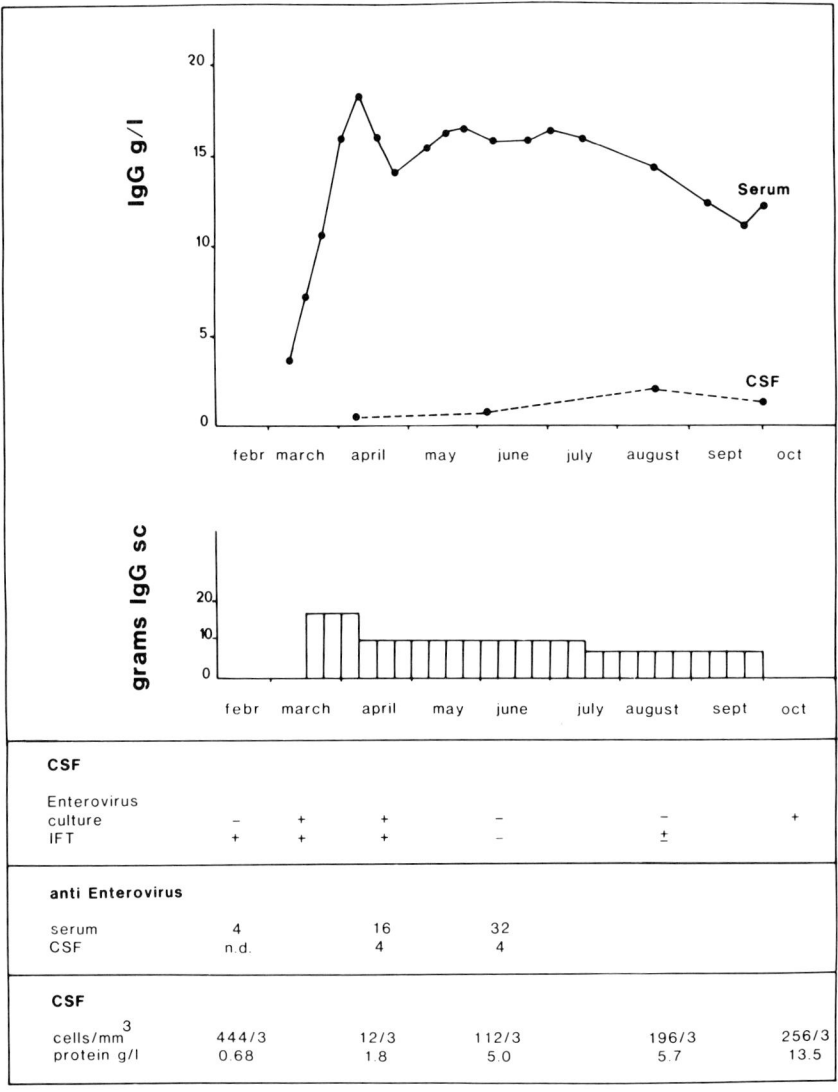

Fig. 3. Course of IgG in serum and cerebrospinal fluid (CSF) in a male patient (12 years of age) with hypogammaglobulinemia and persistent enterovirus infection of the CNS. 16% immunoglobulin (IgG) was administered subcutaneously. Enterovirus was detected in CSF by culture and indirect immunofluorescence test (IFT). Anti-enterovirus antibody concentrations are represented as the reciprocal of the titer.

ally, a local tender area was noted at the infusion site which could be quickly alleviated by gentle massage. During a period of 4 to 20 months only a few minor upper airway infections developed in 20 patients that were instructed and followed by us [19]. By increasing the frequency of administration (100 mg IgG/kg daily) a normal serum IgG according to the patient's age can be reached within 1 to 2 weeks, and by weekly administration of 100 mg IgG/kg/bw this level can be maintained [20]. Whether such a high level of substitution is advantageous is uncertain.

Little is known about the effect of high-dose versus low-dose substitution in relation to viral infections, autoimmune diseases, and malignancies. High gamma globulin substitution has been reported to be beneficial in patients with persistent ECHO-virus infection of the CNS [21]. We have treated a 12-year-old boy with hypogammaglobulinemia, who developed an enterovirus infection of the CNS while on im replacement therapy. By daily sc administration of the im preparation—containing virus-specific antibody—we could obtain a serum IgG of 20 gm/L (Fig. 3). Despite the fact that virus-specific antibodies could be demonstrated in the serum (titer 1:32) and in the cerebrospinal fluid (CSF) (titer 1:4), only a temporary improvement was observed, and the success reported by Mease et al [21] with respect to the virus infection could not be reproduced. However, another interesting phenomenon was observed. The signs of juvenile rheumatoid arthritis in this patient—present since the age of 6 years—disappeared completely and the antirheumatic medication could be stopped. A similar observation was made in an 8-year-old hypogammaglobulinemic boy with a severe form of juvenile rheumatoid arthritis (dry arthritis): a marked improvement was seen when he was started on high-dose sc gamma globulin administration. In both patients the clinical improvement was observed as the serum IgG reached a concentration of 5–6 gm/L. At this serum concentration, IgG could also be demonstrated in the saliva of these patients. In another study, no beneficial effect of a high-dose substitution regimen (50 mg IgG versus 25 mg IgG/kg/week) was observed on the incidence of rheumatoid arthritis, but that dose might have been too low [1]. However, prospective, randomized trials will be needed to compare the different routes of administration, as well as IgG dosages with respect to the various clinical manifestations (bacterial infections, viral infections, autoimmune diseases, and malignancies), to patient compliance, to side effects, and to cost-benefit.

REFERENCES

1. Hill LE, Mollison PL: Conclusions. In "Hypogammaglobulinaemia in the United Kingdom." Spec Rep Ser Med

Res Coun 1971, no. 310.
2. Wyatt HV: Poliomyelitis in hypogammaglobulinemics. J Infect Dis 128:802, 1973.
3. Wilfert CM, Buckley RH, Mohanakumar T, Griffith JF, Katz SL, Whishnant JK, Eggleston PA, Moore M, Treadwell E, Oxman MN, Rosen FS: Persistent and fatal central nervous system echovirus infections in patients with agammaglobulinemia. N Engl J Med 296:1485, 1977.
4. Bruton OC: Agammaglobulinemia. Pediatrics 9:722, 1952.
5. Stiehm ER, Vaerman J-P, Fudenberg HH: Plasma infusions in immunologic deficiency states: Metabolic and therapeutic studies. Blood 28:918, 1966.
6. Stiehm ER: Plasma therapy: An alternative to gamma globulin injections in immunodeficiency. In Bergsma D (ed): "Immunodeficiency in Man and Animals." Sunderland, MA: Sinauer Associates for The National Foundation-March of Dimes, BD:OAS XI (1):343–344, 1975.
7. Buckley RH: Plasma therapy in immunodeficiency diseases. Am J Dis Child 124:376, 1972.
8. Barandun S, Kistler P, Jeunet F, Isliker H: Intravenous administration of human gamma globulin. Vox Sang 7:157, 1962.
9. Ochs HD, Buckley RH, Pirofsky B, Fischer SH, Rousell RH, Anderson CJ, Wedgwood RJ: Safety and patient acceptability of intravenous immune globulin in 10% maltose. Lancet 2:1158, 1980.
10. Koblet H, Barandun S, Diggelmann H: Turnover of standard-gamma globulin, pH-4-gamma globulin and pepsin desegregated gamma globulin and clinical implications. Vox Sang 13:93, 1967.
11. Sgouris JT: The preparation of plasmin treated immune serum globulin for intravenous use. Vox Sang 13:71, 1967.
12. Nolte MT, Pirofsky B, Gerritz GA, Golding B: Intravenous immunoglobulin therapy for antibody deficiency. Clin Exp Immunol 36:237, 1979.
13. Joller PW, Barandun S, Hitzig WH: Neue Möglichkeiten der Immunglobulin-Ersatz-Therapie bei Antikörpermangel-Syndrom. Schweiz Med Wochenschr 110:1451, 1980.
14. Kobayashi N, Gohya N, Matsumoto S: Clinical trial of sulfonated immunoglobulin preparation for intravenous administration. Eur J Pediatr 136:159, 1981.
15. van Furth R, Leijh PCJ: Functional interactions of various commercial gamma globulin preparations with Staphylococcus aureus and granulocytes. In "Immunochemotherapy." New York: Academic Press, 1981, p 181.
16. van Furth R: The role of macrophages in the immune process. This volume.
17. Fehr J, Hofmann V, Kappeler U: Transient reversal of thrombocytopenia in idiopathic thrombocytopenic purpura by high-dose intravenous gamma globulin. N Engl J Med 306:1254, 1982.
18. Berger M, Cupps TR, Fauci AS: Immunoglobulin replacement therapy by slow subcutaneous infusion. Ann Intern Med 93:55, 1980.
19. Roord JJ, van der Meer JWM, Kuis W, de Windt GE, Zegers BJM, van Furth R, Stoop JW: Home treatment in patients with antibody deficiency by slow subcutaneous infusion of gamma globulin. Lancet 1:689, 1982.
20. Ugazio AG, Duse M, Re R, Mangili G, Burgio GR: Subcutaneous infusion of gamma globulins in management of agammaglobulinaemia. Lancet 1:226, 1982.
21. Mease PJ, Ochs HD, Wedgwood RJ: Successful treatment of Echovirus meningoencephalitis and myositisfasciitis with intravenous immune globulin therapy in a patient with X-linked agammaglobulinemia. N Engl J Med 304:1278, 1980.

Epidemiology and Treatment of Hypogammaglobulinemia

C.S. Hosking, MD, FRACP, FRCPA, and D.M. Roberton, MD, FRACP

Department of Immunology, Royal Children's Hospital, Parkville, Victoria 3052, Australia

Since the description of hypogammaglobulinemia in childhood by Bruton, the delineation of disorders of immunoglobulin production has expanded to reveal a heterogeneous group of conditions with differing genetic implications and clinical manifestations. The clinically significant hypogammaglobulinemias of childhood are relatively rare, but cause major morbidity and mortality. In the absence of disease registers for specific populations the true incidence of these disorders is unknown.

The Clinical Immunology Unit of the Royal Children's Hospital, Melbourne, provides the only pediatric immunodiagnostic and treatment service for the state of Victoria, Australia. The state population is 3.9 million and the mean birth rate for the years 1970–1982 has been 58,000 births per year. From 1972 a comprehensive clinical and in vitro assessment has been provided for all children referred for investigation of recurrent persistent or unusual infections [1]. This has enabled assessment of the prevalence and incidence of classifiable major and minor immunodeficiency (ID) disorders in childhood according to the recommended WHO criteria [2].

PREVALENCE OF SYMPTOMATIC HYPOGAMMAGLOBULINEMIA

Excluding symptomatic IgA deficiency, 38 children have been found to have a classifiable disorder of immunoglobulin production in the population. Eighteen have had sex-linked agammaglobulinemia (SLA) (including 3 with elevated levels of IgM). Two children have had an isolated IgM deficiency, 4 a transient hypogammaglobulinemia of infancy, and 14 have had common variable ID with predominant hypogammaglobulinemia.

Five with SLA have died, all prior to 1976. One died of a pseudomonas septicemia at the time of diagnosis at age 2 years. One died at 6 years of age of cardiac failure secondary to chronic severe pulmonary disease; his affected brother died at 14 years of age, following a protracted dermatomyositis-like illness associated with an ECHO-8 viral encephalitis which was unresponsive to high dose intravenous gamma globulin and fresh frozen plasma. A 4th boy died at age 11 years following a dermatomyositis-like illness associated with a chronic hepatitis and encephalitis. No viral agent was isolated. The 5th death was a 5-year-old boy with hypogammaglobulinemia with elevated IgM. The cause of death was an interstitial pneumonitis of unknown etiology.

The surviving patients with SLA have had few problems with severe acute infections since 1976. The oldest survivor is 31 years of age. Six in late adolescence and early adult life have radiologic evidence of bronchiectasis, although only one has incapacitating recurrent illness. No patients have required admission to hospital in the last 6 years for bacterial infections sited outside the respiratory tract. No surviving patients have developed an arthropathy. However, most have minor-to-moderate chronic secretory otitis media, and several have required middle ear drainage procedures.

The hypogammaglobulinemic children with common variable ID have had a similar spectrum of illness. One has established and progressive bronchiectasis; one died of mediastinal lymphoma; several have recurrent otitis media.

INCIDENCE OF SYMPTOMATIC HYPOGAMMAGLOBULINEMIA

The incidence of diagnosed disorders of immunoglobulin production as defined by the WHO classification [2] has been calculated for children born in Victoria between January 1970 and June 1982 (Table 1). During this time, the commonest major classifiable ID disorder has been SCID (14 per million live births).

The overall incidence of significant symptomatic Ig deficiency was 1:11,000 live births. Most children in this category have had selective IgA deficiency, defined as absolute or partial deficiency (the latter characterized by unmeasurable levels by nephelometry and a trace only of protein detected by immunodiffusion) in children over the age of 6 months in association with significant recurrent symptomatic infection. The predominant features at presentation in children with absolute or partial IgA deficiency were recurrent upper and/or lower respiratory tract infections. Ten percent had recurrent skin infections and abscesses; 7% had an associated neutropenia. The true incidence of symptomatic IgA deficiency is almost certainly under-represented in this study, as

TABLE 1. Incidence of Diagnosed Immunodeficiency Disorders per Million Live Births, January 1970–June 1982, Victoria, Australia

Immunodeficiency Disorders	Incidence per 10^6 Live Births
SLA	7
SLA with elevated IgM	3
Common variable immunodeficiency (predominantly immunoglobulin)	12
Isolated IgM deficiency	1.5
Symptomatic absolute IgA deficiency	24
Symptomatic partial IgA deficiency	42

only children with significant recurrent symptomatic infection with normal results for phagocytic cell and lymphocyte function studies have been included. Many other children with relatively minor symptoms have been found to have absent or low levels of IgA, but these symptoms have not been of sufficient severity to justify more extended investigation.

The diagnosis of SLA has been made with a frequency of 10 per million live births. Three of these 10 have SLA with increased IgM levels. Common variable ID, predominantly immunoglobulin in nature, has been diagnosed with an incidence of 12 per million live births. In our population, the congenital X-linked and "acquired" hypogammaglobulinemic disorders have been found to have similar incidence in the first 12 years of life.

TREATMENT

Treatment of hypogammaglobulinemia was studied initially in the United Kingdom MRC trial, with the demonstration that intramuscular injections of gamma globulin offered significant protection from infections [3]. Intramuscular preparations have been used in our patients from 1964. These injections were of large volume in older children, were painful, and often required administration at weekly intervals to control susceptibility to infection.

An experimental IV preparation was prepared by Commonwealth Serum Laboratories and made available for use in 3 patients with hypogammaglobulinemia, and 3 patients with AT in 1968 [4,5]. Pooled human gamma globulin was treated at pH 4 in the presence of trace amounts of pepsin for 24 hours. The mean half-life following IV infusion of this preparation was 25 days [5].

Quantities of gamma globulin for IV use became more readily available in 1972, and since then IV gamma globulin has been used for all patients referred for management. In the last 5 years, pepsin digestion of the gamma globulin has been omitted. Thirty-four children have now received regular IV gamma globulin replacement therapy. Eight of these were children with SCID awaiting bone marrow transplantation. The remaining 26 have had predominantly immunoglobulin deficiency syndromes.

Currently, 18 children attend a day transfusion clinic at monthly intervals for treatment. Many had received treatment with the im preparation prior to referral. Without exception, the IV preparation has been the method of administration preferred by the patients. The amount given each month is 5–7.5 ml/kg of a 6% solution (300–450 mg/kg) after an initial loading dose of 10–15 ml/kg (600–900 mg/kg). IgG trough levels are maintained above 25 IU/ml (200 mg/dl) and are usually in the range 30–40 IU/ml (240–320 mg/dl). The median trough IgG level over a 12-month period in the treated children for 1981–82 was 37 IU/ml (297 mg/dl).

The clinical course of 14 boys with SLA is shown in Figure 1. Thirteen have received prolonged courses of treatment with IV gamma globulin; 5 have received *only* IV gamma globulin. Hospital admissions for acute infection have been less frequent with the use of the IV preparation since late 1975, when the dose administered was increased and regular outpatient infusion services became available. Since that time only 2 of 10 treated males have required hos-

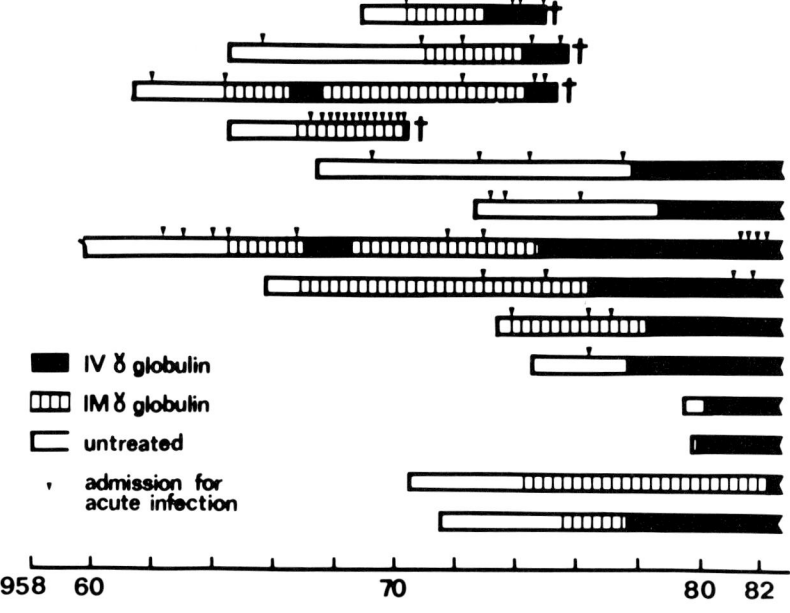

Fig. 1. Clinical course during treatment of 14 males with SLA.

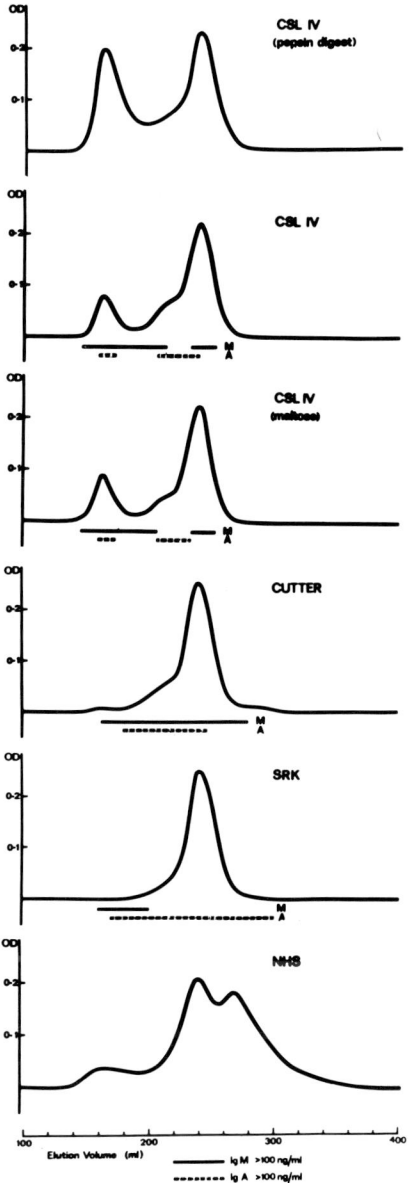

Fig. 2. Gel filtration of gamma globulin preparations through 98 × 2.5 cm column packed with Sephacryl S 300 and run in pH 7.4 Tris/HCl buffer.

pital admission for control of acute infections; these 2 are brothers with established bronchiectasis who have each had infective exacerbations of their lower respiratory tract disease.

Acute otitis media, otitis externa, and conjunctivitis have also become uncommon, as have other minor infections. No patients with SLA or common variable ID receiving IV gamma globulin since late 1975 have had significant infections of body tissues outside the respiratory tract. However, a mild purulent rhinitis and chronic secretory otitis media persist in several.

REACTIONS TO INTRAVENOUS GAMMA GLOBULIN

Early attempts at administration of gamma globulin by the intravenous route resulted in reports from other centers of reactions which were often severe and life-threatening [6]. These reactions were thought to be related to the complement fixing properties of the aggregated IgG present in the preparations [7]. Attempts have been made by several groups to prevent aggregation by incubation at low pH and/or enzyme digestion. Recently, other preparations have been used which have been treated by reduction or sulfonation, and which contain lower proportions of aggregated IgG and lower levels of anticomplementary activity [8,9].

Gel filtration results for CSL preparations and for the SRK and Cutter preparations are shown in Figure 2. The initial Commonwealth Serum Laboratories (CSL) pepsin digest available from 1972 contained large amounts of aggregated IgG when tested. Modifications of the preparative process in 1977 with the omission of pepsin digestion allowed a reduction in the amount of aggregate present. Treatment of this preparation with maltose did not alter significantly the proportion of aggregated IgG. The SRK preparation appears to contain no aggregate after reconstitution, and the Cutter IV gamma globulin has relatively little aggregate, most of which is probably dimeric. Each of the preparations was shown to contain trace amounts of IgA and IgM by ELISA assay. Some of the IgA was found in elution fractions suggestive of aggregation and some IgM eluted in positions which suggested it was present in trace amounts in monomeric and dimeric forms.

Two of 34 children have had reactions to the CSL preparations of sufficient severity to terminate further treatment. One child with SCID, who was awaiting transplantation, had a severe anaphylactic reaction to the pepsin-treated preparation. The second has common variable ID and had repeated severe reactions to both CSL preparations. He is now receiving regular subcutaneous infusions and is tolerating these without incident. A double-blind crossover trial of the maltose-treated preparation over an 8-month treatment period in 11 patients did not significantly alter the incidence or severity of reactions, although there was a trend toward less symptomatology with the treated preparations (Table 2). During this trial the incidence of reactions, almost always minor, was 50% with the standard preparation, and 35% with the maltose-treated preparation.

TABLE 2. Symptom Scores During Treatment With Maltose-Treated/Nonmaltose-Treated IV Gamma globulin (CSL)

Patients	Diagnosis	Nonmaltose-Treated IV Gamma globulin	Maltose-Treated IV Gamma globulin
1	SLA	1	0
2	CVI	2	2
3	CVI	0	1
4	SLA	4	3
5	SLA	2	0
6	SLA, IgM	2	2
7	CVI	4	3
8	SLA, IgM	5	8
9	SLA	3	1
10	CVI	5	0
11	CVI	9	6

Wilcoxon matched-pairs signed ranks test: not significant

The commonest reactions have been rigors and chest discomfort. These abate when the infusion is ceased for a few minutes and do not recur when the infusion is recommenced. The mechanism of reaction is unclear. Complement activation can be demonstrated by immunoelectrophoresis of EDTA-treated plasma samples followed by staining for C3 and its breakdown products in samples taken serially during infusion in children experiencing reactions. However, the appearance of complement conversion products does not coincide with the time of reaction, and complement conversion persists during the later asymptomatic period. During and following reactions, the direct and indirect Coombs tests are negative using anti-IgG, and anti-C3b, and no hemolysis of red cells is seen microscopically. However, the CSL IV preparations in vitro do cause agglutination of human group O, A, and B cells in the presence of patient serum, pooled human serum, and human serum albumin, but not in the presence of bovine serum albumin. Agglutination of group A and B cells was detected with the Cutter and SRK preparations, but group O cells were not agglutinated in vitro.

DISCUSSION

There is very little data available which allow determination of the incidence of hypogammaglobulinemic disorders in pediatric populations. Two recent studies from Sweden and Japan demonstrate that antibody deficiencies account for approximately half of all primary ID syndromes [10,11]. The study from Sweden described an incidence of SCID of 14 per million live births, identical to the figure described for our population in Victoria, Australia. In this same study, the prevalence in Sweden of congenital agammaglobulinemia (including hyper-IgM syndrome) was 8 per million children, for common variable ID 6 per million, and for symptomatic selective IgA deficiency 19 per million. The incidence figures for the Victorian population from 1970 to 1982 were 10 per million, 12 per million, and 66 per million, respectively. If only symptomatic absolute IgA deficiency were considered, this latter figure falls to 24 per million. The corresponding data from Japan have not been reported in sufficient detail to allow comparison for the pediatric population, but the reported prevalence in that community appears to be much lower. In our population, the overall incidence of symptomatic immunoglobulin deficiency disorders is 1:11,000 births, or 90 per million.

Our experience with the use of IV gamma globulin for the therapy of congenital agammaglobulinemia and common variable ID in childhood during a 10-year period has been similar to that reported by others with respect to patient acceptability [12, 13]. In the last 6 years, while using a higher dosage regimen, we have noted a decrease in morbidity from infection, in comparison with im treatment. This has been noted by others [14], particularly when using a dosage regimen giving more than 100 mg/kg/month.

Ammann et al [8] and Buckley [13] have demonstrated that treatment with the IV preparations was at least as good (apart from the incidence of URIs) as the use of im preparations at equivalent monthly dose rates. The median trough level of IgG in our patients has been maintained at higher levels than those reported by Buckley [13]. It is interesting to note that Magilavy et al [15], using plasmin-treated IV gamma globulin to maintain serum IgG levels above 250 mg/dl were able to achieve these levels by using 3 ml/kg of a 5.5% preparation (165 mg/kg) at 2–4 weekly intervals. Our own patients receive 300–450 mg/kg at 4-weekly intervals to maintain preinfusion levels of almost 300 mg/dl. The difference in dosage requirement may represent less frequent infusions, but could also be related to more rapid clearance of aggregated IgG in preparations such as ours, which contain considerable quantities of aggregate. However, Simons et al [5] found the half-life of an IV preparation containing large amounts of aggregate to still be 25 days. We suspect that higher doses may allow proportionately smaller incremental rises in trough IgG levels due to an increased catabolism.

At the higher dose, Magilavy et al [15] noted an improvement in morbidity from infection, but 3 patients developed chronic oligoarthritis and one developed Giardiasis while on treatment. None of our patients has developed either of these complications while on higher dose IV therapy in the last 6 years. In agreement with others [16], we are concerned that bronchiectasis still occurs and may become progressive. We have also found, as have others [14], that different patients require different dosage regimens to provide adequate trough IgG levels.

Success has been reported in the treatment of an Echovirus-related encephalopathic illness in an agammaglobulinemic patient with high dose IV gamma globulin [17]. Others have reported an arrest of progression of symptoms but persistence of virus excretion in the cerebrospinal fluid [13]. Asherson and Webster used immune animal serum with poor results in 2 of their 3 patients [18]. Our patient failed to respond to either high-dose IV gamma globulin or to plasma infusions.

Reactions to IV infusions occur in 50% of our patients, without a significant reduction in symptoms with the addition of maltose. Others have found a decrease in the incidence of reactions from 59% to 3% of infusions [12]. Certainly, the addition of maltose has not decreased the amount of aggregate in the CSL preparation used by us. We have also experienced a severe reaction in a patient with SCID; this has also been reported by others [19]. The nature of the reactions remains unclear. In our patients complement activation does occur, apparently independently of symptoms. In vitro agglutination of red cells of all groups is also seen, through mechanisms which remain to be elucidated. Subcutaneous infusions of gamma globulin offer benefits in patients experiencing reactions to IV preparations, and also may allow much higher maintenance serum IgG levels [20,21]. This approach requires further study.

ACKNOWLEDGMENTS

We are grateful for the assistance of Sr. M. Kent-Hughes, J. Hutchinson, E. Wakefield, J. Dix, M. Fitzgerald, M. Shelton, Dr. A. Pereira, and to the Commonwealth Serum Laboratories (CSL) for making the preparations available for trial.

REFERENCES

1. Hosking CS, Fitzgerald MG, Shelton MJ: The immunological investigations of children with recurrent infections. Aust Paediatr J 13 (Suppl):61–69, 1977.
2. World Health Organization: Immunodeficiency. Report of a WHO scientific group. Clin Immunol Immunopathol 13:296–359, 1979.
3. Medical Research Council Working-Party: Summary report: Hypogammaglobulinaemia in the United Kingdom. Lancet 1:163–168, 1969.
4. Schiff P, Sutherland SK, Lane WR: The preparation, testing, and properties of human gammaglobulin for intravenous administration. Aust Paediatr J 4:121–126, 1968.
5. Simons MJ, Schumacher MJ, Fowler R: Intravenous gammaglobulin therapy of immunoglobulin deficiency diseases. Aust Paediatr J 4:127–133, 1968.
6. Barundun S, Kistler P, Jeunet F, Isliker H: Intravenous administration of human γ-globulin. Vox Sang 7:157–174, 1962.
7. Ishizaka T, Ishizaka K, Borsos T: Biological activity of aggregated gammaglobulin. J Immunol 87::433–438, 1961.
8. Ammann AJ et al: Use of intravenous γ-globulin in antibody immunodeficiency: Results of a multicenter controlled trial. Clin Immunol Immunopathol 22:60–67, 1982.
9. Kobayashi N, Gohya N, Matsumoto S: Clinical trial of sulfonated immunoglobulin for intravenous administration. I. Replacement therapy for primary immunodeficiency syndromes. Eur J Pediatr 136:159–165, 1981.
10. Foster A: Primary immunodeficiency disorders in Sweden: Cases among children, 1974–1979. J Clin Immunol 2:86–92, 1982.
11. Nayakawa H, Iwata T, Yata J, Kobayashi N: Primary immunodeficiency syndrome in Japan I: Overview of a nationwide survey on primary immunodeficiency syndrome. J Clin Immunol 1:31–39,1981.
12. Ochs HD, Buckley RH, Pirofsky B, Fischer SH, Rousell RN, Anderson CJ, Wedgwood RJ: Safety and patient acceptability of intravenous immune globulin in 10% maltose. Lancet 2:1158–1159, 1980.
13. Buckley RH: Long-term use of intravenous immunoglobulin in patients with primary immunodeficiency diseases: Inadequacy of current dosage practices and approaches to the problem. J Clin Immunol 2 (Suppl):15S–20S, 1982.
14. Pirofsky B, Campbell SM, Montanaro A: Individual patient variations in the kinetics of intravenous immune globulin administration. J Clin Immunol 2 (Suppl):7S–11S, 1982.
15. Magilavy DB, Cassidy JT, Tubergen DG, Petty RE, Chisholm R, McCall K: Intravenous gammaglobulin in the management of patients with hypogammaglobulinaemia. J Allergy Clin Immunol 61:378–383, 1978.
16. Ochs HD, Fischer SH, Wedgwood RJ: Modified immune globulin: Its use in the prophylactic treatment of patients with immune deficiency. J Clin Immunol 2 (Suppl):22S–29S, 1982.
17. Mease PJ, Ochs HD, Wedgwood RJ: Successful treatment of Echovirus meningoencephalitis and myositis-fasciitis with intravenous immune globulin therapy in a patient with X-linked agammaglobulinaemia. N Engl J Med 304:1278–1281, 1981.
18. Asherson GL, Webster ADB: In "Sex-Linked Hypogammaglobulinaemia, in Diagnosis and Treatment of Immunodeficiency Diseases." London: Blackwell Scientific Publications, 1980, pp 7–36.
19. Matsumoto S, Kobayashi N, Gohya N: Clinical trials of sulfonated immunoglobulin preparation for intravenous administration: II; adverse reactions. Eur J Pediatr 136:167–171, 1981.
20. Ugazio AG, Duse M, Re R, Mangili G, Burgio GR: Subcutaneous infusion of gammaglobulins in management of agammaglobulinaemia. Lancet 1:226, 1982.
21. Roord JJ, van der Meer JWM, Kuis W, de Windt GE, Zegers BJM, van Furth R, Stoop JE: Home treatment in patients with antibody deficiency by slow subcutaneous infusion of gammaglobulin. Lancet 1:689–690, 1982.

Oral Administration of Secretory Immunoglobulin A and Its Clinical Significance*

Shuzo Matsumoto, MD, Tohru Watanabe, MD, Shunzo Chiba, MD, Wataru Abo, MD, and Tooru Nakao, MD

Department of Pediatrics, Hokkaido University School of Medicine, Sapporo, Japan (S.M., T.W.); Department of Pediatrics, Sapporo Medical College, Sapporo, Japan (S.C., W.A., T.N.)

INTRODUCTION

Secretory IgA antibodies are believed to comprise an important defense mechanism against local infections of the mucous membranes [1] of the body. In man, perhaps related to the presence of the covalent linkage between the secretory pieces and the majority of other molecules, there appears to be significant resistance of a large part of the secretory IgA (S-IgA) molecules to proteolysis as compared to their serum counterpart [2–5]. This resistance could be of some benefit both in regard to mucosal transport, and also in the exertion of its biologic function in fluids which contain proteolytic enzymes, although this thesis is still speculative. The manner in which the IgA antibody molecule exerts its biologic function is also not entirely clear. It has been well shown in viruses that S-IgA inhibits growth. While the role of secretory antibodies in aiding resistance of the GI tract to certain enteroviruses seems well established, efficacy of its replacement therapy in patients with certain kinds of immunodeficiency has not been adequately evaluated at the present time.

We have applied orally purified S-IgA as a form of replacement therapy in 2 patients with immunodeficiency disease who lack an IgA system. In the first patient, an infant with SCID with no histocompatible sibs, S-IgA was applied in an attempt to manage intractable diarrhea and weight loss. The second patient was a boy with congenital agammaglobulinemia [6] who developed paralytic poliomyelitis 18 months after an inadvertent second administration of polio vaccine. Although paralysis was not progressive, the patient continued to excrete type 2 polioviruses for more than 2 years after the onset of paralysis. Oral administration of S-IgA was used in an attempt to terminate the persistent replication and excretion of the virus in the gut. The results of the use of S-IgA in these patients are reported here in comparison with those of using enteric-coated or noncoated serum IgA, or breast milk alone.

IgA PREPARATIONS USED IN THE STUDY

Secretory IgA

S-IgA was prepared from normal human colostrum and breast milk in the first puerperal month by the method of Tomasi et al, with a slight modification [7]. Whey was prepared from the pooled colostrum, transitional milk, and breast milk within a month after delivery by centrifuge at 20,000 rev/min for 2 hours to remove fat, then acidified to pH 4.6 with 1 N acetic acid to precipitate casein. The prepared whey was chromatographed on a DEAE cellulose column by stepwise elution using 2 Na-phosphate buffers of a) 0.01M, pH 7.6, and b) 0.1M, pH 6.4. The fraction containing IgA was concentrated and applied to gel filtration of Sephadex G-200 with a 0.05 Tris-HCl buffer, pH 8.0, containing 1M NaCl. The fraction of the first peak containing the S-IgA was rechromatographed on the same Sephadex column, dialyzed exhaustively against 0.9% NaCl as described in Figure 1, and its concentration was adjusted to 25 mg/ml. After filtration through a millipore membrane, it was stored frozen at −20°C until used.

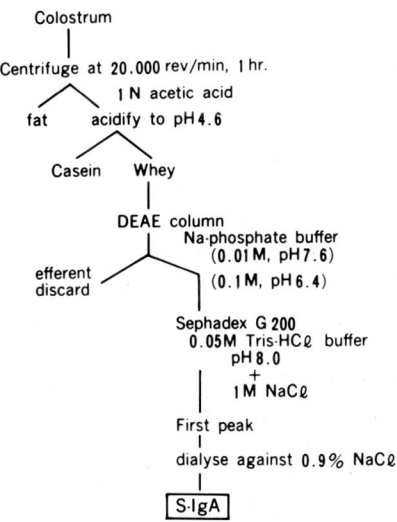

Fig. 1. Method of preparation of secretory IgA.

Serum IgA

IgA-rich human serum globulins were prepared by the laboratory of Green Cross Pharmaceutical Company, Osaka. IgA content was more than 45% of their total protein constituents. The preparation was used in the original solution or in the form

*This work was supported in part by research grants for immunodeficiency diseases from the Ministry of Health and Welfare of Japan.

of enteric-coated pellets (diameter of the particles was 0.8 mm). One gram of the IgA-rich serum globulin in an enteric-coated pellet contained 50 mg of serum IgA.

Colostrum

It was obtained from breast milk of healthy mothers within 7 days after delivery and stored frozen.

CASE REPORTS

Patient A

Male, 11 months old: SCID with B lymphocytes. The patient showed no abnormalities during his first 4 months of life except poor weight gain. At 5 months of age his weight was 3,600 gm (birthweight: 3,200 gm), and intermittent diarrhea developed. Upon admittance into Hokkaido University Hospital, he was in an advanced state of malnutrition. The patient was given milk without lactose or modular formula for 3 weeks, but the diarrhea was not improved. He had no palpable lymph nodes or tonsillar tissue, and the absolute lymphocyte counts ranged from 400 to 1,000/mm^3. T cells (E rosette-forming cells [E-RFC]) and B cells (lymphocytes with membrane-bound Ig) were 5% and 36.2%, respectively. Serum level of IgG was 135 mg/dl, IgM was 20 mg/dl, and IgA was not detectable. Lymphocyte response in vitro was negative to both PHA and PPD. When stimulated with allogeneic cells in one-way MLC, the stimulation index of the patient's lymphocytes was 1.7. ADA and PNP were present in the erythrocytes in normal amounts.

Based on the above results, the patient was diagnosed as having SCID with B lymphocytes. However, as his diarrhea was unresponsive to any treatment, complete IV hyperalimentation was conducted from 6 months of age to prevent further loss of body weight, and continued for a 7-month period. In spite of the IV feedings, the diarrhea was not improved at all. Specific pathogenic bacterias were not detected by cultures of fecal specimens. By negative-contrast stain electron microscopy, a large number of small round virus particles, as shown in Figure 2, were seen in the supernatant of the feces. These, however, were not identified as any of the known etiologic viral agents associated with gastroenteritis.

As the search for an HLA identical and/or MLC nonreactive donor was unsuccessful, transplantations of fetal liver cells and fetal thymus were tried twice, but they failed to engraft. As the patient's weight was 3,300 gm at 11 months of age and the chronic diarrhea was still uncontrollable, treatment of the IgA preparations by oral administration was considered as a last resort.

Evaluation of the antidiarrheal effect of the oral administrations of S-IgA or other IgA preparations was made by noting increases of body weight and urine volume, and decreases in the number of times of stool elimination, and stool weight. During IgA treatment, the patient fasted under IV hyperalimentation and was not administered any other antidiarrheal drug. IgA-rich human serum globulin in the enteric-coated pellet was given first by mouth, 3 times a day. Daily dose of the enteric-coated IgA was 100 mg/day as pure serum IgA. This treatment seemed to be effective in controlling the persistent diarrhea, as shown in Figure 3, but no beneficial effect was seen during the second period of administration of the same preparation at the same dose (Fig. 4). Noncoated serum IgA of the same dose had no effect at all as seen in Figure 5. During the period of colostrum administration (Fig. 4: 40 ml/day), the patient's diarrhea worsened and his body weight decreased.

S-IgA, on the other hand, worked effectively to control diarrhea after each administration. The first period of S-IgA (150 mg/day) treatment is shown in Figure 4 and the second and third periods (100-50 mg/day) in Figure 5. During all of these periods, the times of stool elimination and stool weight decreased with an increase of urine volume. But, as seen in Figure 5, when the dosage of S-IgA was reduced to as little as 25 mg/day, the diarrhea reappeared.

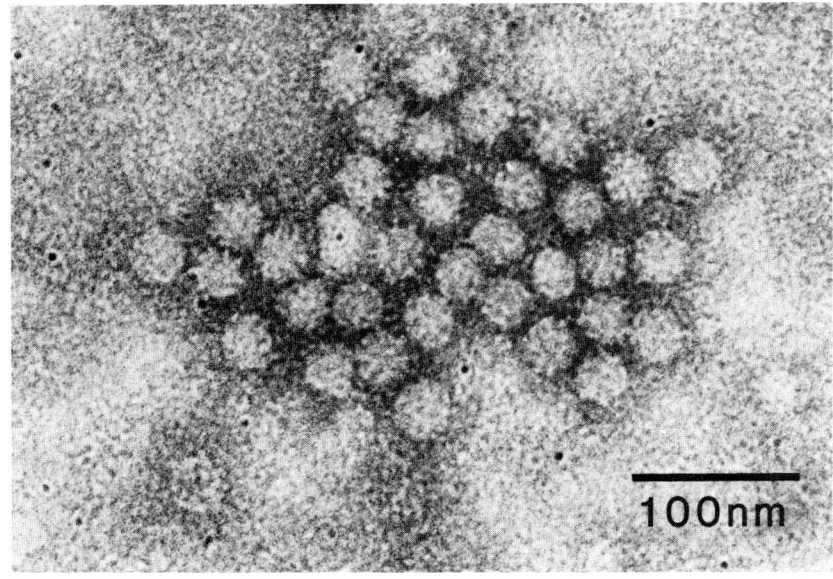

Fig. 2. A large number of small round virus particles in the supernatant of the feces of *Patient A*. (Negative-contrast stain electron microscopy).

Patient B

Male, 4 years old: Congenital agammaglobulinemia with paralytic poliomyelitis. The patient had no sibs, and there was nothing unusual in the family history. He appeared to be well before one year of age, but episodes of infections such as otitis media, URI, and diarrhea began between the period of 1 and 2 years. At the age of 2 years, the boy was admitted to Sapporo Medical College Hospital and a diagnosis of agammaglobulinemia was made. Although he had no serum immunoglobulins (IgG and IgA were undetectable, IgM 10 mg/dl), and no surface Ig+ cells were detected, there were an abnormal number of T cells and EAC rosette-forming cells. The patient subsequently received replacement therapy with S-sulfonated immune serum globulin (ISG) (100 mg/kg/3-4 weeks) with good results. At the age of 2 years, 10 months, he developed serous meningitis, followed by paralysis in his left arm and right leg, at which time poliovirus type 2 was isolated from the stool. His past history revealed that he had received 2 doses of trivalent oral polio vaccine at 5 and 16 months of age. Type 2 poliovirus was also isolated from a stool specimen tested at age 22 months (1 year before the onset of paralysis). The strain of these polioviruses was classified as nonvaccine-like type 2, based on the results of the Wecker and McBride tests [6]. It was concluded that the nonvaccine-like virus was derived from the Sabin vaccine by antigenic variation that occurred during long-term multiplication in the intestinal tract of the patient, who obviously possessed an immunodeficiency [8]. The patient excreted type 2 poliovirus as long as 1 year and 5 months after the onset of paralysis. As continuation of fecal excretion of the virulent virus raised the possibility of a serious public health problem, oral use of IgA preparations was considered.

Oral administration of enteric-coated IgA-rich human serum globulin (100 mg serum IgA/day) was tried for 5 days, 1½ years after the onset of paralysis (Fig. 6). Neutralizing antibodies against the type 2 poliovirus contained in a 10% solution of the IgA-rich serum globulin were 128 units/0.25 ml. Subsequently, 300 ml of transitional breast milk were given for 7 days. These attempts, however, failed to halt the fecal shedding of the virus (Fig. 6).

Next, purified S-IgA (Fig. 1) was administered orally (150 mg S-IgA/day) for 7 days (Figs. 6 and 7). This 5% preparation contained neutralizing antipolio type 2 antibodies of 6 U/0.25 ml. Type 2 poliovirus was isolated from all of the 14 stools collected within 54 days after S-IgA treatment, but its collection was negative for the first time in the stool at 69 days after S-IgA use. The virus has not been isolated during the follow-up period of about 2½ years. Although the amount of virus excreted in the stool was $10^{4.2}$ PFU/ml in a 10% suspension at 20 days after the therapy, it was markedly reduced to $10^{2.5}$–$10^{3.0}$ PFU/ml at 30 days after therapy. Fecal shedding of the virus ceased completely between 54 and 69 days after the treatment.

DISCUSSION

SCID is an immunodeficiency that manifests itself in serious vulnerability to infection caused by congenital functional defects of T and B cells [9]. In many cases, the onset occurs within 3 months after birth with fever, respiratory infection, diarrhea

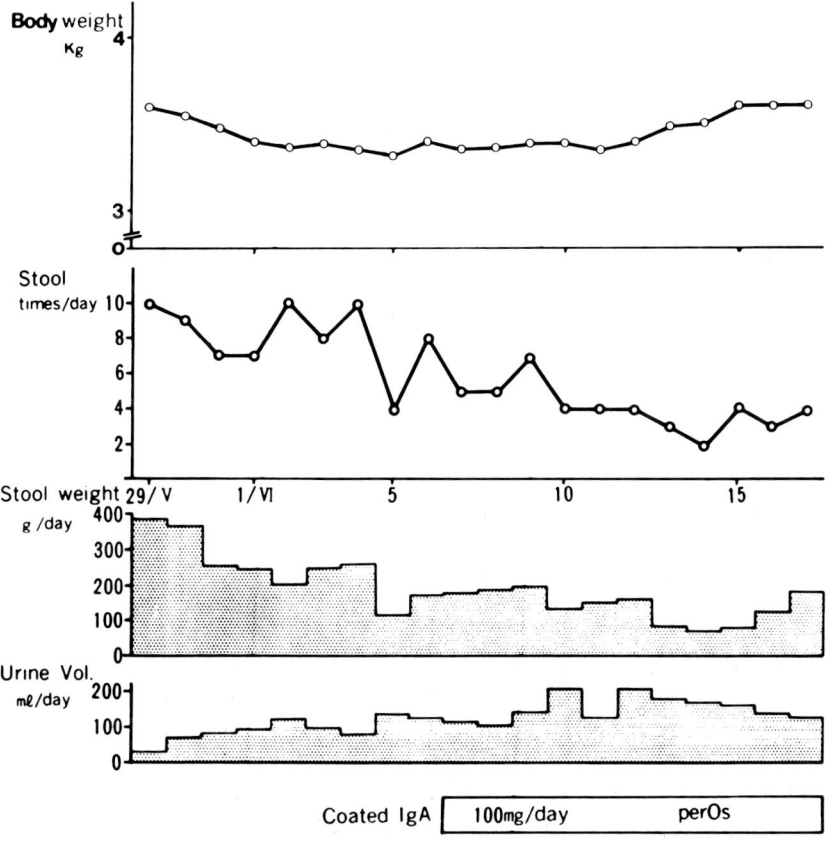

Fig. 3. Clinical response of *Patient A* to oral administration of enteric-coated preparations of IgA-rich human serum globulin, which was given 3 times a day (daily dose: 100 mg as pure serum IgA) for 11 days. Between the 4th and 8th day of administration, this treatment seemed to be effective in controlling the persistent diarrhea, but after the 9th day of administration, the diarrhea worsened again.

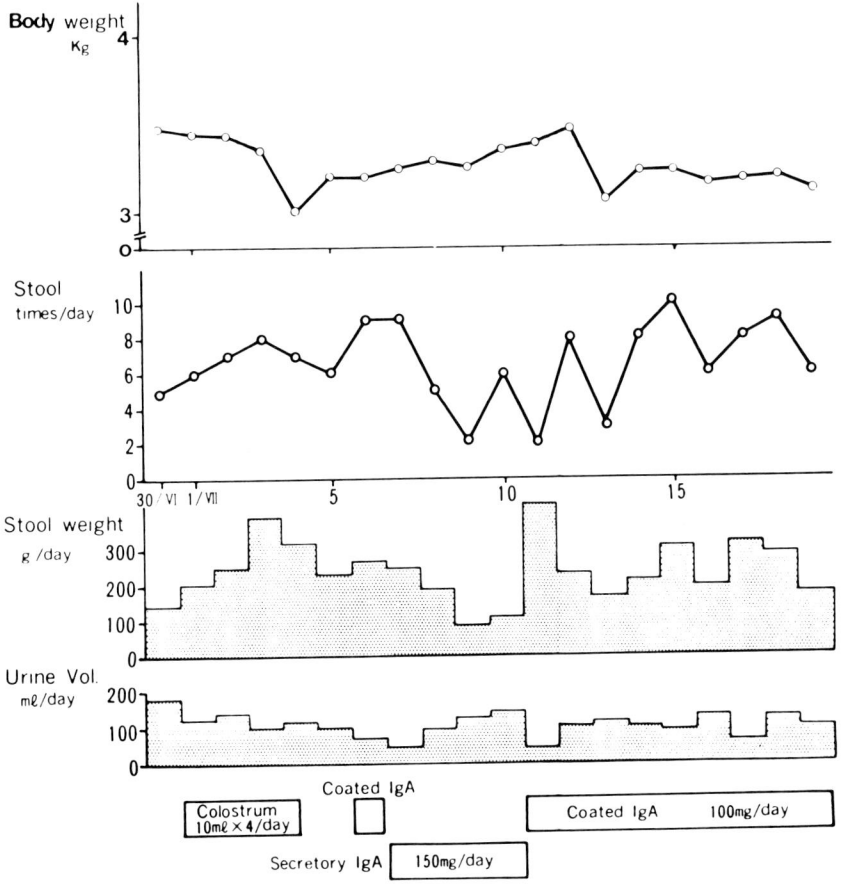

Fig. 4. Clinical response of *Patient A* to oral administration of colostrum, enteric-coated serum IgA and secretory IgA. During colostrum administration, the patient's diarrhea worsened and his body weight decreased. No beneficial effect was seen during the second and third periods of administration of IgA-rich human serum globulin by the enteric-coated pellet. On the other hand, administration of S-IgA (150 mg/day) was effective in controlling the diarrhea. Body weight and urine volume increased and frequency of diarrhea and weight of stool decreased during the 4 days of treatment.

and other digestive tract symptoms, along with thrush or other infections. If not properly treated, death usually occurs before the victim reaches the age of one year. In some cases total normal immunity was obtained through such radical therapy as transplantation of bone marrow, fetal liver stem cells, and fetal thymus glands which have been reported in recent years [10,11]. More than half of all SCID cases, however, present symptoms of intractable diarrhea, for which administration of antidiarrheals and antibiotics is ineffective. As a result, such patients often develop severe malnutrition. For this reason, management of nutrition and alleviation of diarrhea during the period prior to undertaking the aforementioned radical therapy often become important issues. The experimental oral administration of S-IgA reported in this study brought about marked improvement of the diarrhea symptoms in this disorder.

S-IgA plays an important role in local immunity and is known to possess antibody activities, such as agglutinating and neutralizing capacity against various viruses, bacterias and toxins [12, 13]. The activities of S-IgA on the surface of the intestinal mucosa can be illustrated, as shown in Figure 8. S-IgA present within the intestinal canal forms complexes with the majority of pathogenic microorganisms invading the GI tract, and thus results in their excretion [14]. It is assumed that S-IgA within the mucin layer, which covers the mucous surface layer, acts against invaders near the mucous surface to create a state of aggregation immediately, and thus prevents the infection from spreading to the epithelial layer [14,15]. It is also assumed that the S-IgA in the intestinal canal and in the mucin layer acts according to a similar mechanism in preventing sensitization by the organism or the high-molecular-weight antigens taken by mouth [16-19]. In the cases presented herein, antibiotics were ineffective for the treatment of diarrhea of the SCID patients, stool cultures failed to isolate specific pathogenic bacteria, and no improvement of symptoms was noted, even when oral intake of nutrition was totally discontinued. Futhermore, electron microscopic examination of the stools revealed a large amount of small round viruses (Fig. 2). These findings indicate the strong possibility that the diarrhea was induced by viral infection.

Barnes et al [20] recently reported that oral intake of human gamma globulin containing rotavirus antibodies modified the course of infection and disease caused by rotavirus in low-birthweight babies by delaying excretion of rotavirus, and slightly reducing the duration and quantity of rotavirus excretion. As symptoms of infection were also milder than in the placebo group, it appeared that oral administration of ISG was effective in protecting low-birthweight infants from diarrhea caused by rotavirus.

Rapid degradation of IgG in the GI tract is considered to be a cause of gamma globulin ineffectiveness. However, Snodgrass et al demonstrated [21] that, given orally, gamma globulin was an effective treatment in rotavirus-infected lambs, and Blum et al [22] recently demonstrated that human ISG retains activity after passage through the GI tract of low-birthweight infants. This phenome-

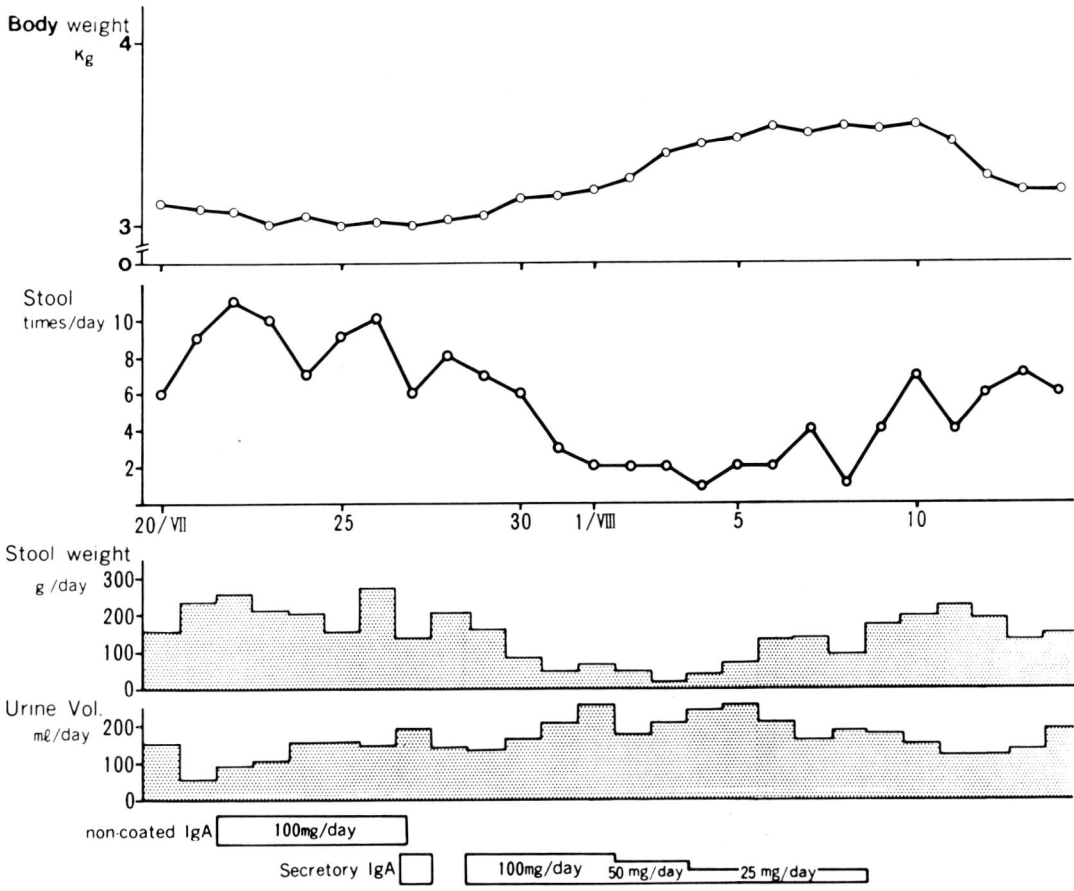

Fig. 5. Clinical response of *Patient A* to oral administration of noncoated serum IgA and secretory IgA in 3 different doses. Noncoated serum IgA (100 mg/day) showed no effect at all. However, during the second and third administrations of 100 mg or 50 mg/day of S-IgA, frequency of diarrhea and stool weight decreased, and body weight and urine volume increased. When the dosage of S-IgA was reduced to as little as 25 mg/day, the diarrhea reappeared.

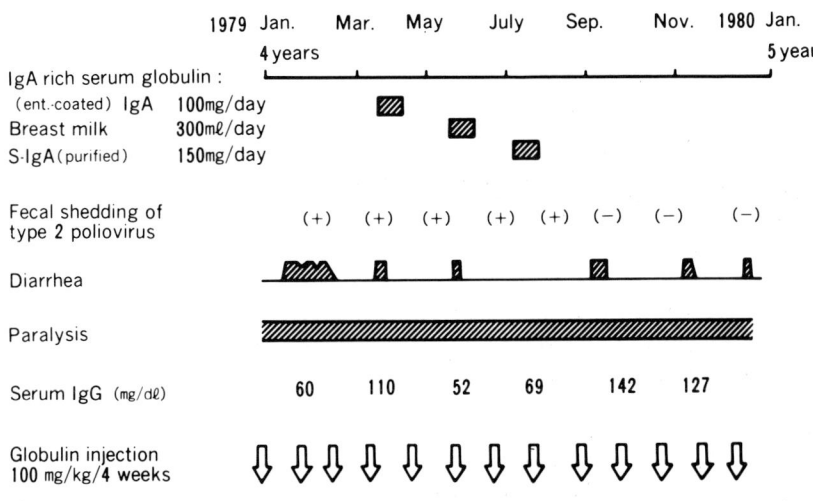

Fig. 6. Relationship between administrations of IgA preparations and fecal shedding of type 2 poliovirus in *Patient B*.

non is observed usually in newborn infants. However, in our 11-month-old patient, while the antidiarrheal effects of S-IgA as well as the stability of its effects were apparent, the efficacy was not clear in most periods in which serum IgA was employed. S-IgA is not readily broken down, and its activity is also not easily lost, even when it encounters digestive enzymes [3,4]. This assumption is verified by the fact that while nonenteric-coated serum IgA, which was also administered, was totally ineffective, S-IgA always showed stable efficacy.

The exact reason why S-IgA was markedly effective against diarrhea is not known; however, considering that a large number of small round virus particles were found in the stools of patients to whom S-IgA was being administered orally as observed by electron microscopy, the possibility that the agglutination capacity of S-IgA [23] effectively acted against the viral infection of the intestines and thus achieved the ability to improve the inflammation of the intestines, can be assumed. The possibility also exists that S-IgA demonstrated more stable effects than enteric-coated serum IgA due to the higher agglutination capacity of S-IgA than that of serum IgA.

The antidiarrheal effects of S-IgA disappeared immediately after discontinuation of the administration, and the diarrhea became aggravated. This finding suggests that the effects of orally administered S-IgA are limited to the intestinal mucosa. S-IgA is synthesized within the epithelial cells of the intestine from IgA produced in the plasma cells under the intestinal mucosa, and is secreted onto the surface of the mucosa [18]. It is believed to exhibit local immune activity also during the process of its production and secretion. Although orally ad-

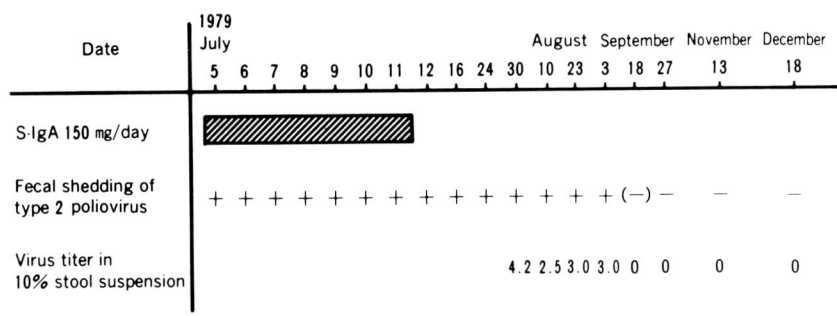

Fig. 7. Change in the amount of type 2 poliovirus excreted in the stool of *Patient B* after S-IgA treatment.

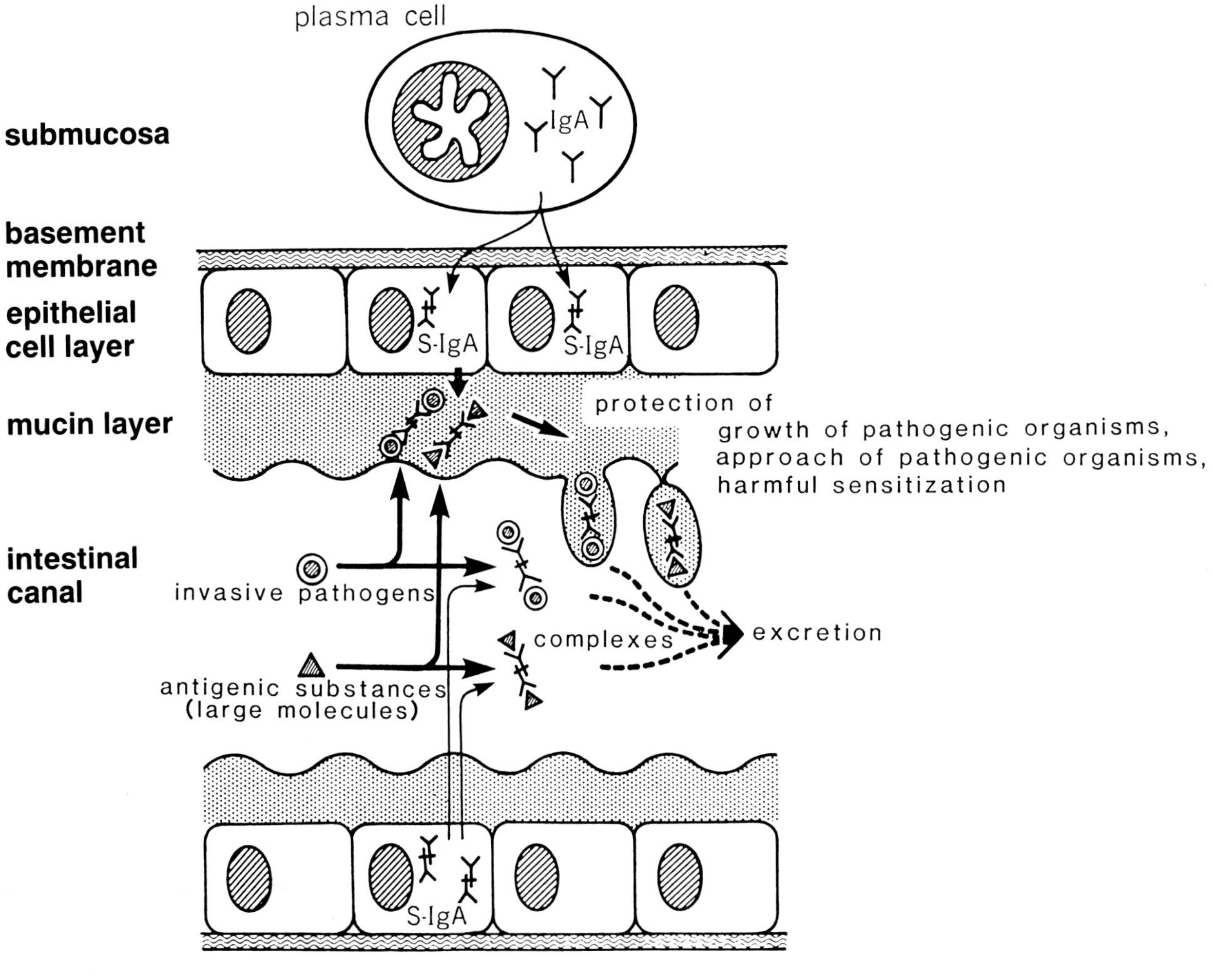

Fig. 8. The supposed activities of S-IgA on the surface of the intestinal mucosa.

ministered S-IgA may not extend its effects into the intestinal mucosa, it is believed to contribute to local immunity in the area above the mucous epithelium, with an efficacy similar to that of S-IgA produced and secreted physiologically in vivo. The antidiarrheal effects of orally administered S-IgA thus appear to be related to one of the above-mentioned factors.

Thus considered, oral administration of S-IgA is highly useful as a replacement therapy for various immunodeficiencies manifesting reduced secretion of S-IgA. It is particularly valuable in the treatment of intractable diarrhea found in patients with these immunodeficiencies, and moreover, when administered at an early stage, it appears to aid in the prevention of such diarrhea.

On the other hand, colostrum, which contains a large amount of S-IgA, had no antidiarrheal effect. On the contrary, it aggravated the diarrhea. This result is believed to have been caused by lactose intolerance which developed secondarily because of the persistent diarrhea. Therefore, it is necessary to administer isolated S-IgA when intractable diarrhea is treated with the intention of assisting the local immunity.

Intravenous hyperalimentation should probably be undertaken if the patient suffers from severe malnutrition due to prolonged diarrhea, as in the case of *Patient A* in the present report. The table of nutrients by Dudrick [24] and Nelson [25] is usually referred to in adjusting the contents of nutrient fluid. The authors prepared this fluid on the basis of Nelson's suggestions and had no problems with the adjustments. The silicone-type catheter was inserted from the great saphenous vein, the femoral vein, or the subclavian vein, to the superior or inferior vena cava. Changes in the flow rate were minimized by using a transfusion pump.

It is well known that local immunity mediated by the secretory antibody response in the alimentary tract plays an important role in the defense mechanism of the body against poliovirus infection [26]. Experiments by Ogra [26] indicate that the presence of neutralizing antibody in the secretions of the intestine is associated with eradication of the infection and resistance to reinfection with poliovirus. In fact, agammaglobulinemic patients [27] have been reported to experience paralytic poliovirus infections caused by wild strain viruses; furthermore, 2 reports [28, 29] have suggested that hypogammaglobulinemic patients may experience paralytic poliomyelitis caused by vaccine-derived strains. Wyatt [30] suggested that patients with hypogammaglobulinemia constitute about 9% of vaccine-associated poliomyelitis. On the other hand, Lopez and co-workers [31] reported 4 patients with SCID who developed nonparalytic poliovirus infection after immunization with oral polio vaccine, and demonstrated that persistent intestinal poliovirus infection frequently develops in patients with CID by routine immunization. Two of these patients stopped excreting poliovirus in their stools shortly after the first evidence of acceptance of the immunocompetent cells by allogeneic BMT. This observation indicates that CMI might play an important role in the eradication of intestinal poliovirus infections. In general, CMI and infection must also be considered to play a possible role in the defense against intestinal virus infections, in addition to local secretory immunity.

In our *Patient B*, however, deficiency of the IgA system may be essentially responsible for the reversion of the type 2 vaccine virus to a virulent virus during its extensive replication and persistence in the intestinal tract for a few years [8].

The mass polio vaccine of children in the susceptible age group in Japan, started in 1962, was believed to have eliminated the possibility of infection by wild poliovirus during the past 20 years [6]. Therefore, the occurrence of persistent fecal shedding of the virulent poliovirus in *Patient B* presented a potentially serious public health problem. Consequently, in order to disrupt the cycle of viral replication in the intestinal mucosa, oral administration of the purified S-IgA containing neutralizing antibody against type 2 poliovirus was conducted.

The cessation of fecal poliovirus shedding 2 months after local treatment with S-IgA could be simply coincidental. However, the following 2 points may provide evidence that this immunologic treatment had a favorable effect on the chronic poliovirus infection in this patient: 1) the fecal shedding of type 2 poliovirus, which had continued for almost 2 years after the onset of paralysis, and for more than 3 or 4 years after the second or first polio vaccination, was stopped as early as 2 months after the start of treatment; and 2) immunologically competent patients with poliomyelitis frequently shed poliovirus for 2 months [32]. Weiner et al [33] reported a case of chronic echovirus type 5 encephalitis in a hypogammaglobulinemic patient in whom the IV administration of hyperimmune plasma improved the neurologic status and eliminated detectable virus from the blood and cerebrospinal fluid. In our patient, ordinary replacement therapy of ISG continued for more than 2 years before S-IgA treatment was begun, but it had no effect on excretion of the poliovirus. After the oral administration of S-IgA, the virus population was changed to a dramatic degree, and type 2 poliovirus became undetectable. The disappearance of the virus may be due to some effect of S-IgA; however, this assumption cannot be proven at the present time, because it took about 60 days before the virus shedding finally ceased.

In conclusion, oral administration of S-IgA might be useful as a part of replacement therapy in various types of immunodeficiencies associated with reduced secretion of S-IgA, especially in the management of persistent infection of enteroviruses.

CONCLUSIONS

1) Oral administration of secretory IgA (S-IgA) may be effective in the control of intractable diarrhea complicated by the lack of a functional IgA system in some patients.

2) In the cases examined herein, enteric coating was not essential to obtain the effects of S-IgA, the appropriate dose of which was considered to be 50–150 mg/day for infants.

3) Possibly S-IgA administered orally has some effect on persistent intestinal infection of poliovirus which develops accidentally in patients with immunodeficiency.

ACKNOWLEDGMENTS

We are indebted to Dr. K. Kobayashi (University of Yamaguchi) for collaboration and advice in preparation of secretory IgA, to Dr. K. Horino (Teishin Hospital, Sapporo) for electron microscopic examination of virus particles in the stool of *Patient A*, and to Dr. M. Hara (Department of Enteroviruses, National Institute of Health, Tokyo) who kindly performed the virologic investigation of *Patient B*.

REFERENCES

1. Dayton DH Jr, Small PA Jr, Tomasi TB Jr et al: "The Secretory Immunologic System." National Inst Child Health and Hum Dev, Bethesda. Washington: U.S. Government Printing Office, 1971.
2. Brown WR, Newcomb RW, Ishizaka K: Proteolytic degradation of exocrine and serum immunoglobulins. J Clin Invest 49:1374–1380, 1970.
3. Shim BS, Kang YS, Kim WJ et al: Self-protective activity of colostral IgA against tryptic digestion. Nature 222:787, 1969.
4. Tomasi TB Jr, Czerwinski DS: The secretory IgA system. In Bergsma D, Good RA (eds): "Immunologic Deficiency Diseases in Man." New York: The National Foundation - March of Dimes, BD:OAS IV(1):270–282, 1968.
5. Lawton AR: Proteolytic fragments of rabbit colostral IgA. Supra #1, pp 55–70.
6. Abo W, Chiba S, Yamanaka T et al: Paralytic poliomyelitis in a child with agammaglobulinemia. Eur J Pediatr 132:11–16, 1979.
7. Kobayashi K: Studies on human secretory IgA comparative studies of the IgA-bound secretory piece and the free secretory piece protein. Immunochemistry 8:785–800, 1971.
8. Yoneyama T, Hagiwara A, Hara M et al: Alteration in oligonucleotide fingerprint patterns of the viral genome in poliovirus type 2 isolated from paralytic patients. Infect Immun 37:46–53, 1982.
9. Asherson GL, Webster ADB: "Diagnosis and Treatment of Immunodeficiency Diseases." Oxford, London: Blackwell Scientific Publications, 1980, pp 157–174.
10. Advisory Committee of the International Bone Marrow Transplant Registry (Bortin MM, Rimm AA): Severe combined immunodeficiency disease. JAMA 238:591–600, 1977.
11. Kenny AB, Hitzig WH: Bone marrow transplantation for severe combined immunodeficiency disease. Reported from 1968 to 1977. Eur J Pediatr 131:155–177, 1979.
12. Goldman AS, Smith CW: Host resistance factors in human milk. J Pediatr 82:1082–1090, 1973.
13. Walker WA: Antigen absorption from the small intestine and gastrointestinal disease. Pediatr Clin North Am 22:731–746, 1975.
14. Gibbons RJ: Bacterial adherence of mucosal surface and its inhibition by secretory antibodies. Adv Exp Med Biol 45:315–325, 1974.
15. Williams RC, Gibbons RJ: Inhibition of bacterial adherence by secretory immunoglobulin A: A mechanism of antigen disposal. Science 177:697–699, 1972.
16. Brandtzaeg P, Fjellanger I, Gjeruldsen ST: Adsorption of immunoglobulin A onto oral bacteria in vivo. J Bacteriol 96:242–249, 1968.
17. Walker WA, Isselbacher KJ, Bloch KJ: The role of immunization in controlling antigen uptake from the small intestine. Adv Exp Med Biol 45:295–283, 1974.
18. Bienenstock J: The physiology of the local immune response and the gastrointestinal tract. In Brent L, Holborow J (eds): "Progress in Immunology II." Amsterdam: North Holland Publishing Co, 1974, vol 4, pp 197–208.
19. Buckley RH, Dees SC: Correlation of milk precipitins with IgA deficiency. N Engl J Med 281:465–469, 1969.
20. Barnes GL, Doyle LW, Hewson PH et al: A randomised trial of oral gamma-globulin in low-birth-weight infants infected with rotavirus. Lancet 1:1371–1373, 1982.
21. Snodgrass DR, Madeley CR, Wells PW et al: Human rotavirus in lambs: Infection and passive protection. Infect Immun 16:268–270, 1966.
22. Blum PM, Phelps DL, Ank BJ et al: Survival of oral human immune serum globulin in the gastrointestinal tract of low birth weight infants. Pediatr Res 15:1256–1260, 1981.
23. Newcomb RW, DeVald BL: Protein concentrations in sputa from asthmatic children. Albumin, lactoferrin, γA and G. J Lab Clin Med 73:734–743, 1969.
24. Dudrick SJ: General principles and technique of administration in complete parenteral nutrition. In Wilkinson AW (ed): "Parenteral Nutrition." Edinburgh: Churchill and Livingstone, 1972, 222 pp.
25. Nelson R: Parenteral nutrition. In McLaren DS, Burman D (eds): "Textbook of Pediatric Nutrition." Edinburgh: Churchill and Livingstone, 1976, 221 pp.
26. Ogra PL: The secretory immunoglobulin system of the gastrointestinal tract. Supra #1, pp 259–279.
27. South MA, Figueroa M, Rossen R et al: The biologic significance of IgA in mucous secretions: Response to oral polio vaccine in IgA deficient subjects, protides of the biological fluids. "Proceedings of the Sixteenth Colloquium." New York: Pergamon Press, 1969, pp 315–318.
28. Changs T, Weinstein L, MacMahon HE: Paralytic poliomyelitis in a child with hypogamma-globulinemia: Probable implication of type I vaccine strain. Pediatrics 37:630–636, 1966.
29. Feigin RD, Guggenheim MA, Johnson SD: Vaccine-related paralytic poliomyelitis in an immunodeficient child. J Pediatr 79:642–647, 1971.
30. Wyatt HV: Poliomyelitis in hypogammaglobulinemics. J Infect Dis 128:802–806, 1973.
31. Lopez C, Biggar WD, Park BH et al:

Nonparalytic poliovirus infections in patients with severe combined immunodeficiency disease. J Pediatr 84:497–502, 1974.
32. Krugman S, Katz SL: Enteroviral infections. In "Infectious Diseases of Children," 7th Ed. St. Louis, London: Mosby Co, 1981, pp 35–56.
33. Weiner LS, Howell JT, Langford MP et al: Effect of specific antibodies on chronic echovirus type 5 encephalitis in a patient with hypogammaglobulinemia. J Infect Dis 140:858–863, 1979.

Dietary Protein Antigenemia in Hypogammaglobulinemia: Relationship to Splenomegaly*

Charlotte Cunningham-Rundles, MD, PhD, Ronald I. Carr, MD, PhD, and Robert A. Good, MD, PhD

Memorial Sloan-Kettering Cancer Institute, New York, NY 10021 (C.C.-R.), National Jewish Hospital, Denver CO 80206 (R.I.C.), Oklahoma Medical Research Foundation, Oklahoma City, OK 73104 (R.A.G.)

INTRODUCTION

In neonates, the epithelial cells of the immature GI tract display an extensive capacity for pinocytosis which results in a substantially greater absorption of a range of macromolecules than can be normally demonstrated for older infants and adults [1,2]. However, other factors besides immaturity can result in excessive GI absorption of luminal antigens. Examples of these factors are a variety of mucosal lesions [3], allergy [4], and selective IgA deficiency [5]. Because IgG and IgM antibody responses are usually normal in these latter conditions, the excess absorption which occurs under these circumstances can result in the periodic circulation of antigen-antibody complexes [3–5]. In the present studies, we have quantitated the amounts of bovine food protein which is present in the sera of patients with panhypogammaglobulinemia and agammaglobulinemia. These individuals are not only IgA deficient, but also do not produce the antibody necessary for immune complex formation; this study investigates the possibility that the presence of such foreign proteins could be linked to specific clinical or laboratory observations.

*This work was aided by grants from the USPH-AI-18509, CA-19267, CA-29502, The American Cancer Society Grant, ACS-IM-245, and the Zelda R. Weintraub Cancer Fund.

MATERIALS AND METHODS

Patients

The sera of 17 patients with panhypogammaglobulinemia (common varied immunodeficiency) and 3 patients with X-linked (Bruton-type) agammaglobulinemia (SLA) were studied after a 16-hour overnight fast. All patients were completely evaluated by radiographic, medical, and immunologic testing; and each had a complete physical examination. The hypo- and agammaglobulinemic patients were treated with im gamma globulin (60 mg/kg/2 weeks).

Detection and Quantitation of Dietary Proteins in Serum

Radioimmunoassay (RIA). Serum samples were tested for the presence of bovine gamma globulin (BGG) and bovine casein by RIA [6]. In brief, the amount of dietary protein in each serum was calculated from the inhibition the patient's serum produced on the binding of rabbit anti-casein or anti-BGG to ^{125}[I]-casein or ^{125}[I]-BGG as compared to a standard curve prepared using the same reagents.

Antigens. Cow's milk casein and BGG were purchased from Pentex (Kankakee, IL) and used without further purification. Proteins were labeled with ^{125}[I] using the lactoperoxidase procedure [7] to a specific activity of about 0.4 μCi/μg. The labeled proteins were stored in small aliquots at −70°C. These labeled proteins were stable with a trichloroacetic acid precipitability of >90% for at least 3 months.

Molecular Weight Analyses

The apparent molecular weight of casein antigen in the sera of 2 patients (Cases 1 and 3) was estimated from filtration of 100 μl aliquots of sera on a Sephadex G-200 column (30 × 1 cm) equilibrated in phosphate buffered saline, and analysis of 300 μl aliquots for capacity to block the interactions of anti-casein and labeled casein. These results were compared to the molecular weight calibrations of this column performed using dextran blue, ε-DNP lysine, purified bovine serum albumin, casein, chymotrypsin, and RNA-ase.

RESULTS

Quantitation of Dietary Proteins

In order to assess the range of levels of food antigens which might be present in the sera of these patients, we quantitated the level of casein and BGG in the sera of 17 patients with hypogammaglobulinemia, and 3 with SLA (Table 1). All patients with hypogammaglobulinemia were found to have detectable casein (range 80–1600 ng/ml serum), and 7 (41%) had detectable BGG (range 250-800 ng/ml). In contrast, of the 3 patients with SLA, only one had trace amounts of casein and none had detectable BGG. Normal sera analyzed under these conditions contained no detectable bovine antigens.

TABLE 1.

	Patient	ng Casein/ml Serum	ng BGG/ml Serum	Spleen†	Lymphoid Hypertrophy
Hypogamma-globulinemia	1	1,600	650	+++	Cervical lymphadenopathy nodular lymphoid hyperplasia
	2	1,200	500	++	lymphoid pulmonary infiltration
	3	1,280	300	++	
	4	1,080	250	+	
	5	1,000	ND*	++	
	6	980	700	++	nodular lymphoid hyperplasia
	7	980	ND	0	cervical lymphadenopathy
	8	970	ND	0	
	9	690	ND	0	
	10	960	ND	+	
	11	930	260	+	
	12	900	ND	0	
	13	900	800	+++	
	14	400	ND	0	
	15	400	ND	0	
SLA	16	300	ND	0	
	17	80	ND	0	
	18	ND	ND	0	
	19	trace	ND	0	
	20	ND	ND	0	

*ND = not detectable
†Spleen: +++ = enlarged by 4 cm or greater
++ = enlarged by 2–3 cm
+ = just palpable or 1 cm enlarged
0 = not palpable or enlarged by examination

Clinical Correlations

To ascertain what correlation the level of these foreign proteins might have to clinical status, the medical history, physical examination, and extensive medical and immunologic analyses of each patient were scrutinized. Most particularly, we sought relationships between the presence of food proteins in the serum and evidence of current or previous GI disease (including frequent diarrhea, malabsorption, giardiasis, liver disease, or gallbladder dysfunction), level of serum Igs, and evidence of T-cell defects (lymphocyte proliferation, lymphocyte-surface marker analyses, thymic hormones, and leukocyte migration inhibition). Although correlations between these factors and dietary protein antigenemia were not found, greater amounts of bovine casein and the presence of BGG in the serum were both strongly correlated with the presence of chronic splenomegaly as repeatedly noted by the examining physicians ($p<0.01$, 2-sample T test, Table 1).

In addition, 4 patients, each with substantial amounts of bovine antigen in his or her sera, had lymphoid hypertrophy elsewhere. *Patient 1* had (in addition to a large spleen) cervical lymphadenopathy and nodular hyperplasia in the intestinal tract; *Patient 2* had lymphoid pulmonary infiltrations on lung biopsy and *Patients 6 and 7* had nodular lymphoid hyperplasia and cervical lymphadenopathy. The 3 patients with SLA had no evidence of lymphoid hypertrophy or splenomegaly.

DISCUSSION

We demonstrate here that many patients with hypogammaglobulinemia have large amounts of antigenically intact foreign protein of food origin in their sera, while the sera of 3 patients with SLA do not appear to contain these proteins. In 2 patients, the molecular weight of the casein antigen was found to be similar to isolated purified bovine casein. We also found that the presence of large amounts of such protein was correlated with lymphoid hypertrophy, particularly splenomegaly.

The amount of such proteins present in these sera is quite large. Values for fasted human subjects (similar to those studied here) are lacking, but Paganelli and Levinsky [8] found that 3 adults had a maximum of 3 ng β-lactoglobulin/ml in their serum after ingesting 1.2 liters of milk. Block et al [9] found that feeding 4 gm bovine serum albumin (BSA)/kg/bw to rats resulted in 170 ng BSA/ml serum at 6 hours. The human sera studied here had levels of 80–1,600 ng food antigen/ml serum after a 16-hour fast. The clearance of a single dose of parenterally administered ^{125}[I]-BSA from the circulation can take 10–15 days in normal rabbits [10], but, the length of time required for a hypogammaglobulinemic individual, who cannot make antibody or immune complexes, to clear such antigens is unknown.

The exact factor(s) responsible for the excessive absorption of food antigens in the hypogammaglobulinemic patients remains to be clarified. The lack of secretory IgA should affect patients with SLA as much as those with hypogammaglobulinemia, but we did not find evidence of this in the sera of the 3 SLA patients studied here. Further evaluation of the GI differences between these 2 groups of patients is required to explain these findings.

Our data establish a strong statistical relationship between food protein antigenemia and lymphoid hypertrophy—particularly splenomegaly. Although a causative role cannot be established, it is possible that a leaky GI mucosa is linked to chronic lymphoid stimulation. It is known that about 20% of patients with hypogammaglobulinemia have splenomegaly, nodular lymphoid hyperplasia, and/or dramatic peripheral lymphadenopathy [11,12]. Again, the SLA patients differ—lymphoid hyperplasia is rarely seen in this group of patients. Of importance, is the 15% incidence of lymphoid malignancies in the hypogammaglobulinemic, (but not the SLA) population [11,12]. Could chronic GI leakage of luminal antigens of food, bacterial, and viral origin be linked to lymphoid hypertrophy and the possible development of lymphoma in hypogammaglobulinemia?

Our data indicate a need for a better understanding of the mucosal lesions present in the immunodeficient population. Such work may help to clarify the role of the immune system in antigen clearance.

REFERENCES

1. Schloss OM, Worthen TW: The permeability of the gastrointestinal tract of infants to undigested protein. Am J Dis Child 11:342, 1916.
2. Gruskay FL, Cooke RE: The gastrointestinal absorption of unaltered protein in normal infants and in infants recovering from diarrhea. Pediatrics 16:763–768, 1955.
3. Walker WA: Antigen absorption from the small intestine and gastrointestinal disease. Pediatr Clin North Am 22:731–747, 1975.
4. Cunningham-Rundles C, Kirkwood EM, Ferguson A, Parrott D, Good RA: Circulating immune complexes in sera of allergic patients. Clin Res 28:343, 1980.
5. Cunningham-Rundles C, Brandeis WE, Good RA, Day NK: Bovine antigens and the formation of circulating immune complexes in selective IgA deficiency. J Clin Invest 64:270–272, 1979.
6. Carr RI, Wold RT, Farr RS: Antibodies to bovine gammaglobulin and the occurrence of a BGG-like substance in systemic lupus erythematosus. J Allergy Clin Immunol 50:18–25, 1972.
7. Vitetta ES, Baur S, Uhr JW: Cell surface immunoglobulin isolation and characterization of immunoglobulin from mouse splenic lymphocytes. J Exp Med 134:242–264, 1971.
8. Paganelli R, Levinsky RJ: Solid phase radioimmunoassay for detection of circulating food protein antigens in human sera. J Immunol Methods 37:333–341, 1980.
9. Block KJ, Bloch DB, Stearns M, Walker WA: Intestinal uptake of macromolecules. VI. Uptake of protein antigen *in vivo* in normal rats and rats infected with *Nippostrongylus brasiliensis* or subjected to mild systemic anaphylaxis. Gastroenterology 77:1039–1044, 1979.
10. Griswold WR: Studies of the integrity of iodinated bovine albumin after circulation in vivo. Immunol Commun 9:297–308, 1980.
11. Asherson GL, Webster AD: "Diagnosis and Treatment of Immunodeficiency Disease." Oxford:Blackwell Scientific Publication, 1980, p 22.
12. Good RA: Immunodeficiency, common variable. In Bergsma D (ed): "Birth Defects Compendium," 2nd Ed. New York: Alan R Liss for the National Foundation-March of Dimes, 1979, p 574.

SECTION 4
THE ROLE OF THE THYMUS

The Thymus in Immunodeficiency Diseases: New Therapeutic Approaches

Jean-François Bach, MD

Hôpital Necker, INSERM U 25, 75015 Paris Cedex 15, France

The role of the thymus in the differentiation of lymphoid cells is well established. The thymic epithelium transforms blood-borne precursor cells into mature T cells. The question of the respective involvement of an intrinsic defect of T-cell lineage and a failure of the thymic epithelium in the pathogenesis of immunodeficiency (ID) diseases associated with T-cell defect has not been resolved. Before reviewing the main clinical conditions where thymus failure is assumed to explain peripheral T-cell abnormalities, we shall briefly discuss the present state of our knowledge of intrathymic T-cell differentiation. Particular attention will be given to the signals promoting such differentiation, inasmuch as one may expect anomalies in T-cell differentiation to relate to abnormal signals, and considering that some of these signals could be used therapeutically.

THE DIFFERENTIATION FUNCTIONS OF THE THYMIC EPITHELIUM

The differentiation of T cells from hemopoietic stem cells takes place in a number of steps that have been progressively characterized. It is well established that T cells derive initially from hemopoietic stem cells (CFU-S) which transform into lymphoid stem cells. The latter are found in fetal liver and in adult bone marrow. It is not yet known whether the lymphoid progenitor cells differentiate into pre-T and pre-B cells before undergoing the influence of the thymus and the bursa of Fabricius (or its cellular equivalent in mammals). Experiments by Le Douarin and Jotereau [1] showing the migration of precursor cells from bursa to thymus would suggest the absense of pre-commitment. However, it cannot be excluded that in these experiments pre-T cells may contaminate the bursa or that among CFU-S reaching the bursa, only those that transform spontaneously into pre-B cells give rise to B cells under bursal influence, whereas those which ultimately give rise to pre-T cells die locally or leave the bursa. Furthermore lymphoid cells present in nude mouse spleen are known to express a small amount of T-cell antigens (Thy-1 antigen [2] or brain-associated antigen [3]), and these antigens can be induced in vitro and in vivo on a fraction of Ig$^-$ spleen cells by treatment with thymic hormones [4, 5].

Whether or not the pre-T cells appear before undergoing thymic influence, they mature within the thymus into Lyt 1+ and Lyt 123+ cells—the so-called postthymic precursor cells [6]. These postthymic cells eventually leave the thymus without entering the medulla and seed in the periphery where they give rise to 2 cell subsets: Lyt 1+ helper/inducer T cells and Lyt 123+ suppressor/cytotoxic T cells. In this scheme, the medulla of the thymus does not represent a necessary site of differentiation, as was initially thought. In fact, recent results indicate that thymic emigrant cells may derive directly from the thymic cortex [7]. Several signals promote the various steps of T-cell maturation just mentioned.

Migration of T-Cell Precursors to the Thymus

The thymic epithelial rudiment is seeded with blood-borne stem cells that originate in the yolk sac. Migration to the thymus is an active phenomenon in which stem cells are sensitive to a concentration gradient of chemotactic factors of thymic origin. In vitro experiments using Millipore filters and showing direct migration of stem cells to the thymic rudiment [1] support this hypothesis. Less information is available on the migration of T-cell precursors in mammals. Results from our laboratory indicate that migration of hemopoietic precursors proceeds through chemotactic mechanisms similar to those described in avian embryos. Using a migration technique under agar, we demonstrated the attraction of fetal liver cells to mouse thymic rudiments [8].

Intrathymic Differentiation

The maturation of T cells within the thymus is a complex event. It was initially assumed that the main maturational effect of the thymus was mediated by humoral thymic factors [9]. It was then thought that direct contact with the epithelial microenvironment played the major role [10]. It is now believed that both these signals operate and that, in addition, exposure of T-cell precursors to major histocompatibility complex (MHC) products on thymic epithelial cells, and the

TABLE 1. Chemically Defined Thymic Peptides

	Molecular weight	N°aa	PI	Synthesis
Thymosin 1 (A.L. Goldstein)	3,108	28	4.2	Yes
Thymopoietin (G. Goldstein)	5,562	49	5.5	Yes
Thymulin (FTS-Zn) (J.F. Bach)	847	9	7.5	Yes
Thymic humoral factor (THF) (N. Trainin)	3,200	aa sequence not determined	5.8	No

aa = amino acid

action of lymphokines produced by medullary T cells, also play a part.

Thymic Hormones

The production of various factors by the thymus gland is now well established [11]. Several peptides have been isolated from thymic extracts, characterized, and then sequenced and synthesized (Table 1). Thymosins represent a set of polypeptides found in fraction 5, such as thymosin $\alpha 1$ or $\beta 4$, which have immunomodulatory properties and are responsible part of the biologic activity of the whole fraction 5. Thymopoietin, initially isolated on the basis of its capacity to depress neuromuscular conduction, has been shown to induce T-cell maturation in vitro and in vivo. Thymic humoral factor (THF) is a polypeptide shown to enhance graft-versus-host (GVH) reactions and to increase cyclic AMP (cAMP) synthesis in lymphocytes of neonatally thymectomized (NTx) mice. The serum thymic factor (FTS) (Facteur Thymique Sérique) is a nonapeptide, recently given the name of thymulin, after the presence of zinc in the molecule was demonstrated.

No homology in amino acid sequences has yet been observed among the peptides whose sequences have been established (thymosins $\alpha 1$ and $\beta 4$, thymopoietin, and FTS). Finally although the homogeneity and the biologic significance of some of the materials mentioned above remain to be established, the diversity of physical and chemical properties suggests the existence of a family of thymic hormones.

The problem of the exclusively thymic origin of each of these factors must be considered. Most of them have been isolated from the thymus and thus may be considered a priori as thymus-derived. In fact, it remains to be proven that they are not also produced in other organs and, if so, are not authentic thymic hormones. Such proof is available for thymosin $\alpha 1$ and thymulin, since antisera or monoclonal antibodies for thymulin produced against the purified hormones have been shown to bind to the thymic epithelium [12–14].

The results obtained with purified or synthetic thymic factors suggest that they act on the so-called postthymic cell. There are some reports that thymic factors might act in nude mice or in mice totally deprived of T cells (thymectomized, irradiated, and reconstituted with anti-Thy 1 serum-treated bone marrow cells). However, these studies either deal with T-cell markers [15, 16] and therefore cannot be extrapolated to T-cell activity, or relate to T-cell functions [17] but have not been confirmed. Most results, obtained in vitro or in vivo, derive from studies in normal adult thymectomized (ATx) or partially T-cell-deprived NZB or aged mice, which may show some degree of T-cell deficiency but share the property of possessing postthymic cells.

Most T-cell functions have been reported to be induced or enhanced by thymic factors (provided an adequate recipient is used). Thus, thymulin enhances T-cell-mediated cytotoxicity in thymectomized mice [18]. This effect is quite clearly shown in adult thymectomized mice by the Brunner assay. It is not known whether thymulin directly stimulates the generation of cytotoxic cells or enhances the function of a regulatory cell that could be the Lyt 123+ spleen cell. Similarly, thymulin also acts on T cells involved in delayed type hypersensitivity induced by dinitrofluorobenzene (DNFB). It restores a normal response in ATx mice. Its effect on helper T (Th) cells, as studied on the production of anti-sheep red blood cell (SRBC) antibody, is much less clear (we have not reproducibly obtained major effects, perhaps because of a simultaneous action on T suppressor (TS) cells). In fact, thymulin has recently proven to be remarkably active on TS cells in various in vitro and in vivo systems. When given to normal mice, thymulin suppresses the generation of alloantigen-reactive T cells or DNFB-sensitive T cells. Given in doses of 10–100 ng, it prolongs skin allograft survival or enhances the growth of Moloney sarcoma virus (MSV)-induced sarcoma in T-cell-deprived mice, while at lower doses it stimulates its rejection [11].

We have recently demonstrated specific thymulin receptors on T-cell lines derived from patients with acute lymphoblastic leukemia [19]. Cultured lymphocytes were incubated with labeled thymulin for 90 min: 12–15% thymulin bound to the cell line. The specificity of the binding was assessed by inhibition of binding obtained by adding unlabeled thymulin (10^{-8}M), as well as by the absence of displacement by close (but inactive) chemical thymulin analogs. Scatchard analysis demonstrated the high affinity of the receptors (K_D or $10^{-8}M$). The fact that some T-cell lines did not bind thymulin indicates that T cells do not express thymulin receptors at all stages of their differentiation.

Three assay systems have been described to evaluate the level of circulating thymic hormone. The rosette assay was the first described. It is based on the induction of sensitivity to anti-Thy-1 serum or azathioprine of the rosette-forming cell (RFC) present in the spleen of ATx mice [20]. This rosette assay is sensitive and quantitative and has now been successfully reproduced in more than 10 different laboratories notably that of Drs. Incefy and Good, who have published several studies based on this assay. The second assay is also of a biologic nature. It consists in the induction of Thy-1 antigen in Thy-1 negative nude mouse spleen cells [21]. Results are expressed as ng of thymopoietin equivalent, but there is no evidence for the direct responsibility of thymopoietin in the activity detected, and other peptides such as thymosin α1 and thymulin-FTS could also contribute to this activity. The third assay is a radioimmunoassay for thymosin α1 [22]. The level of serum thymosin α1 thus detected is age-dependent with a very rapid decline, as early as 5 years of age. In fact, few data are yet available on the specificity of the assay (in particular, no clear data have been published concerning thymus-deprived subjects or animals).

Maturation Signals Provided by Direct Contact or Precursor Cells With the Thymic Epithelium

Thymic hormones are apparently less effective in nude mice than in neonatally thymectomized (NTx) mice [6]. Grafting a thymus within a Millipore chamber restores the immunocompetence of the Tx but not of the nude mouse. The above discussion suggests that thymic hormones intervene only at late stages of intrathymic differentiation, with the probable exception of differentiation antigen induction. This induction may take place under the sole influence of thymic hormones (achieving a paradoxical "nonfunctional" differentiation). In the early stages of maturation, the thymic epithelium probably operates by direct contact with the stem cells, whatever the events associated with this contact may be (action of high local concentrations of thymic hormones, cell-to-cell interaction, etc). The need for direct contact would explain why stem cells have to migrate into the thymus to benefit from the thymic influence (which they could receive in the periphery if thymic hormones alone were effective). The role of direct contact of stem cells with the thymic epithelium has been supported by the demonstration with chromosome markers of fetal liver cell migration to the thymus at a time in development when the influence of thymic hormones is not yet sufficient to achieve T-cell maturation [6].

Zinkernagel and others have convincingly shown that T cells recognize conventional antigens only when they are associated with MHC products shared with those present on their own membrane [23]. Recent results indicate that the capacity to recognize self-MHC products is acquired within the thymus [24]. Although it may not be as general as was initially thought, the intrathymic acquisition of H-2 restriction on contact with radio-resistant thymic epithelium implies that early T cells are selected within the thymus. One may assume that self-MHC recognition represents one of the signals provided by the direct contact of precursor cells with the thymic epithelium. There is no evidence yet, however, that this signal promotes the metabolic processes of T-cell differentiation, by which the T cell that has recognized the antigen or bound a lectin becomes capable of proliferating and eventually mounting an immune response.

T-Cell Growth Factors: Role of Intrathymic Lymphocytes as Amplifiers of T-Cell Maturation

The thymic reticulum is made up of entodermal epithelial cells and mesenchymal reticular cells. It contains lymphocytes and a few macrophages. Recent developments in the study of lymphokines secreted by activated mature T cells, and the demonstration of their role in T-cell triggering, have led to investigating the possible involvement of mature intrathymic medullary lymphocytes in the maturation of T-cell precursors.

Thymic medullary cells can produce Interleukin-2 (Il-2) [25]. Conversely, cortical thymocytes, which do not produce Il-2, respond to it [25]. These two observations have led to the hypothesis that the Lyt 1+ thymic medullary cells present in the reticular network of the thymic microenvironment (which appear very early in ontogeny) could represent an important amplification circuit of T-cell differentiation. This could occur through the secretion of Il-2, perhaps triggered by self-MHC products.

Recent experiments (our unpublished results) have shown that thymic medullary cells activated by allogeneic, irradiated cells can induce spleen cells from nude mice or from T-cell-deprived mice to respond to Con A or to allogeneic cells. These results confirm the possibility that thymic medullary cells may promote the differentiation of immature T cells. However, it should be remembered that Il-2 is produced only by T cells which, themselves, have had to differentiate from precursor stem cells (with epithelial contact and under the influence of thymic hormones). In other words, Il-2-induced T-cell maturation represents, at best, an amplification circuit of T-cell maturation and may not be an obligatory maturation stimulus.

IMMUNODEFICIENCY (ID) DISEASES DUE TO ABNORMAL THYMIC DEVELOPMENT

A considerable role is attributed to T-cell anomalies in a number of ID diseases. In most cases it is not known, however, which are secondary to a T-cell precursor defect, and which to abnormal development of the thymus gland itself (more precisely, of the epithelium, which is the main element inducing intrathymic T-cell differentiation). Three main ID diseases will be discussed here, as putatively due to abnormal thymic development: the DiGeorge (DiG) syndrome, ataxia telangectasia, and some cases of severe combined immunodeficiencies (SCID) with circulating B cells. We do not intend to imply that the thymus may not be abnormal in other ID diseases associated with T-cell abnormalities. Such abnormalities could arise within the thymus (rather than be genetically programmed in the pre-T cell), notably in some cases of common variable ID and selective T-cell deficiency, but positive evidence is lacking.

The DiGeorge Syndrome

Converging arguments indicate that the DiG syndrome is secondary to thymic aplasia. More precisely, it is due to abnormal development of the 3rd and 4th pharyngeal pouches, which explains the association of hypoparathyroidism and malformations of the aortic arch and of the face. The absence of familial cases (with one published exception) suggests that the disease is secondary to fetal insult. On postmortem examination the thymus may be absent or distributed into several small ectopic glands [26]. Importantly, when present, the thymic tissue is not morphologically abnormal with distinct cortico-medullary differentiation or the presence of lymphocytes and of Hassall corpuscles [26]. No thymic hormone has been found in the circulating blood in all cases where it was studied, either by the rosette assay [27, 28] or the Thy-1 antigen induction assay [29]. Major abnormalities of peripheral T-cell markers and functions essentially involving cell-mediated immunity (CMI) are observed. Antibody production and serum Ig levels (in particular those of the highly thymus-dependent isotypes IgA and IgE) are grossly normal [26], with rare exceptions [30]. Although one may argue that antibody production has essentially been investigated against thymus-independent antigens, it remains that Th cells are probably not totally deficient in the DiG syndrome, as is observed in nude mice completely deprived of thymus [31], or in NTx mice or rabbits [6, 32]. Furthermore, the rapid immunologic restoration (within a few hours) after grafting a thymus [33, 34] (eventually placed in a Millipore diffusion chamber [35]) strongly suggests that the reconstitution is due to thymic hormones and operates on not totally immature T cells. This assumption is based on the difficulty and the interval of several weeks required to restore the immunocompetence of nude or NTx mice [6]. All these arguments suggest that thymic aplasia occurs at a late stage of development, after pre-T cells have come into contact with the thymic epithelium, and, at least in incomplete cases, that the thymic anomaly is essentially quantitative. This hypothesis is strengthened by the observation that incubation with thymic extracts of lymphocytes from patients with the DiG syndrome increases the number of cells forming E rosettes and expressing T-cell-specific xenoantigens [36, 37]. These T cells, which can be "induced" rather than "differentiated" by thymic hormones, are initially null cells which coexist with T cells expressing normal T-cell markers (not totally absent in the DiG syndrome, and even close to normal values in incomplete forms [38]). This observation is reminiscent of marker induction experiments in mice. It has indeed been our experience that T-cell markers can be induced with thymic hormones at much lower concentrations on spleen cells from ATx mice, which are not deprived of postthymic cells, than on nude mouse spleen cells, which lack them [39]. These data are also in keeping with the fact that NTx mice which, at least early in life, possess postthymic cells have a limited but significant number of Thy-1 positive cells, which nude mice do not have at a similar level.

Spontaneous recovery of immunocompetence has been reported in several cases of the DiG syndrome [40]. This phenomenon could relate to the stimulation of relatively mature postthymic cells by nonspecific agents such as prostaglandins or Il-2 (produced by the few mature T cells present in these patients), known to promote T-cell differentiation. Recent (unpublished) data from our laboratory indicate that a depletion of thymic hormone (experimentally induced by injection of monoclonal antibody against thymic hormone) may induce a compensatory hyperfunction of the thymus (as assessed by the number of thymic hormone-containing cells).

Ataxia Telangiectasia (AT)

AT is a complex autosomal recessive disease involving several systems in addition to lymphoid cells. Such a diversity of anomalies for one single genetic disease suggests the existence of a common basic cellular lesion. Anomaly of DNA repair (sensitivity to irradiation) and abnormal entoderm-mesenchyme interaction have often been suggested [41]. Whatever the putative common underlying mechanism, AT patients have profound alterations of humoral and cell mediated immunity (CMI) whose mechanisms should be discussed in terms similar to those for other ID diseases. The alterations predominate on T cells: delayed-type reactions are depressed, skin allograft rejection is delayed, and T-cell proliferative responses to mitogens and alloantigens are decreased [41]. Serum IgA and IgE are undetectable in a majority of cases (with normal levels of IgG and IgM). The production of antibodies against deliberately injected antigens is variable depressed, whereas IgA response to vaccine is often low or absent. If there is little doubt as to the existence of a T-cell defect, one may question the existence of a B-cell defect. In fact, several pathogenetic hypotheses may be considered to explain the anomaly of antibody production: 1) intrinsic B-cell defect; 2) Th cell deficiency; 3) increased Ts cell function; and 4) lymphocyte inhibitory serum factor. Well-documented data have been presented in support of each of these hypotheses [42–44]. In fact it might be, as suggested by several studies, that no single mechanism explains the ID observed in all AT patients who, immunologically speaking, could represent a fairly heterogeneous group. A similar comment applies to selective IgA deficiency, with the double and important reservation that in most investigations T-cell number and functions are normal in such patients (whereas they are regularly abnormal in AT), and that excessive IgA-specific Ts cell function is often found in selective IgA deficiency and has not been reported in AT. In any case, it remains that a major T-cell deficit exists in AT. Since the IgA deficiency is far from being regularly associated with increased sinopulmonary infections, one may wonder whether infections observed in AT are not more directly related to the T-cell defect, rather than to the IgA deficiency.

Three arguments strongly suggest that the AT-associated T-cell defect is due to a primitive failure of the thymic epithelium. First, available histologic data show that the thymus of AT patients is deeply immature, reduced to its stromal reticular compartment, with only few mature lymphocytes and a total absence of Hassall corpuscles [45, 46]. This situation is significantly different from the incomplete DiG syndrome where the thymus mass is reduced, but morphologically grossly normal. Second, circulating levels of thymic hormone have been repeatedly found to be low in most cases of AT, whatever the technique used to evaluate the hormone [27–29, 47]. Finally, we have recently reported that thymulin treatment of 4 patients with AT totally restored CMI, T-cell number (and markers), IgA levels and deficient IgA antibody production against vaccines and Epstein-Barr virus (EBV), and also suppressed chronic sinopulmonary infections [47]. It would thus appear that a deficiency of the thymic epithelium may lead concomitantly to a major failure of CMI and of IgA (and IgE) production. This interpretation fits with experimental data mentioned above, showing the selective thymus dependence of IgA synthesis. It is not yet understood, however, why other T-cell deficiencies, such as complete DiG syndrome, do not lead to IgA deficiency, or why thymus grafting was not effective in the few AT cases where it was tried, as it is in the DiG syndrome.

The very inconstant and, generally, very modest therapeutic effect of Thymosin fraction V [48] (bearing only on T-cell functions and markers not on IgA level) is puzzling as well, since fraction V contains thymulin [49] and has shown some effect in the DiG syndrome [48]. One may hypothesize that higher doses of active thymic hormone are needed in AT than in the DiG syndrome, and that Thymosin fraction V, which represents a relatively ill-defined mixture of thymic peptides, does not allow administration of sufficient amounts of active peptides in AT. Our studies indicate that Thymosin fraction V contains about 5 μg of thymulin per 100 mg of protein weight [49] which, as far as thymulin is concerned, implies that AT patients received about 1 μg/kg/day thymulin, which is significantly less than the dose given in synthetic form to our patients (10 μg/kg/day).

At any rate, our clinical data provide the first example of therapy capable of significantly altering AT evolution, both immunologically and clinically. Whether or not thymulin-FTS treatment will influence the long-term outcome of the disease, notably the onset of malignancy observed in up to 15% of these patients and autoimmune manifestations, is open to speculation. The effect on autoimmunity will be particularly interesting to follow, since in NZB mice thymulin-FTS has proven capable of either preventing or accelerating autoimmunity, according to the manifestations and to the recipient (male or female, NZB or B/W mice) [11].

Severe Combined Immunodeficiency Diseases (SCID)

It is commonly accepted that the majority of SCID are secondary to a lymphoid precursor cell defect, which explains that both B- and T-cell lineages are usually involved. There are cases, however, with normal numbers of circulating B cells (and sometimes normal function). Such B cells have been shown in co-culture experiments to collaborate normally with normal T cells to produce antibody [50]. Several factors indicate that these SCID might be related to an anomaly of thymic development. Here again the problem is to discriminate between an intrinsic defect of the T-cell lineage (probably at the pre-T-cell level, supposed to be distinct from pre-B cells), and a deficiency of the thymic epithelium. A number of factors may be mentioned in favor of the latter hypothesis. First, the circulating level of thymic hormone is low in some SCID cases [28, 29, 36].

Second, thymus grafting performed after fetal liver grafting [36], or grafting a thymic epithelium obtained after 2–3 week culture [51], has been shown to restore immunocompetence, although in a limited number of cases. Lastly, Pyke and Gelfand [52] have shown that in vitro cultured thymic epithelium induces peripheral blood lymphocytes from a SCID patient to form E rosettes and to respond to phytohemagglutinin, a finding confirmed by Pahwa and Good [33]. Pyke has shown that the supernatant from the culture obtained with the patient's thymus was unable to attract mouse fetal liver cells in an in vitro migration assay; this observation contrasts with results with normal epithelium [8].

It is interesting that in some SCID cases bone marrow grafting is associated with the appearance of significant thymic hormone levels in the blood [36], indicating that the contact of normal stem cells with a nonthymic hormone-secreting thymic epithelium may induce thymic hormone synthesis. It also indicates that a nonsecreting epithelium in SCID may be potentially capable of normal function when a normal influx of stem cells is provided.

THERAPEUTIC CONSIDERATIONS

ID disease due to abnormal thymic development may be treated specifically, either by thymus grafting or by injection of humoral thymic products. Thymus grafting has the advantage of simultaneously providing all the cellular and humoral components responsible for the differentiating capacity of the thymus. However, it poses a number of unsolved problems linked to the difficulties in finding an organ to graft, and to the uncertainties of the long-term graft survival. Injection of thymic products, practical thymic hormones, is easier and can be used for long-term treatment. Uncertainties persist, however, as to the nature of the physiologically significant hormones and the potential indications of the peptides which, in any case, cannot substitute for the thymus at all stages of T-cell differentiation.

Thymus Grafts

Most grafts in patients with DiG syndrome have been made with fetal thymus glands (reviewed by Pahwa and Good [33]). The age of the fetus and the route of grafting (ip or sc) do not seem to be major factors affecting graft success. Hong et al [51] have proposed the use of thymic epithelium obtained after 2–3 weeks of in vitro culture. However, with the exception of a successful initial case [51], clinical reconstitution has been only modest or null, both in Hong's experience and in that of others [33]. In one case, the thymus was grafted within a diffusion chamber in order to avoid GVH reaction [35], but unfortunately the recipient died after a few days so that the long-term benefit of the graft could not be fully evaluated.

Thymus grafting has not been widely used in ID secondary to thymus failure. Presumably most successful grafts are reported in the literature, essentially in DiG syndrome and in a few cases of selective T-cell deficiency [53]: their number so far is limited. This can be explained by a series of practical and more basic difficulties inherent in thymus grafting. The thymus gland must survive long enough but not induce a GVH reaction. It must also provide adequate education of pre-T cells on the thymic epithelium [24], all conditions prompting the selection of HLA compatible grafts, which is very difficult, if not impossible. It should be remembered, however, that the use of fetal grafts prevents potential GVH reactivity, and that HLA compatibility is probably not mandatory in most cases. In addition, in the DiG syndrome, thymus failure is likely to occur after the first phase of intrathymic pre-T-cell education in the epithelium. In fact, such intrathymic education is not obligatory, since nude mice, which are more T-cell-deficient than any of these patients, may be restored by Il-2 injections [54]. The rejection problem is probably more serious. Patients with T-cell deficiency are not always totally T-cell-deficient and, in any case, they recover their competence under the effect of the graft, becoming capable of rejection if some tolerance or adaptation does not occur. The demonstration of H-2 and Ia antigens on the thymic epithelium indicates that the epithelium is indeed an excellent potential target for allogeneic reactions. It could be argued that a short-term graft could suffice for restoration, as in the long-term reconstitution of NTx mice [6]. However, our experience with thymulin-FTS indicates that substitutive long-term treatment is necessary to maintain immunocompetence. All of these factors added to the difficulty of obtaining fetal thymuses for grafting, and the possible technical failures due to necrosis explain the present limited use of thymus grafts.

Thymic Hormones

Several thymic preparations are now available for clinical use. Thymic extracts have been used in children with ID [55–57]. The mode of extraction is different for each preparation. Practically, one may distinguish trials performed with Thymosin fraction V and extracts prepared along the same line (which contain most thymic proteins and polypeptides with molecular weight between 500 and 15,000 daltons) and those made with thymic extract dialysates, as used by Trainin et al [58], which contain only molecules with molecular weight below 5,000 daltons. In any case, all these extracts

TABLE 2. Classification of Substances Present in Thymic Extracts or Thymic Epithelial Supernatants

1. Lymphocyte-differentiating factors
   a) produced by the epithelium (thymic hormones)
   b) produced by macrophages (eg Il-1)
   c) produced by lymphocytes (eg Il-2)
2. Immunoactive substances not specific of the thymus
   a) prostaglandins and cAMP
   b) proteins
      - xenogeneic stimuli
      - immunologic activity (eg lymphokines present in thymocytes)
      - nonspecific pharmacologic activity on cell membranes (eg ubiquitin)
   c) endotoxins (issued from bacterial contamination)
   d) nucleic acids (known as possible immunoadjuvants)
3. Inhibitors of thymic hormones
4. Nonimmunoactive substances

are heterogeneous and contain many undesirable molecules (Table 2) which can produce side effects (notably anaphylaxis) or nonspecific immunologic or pharmacologic stimulation. In addition, the efficacy of these extracts is poorly controlled. Their content in putatively active hormones is unknown, which limits the theoretic advantage of including all potentially active peptides. A given factor may be present at low concentrations or mixed with an inhibitor. These extracts have been useful, however, both experimentally and clinically by revealing the biologic properties of thymic humoral products. The time has probably come when synthetic peptides should be substituted for them. Three thymic peptides are now available in synthetic form: thymopoietin, thymosin $\alpha 1$, and thymulin-FTS. Thymopoietin is used as a pentapeptide (TP-5) and has been shown to possess the immunologic activity [59]. Thymulin-FTS, initially used as a nonapeptide bound to patient's plasma (to increase life-span), is now used coupled to zinc [60] and directly injected subcutaneously without vehicle. Doses used vary with each peptide: 1 mg/kg for TP5, 20 mg/kg for thymosin [56], and 10 μg/kg for thymulin-FTS [47]. As mentioned above, the treatment is essentially substitutive and cannot be stopped without risking loss of immunocompetence. The spacing of injection is still a matter of debate. Studying the effect of FTS on T-cell markers, we have shown that a single injection of the peptide-induced marker expression for a 2–3-day period when 0+ RFC from ATx mouse spleen were considered [39], but for a much longer time (2–3 weeks) with regard to the number of sheep erythrocyte binding cells and Thy-1 positivity in thymocytes from normal mice [61]. Similarly, G. Goldstein (personal communication) has reported that a single injection of TP-5 induces a long-lasting effect (1 week) although the peptide is degraded within 1 minute. Practically, our policy is to start treatment with daily doses and then space the injections to once or twice a week. We adapt the dosage to serum levels (evaluated by the rosette assay and compared to biologically efficient levels in mice) and to change induced in immunologic parameters (OKT phenotype, mitogen responses, E rosettes). Selection of a useful dosage remains quite arbitrary, however. So far, no side effects have been reported with any of the synthetic peptides used in man. It will be important to follow up possible sensitization against the injected hormones (although it is unlikely in view of their small molecular weight), and, especially, induction of autoimmunity (since in some settings thymic hormone can promote or enhance autoimmune reactions [11]).

Thymulin-FTS has been administered to various patients with ID disease. It has been shown to increase the number of E rosettes in the DiG syndrome (2 cases) and especially (in collaboration with P. Bordigoni and D. Olive) to restore IgA production and CMI in 6 cases of IgA deficiency (4 cases of AT, 1 of common variable immunodeficiency, and 1 unclassified ID [47]). Importantly, thymulin (FTS-Zn) given sc without vehicle has proven to be as efficient as FTS (without zinc) bound to patients' plasma or albumin. In one SCID child who had received a bone marrow transplant from her mother, thymulin was given at 5 months of age. Within a week, the treatment induced a GVH reaction due to activation of chimeric cells of the mother, as assessed by skin rash, and the appearance of blast cells in the circulation. Fortunately, the reaction stopped as soon as thymulin treatment was interrupted (Griscelli and Bach, unpublished data).

Lastly, it should be mentioned that thymulin has been successfully given to a patient with generalized herpes secondary to a major T-cell deficiency. All these data are promising and argue for further clinical trials of thymulin and other synthetic thymic hormones in ID diseases with T-cell defect, whether or not they are due to a failure of the thymic epithelium.

REFERENCES

1. Le Douarin N, Jotereau FV: Homing of lymphoid stem cells to the thymus and the bursa of Fabricius studied in avian embryo chimeras. In Fougereau M, Dausset J (eds): "Immunology 80." Progress in Immunology IV. London: Academic Press, 1980, pp 285–302.
2. Loor R, Roelants GE: High frequency of T lineage lymphocytes in nude mouse spleen. Nature 251:229–230, 1974.

3. Sato VL, Waksal SD, Herzenberg LA: Identification and separation of pre T cells from nu/nu mice: Differentiation by preculture with thymic reticuloepithelial cells. Cell Immunol 24:173–185, 1976.
4. Bach JF, Dardenne M, Goldstein AL, Guha A, White A: Appearance of T cell markers in bone marrow rosette forming cells after incubation with purified thymosin, a thymic hormone. Proc Natl Acad Sci USA 68:2734–2738, 1971.
5. Komuro K, Boyse EA: In vitro demonstration of thymic hormone in the mouse by conversion of precursor cells into lymphocytes. Lancet 1:740–743, 1973.
6. Stutman O: Intrathymic and extrathymic T cell maturation. Immunol Rev 42:138–184, 1978.
7. Weissman IL, Baird S, Gardner RL, Papaioannou VE, Raschke W: Normal and neoplastic maturation of T lineage lymphocytes. Cold Spring Harbor Symp Quant Biol 41:9–21, 1977.
8. Pyke KW, Bach JF: In vitro migration of potential haemopoietic precursors from the murine thymus. Thymus 3:1–7, 1981.
9. Miller JFAP, Osoba D: The role of the thymus in the origin of immunological competence. In "The Immunologically Competent Cell: Its Nature and Origin." (Ciba Found Study Gp 16) London: Churchill, 1963, pp 62–70.
10. Davies AJS: The thymus and the cellular basis of immunity. Transplant Rev 1:43–91, 1969.
11. Bach JF: Thymic hormones. J Immunopharmacol 1:277–310, 1979.
12. Hirokawa K, McClure MC, Goldstein AL: Age related changes in localization of thymosin $\alpha 1$, in the human thymus. Thymus 4:19–26, 1982.
13. Jambon B, Montagne B, Bene MC, Brayer MP, Faure G, Duheille J: Immunohistologic localization of "facteur thymique sérique" (FTS) in human thymic epithelium. J Immunol 127:2055–2059, 1981.
14. Savino W, Dardenne M, Papiernik M, Bach JF: Thymic hormone containing cells. Characterization and localization of serum thymic factor in young mouse thymus studied by monoclonal antibodies. J Exp Med 196:628–634, 1982.
15. Bach MA, Fournier C, Bach JF: Regulation of theta antigen expression by agents altering cyclic AMP level and by thymic factor. Ann NY Acad Sci 249:316–327, 1975.
16. Scheid MP, Goldstein G, Boyse EA: Differentiation of T cells in nude mice. Science 190:1211–1213, 1975.
17. Ikehara S, Hamashima Y, Masuda T: Immunological restoration of both thymectomized and athymic nude mice by a thymus factor. Nature 258:335–337, 1975.
18. Bach MA: Lymphocyte-mediated cytotoxicity: Effects of ageing on adult thymectomy and thymic factor. J Immunol 119:641–648, 1977.
19. Pléau JM, Fuentes V, Morgat JM, Bach JF: Specific receptor for the serum thymic factor (FTS) in lymphoblastoid culture cell lines. Proc Natl Acad Sci USA 77:2861–2865, 1980.
20. Bach JF, Dardenne M: Studies on thymus products. II. Demonstration and characterization of a circulating thymic hormone. Immunology 25:353–366, 1973.
21. Twomey JJ, Goldstein G, Lewis VM, Bealmear PM, Good RA: Bioassay determinations of thymopoietin and thymic hormone levels in human plasma. Proc Natl Acad Sci USA 6:2541–2545, 1977.
22. McClure JE, Lameris N, Wara DW, Goldstein AL: Immunochemical studies of thymosin; Radio immunoassay of thymosin α_1. J Immunol 128:368–375, 1982.
23. Zinkernagel RM: H-2 restriction of virus specific T cell mediated effector functions in vitro. II. Adoptive transfer of delayed type hypersensitivity to murine lymphocytic choriomeningitis virus is restricted by the K and D regions of H-2. J Exp Med 144:776–787, 1976.
24. Zinkernagel RM, Althage A, Waterfield E, Kindred B, Welsh RM, Callahan G, Pincetl P: Restriction specificities, alloreactivity and allotolerance expressed by T cells from nude mice reconstituted with H-2 compatible or incompatible thymus grafts. J Exp Med 151:376–399, 1980.
25. Wagner H, Hardt C, Heeg K: T-T cell interactions during cytotoxic T lymphocytes (CTL) responses: T cell derived helper factor (Interleukin 2) as a probe to analyze CTL responsiveness and thymic maturation of CTL progenitors. Immunol Rev 51:215–255, 1980.
26. Lischner HW, Huff DS: T-cell deficiency in DiGeorge syndrome. Birth Defects*, 11(1):16–21, 1975.
27. Bach JF, Dardenne M, Pléau JM, Bach MA: Isolation, biochemical characteristics and biological activity of a circulating thymic hormone in the mouse and in the human. Ann NY Acad Sci 249:186–210, 1975.
28. Iwata T, Incefy GS, Cunningham-Rundles S, Cunningham-Rundles C, Smithwick E, Geller N, O'Reilly R, Good RA: Circulating thymic hormone activity in patients with primary and secondary immunodeficiency diseases. Am J Med 71:385–394, 1981.
29. Lewis V, Twomey JJ, Goldstein G, O'Reilly R, Smithwick E, Pahwa R, Pahwa S, Good RA, Schulte-Wisserman H, Horowitz S, Hong R, Jones J, Sieber O, Kirkpatrick C, Polmar S, Bealmear P: Circulating thymic hormone activity in congenital immunodeficiency. Lancet 2:471–475, 1977.
30. Gatti RA, Gershanik JJ, Levkoff AH, Wertelecki W, Good RA: Thymic activity in severe combined immunodeficiency diseases. Proc Natl Acad Sci USA 74:1250–1253, 1977.
31. Nomura T, Ohsawa N, Tamaoki N, Fugiwara K: The potentialities and limitations of the Nude mice. In Proc Sec Intern Workshop on Nude Mice. Stuttgart, New York: Gustav Fischer Verlag, 1977, p 600.
32. Clough JD, Mims LH, Strober W: IgA antibody responses to arsanilic acid bovine serum albumin (BSA) in neonatally thymectomized rabbits. J Immunol 106:1624–1629, 1971.
33. Pahwa R, Pahwa S, O'Reilly R, Good RA: Treatment of the immunodeficiency diseases. Progress toward replacement therapy emphasizing cellular and macromolecular engineering. In Cooper MD, Lawton AR, Miescher PA, Mueller-Huebach E (eds): "Immunodeficiency." Berlin: Springer Verlag, 1975, pp 121–170.
34. August CS, Rosen FS, Filler RM, Janeway CA, Mackowski B, Kay HEM: Implantation of a foetal thymus restoring immunological competence in a patient with thymic aplasia (DiGeorge's syndrome). Lancet 2:1210–1211, 1968.
35. Steele RW, Limas C, Thurman GB, Schulein M, Bauer H, Bellanti JA: Familial thymic aplasia. Attempted reconstitution with foetal thymus in a Millipore diffusion chamber. N Engl J Med 287:787–791, 1972.
36. Incefy GS, Dardenne M, Pahwa S, Grimes E, Pahwa RN, Smithwick E, O'Reilly R, Good RA: Thymic activity in severe combined immunodeficiency diseases. Proc Natl Acad Sci USA 74:1250–1253, 1977.
37. Touraine JL, Touraine F, Dutruge J, Gilly J, Colon S, Gilly R: Immunodeficiency diseases. I. T-lymphocyte precursors and T lymphocyte differentiation in partial DiGeorge syndrome. Clin Exp Immunol 21:39–46, 1975.
38. Reinherz EL, Cooper MD, Schlossman SF, Rosen FS: Abnormalities of T cell maturation and regulation in human beings with immunodeficiency disorders. J Clin Invest 68:699–705, 1981.

*Birth Defects: Original Article Series, published for the March of Dimes Birth Defects Foundation.

39. Dardenne M, Bach JF: Studies on thymus products. I. Modification of rosette-forming cells by thymic extracts. Determination of the target RFC subpopulation. Immunology 25:343–352, 1973.
40. Sieber OF, Durie BC, Hattler BC: Spontaneous evolution of immune competence in DiGeorge syndrome. Pediatr Res 8:418, 1974.
41. Gatti RA, Bick M, Tam CE, Medici MA, Oxelius V-A, Holland M, Goldstein AL, Boder E: Ataxia-telangiectasia: A multiparameter analysis of eight families. Clin Immunol Immunopathol 23:501–516, 1982.
42. Mitsuya H, Matsukura M, Tomino S, Fujiwara H, Kishimoto S: T cell suppression of immunoglobulin synthesis in ataxia-telangiectasia: Restriction of suppressor activity to B cell from unrelated donors. Clin Immunol Immunopathol 19:383–393, 1981.
43. McFarlin DE, Oppenheim JJ: Impaired lymphocyte transformation in ataxia-telangiectasia in part due to a plasma inhibitory factor. J Immunol 103:1212–1222, 1969.
44. Waldmann T: Immunological abnormalities in ataxia-telangiectasia: A cellular and molecular link between cancer neuropathology and immune deficiency. In Bridges BA, Harnden DE (eds): "Ataxia Telangiectasia: A Cellular & Molecular Link Between Cancer, Neuropathology & Immune Deficiency. New York: J. Wiley & Sons, 1982, pp 37–51.
45. Peterson RDA, Cooper MD, Good RA: Lymphoid tissue abnormalities associated with ataxia-telangiectasia. Am J Med 41:342–359, 1966.
46. Biggar WD, Good RA: Immunodeficiency in ataxia-telangiectasia. Birth Defects* 11(1):271–274, 1975.
47. Bordigoni P, Bene MC, Bach JF, Faure G, Dardenne M, Duheille J, Olive D: Improvement of cellular immunity and IgA production in immunodeficient children after treatment with synthetic serum thymic factor (FTS). Lancet 2:293–297, 1982.
48. Wara DA, Ammann AJ: Thymosin treatment of children with primary immunodeficiency disease. Transplant Proc 203:10–14, 1978.
49. Dardenne M, Pléau JM, Blouquit JY, Bach JF: Characterization of facteur thymique sérique (FTS) in the thymus. II. Direct demonstration of the presence of FTS in thymosin Fraction V. Clin Exp Immunol 42:477–482, 1980.
50. Waldmann TA, Broder S, Krakauer R, Durm H, Meade B, Goldman C: Defect in IgA secretion and in IgA specific suppressor cells in patients with selective IgA deficiency. Trans Assoc Am Physicians 89:219–224, 1976.
51. Hong R, Santosham M, Schulte-Wissermann HW, Horowitz S, Han S, Winkelstein J: Reconstitution of B and T lymphocyte function in severe combined immunodeficiency disease after transplantation with thymic epithelium. Lancet 2:1270–1272, 1976.
52. Pyke KW, Dosch HM, Ipp MM, Gelfand EW: Intrathymic defect in severe combined immunodeficiency disease. N Engl J Med 293:424–428, 1975.
53. Aiuti F, Businco L, Gatti RA: Reconstitution of T-cell disorders following thymus transplantation. Birth Defects*11(1): 370–376, 1975.
54. Gillis S, Union NA, Baker PE, Kendall A: The in vitro generation and sustained culture of nude mouse cytolytic T lymphocytes. J Exp Med 149:1460–1479, 1979.
55. Wara DW, Goldstein AL, Doyle NE, Ammann AJ: Thymosin activity in patients with cellular immunodeficiency. N Engl J Med 292:70–74, 1975.
56. Wara D: Thymic hormones in primary immunodeficiency. In "Clinics in Immunology and Allergy." New York: WB Saunders (In press).
57. Aiuti F, Ammirati P, Fiorilli M: Immunologic and clinical investigation on a bovine thymic extract: Therapeutic applications in primary immunodeficiencies. Pediatr Res 13:797–802, 1979.
58. Trainin N, Small M, Sipori D, Umiel T, Kook AI, Rotter V: Characteristics of THF, a thymic hormone. In Van Bekkum DW (ed): "The Biological Activity of Thymic Hormones." Rotterdam: Kooyter Scientific, 1975, pp 117–144.
59. Goldstein G, Scheid MP, Boyse EA, Schlesinger DH, Van Wauwe J: A synthetic pentapeptide with biological activity, characteristic of the thymic hormone thymopoietin. Science 204:1309–1312, 1979.
60. Dardenne M, Nabarra B, Lefrancier P, Derrien M, Choay J: Contribution of zinc and other metals to the biological activity of the serum thymic factor (FTS). Proc Natl Acad Sci USA 79:53–70, 1982.
61. Dardenne M, Charreire J, Bach JF: Alterations in thymocyte surface markers after in vitro treatment by serum thymic factor. Cell Immunol 39:47–54, 1978.

Demonstration of Abnormalities in Expression of Thymic Epithelial Surface Antigens in Severe Cellular Immunodeficiency Diseases*

Barton F. Haynes, MD, Robert W. Warren, MD, PhD, Rebecca H. Buckley, MD, John E. McClure, PhD, Allan L. Goldstein, PhD, Frederick W. Henderson, MD, Lucinda L. Hensley, MT, and George S. Eisenbarth, MD, PhD

Departments of Medicine, Microbiology, and Immunology, Duke University School of Medicine, Durham, NC 27710 (B.F.H.), Duke University Medical Center, Durham, NC 27710 (R.W.W., R.H.B.), Department of Biochemistry, George Washington University, Washington, DC 20037 (J.E.M, A.L.G.), Pediatric Infectious Diseases, North Carolina Memorial Hospital, Chapel Hill, NC 27514 (F.W.H), 5011 Timmons Dr., Durham, NC 27713 (L.L.H.), Research Department, Joslin Diabetes Center, Boston, MA 02215 (G.S.E.)

Severe cellular immunodeficiency diseases comprise a spectrum of heterogeneous disorders characterized by profound T- and B-lymphocyte dysfunction and are complicated by bacterial and viral infections, usually leading to death within the first 2 years of life [1]. SCID and cellular immunodeficiency with normal serum Ig (Nezelof syndrome) are 2 clinical syndromes within this spectrum of diseases [1–3]. In these conditions the thymus is frequently dysplastic; histopathologic study usually has revealed a small thymic rudiment, with scanty lymphoid cells and islands of thymic epithelium scattered throughout a fibrofatty stroma [4].

We have recently developed a number of novel probes for the study of human thymic epithelium [5]. We have reported that a GQ ganglioside antigen (defined by monoclonal antibody A2B5), and GD and GT ganglioside receptors for tetanus toxin (TT) selectively identified the neuroendocrine thymopoietin and thymosin α_1-containing portion of epithelium in normal thymus [5]. In this study, we describe the use of these probes to study the surface antigen characteristics and thymic hormone content of thymus tissue from 3 children with severe cellular immunodeficiency disease.

MATERIALS AND METHODS

Patients and Control Subjects

In October 1981 and March 1982, 2 infants with SCID expired at Duke University Medical Center (*Patients 1* and *2*, Table 1). A child with cellular immunodeficiency and normal serum Ig (Nezelof syndrome) expired at Memorial Hospital at the University of North Carolina, Chapel Hill, during the same time period (*Patient 3*, Table 1). All 3 children's erythrocytes contained adenosine deaminase (ADA) and nucleoside phosphorylase (NP). The clinical characteristics of each patient are shown in Table 1. The immunologic criteria upon which the diagnosis of severe cellular immunodeficiency disease was based are shown in Table 2.

Assay for Lymphocyte or Thymus Epithelium Cell-Surface Markers Using Monoclonal Antibodies

Acetone fixed 4μ tissue sections were incubated with a saturating amount of monoclonal reagent for 30 minutes at 25°C, washed in PBS and then incubated with a saturating amount of fluoresceinated goat anti-mouse Ig (F/P–6.0) (TAGO, Inc., Burlingame, CA). After 30 minutes incubation and washes in PBS and water, the tissue sections were overlaid with 30% glycerol in saline and a coverslip, and viewed on a Nikon Optiphot fluorescent microscope [6].

Monoclonal Antibodies

For the study of surface markers of thymic epithelium, monoclonal antibody A2B5 binds to a GQ ganglioside antigen found on normal and malignant neural crest-derived or neuroendocrine tissue [7,8]. Human Thy-1 antigen, as defined by a monoclonal antibody produced by McKenzie and Fabre [9], is the homolog of the mouse Thy-1 antigen. In the human, Thy-1 is not expressed on thymocytes, but is selectively expressed on normal subcapsular cortical thymic epithelial cells [10].

For the study of thymocyte or lymphoid cell-surface antigens, monoclonal antibodies recognizing the panleukocyte T-200 antigen [11], the early thymocyte antigen T6 [12], the 3A1 T-cell antigen [13], the E-rosette receptor [14], the mature T-cell antigens T1, T3, T4, T8 [12], and the thymus medullary-specific antigen A3D8 [15] were used as described previously [16].

---

*This article will appear in the March 1983 issue of J Immunol in extenso.

TABLE 1. Clinical Features of Patients With Severe Cellular Immunodeficiency Diseases

Patient	Diagnosis	Sex	Age at Presentation	Age at Death	Cause of Death	X-ray Thymus Shadow	Thymus Histopathology
1	SCID	M	8 mo	21 mo	Aspergillus, parainfluenza pneumonias	Absent	Fibrofatty rudiment with lobules of epithelial cells. No Hassall bodies present
2	SCID	M	8 mo	21 mo	Disseminated parainfluenza 3 infection	Absent	Fibrofatty rudiment with lobules of epithelial cells. No Hassall bodies present
3	Nezelof syndrome	F	6 mo	7 mo	Disseminated polio type 2 infection, Pneumocystis carinii pneumonia	Absent	Fibrofatty rudiment with lobules of epithelial cells. No Hassall bodies present. Occasional lymphocytes seen among epithelial cells

TABLE 2. Immunologic Characteristics of Patients With Severe Cellular Immunodeficiency Diseases*

Patient	Diagnosis	Serum Ig (mg/dl)[a] IgG	IgM	IgA	Lymphocytes (cells/mm^3)	T Cells[b] (cells/mm^3) Total	T4$^+$	T8$^+$	B Cells (cells/mm^3)	Isoagglutinins	Anti-TT[c] or Anti-Polio Virus Titer	Mitogen Response PHA	CON A	MLR
1	SCID	38	0	0	736	301	165	226	0	Absent	Anti-TT negative	Absent	Absent	Present[d]
2	SCID	<10	7.0	<1	1424	199	149	0	1053	Absent	Anti-TT negative	Absent	Absent	Absent
3	Nezelof syndrome	381	49	14	1200	480	48	144	144	Absent	Anti-polio negative	Absent	Absent	Absent

*Data taken at time of clinical presentation.
[a]Normal serum Ig levels for age = IgG = 314–799 mg/dl, IgM = 12–24 mg/dl, IgA = 27–73 mg/dl.
[b]Total T lymphocytes as determined by ability of lymphocytes to rosette with neuraminidase-treated sheep erythrocytes.
[c]TT=tetanus toxoid. Normal anti-TT antibody titers > 10,000.
[d]Allogeneic mixed lymphocyte reaction (MLR) induced tritiated thymidine incorporation but at 25% of the level of the normal subject assayed concurrently.

Assay for Thymic Tissue Reactivity With Anti-Thymic Hormone Antisera

Monospecific rabbit anti-thymosin α_1 and anti-thymosin β_4 were prepared as previously described [17,18]. Rabbit anti-thymopoietin antisera was the generous gift of Dr. G. Goldstein, Ortho Pharmaceuticals, Raritan, NJ [19]. Normal rabbit serum (NRS) was used as a control. Reactivity of normal or severe cellular immunodeficiency disease tissue with NRS, anti-thymopoietin, anti-thymosin α_1, or thymosin β_4 was determined by incubation of tissue sections with saturating amounts of antisera for 45 minutes as above and developed with saturating amounts of fluoresceinated or rhodaminated goat anti-rabbit Ig. Thymus tissue levels of thymosin α_1 were assayed by a sensitive RIA [17].

RESULTS

Thymic Epithelial Surface Antigens and Thymic Hormone Distribution in Normal Human Thymus

The neuroendocrine epithelial component of the human thymus is present in 2 definable compartments—the subcapsular cortical, and medullary thymic epithelium. Thymic lymphocytes teased from normal thymus tissue did not react with any of the rabbit anti-thymic hormone antisera, bind TT or monoclonal antibodies A2B5 or anti-Thy-1. The normal subcapsular cortical thymic epithelial region differed from the medullary region by reactivity with anti-Thy-1 and anti-thymosin β_4. Otherwise the subcapsular cortical and medullary thymic epithelium were identical in their reactivity with A2B5, TT, and anti-thymosin α_1 and anti-thymopoietin. We have previously shown (using double indirect immunofluorescence) that all

A2B5+, TT+ subcapsular cortical and medullary thymic epithelial cells contain thymosin α_1 and thymopoietin [5].

Thymic Epithelial Surface Antigens in Thymic Rudiments From Patients With Severe Cellular Immunodeficiency Diseases

While the reactivity patterns of A2B5 and TT were identical on the thymic epithelium from both patients with SCID (*Patients 1* and *2*), reactivity of these probes with Nezelof syndrome (*Patient 3*) thymic rudiment was different from the pattern seen on SCID thymus. Both SCID thymus rudiments were entirely A2B5+ and Thy-1+. Unlike normal subcapsular cortical or medullary thymic epithelium, however, epithelial islands in both SCID thymuses did not bind TT.

In contrast to the reactivity pattern of SCID thymus, thymic tissue from the Nezelof syndrome patient (*Patient 3*) bound TT and anti-Thy-1 but was unreactive with antibody A2B5. The thymic epithelial antigen patterns in SCID and Nezelof syndrome are contrasted in Table 3.

Reactivity of Anti-Thymic Hormone Antisera With Severe Cellular Immunodeficiency Disease Thymic Rudiment Tissue

To determine if the thymic epithelium remnants present in our patients with severe cellular immunodeficiency diseases contained thymic hormones, reactivity of anti-thymosin α_1, anti-thymosin β_4 and anti-thymopoietin was determined by indirect immunofluorescence, and thymosin α_1 levels per gram of wet thymic tissue were determined by RIA.

All 3 patients' entire thymic epithelium reacted with antisera against thymosin α_1, thymosin β_4, and thymopoietin. When thymosin α_1 levels were measured in extracts of normal or patient thymus tissue, we found that whereas the 4 normal thymuses contained a mean ($\pm$SEM) of 14.3$\pm$3.4 μg thymosin α_1/gm of tissue, the SCID thymus (*Patients 1* and *2*) contained low but detectable (1.0, 1.2 μg thymosin α_1/gm of tissue, respectively) amounts and the Nezelof thymus (*Patient 3*) contained an intermediate amount of thymosin α_1 (6.9 μg/gm tissue).

Correlation of Thymic Epithelial Antigen Pattern and Thymic Thymosin α_1 Content With Intrathymic T-Cell Maturation

Using a panel of monoclonal antibodies that recognize cell-surface antigens of either mature or immature thymocytes [reviewed in 20,21], we next looked for the presence of intrathymic leukocytes as defined by expression of the panleukocyte marker T-200, and when present, determined the stage of T-cell maturation as defined by surface T-cell antigen expression.

Both SCID thymus rudiments contained only scattered T-200+ lymphocytes. Lymphocytes that were present expressed only the T-cell antigens 3A1 and 9.6 (E-rosette receptor) (*Patient 1*) or, in the case of *Patient 2*, antigens 3A1 and T1. Of the few lymphocytes present in SCID thymus, none expressed mature T-cell antigens (T4, T8, A3D8). In contrast to both SCID thymuses, the Nezelof syndrome thymus contained many T-200+ lymphocytes—all of which were 3A1+, T3+, T1+ and 9.6+ (E-rosette receptor). In addition, approximately 80% expressed the T4 antigen, 20% the T8 antigen and all expressed the medullary (mature) thymocyte-specific antigen defined by antibody A3D8. Thus, the Nezelof thymus, although dysplastic and devoid of a normal cortical-medullary architecture, was able to induce some T cells to mature.

Further evidence that some intrathymic T-cell division (and therefore maturation) was occurring in the Nezelof thymus came from the observation that 10–20% of intrathymic lymphocytes in the thymus of *Patient 3* expressed transferrin receptors and T10 antigen, both markers of rapidly dividing cells [12,20]. Neither of the SCID thymuses had transferrin-receptor bearing or T10-positive cells.

DISCUSSION

Using probes that bind complex gangliosides (TT or antibody A2B5), our study for the first time demonstrates abnormalities in thymic epithelium surface antigens in patients with severe cellular immunodeficiency diseases. Limited intrathymic T-cell maturation was shown to occur in dysplastic thymus tissue from a Nezelof syndrome patient but not in SCID thymic rudiments. By indirect immunofluorescence thymosin α_1, thymopoietin, and thymosin β_4 thymic hormones were all present in thymic epithelial cells of all 3 pa-

TABLE 3. Thymic Epithelial Antigen Expression in Severe Cellular Immunodeficiency Diseases*

Patient	Diagnosis	Receptors for Tetanus Toxin (GD/GT Gangliosides)	Receptors for Antibody A2B5 (GQ Gangliosides)	Thy-1
1	SCID	Absent	Present	Present
2	SCID	Absent	Present	Present
3	Nezelof syndrome	Present	Absent	Present

*In addition to the above markers, similar to normal thymic epithelium, all 3 patients' thymic epithelium expressed nonpolymorphic HLA A, B, and C and Ia-like antigens as determined by monoclonal antibodies 3F10 (anti-HLA) and L-243 (anti-Ia-like).

tients. By RIA, thymosin α_1 levels per gram of tissue were markedly decreased in both SCID thymuses, whereas thymosin α_1 was present at approximately one-half normal level in the Nezelof patient's thymus.

The importance in our study lies in the observations that a) in SCID and Nezelof thymus, abnormalities in surface antigens (presumably gangliosides) are present—these abnormalities are different in SCID (TT−, A2B5+) versus the Nezelof syndrome (TT+, A2B5−); b) various thymic hormones appeared to be present in the thymic epithelium, indicating that the inability of thymic epithelium to synthesize thymic hormones at a cellular level is not a factor in the pathogenesis of immunodeficiency in these diseases. However, these data do not rule out the possibility that there may be a secretory defect in thymic epithelium of one or more of the thymic hormones, or that the hormones, though antigenically recognized by rabbit antisera, may be functionally inactive. The lower levels of thymosin α_1 in SCID thymus compared to Nezelof and normal thymic tissue most likely reflect a smaller volume of thymic epithelium in SCID per gram of tissue. Evidence for defect in secretion of thymopoietin comes from Lewis et al who demonstrated near-absent plasma levels of thymopoietin in both ADA+ and ADA-SCID [21]. Successful reconstitution of these patients with thymus or bone marrow grafts and with RBC transfusions was associated with rises in plasma thymopoietin [21]. These data suggested that interaction of normal bone marrow stem cells with either primary or secondary abnormal thymic epithelium resulted in elevation of plasma thymopoietin levels postreconstitution [21]. We do not have preplasma infusion plasma samples for thymosin α_1 levels in our 2 SCID patients, but RIA determination of plasma thymosin α_1 levels in 4 patients with SCID (D. Wara and A.L. Goldstein, unpublished data) demonstrated low-to-normal levels in all 4 patients. Finally, the observation of normal (1430 ± 145 pg/ml in *Patient 3* versus 1465 ± 210 pg/ml in the normal newborn) serum thymosin α_1 levels in our patient with Nezelof syndrome rules out a secretory defect of thymosin α_1 in this patient.

Thus, this battery of probes used in our study of normal and abnormal thymic epithelium, coupled with assays of thymic epithelial and lymphocyte function should prove useful in elucidating precise pathophysiologic defects in severe cellular immunodeficiency diseases, and therefore in planning immunologic reconstitution therapy for these patients.

REFERENCES

1. Buckley RH: Primary immunodeficiency diseases. In Wyngaarden JB, Smith LH (eds): "Cecil Textbook of Medicine." Philadelphia: WB Saunders, 1982, pp 1789–1796.
2. Dosch HM, Lee JWW, Gelfand EW, Falk JA: Severe combined immunodeficiency disease: A model of T cell dysfunction. Clin Exp Immunol 34:260–267, 1978.
3. Lawlor GJ, Ammann AJ, Wright WC, LaFranchi SH, Bilstrom D, Stiehm ER: The syndrome of cellular immunodeficiency with immunoglobulins. J Pediatr 84:183–192, 1974.
4. Borzy MS, Schulte-Wisserman H, Gilbert E, Horowitz SD, Pellett J, Hong R: Thymic morphology in immunodeficiency diseases: Results of thymic biopsies. Clin Immunol Immunopathol 12:31–51, 1979.
5. Haynes BF, Shimizu K, Eisenbarth GS: Identification of human and rodent thymic epithelium using tetanus toxin and monoclonal antibody A2B5. J Clin Invest (In press)
6. Haynes BF, Hensley LL, Jegasothy BV: Phenotypic characterization of skin infiltrating T cells in cutaneous T cell lymphoma. Comparison with benign cutaneous T cell infiltrates. Blood 60:463–473, 1982.
7. Eisenbarth GS, Walsh FS, Nirenberg M: Monoclonal antibody to a plasma membrane antigen of neurons. Proc Natl Acad Sci USA 76:4913–4917, 1979.
8. Eisenbarth GS, Shimizu K, Bowring MF, Wells S: Expression of receptors for tetanus toxin and monoclonal antibody A2B5 by pancreatic islet cells. Proc Natl Acad Sci USA 79:5066–5070, 1982.
9. McKenzie JS, Fabre JW: Human Thy-1: Unusual localization and possible functional significance in lymphoid tissue. J Immunol 126:843–850, 1981.
10. Ritter MA, Sauvage CA, Cotmore CF: The human thymus microenvironment: In vivo identification of thymic nurse cells and other antigenically distinct subpopulations of epithelial cells. Immunology 44:439–446, 1981.
11. Dalchau R, Kirkley J, Fabre J: Monoclonal antibody to a human leucocyte specific membrane glycoprotein probably homologous to the leucocyte common (LC) antigen of the rat. Eur J Immunol 10:737–744, 1980.
12. Reinherz EL, Schlossman SF: Regulation of the immune response-inducer and suppressor T lymphocyte subsets in human beings. N Engl J Med 303:370–373, 1980.
13. Haynes BF: Human T lymphocyte antigens as defined by monoclonal antibodies. Immunol Rev 57:127–161, 1980.
14. Kamoun M, Martin PJ, Hansen JA, Brown MA, Siatek AW, Novinshi RC: Identification of a human T lymphocyte surface protein associated with the E-rosette receptor. J Exp Med 153:207–211, 1981.
15. Telen MJ, Eisenbarth GS, Haynes BF: Characterization and distribution of a Lutheran erythrocyte antigen as defined by a monoclonal antibody. (Abstract) Clin Res 30:331A, 1982.
16. Haynes BF, Metzgar RS, Minna JD, Bunn PA: Phenotypic characterization of cutaneous T cell lymphoma. Use of monoclonal antibodies to compare with other malignant T cells. N Engl J Med 304:1319–1323, 1981.
17. McClure JE, Lameris N, Wara DW, Goldstein AL: Immunochemical studies of thymosin: Radioimmunoassay of thymosin 1. J Immunol 128:368–375, 1982.
18. Hirokawa K, McClure JE, Goldstein AL: Age-related changes in localization of thymosin in human thymus. Thymus 4:19–29, 1982.
19. Goldstein G: Radioimmunoassay for thymopoietin. J Immunol 117:690–692, 1976.
20. Terhorst C, van Agthoven A, LeClair K, Snow P, Reinherz E, Schlossman S: Biochemical studies of the human thymocyte cell surface antigens T6, T9 and T10. Cell 23:771–780, 1981.
21. Lewis V, Twomey J, Goldstein G et al: Circulating thymic hormone activity in congenital immunodeficiency. Lancet 2:471–475, 1977.

Thymus Transplantation*

Richard Hong, MD

Division of Immunology, Center for Health Sciences, University of Wisconsin, Madison, WI 53792

Attempts to define a role for the thymus gland in the immune response relied upon a classic embryologic approach, namely that of extirpation. MacLean and Good [1] removed the gland from adult rabbits without any effect upon the immune system, leading them to conclude that the thymus gland did not play a significant role in the development of the immune response. Of course, they were simply demonstrating what is now a well-known fact of the T-cell system, viz that T lymphocytes peripheralize and accomplish their function (at least in part) by long-lived cell populations. It was some years before Good et al [2], Miller [3], and Waksman et al [4] were able to pinpoint the thymus role. Extirpation experiments in newborn animals, or in thymectomized irradiated adults produced a defect of the T-cell system which was lethal and corrected by thymus transplantation.

This discovery was applied in the clinical setting by Rosen et al in 1962 [5], and Hitzig et al in 1965 [6]. Unfortunately, the full delineation of T- and B-cell roles had not been accomplished at that time and therefore, thymus transplantation was not in all cases the appropriate reconstitution modality. For this and other reasons, early attempts with thymus transplantation met with failure.

FETAL THYMUS

Originally, fetal thymus slices were inserted into the rectus abdominus muscle, perhaps, in part, because of the success observed when parathyroid glands are reimplanted in muscles should they inadvertently be removed at surgery. Whether this subliminally presaged the later appreciation of hormonal function of the thymus is unknown. The intramuscular site should have worked, for the route of transplantation of thymus seemed not to make a difference in mouse studies [7]. However, the exhaustive testing used today was not available originally and it seems possible that some differences might be discernible by modern evaluation of transplanted animals. If one examines the histology of transplanted thymuses, one is impressed with the tremendous amount of necrosis which occurs prior to establishment of the graft as a viable organ [8]. Also, the possibility of a local graft-versus-host (GVH) reaction, wherein T cells of the thymus would react against the host, either within or near the gland, seems very likely. I believe that this local reaction could have harmed the gland sufficiently to impair its function. In the older literature, it was concluded that allogeneic grafts could not reconstitute athymic nude mice. We know today that cultured grafts (devoid of mature T cells) are very effective in this regard [9]. Therefore, it is possible that a large number of mature T cells persisting in the graft prior to transplant are not biologically insignificant and that the route of transplant was important in the early failures in man.

A major event in the resurgence of interest in thymus transplantation occurred when Ammann et al [10] showed T-cell benefit following fetal thymus transplantation into a patient with SCID. The major departure from standard protocols was that Ammann injected his tissues intraperitoneally instead of intramuscularly. In following our in vitro thymus cultures, we see a tremendous outpouring of thymocytes from small fragments. Small thymus cultures appear to be fountains, raining thymocytes into the surrounding medium. The Ammann transplant can be likened to the delayed-release medication capsules, spraying millions of thymocytes into the peritoneal cavity. As an aside, I mention that fetal liver cell transplants likewise resulted in no benefit until an intraperitoneal route was employed. It may be that special routes of traffic are favored by an intraperitoneal route. In examining the results of the Ammann experience, the striking characteristic seen was that T cells of the donor were easily found and apparently demonstrated PHA responsiveness. Therefore, basically this form of reconstitution was in fact a small allogeneic T-cell infusion which did not produce fatal GVH disease. (Subsequent experience did indicate that thymuses from fetuses over 14 weeks of age could cause fatal GVH disease.) Three published reports of fetal thymus transplants in SCID all showed the same characteristics: T-cell engraftment, some functional responses, and no B-cell reconstitution [10-12]. Two of the patients have died, one of overwhelming cytomegalovirus infection and one of varicella [13]. Seven years after transplant, the third is alive, but suffers from chronic encephalitis. The results of fetal thymus transplantation can be considered in the framework of having achieved a small infusion of allogeneic T cells, producing a lym-

*Supported by NIH grant AI 14354.

phoid chimera. The result of that infusion is acquisition of positive responses to some T-cell mitogens; however, full and complete T-cell reconstitution is not seen because a site for maturation has not been engrafted, and whatever T-cell benefit is obtained results from the small numbers of T cells which have survived the transplantation procedure. It is assumed, but not proven, that replication of the infused cells occurs, since chimerism persists for many years. Persistent lymphopenia, however, suggests that long-lived T cells may account for the observed phenomena, rather than proliferation. What is clear, nevertheless, is that a gradual increase in T-cell capability does not seem to occur and the amount of T-cell reconstitution is fixed at the level attained shortly after transplant and consistent with a rather restricted population of T cells. The failure of B-cell benefit can be explained on the basis of genetic restriction which prevents full and vigorous T-B-macrophage cooperation necessary for complete antibody responses [14].

The attractiveness of fetal thymus as a therapeutic modality was based upon hope that fetal T cells were less capable of causing GVH disease and that fetal tissue might be tolerized to the host. Unfortunately, as mentioned above, cells from older fetuses are potentially lethal. Further, the mass of a less than 14-week-old thymus is simply not enough to effect a vigorous reconstitution. In any event, in my judgment, unless it becomes engrafted as a solid intact organ, fetal thymus tissue cannot become an effective form of treatment for T-cell deficiency. Recent experiences with cultured organs offer hope for the use of fetal tissues, older than 14 weeks, as will be described below.

CULTURED THYMUS FRAGMENTS (CTF)

In 1975, Lafferty et al [15] showed that organ culture permitted prolonged acceptance of allogeneic thyroid grafts. Furthermore, the grafts functioned very well and were able to restore thyroidectomized recipients. We did not have to contend with allograft rejection in T-cell deficiency, but nevertheless, we thought that cultured thymus fragments should be of interest to study, because it seemed likely that the epithelial cells of the thymus were important in differentiation, possibly as sources of hormone monolayers were being studied by others [16,17]. The in vitro changes which Pyke et al [16] had shown in SCID were extremely provocative in this regard. However, because of the local influence of Robert Auerbach, a pioneer in organ culture and in developmental biology of the thymus, we began our studies with thymus fragments, rather than monolayers.

Culture of the small organ fragments (approximately 2 mm in the greatest diameter) caused a marked egress of the thymocytes leaving only scattered islands of epithelial cells. Macrophages also remained. When the fragments were teased apart, only a few thymocytes were found (approximately 2–3000/fragment) and nearly all were nonviable, as defined by failure to exclude trypan blue. Thus, the transplants consisted primarily of epithelial cells and macrophages. Though we did not know at that time, present knowledge suggests that nurse cells are probably also included.

We used athymic nude mice as our experimental model and were extremely gratified to find an excellent reconstitution when the mice were subjected to exhaustive immunologic characterization. Of special interest was the fact that fully allogeneic thymuses reconstituted the nudes in every parameter, as well as syngeneic thymuses. This latter finding was of extreme importance in our ultimate determination to not attempt matching donor and recipient. Animals reconstituted by allogeneic thymuses have been challenged by vaccinia virus, have survived the challenge and later showed the ap-

TABLE 1. Thymus Transplantation in ADA+ SCID*

Good health when transplanted (N=24)	
Alive	8
T-cell benefit	16
B-cell benefit	14
Chronically ill when transplanted (N=10)	
Alive	0
T-cell benefit	4±
B-cell benefit	0
Moribund when transplanted (N=4)	
Alive	0
T-cell benefit	0
B-cell benefit	0

*From Hong R: Present and future status of thymus transplantation. Ann Clin Res 13:350–357, 1981, with permission.

propriate in vitro cytotoxic T-cell responses. These findings are somewhat different from earlier reports [18], but later studies by these same workers agree with ours [19]. The reason for the difference is not clear, but I feel that one element might be that the culture technique, by depleting the CTF of thymocytes may prevent a local GVH reaction, as alluded to above.

The reconstituted animals show levels of lymphocytes which are only about 50% of that seen in normal controls of the same strain, but this lymphopenia is not clinically significant. The mice show normal longevity and do not show undue susceptibility to any infections.

We transplanted our first patient with SCID in 1976 [20]. At that time, the prevailing concept of the cause of SCID was that a stem-cell fault was the most likely cause. Therefore, we expected, at best, only a T-cell response. To our pleasant surprise, a remarkable T- and B-cell response occurred. This observation provided clinical confirmation at a functional level, for notions set forth by the observations of Pyke et al [16] and Seeger et al [21], wherein a major T-cell defect was observed in SCID.

Since that time, a total of 38 patients with adenosine deaminase positive (ADA+) SCID have been transplanted. Results of those transplants are shown in Table 1. From review of those data, we can see that approximately 30% of the patients in good health at the time of transplant are now living at home in a reasonably normal environment. If there is a significant illness present at the time of transplant, we usually cannot reverse the process and effect any significant reconstitution. It should be remembered that one must create immunity from the ground zero state, and this requires time. It is usually about 4 months before one sees any appreciable change in lymphocyte tests. Often, one can see a reversal of wasting and freedom from further infections as early as a few weeks following the transplant.

Detailed immunologic testing, shown in Figures 1-5, shows that variable degrees of reconstitution are achieved. Certainly 100% normality is not the rule. Nevertheless, it is important to emphasize that the children are home and, except for those to be mentioned later, come to us only for routine follow-up twice a year. They are not suffering from chronic candidiasis or recurrent severe infections. This clinical response tells us that one does not have to achieve 100% immune response to be essentially free of infections and wasting disease. An interesting parallel can be drawn between these patients and those with hemophilia or thrombocytopenia. Patients with those 2 latter disorders will not bleed if their antihemophiliac globulin or platelet values are 20% of normal. In the same way, our patients do amazingly well with values only 20% of normal. Values found in some of our untreated patients with such disorders as cartilage hair hypoplasia (CHH) are quite similar to those seen in these partially reconstituted SCID patients. Those CHH patients also are essentially free of infection. I should emphasize that I do not believe these children are completely free of risk from overwhelming disease. I feel quite certain that varicella would be fatal in the SCID children.

Another interesting point in evaluation of the responses is that functional IgA responses as measured by

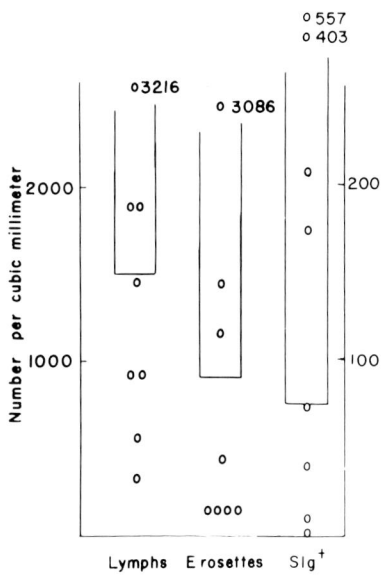

Fig. 1. Lymphocyte count, E-rosette number and SIg+ cells in 8 surviving patients after CTF transplant. The lower limits of normal values are shown by the bottom portion of the open bar. The same patient population is illustrated in Figs. 1-5. (Figs. 1-4 from "Proceedings of the 8th International Convocation on Immunology." Basel: S. Karger, 1983, reproduced with permission.)

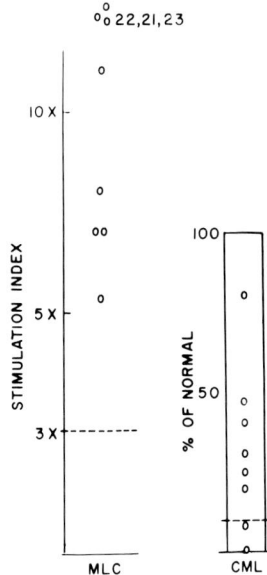

Fig. 3. Responses to allogeneic cells. Mixed leukocyte culture (MLC) responses shown as stimulation indices, defined as counts/minute of stimulated cultures/counts/minute of resting cultures. Values over 3× are in normal range. Cell-mediated lympholysis (CML) is the percent of specific release from chromium labeled targets of the same individual used to stimulate a given responder (the transplanted patient). Normal values vary from day to day. The patients' values shown are expressed as a percentage of a normal individual's response to the same target on the day of the test. Dotted line shows 10% of a normal response.

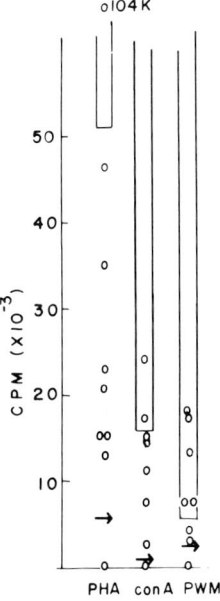

Fig. 2. Proliferation responses. The lower limits of normal responses are indicated by the bottom of the open bar. The horizontal arrow shows the highest value ever attained by any SCID patient studied over the past 8 years (N=43).

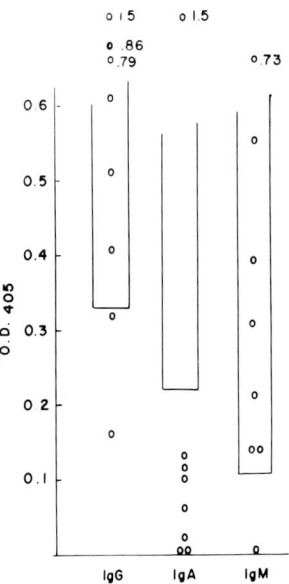

Fig. 4. Isotype responses to E. coli determined by ELISA assay. Values are expressed as OD_{405} units. The lower limits of the normal range are shown by the bottom portions of the open bars.

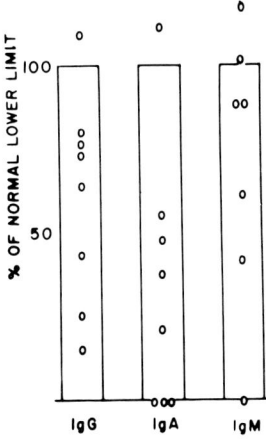

Fig. 5. IgG, IgA, and IgM responses expressed as percent of age-matched controls.

TABLE 2. Results With Fetal Thymus (Cultured)

	3/4/81		10/31/81	7/21/82
Lymphs	1,058	↓*	3,350	5,096
T6	5		ND	0
T3	5		41	53
T4	0		1	10
T8	0		32	43
SIg+(μ)	37		40	12
PHA	5X		17X	123X
Con A	2X		51X	6X
PWM	6X		3X	6X
MLC	1X		34X	27X
Cand	1X		ND	4X
CML	0		42.7%	31.1%
IgG	265		313	871
IgA	4		15	11
IgM	26		65	76

*CTF transplant.

E. coli isotype responses, are virtually nil in these patients. This would be consistent with the extreme dependence of IgA upon T-helper activity, and with previous suggestions that sometimes selective IgA deficiency could be a manifestation of a primary T-cell defect [22]. The high association of IgA deficiency in ataxia telangiectasia would be a case in point [23].

As these children have been followed for longer periods of time, the suggestion of decrease in thymic function has been observed. One patient, cared for in collaboration with Dr. E.R. Stiehm, was transplanted in 1978. He showed a marvelous response at first; he even recovered from hepatitis A infection and demonstrated an appropriate antibody response. In recent months, however, he has experienced a chronic diarrheal state. Finally, intravenous hyperalimentation was necessary to achieve reasonable nutrition. Repeat thymus transplants did not seem effective. At the present time he is extremely lymphopenic and his thymic function appears to be gone. Another child, first transplanted in 1979, appears to be entering this same phase. Thus, it is possible that the thymus transplants are unable to provide sustained benefit.

In the light of recent reports of successful transplantation from haploidentical donors using lectin separation of mature T cells from the marrow, cultured thymus fragments for the treatment of SCID may become a treatment of the past [24]. The efforts have not all been for naught, however. The CTF transplants have provided insight into the effect of the thymus gland upon the T- and B-cell system in man, and for a number of children they have brought precious years. CTF does not preempt other therapeutic attempts. There seems to be no reason that the children who have received cultured thymus and are not progressing well cannot have a prepared bone marrow transplant.

A recent observation in one of our patients is of interest. We had the opportunity of using thymus tissue obtained from a 22-week-old fetus for transplant. It is theoretically possible that such glands might behave differently from portions of whole glands obtained from older children. These differences could be due to the fact that a whole gland is employed, and there might not be any selection problem as there could be with only a portion of the gland employed. Metcalf and Brumdy [25] showed that thymus transplants consisting primarily of cortex were less effective than medullary transplants. Also fetal tissue might have different growth potential. Data from this child are shown in Table 2. Although there was virtually no response for nearly a year, we are now seeing a progressive improvement in his functions. Clinically, he has had no infections since the original hospitalization which was for pneumocystis pneumonia. He had chronic diarrhea when transferred to us and was malnourished. It is too early to make any judgments as to whether this child will fare differently from the others, but his course and the kinetics of his reconstitution are of interest.

One of the main reasons for an unsustained response is the basic quality of the thymus transplant. At first, we had no evidence for replication of epithelial cells. It has always been my belief that we were dealing with dying cultures, and that the lymphocytes were dying faster than the other cells. The point of the culture was to go as long as one could to maximize lymphoid depletion and minimize epithelial cell death. More recently, influenced strongly by the quality of thymus cultures produced by Australian workers [26], we have altered our culture techniques. As can be seen in Figures 6–8, there is much less fibrosis and evidence of replication. Thus, in future transplants, we anticipate a much more salutory response.

Thymus transplants should be effective in the less severe T-cell deficiency states. We have utilized CTF transplantation in a man who suffered from chronic candidiasis and acquired a buccal carcinoma in the area of the chronic and repeated infection. The lesion was so severe that a complete excision of his buccal mucosa was required. At that time, we transplanted him with CTF. He showed a marked return of responsiveness to Candida antigen in in vitro stimulation tests. Minor decreases of other T-cell parameters also improved [27]. He has remained free of carcinoma and his Candida is controlled on minimal therapy.

We have also employed CTF transplantation in ADA-SCID. The benefit which Polmar et al [28] observed with blood transfusion enzyme replacement therapy does not seem to occur with all patients [29]. We studied the effect of toxic metabolites on CTF and found that the nonlymphoid elements of the thymus were also affected by the ADA deficiency [30]. Accordingly, we have used CTF in 2 patients with ADA-SCID. Although the lymphopenia persists, the children are free of infection and have not shown the progressive downhill course reported by others [29].

Another disease which has piqued our interest in recent years has been

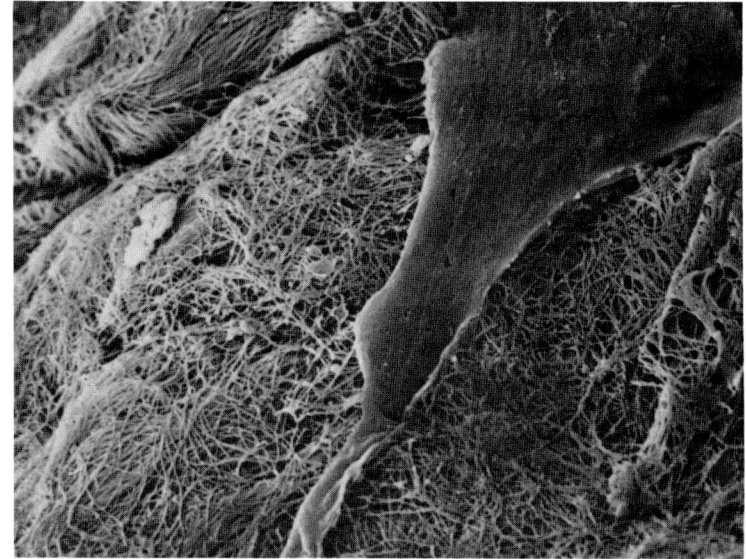

6

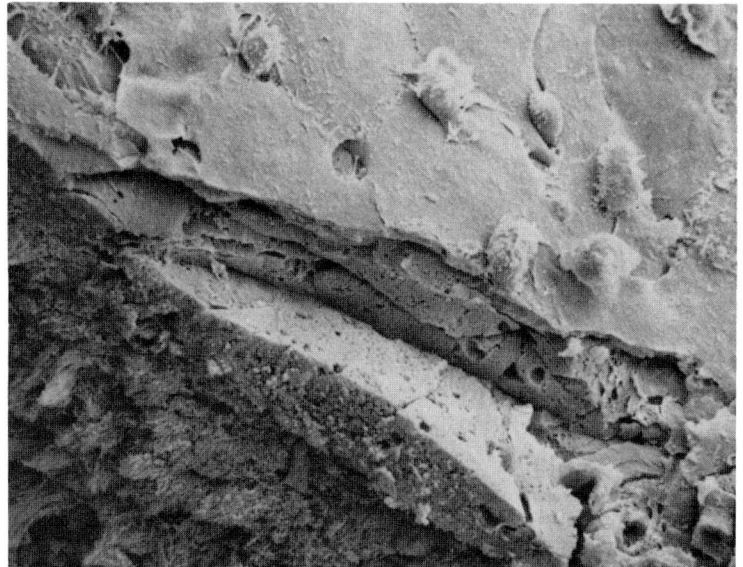

7

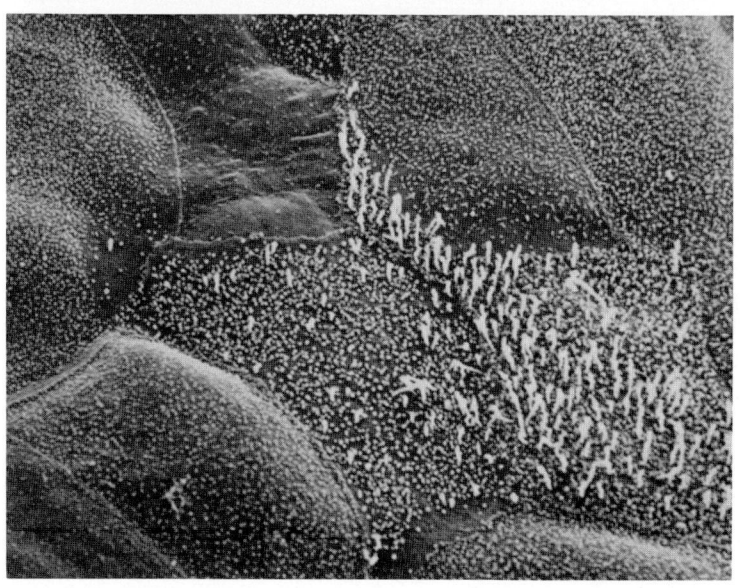

8

Fig. 6. Scanning electron micrograph of thymus culture after 3 weeks, present techniques. The healthy state of the epithelium is evident from the cellular margins and the villous structures.

Fig. 7. Scanning electron micrograph of thymus culture after 3 weeks, previous culture technique. Most of the surface is fibrous tissue.

Fig. 8. Freeze-fracture of culture shown in Fig. 6; at least 3 cell layers thick, suggesting replication.

chronic lymphocytic leukemia. Although at first considered a B-cell disease, recent reports demonstrate a significant T-cell abnormality as well [30–32]. We tested the response of mononuclear cells from patients with chronic lymphatic leukemia to pokeweed mitogen. In the presence of cultured thymic fragments, augmented production of IgG and/or IgA was seen. Encouraged by this response, we have recently transplanted our first chronic lymphatic leukemia patient with extremely gratifying results. Plagued by repeated infections, he is now symptom free with acquisition of significant T-cell capability.

We do not know of any complications unique to this transplant. Some years ago, we reported the occurrence of immunoangioblastic lymphoma in 3 patients following CTF transplantation [33]. Similar tumors occur in SCID patients both with and without any therapeutic intervention [34]. I believe that immunodeficient patients are at high risk for this complication. It may be that CTF or other types of therapy accelerate the rate of development or provide one of the necessary elements to produce the malignant change. In some cases, Epstein-Barr virus appears to be the direct causative agent. In any event, I do not believe that CTF is any more or less likely to induce the event than any other treatment which does not provide a rapid and high-grade reconstitution. This type of lymphoma has even been recorded after bone marrow transplantation for leukemia [35]. We have not observed this complication in any of our transplants since 1978.

A theoretic complication, that of autoimmune disease, which would be predicted according to the theory of Jerne [36], has not been observed. According to Jerne, clones capable of reacting with self-histocompatibility antigens are eliminated according to the histocompatibility expressed by the nonlymphoid cells of the thymus. Thus, the killer cells generated by the allogeneic transplanted thymus would spare the thymus, but not realize that the host was really self. Emergent cytotoxic T cells could potentially wreak havoc on the host. This has not been observed in nearly 50 human transplants or in over 400 animal transplants. This sparing of self is probably due to the fact that self appears to be defined prethymically [37]. Therefore, although the thymus modulates killer-cell behavior, it does not create self-destructing populations. This is an extremely fortunate happenstance for our transplantation efforts.

CONCLUSION

This brief review traces the history of thymus transplants as employed over the past several years. Benefits and problems of cultured thymus transplants have been considered in detail. It seems likely that superior treatment of SCID is near if not already at hand, and CTF for that disorder may no longer be indicated. For a number of milder T-cell disorders, however, CTF offers hope and should provide reasonable benefit.

REFERENCES

1. MacLean LD, Zak SJ, Varco RL, Good RA: The role of the thymus in antibody production. An experimental study of the immune response in thymectomized rabbits. Transplant Bull 4:21–22, 1957.
2. Good RA, Dalmasso AP, Martinez C, Archer OK, Pierce JC, Papermaster BW: The role of the thymus in development of immunologic capacity in rabbits and mice. J Exp Med 116:773–796, 1962.
3. Miller JFAP: Immunological function of the thymus. Lancet 2:748–749, 1961.
4. Waksman BH, Arnason BG, Jankovic BD: Role of thymus in immune reactions in rats. III. Changes in the lymphoid organs of thymectomized rats. J Exp med 116:187–205, 1962.
5. Rosen FS, Gitlin D, Janeway CA: Alymphocytosis, agammaglobulinemia, homografts and delayed hypersensitivity; Study of a case. Lancet 2:380–381, 1962.
6. Hitzig WH, Kay HEM, Cottier H: Familial lymphopenia with agammaglobulinemia (Swiss type of agammaglobulinemia): Attempt of treatment by implantation of foetal thymus. Lancet 2:151–154, 1965.
7. Metcalf D: The nature and regulation of lymphopoiesis in the normal and neoplastic thymus. In Wolstenholme GEW, Porter R (eds): "Ciba Foundation Symposium on the Thymus, Experimental and Clinical Studies." London: Churchill, 1966, pp 242–263.
8. Dukor P, Miller JFAP, House W, Allman V: Regeneration of thymus grafts. I. Histological and cytological aspects. Transplantation 3:639–668, 1965.
9. Hong R, Schulte-Wissermann H, Jarrett-Toth E, Horowitz SD, Manning DD: Transplantation of cultured thymic fragments II. Results in nude mice. J Exp Med 149:398–415, 1979.
10. Ammann AJ, Wara D, Salmon S, Perkins H: Thymus transplantation: Permanent reconstitution of cellular immunity in a patient with sex-linked combined immunodeficiency. N Engl J Med 289:5–9, 1973.
11. Rachelefsky GS, Stiehm ER, Ammann AJ, Cederbaum SD, Opelz G, Terasaki P: T-cell reconstitution by thymus transplantation and transfer factor in severe combined immunodeficiency. Pediatrics 55:114–118, 1975.
12. Shearer WT, Wedner J, Strominger DB, Kissane J, Hong R: Successful transplantation of the thymus in Nezelof's syndrome. Pediatrics 61:619–624, 1978.
13. Tanner DD, Buckley PJ, Hong R, Shearer WT: Fatal cytomegalovirus bronchiolitis in a patient with Nezelof's syndrome. Pediatrics 65:98–102, 1980.
14. Katz DH, Hamaoka T, Benacerraf B: Cell interactions between histoincompatible T and B lymphocytes. J Exp Med 137:1405–1418, 1973.
15. Lafferty KJ, Cooley MA, Woolnough J, Walker KZ: Thyroid allograft immunogenicity is reduced after a period in organ culture. Science 188:259–261, 1975.
16. Pyke KW, Dosch HM, Ipp MM, Gelfand EW: Intrathymic defect in severe combined immunodeficiency disease. N Engl J Med 293:424–427, 1975.
17. Willis JI, St. Pierre RL: Immunological reconstitution of neonatally thymectomized rats following implantation of thymic epithelial cells. Adv Exp Med Biol 73A:111–118, 1976.
18. Zinkernagel RM, Callahan GN, Althage A, Cooper S, Streilin JW, Klein J: The lymphoreticular system in triggering virus plus self-specific cytotoxic T cells; Evidence for T help. J Exp Med 147:897, 1978.
19. Zinkernagel RM, Althage A, Waterfield E, Kindred B: Restriction specificities, alloreactivity and allotolerance expressed by T cells from nude mice reconstituted with H-2-compatible or incompatible thy-

mus grafts. J Exp Med 151:376–399, 1980.
20. Hong R, Santosham M, Schulte-Wissermann H, Horowitz S, Hsu SH, Winkelstein JA: Reconstitution of B and T lymphocyte function in severe combined immunodeficiency disease after transplantation with thymic epithelium. Lancet 2:1270–1272, 1976.
21. Seeger RC, Robins RA, Stevens RH, Klein RB, Waldman DJ, Zeltzer PM, Kessler SW: Severe combined immunodeficiency with B lymphocytes: In vitro correction of defective immunoglobulin production by addition of normal T lymphocytes. Clin Exp Immunol 26:1–10, 1976.
22. Horowitz S, Hong R: Selective IgA deficiency—Some perspectives. In Bergsma D (ed): "Immunodeficiency in Man and Animals." Sunderland, MA: Sinauer Associates, for The National Foundation–March of Dimes, BD:OAS XI(1):129–133, 1975.
23. Epstein WL, Fudenberg HH, Reed WB, Bader E, Sedgwick RP: Immunologic studies in ataxia-telangiectasia. I. Delayed hypersensitivity and serum immune globulin levels in probands and first-degree relatives. Int Arch Allergy Appl Immunol 30:15, 1966.
24. Reisner Y, Kapoor N, Kirkpatrick D, Pollack MS, Dupont B, Good RA, O'Reilly RJ: Transplantation for acute leukaemia with HLA-A and B nonidentical parental marrow cells fractionated with soybean agglutinin and sheep red blood cells. Lancet 2:327–331, 1981.
25. Metcalf D, Brumdy M: The role of the thymus in the ontogeny of the immune response. J Cell Physiol 67:(Suppl 1)149–168, 1966.
26. Mandel TE, Kennedy M: The differentiation of murine thymocytes in vivo and in vitro. Immunology 35:317–331, 1978.
27. Hong R, Dibbell DG: Cultured thymus fragment (CTF) transplant in chronic candidiasis complicated by oral carcinoma. Lancet 1:773–774, 1981.
28. Polmar SH, Stern RC, Schwartz AL, Wetzler EM, Chase PA, Hirschhorn R: Enzyme replacement therapy for adenosine deaminase deficiency and severe combined immunodeficiency. N Engl J Med 295:1337–1343, 1976.
29. Dysminski JW, Daoud A, Lampkin BC et al: Immunological and biochemical profiles in response to transfusion therapy in an adenosine deaminase deficient patient with severe combined immunodeficiency disease. Clin Immunol Immunopathol 14:307–326, 1979.
30. Faguet GB: Mechanisms of lymphocyte activation: The role of suppressor cells in the proliferative responses of chronic lymphatic leukemia lymphocytes. J Clin Invest 63:67, 1979.
31. Chiorazzi N, Fu SM, Montazeri G, Kunkel HG, Rai K, Gee T: T cell helper defect in patients with chronic lymphatic leukemia. J Immunol 122:1087, 1979.
32. Ershler WB, Ney P, Britt J, Glynn B, Hong R: Thymic dysfunction in chronic lymphocytic leukemia. Thymus 3:203–212, 1981.
33. Borzy MF, Hong R, Horowitz SD et al: Fatal lymphoma after transplantation of cultured thymus in children with combined immunodeficiency disease. N Engl J Med 301:565–568, 1979.
34. Kersey JH, Filipovich AH, Spector BD: Lymphoma after thymus transplantation (Letter). N Engl J Med 302:301, 1980.
35. Hossett TC, Gale RP, Fleischman H, Austin GE, Sparkes RS, Taylor CR: Immunoblastic sarcoma in donor cells after bone-marrow transplantation. N Engl J Med 300:904–907, 1979.
36. Jerne NK: The somatic generation of immune recognition. Eur J Immunol 1:1–9, 1971.
37. Besedovsky HO, Del Rey A, Sorkin E: Role of prethymic cells in acquisition of self-tolerance. J Exp Med 150:1351–1358, 1979.

Therapy With Thymopoietin Pentapeptide (TP-5) in 26 Patients With Primary Immunodeficiencies*

Fernando Aiuti, MD, Luisa Businco, MD, M. Fiorilli, MD, E. Galli, MD, I. Quinti, MD, S. Le Moli, PhD, R. Seminara, MD, and G. Goldstein, Prof

Department of Clinical Immunology (F.A., M.F., I.Q., S.L.M., R.S.), and Department of Pediatrics I (L.B., E.G.), University of Rome, Italy; Ortho Pharmaceutical Corp., Raritan, NJ (G.G.)

INTRODUCTION

Patients with primary immunodeficiencies suffer from severe infections due to abnormalities of the immune system. Infants with severe combined immunodeficiency (SCID) can only be cured definitely by bone marrow transplantation (BMT) using HLA-identical donors [1]. In other patients with primary T-cell defects such as DiGeorge or Nezelof syndrome, correction of the immunologic disorder has been achieved using thymus transplant [2], thymus cultured epithelium [3] and thymic extracts [4,5]. Abnormalities of the thymus, thymic hormones and the T-cell system have also been described in patients with ataxia telangiectasia (AT), Wiskott-Aldrich syndrome (WAS), and in some cases of common variable hypogammaglobulinemia (CVH) [6–8]. Only a few attempts to correct these immunodeficiencies by using thymic extracts have been reported [9–11]. Thus, it is reasonable to attempt to influence the abnormal T-cell system with thymic hormones in such immunologic disorders.

Recently, several thymic hormone preparations have been described but only a few have been used in clinical trials. These include thymosin fraction 5, a mixture of a number of polypeptides, with a molecular weight between 1,000 and 15,000 daltons [4]; thymostimulin, a crude calf thymic extract [2,5]; thymic humoral factor, a dialyzable fraction of another calf thymic extract [9]. More recently, two additional preparations have been isolated and chemically defined: the serum thymic factor (FTS), a nonapeptide produced by the thymic epithelium, and thymopoietin [12], a pure peptide with a molecular weight of 5,260 daltons. From this molecule a pentapeptide (TP-5) has been synthesized, with the same biologic activity of the whole molecule [13]. FTS and TP-5 have been used recently in some patients with primary T-cell defects [9,14–16]. The purpose of this study was to evaluate the safety and the efficacy of TP-5 treatment in patients with primary immunodeficiencies revealed by absent or defective cell-mediated immunity.

PATIENTS AND METHODS
Cases

Twenty-six patients with various forms of immunodeficiencies were included in the trial: 3 with SCID, 2 with SCID with B cells and 4 with primary severe T-cell defect or Nezelof syndrome, 3 with DiGeorge syndrome, 4 with CVH and associated T-cell defect, 5 with AT, and 5 with hyper IgE syndrome (HypE). The criteria for inclusion in this trial were: evidence of the clinical and immunologic characteristics of one of the diseases reported. The criteria for exclusion were: association or previous therapy with other immunostimulant drugs, or association with steroids or immunosuppressive drugs. The employment of γ globulins, and treatment with antibiotics and chemotherapeutic agents were not criteria for excluding the patients from the trial.

The clinical and immunologic diagnosis was based on WHO criteria [17]. The follow-up during and after TP-5 administration included the following tests:

1) The patients were assessed at weekly intervals using a score from 0 to 12. The score was graded according to severity of infections, with a particular score for candidiasis, on the basis of diarrhea, and weight gain, and, in patients with HypE, on the severity of eczema.

2) Routine laboratory tests (WBC, platelets, liver enzymes, etc) were performed weekly.

3) The following immunologic tests were carried out before starting TP-5 therapy and during the 1st, 2nd, 4th and 12th weeks of therapy: T-cell subset analysis with monoclonal antibodies (OKT3, OKT4, OKT8, OKT9, OKT10, OKT6, OKT11, HNK-1 and OKM1) was assessed by the indirect immunofluorescent method as described in detail by Pandolfi et al [8]; evaluation of T and B lymphocytes by sheep rosette-forming cells (SRFC), surface membrane Ig (SIg) response in vitro to PHA, [18]; NK activity [19] and Ig serum levels with commercial immuno-

---

*Supported in part by a grant from the "Ministero Pubblica Istruzione," 1981, Italy, and in part by a grant from the "Associazione per le Immunodeficienze," Rome, Italy.

TABLE 1. Effect of TP-5 Therapy on Clinical and Immunologic Parameters in 9 Children With ID (Patients No. 1–3 With SCID and Patients No. 4&5 With SCID with B Cells, Patients No. 6–9 With Primary T-Cell Defect)

Patient	Age	Sex	Score Before TP-5	Score After TP-5	L/mm^3	OKT3	OKT4	OKT8	Ratio	PHA	Skin tests	mIg	Serum Ig G	A	M	Observation
1. D.G.F.	3M	M	12	12	—	—	—	—	—	—	—	—	—	—	—	Dead
2. R.M.	6M	M	12	12	—	—	—	—	—	—	—	—	—	—	—	Dead
3. D.F.	3M	M	12	12	—	—	—	—	—	—	—	—	—	—	—	Dead
4. M.S.	12M	M	12	0	↑	↑	↑	↑	=	↑	↑	—	—	—	—	Alive (2Y.)
5. P.A.	4M	M	12	4	—	↑	↑	↑	—	—	—	=	—	—	↑	Dead
6. M.E.	7M	F	12	12	—	—	—	—	—	—	—	=	=	—	=	Bone-marrow reconst.
7. C.L.	13M	F	12	12	—	—	—	—	—	—	—	=	=	=	=	"
8. C.P.	24M	M	4	0	↑	↑	↑	—	↑	↑	↑	=	=	=	=	Alive (3Y.)
9. P.L.	5Y	M	3	1	—	—	—	—	—	—	—	=	=	—	=	Alive (6Y.)

—No variation of the *abnormal* values during and after therapy with TP-5
=No variation of the values when they were *normal* before therapy
↑Significant *increase* during the therapy
↓Significant *decrease* during the therapy

TABLE 2. Effect of TP-5 Therapy on Clinical and Immunologic Parameters in 3 Children With DiGeorge Syndrome

Patient	Age	Sex	Score Before TP-5	Score After TP-5	L/mm^3	OKT3	OKT4	OKT8	Ratio	PHA	Skin tests	mIg	Serum Ig G	A	M	Observation
1. A.F.	1M	M	8	4	↑	ND	ND	ND	ND	↑	—	=	=	—	=	Dead
2. G.F.	1M	M	8	3	↑	↑	↑	↑	=	↑	—	=	=	—	=	Dead
3. C.E.	2M	F	7	2	↑	↑	↑	↑	=	↑	↑	=	=	=	=	Alive

—No variation of the *abnormal* values during and after therapy with TP-5
=No variation of the values when they were *normal* before therapy
↑Significant *increase* during the therapy
↓Significant *decrease* during the therapy

plates. Serum IgE levels were measured by the Phadebas paper disk radioimmunoassay (RIA) technique (PRIST, Pharmacia), which was only performed in patients with HypE. Skin tests against *Candida*, SK-SD, PPD, tetanus toxoid (TT) were carried out before and after 12 weeks of therapy [17]. TP-5 was given daily intramuscularly at the dose of 0.5 mg/kg for the first 2 weeks and then with the same doses 3 times a week for another 10 weeks.

RESULTS

The results of the clinical and immunologic modifications during and at the end of TP-5 treatment are reported in Tables 1, 2, 3, 4, and 5. Before treatment, the 3 infants with SCID (one with ADA deficiency) had markedly depressed immunologic tests. Furthermore, immature and mature thymocytes were completely absent in the peripheral blood. The in vitro incubation of peripheral lymphocytes did not modify the E-rosette percentage (data not published). None of these infants showed any clinical or immunologic variations during therapy. Two of them died of interstitial pneumonia and severe diarrhea one month after treatment had ended.

Three out of 6 patients with SCID with B cells and primary T-cell defect did not show any clinical or immunologic modifications, although immature thymocytes were present in the peripheral blood of 2 patients. The other 3 children showed a marked reduction of infections and clinical improvement in close correlation with an increase in the number of T lymphocytes and T-cell subsets, normalization of PHA response and conversion of skin tests (patients *C.P.* and *M.S.*). In particular, Patient *M.S.* received TP-5 for 6 months. During this period, the number and function of T cells and NK cells were normal, but serum Ig levels did not increase. After 5 months withdrawal from TP-5 therapy, the patient worsened and developed bronchopneumonia with depression of the immunologic data. TP-5 was resumed and the infant's clinical and immunologic data normalized (Fig. 1). At present, the infant is in good health with normal T and NK cells (Fig. 1). The third patient who responded to TP-5 treatment showed weight gain, amelio-

TABLE 3. Effect of TP-5 Therapy on Clinical and Immunologic Parameters in 4 Patients With CVH With T-Cell Defect (OKT4⁺/OKT8⁺ Cell Ratio Inverted)

Patient	Age Yrs	Sex	Score Before TP-5	Score After TP-5	L/mm³	OKT3	OKT4	OKT8	Ratio	PHA	Skin tests	mIg	Serum Ig G	A	M
1. M.M.	5	F	5	1	—	↑	—	—	—	—	—	—	—	—	—
2. P.P.	20	M	9	9	↑	—	—	↓	↑	↑	↑	=	—	—	—
3. V.L.	24	F	9	9	—	—	—	—	—	=	=	=	—	—	—
4. T.M.	24	F	6	6	=	=	—	—	—	=	=	=	—	—	—

—No variation of the *abnormal* values during and after therapy with TP-5
=No variation of the values when they were *normal* before therapy
↑Significant *increase* during the therapy
↓Significant *decrease* during the therapy

TABLE 4. Effect of TP-5 Therapy on Clinical and Immunologic Parameters in 5 Patients With AT

Patient	Age Yrs	Sex	Score Before TP-5	Score After TP-5	L/mm³	OKT3	OKT4	OKT8	Ratio	PHA	Skin tests	mIg	Serum Ig G	A	M	Observation
1. N.E.	13	F	2	2	—	—	—	—	—	—	—	—	=	—	—	Alive
2. M.G.	7	M	3	3	=	=	=	=	=	—	=	=	—	—	—	Alive
3. A.F.	8	M	5	5	—	—	—	—	—	—	—	=	—	—	—	Alive
4. F.A.	7	M	5	5	↓	↓	↓	↓	↓	—	—	=	—	—	—	Dead
5. D.O.A.	13	M	8	8	—	—	—	—	—	—	—	=	—	—	—	Alive

—No variation of the *abnormal* values during and after therapy with TP-5
=No variation of the values when they were *normal* before therapy
↑Significant *increase* during the therapy
↓Significant *decrease* during the therapy

TABLE 5. Effect of TP-5 Therapy on Clinical and Immunologic Parameters in 5 Patients With HypE

Patient	Age Yrs	Sex	Score Before TP-5	Score After TP-5	L/mm³	OKT3	OKT4	OKT8	Ratio	PHA	Skin tests	mIg	Serum Ig G	A	M	IgE	Eos.
1. I.G.	4	F	6	6	—	—	—	—	—	—	—	=	=	=	=	↑	↑
2. P.F.	10	F	6	6	—	—	—	—	—	↓	—	=	=	=	↑	↑	↑
3. A.G.	9	F	6	7	—	—	—	—	—	—	—	=	=	=	=	↑	↑
4. V.G.	6	M	4	1	—	—	—	—	—	—	—	=	=	=	=	↓	↓
5. R.L.	5	M	6	1	↑	↑	↑	—	↑	↑	—	=	=	=	=	↓	—

—No variation of the *abnormal* values during and after therapy with TP-5
=No variation of the values when they were *normal* before therapy
↑Significant *increase* during the therapy
↓Significant *decrease* during the therapy

ration of the interstitial pneumonia and diarrhea, increase of T cells (SRBC) and normalization of T4/T8 ratio during the trial. However, the benefit was only transient and the infant died of severe salmonellosis one month after TP-5 withdrawal.

Three infants with DiGeorge syndrome showed a marked clinical improvement during and after treatment. After 1–2 weeks of therapy, we also noted the disappearance of candidiasis and interstitital pneumonia, normalization of T-cell subsets, and of in vitro responsiveness to mitogens. The in vitro test with TP-5 showed a significant increase in SRBC number and a good correlation with the in vivo response. Furthermore, *Patient C.E.* had an increase of mature T cells associated with a diminution of immature thymocytes in peripheral blood (OKT9, OKT10, OKT6) after 2 months of therapy (Fig. 2). Unfortunately, 2 out of these 3 infants died of heart failure due to severe cardiac malformation.

The immunologic and clinical data of 4 children with CVH, 5 with AT, and 5 with HypE are reported in Tables 3, 4, and 5.

In one patient with CVH (*P.P.*) we observed a diminution of T-cell num-

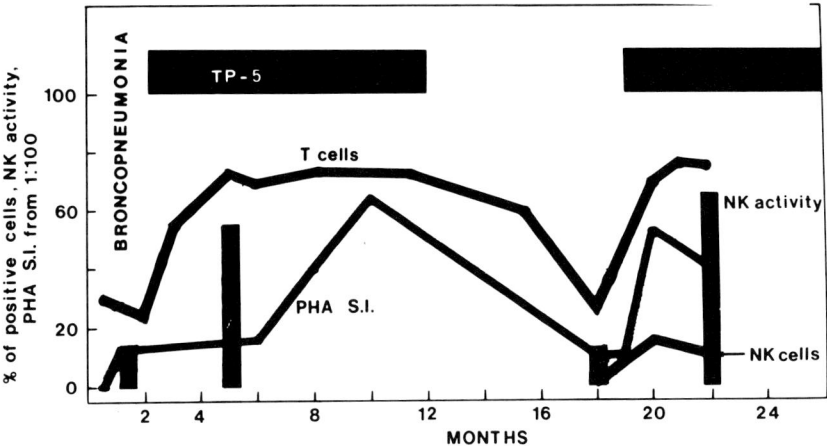

Fig. 1. Immunologic data of *Patient M.S.* (SCID with B cells) during 2 years of follow-up.

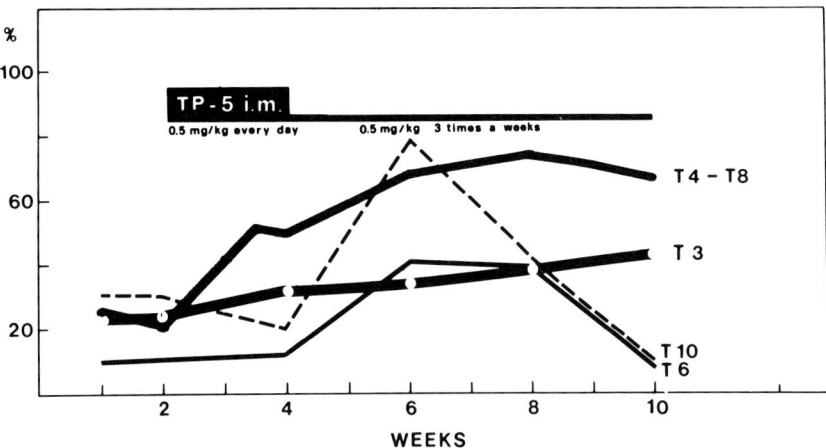

Fig. 2. Lymphocytes detected by monoclonal antibody in a patient with DiGeorge syndrome.

ber, T8 subsets and the conversion from negative to positive of 6 out of 7 skin tests at the end of treatment. In the other 3 patients no modifications were noted. In particular, TP-5 was not capable of modifying the pattern of the T-cell subsets (inversion of OKT4/T8 ratio) nor the function of T cells (ie defective PHA response and Ig synthesis). In 4 patients with AT, the clinical manifestations remained unchanged during and after treatment. On the contrary, one child (*F.A.*) had fever and enlargement of lymph nodes and spleen after one month of therapy with marked diminution of OKT4$^+$ cells and increase of antibodies against EBV. The child died of a reticuloendotheliosis 3 months later.

Finally, 3 children with severe HypE worsened due to increase of itching, eczema, eosinophilic count, IgE levels and infections during the first month of therapy. In 2 children with less severe HypE, a reduction of IgE levels and eosinophil count, and a mild clinical improvement were noted. In all cases the abnormality of T cells (low number of T3 lymphocytes, abnormality of T-cell subsets, defective PHA response, interferon and NK activity) were not corrected by TP-5 treatment.

DISCUSSION

Thymic hormones (TH) have been experimentally shown to promote most T-cell functions when adequate recipients are selected [4,9]. In animals and humans, TH have been reported to enhance alloantigen driven proliferation, deficient cytotoxic T cell, helper and suppressor functions, and NK activity, and to promote skin graft rejection [20–24]. This wide spectrum of actions indicates that they are not selective for a given T-cell subset, but their activity depends upon a variety of factors such as thymic extract preparation, target cell, and dose employed. In this trial we have used a synthetic preparation that is better chemically defined and injected doses can be well controlled in comparison to crude thymic extracts. However, as far as crude thymic extracts are concerned (which are used at present with unquestionably interesting positive effects), it may be said that they are difficult to standardize in pharmacologic terms and, furthermore, side effects were reported in some cases with allergy to bovine protein and in patients with Wiskott-Aldrich syndrome [10]. However, we cannot affirm that TP-5 has the same and all the functions of other thymic preparations. Thymostimulin, for example, is capable of inducing the production of gamma interferon in vitro [25], and shows therapeutic effects in viral diseases in compromised hosts [26]. Such activities were not investigated in this and in other trials with TP-5.

Phase I of our trial with TP-5 was performed in order to establish the safety of the molecule and its immunologic and clinical efficacy in some rare disorders of the immune system. The following conclusions can be drawn from this uncontrolled study:

1) TP-5 was capable of inducing clinical and immunologic improvement in all 3 infants with DiGeorge syndrome, and in 3 out of 6 patients with SCID with B cells and with T-cell defect. In these 6 patients we observed a clear-cut modification of the T-cell number, T-cell subsets and T-cell function. In addition, an increase in IgM synthesis was also observed in one of these infants in agreement with data already reported in animals and man [13,27]. This increase might be due to an improvement in both number and function of T helper cells induced by TP-5. Spontaneous recovery was reported in a few cases with DiGeorge syndrome [28]. However, this occurred only after many months and even years. Furthermore, the patients treated by us showed an immunologic and clinical improvement in correlation with TP-5 therapy.

2) In the 3 infants with SCID, and in 3 out of 6 with SCID with B cells or T-cell defect, we did not observe any response to TP-5 therapy. We speculate that in the patients who did not respond to TP-5 there might have been an absence of T-precursor cells or other mechanism which induces impairment of the immune system and may be operative such as enzyme defects and interleukin abnormalities. However, we cannot exclude the possibility that the dose administered was inadequate to correct some diseases. The administration protocol we used is only preliminary and should be further investigated carefully. In addition, we still do not know how long the therapy should be continued in the responding patients.

3) TP-5 was not capable of modifying the altered ratio of T4/T8 subsets in CVH patients, although TP-5 restored T-cell numbers in compromised host [29], or T-cell subset ratio in older people [30] and in patients with rheumatoid arthritis (Verhagen, personal communication). The Ig synthesis defect of CVH patients might have been due not to a primary abnormality of T helper/suppressor ratio but to an intrinsic impairment of Ig production [17]. However, an increase of T-suppressor cells has been described in one case of CVH which was successfully treated with corticosteroids (Cooper, personal communication), so we cannot exclude that a few patients with Ig synthesis might benefit from TP-5 therapy.

4) The 5 children with AT failed to respond to the therapy. TP-5 may not be able to treat this intriguing disorder. As reported by Waldmann [6], this syndrome is characterized by an abnormality of germ-line interaction that probably explains the failure of organ maturation and the immune defects. The fatal disease which developed in one child may be attributed to the high incidence of tumors, especially of the lymphoid type, reported in AT [17].

5) Three out of 5 children with HypE worsened during therapy. We therefore suggest that these patients should not be treated with thymic extracts. Patients with allergic or autoimmune disorders, as previously recommended, should be treated with thymic extracts exercising great caution [9,10].

6) In regard to the safety of TP-5, it should be emphasized that this drug was shown to be nontoxic and did not induce side effects (except in HypE patients), thus confirming previous data regarding mice and dogs [13,27].

The very short half-life (30″) of TP-5 probably indicates an intravenous route of administration, especially in nonresponding and severely ill patients. Non-covalent binding to several carriers should be tested to increase TP-5's half-life, thus facilitating the treatment of severely ill patients.

In conclusion, TP-5 appears to be a safe molecule for the treatment of patients with DiGeorge syndrome, and primary T-cell defects. This drug seems to be more active on precursors and on mature T-helper cells, as also reported with thymosin [31,32], FTS [9] and thymostimulin [5,10,11] in primary immunodeficiencies. Further double blind trials should be carried out with different doses and in other diseases such as secondary immunodeficiencies.

REFERENCES

1. Good RA, Kapoor N, Pahwa R, West A, O'Reilly R: Current approaches to the primary immunodeficiency. In Fougerau M, Dausset J (eds): "Progress in Immunology IV." New York: Academic Press, 1980, p 906.
2. Businco L, Aiuti F, Giunchi G, Rezza E: Thymic transplantation. Reconstitution of cellular immunity in a four year old patient with T cell deficiency. Clin Exp Immunol 21:32–38, 1975.
3. Horowitz SD, Hong R: Reconstitution of cell-mediated immunity in a patient with SCID after cultured thymus epithelium. Lancet 1:430–432, 1978.
4. Goldstein AL, Thurman GB, Rossio JL: Immunological reconstitution of patients with primary ID diseases and cancer after treatment with thymosin. Transplant Proc 9:1141–1144, 1972.
5. Aiuti F, Ammirati P, Fiorilli M, D'Amelio R, Franchi F, Calvani M, Businco L: Immunologic and clinical investigation of a bovine thymic extract. Therapeutic applications in primary immunodeficiencies. Pediatr Res 131:797–802, 1979.
6. Waldmann T: In Hounde DG, Bridges BA (eds): "Immunological Abnormalities in Ataxia-Telangiectasia." Sussex, England: J Wiley & Sons. (In press)
7. Cooper MD, Seligmann M: B and T lymphocytes in immunodeficiency and lymphoproliferative disorders. In Loor F, Roelants GE (eds): "B and T Cells in Immune Recognition." New York: John B Wiley, 1977, p 323.
8. Pandolfi F, Quinti I, Frielingsdorf A, Goldstein G, Businco L, Aiuti F: Abnormalities of regulatory T cell subpopulations in patients with primary immunoglobulin deficiencies. Clin Immunol Immunopathol 22:323–330, 1982.
9. Bach JF, Dardenne M, Lesaure P, Lefoucier P, Choay J: The clinical case of thymic factors in immunodeficiency diseases. In Seligmann M, Hitzig W (eds): "Primary Immunodeficiencies," Inserm Symposium No. 16. Amsterdam: Elsevier North Holland Biomedical Press, 1980, pp 455–461.
10. Aiuti F, D'Amelio R, Giunchi G: Thymic hormones and their clinical use in immunodeficiency. In Aiuti F, Wigzell H (eds): "Thymus, Thymic Hormones and

10. T Lymphocytes." London: Academic Press, 1980, pp 375–389.
11. Businco L, Rossi P, Quinti I, Perlini R: Therapy of viral disease in immunosuppressed patients with TP-1. Ibid, pp. 295–305.
12. Goldstein G: Isolation of bovine thymosin: A polypeptide hormone of the thymus. Nature 247:11–14, 1974.
13. Goldstein G, Scheid MP, Boyse Ea, Schlesinger DH, Van Wauwe J: A synthetic pentapeptide with biological activity characteristic of the thymic hormone thymopoietin. Science 203:1309–1310, 1979.
14. Aiuti F, Businco L, Rossi P, Quinti I: Response to thymopoietin pentapeptide in a patient with DiGeorge syndrome. Lancet 1: 91, 1980.
15. Fiorilli M, Quinti I, Sirianni MC, Pandolfi F, Businco L, Aiuti F: Immunological reconstitution fo a patient with severe combined immunodeficiency and Zn^+ deficiency after administration of thymopoietin pentapeptide and exogenous Zn. Immunol Clin Sper 2: 141–146, 1982.
16. Fiorilli M, Sirianni MC, Pandolfi F, Quinti I, Tosti U, Aiuti F, Goldstein G: Improvement of natural killer activity after thymopoietin pentapeptide therapy in a patient with severe combined immunodeficiency. Clin Exp Immunol 45:344–351, 1981.
17. WHO Scientific Group: "Immunodeficiency." Technical Report Series. No. 630, 1978.
18. Aiuti F, Cerottini JC, Coombs RA et al: Identification, enumeration and isolation of B and T lymphocytes from human peripheral blood. Scand J Immunol 3:521–532, 1974.
19. Sirianni MC, Fiorilli M, Pandolfi F, Quinti I, Aiuti F: Natural killer activity and lymphocyte subpopulations in patients with primary humoral and cellular immunodeficiencies. Clin Immunol Immunopathol 21:12–19, 1981.
20. Marshall GD, Thurman GB, Low TLK, Goldstein AL: Thymosin: Basic properties and clinical application in the treatment of immunodeficiencies and cancer. Recent Results Cancer Res 75:101–106, 1980.
21. Doria G, D'Agostoro G, Frasca D, Garavini M: Thymic factors enhance T-T cell cooperation in antibody response of ageing. Supra # 10, pp 229–235.
22. Serrou B, Cupissol D, Caraux J, Thiery C, Rosenfield C, Goldstein AL: Ability of thymosin to increase in vivo and in vitro suppressor cell activity in tumour bearing mice and cancer patients. Recent Results Cancer Res 75:110–116, 1980.
23. Kaufman DB: Maturational effects of thymic hormones on human helper and suppressor T cells: Effect of FTS and thymosin. Clin Immunol Immunopathol 39:727–729, 1980.
24. Bardos P, Carmaud C, Bach JF: Augmentation of activity of natural killer cells (NK cells) by serum thymic factor. CR Acad Sci [D] (Paris) 289:1251, 1979.
25. Shoham J, Eskel I, Aboud B, Salzberg S: Thymic hormonal activity on human peripheral blood lymphocytes in vitro. J Immunol 125:54–58, 1980.
26. Tovo PA, Nicola P: TP-1 therapy in patients with secondary immunodeficiencies. Supra # 10, pp 307–311.
27. Lan CY, Goldstein G: Functional effects of thymopoietin pentapeptide (TP-5) on cytotoxic lymphocyte precursor units (CLP-U). J Immunol 124:1861–1872, 1980.
28. Lischner HW, Huff DS: T-cell deficiency in DiGeorge syndrome. In Bergsma D (ed): "Immunodeficiency in Man and Animals." Sunderland, MA: Sinauer Associates, for the National Foundation-March of Dimes, BD:OAS XI(1):16–21, 1975.
29. Di Perri T, Laghi-Pasini F, Auteri A: Immunokinetics of a single dose of thymopoietin pentapeptide. J Immunopharmacol 2:567–572, 1981.
30. Verhagen H, De Cock W, De Cree J, Goldstein G: Restoration of the impaired lymphocyte stimulation in old people by thymopoietin pentapeptide. J Clin Lab Immunol 6:103–109, 1981.
31. Wara DW, Ammann AJ: Thymosin treatment of children with primary immunodeficiency diseases. Transplant Proc 10:203–209, 1978.
32. Mcwhinney H, Gleahill VFD, McCrea S: In vitro and in vivo responses to thymosins in severe combined immunodeficiency. Clin Immunol Immunopathol 14:196–209, 1979.

Effect of Synthetic Thymic Hormone (TP5) in Children With T-Cell Immunodeficiencies

Roland J. Levinsky, MD, FRCP, E. Graham Davies, MRCP,* and Gideon Goldstein, MD

Department of Immunology, Institute of Child Health, London, WC1N 1EH, England (R.J.L., E.G.D.), Ortho Pharmaceutical Corporation, Raritan, NJ 08869 (G.G.)

INTRODUCTION

A functional thymus is necessary for the normal maturation of immunocompetent T cells, and at least part of this thymic processing is mediated by humoral factors [1]. Several preparations have been found to have thymic hormone activity and in some cases, the active molecule has been purified and sequenced. One such molecule is thymopoietin, a 49 amino acid peptide [2]. Recently, the active moiety consisting of a pentapeptide chain (TP5) has been synthesized and shown to have all the biologic functions of the parent molecule [3].

Our initial experience [4] with thymic hormone therapy of 8 immunodeficient children was with the calf thymic extract TP1 (Serono Laboratories) [5]. We found that 3 out of the 8 showed benefit from therapy and that in one child with SCID this benefit was pronounced (Fig. 1). The child had persistent candidiasis and failure to thrive. At 6 months she was treated with TP1 and subsequently her candidiasis disappeared, diarrhea ceased, and she began to grow. Before treatment she had very low T-cell numbers, no B cells, and very low Ig levels. Following therapy, T-cell numbers increased, she developed B cells and produced Igs of all classes. Her lymphocyte mitogenic responses to PHA showed some improvement, though it remained suboptimal (Table 1). She is now 2½ years old, and although not growing at a normal rate, she is relatively free from infections. However, her most recent tests do show deterioration in the immunologic parameters.

More recently, we have started using the synthetic hormone TP5. In this report, the results of the first 4 patients treated are shown.

MATERIALS AND METHODS
Patients

Two children with common variable hypogammaglobulinemia (CVH), one with SCID (with B cells), and one with partial T-cell deficiency were treated.

TP5

After pretreatment assessment, the children were given TP5 by subcutaneous injection 3 times a week for 3 months. The children were assessed at 1 month and 3 months. TP5 was then stopped for 1 month before reassessment. The dosage given was 0.25 mg/kg for the children with CVID, and 1 mg/kg for the other 2. All the children were given prophylactic antibiotics and all but *Case 1* were given Ig replacement therapy. Immunologic tests were performed by methods previously described [6,7]. They included E-rosette-forming cell numbers, B cells, PHA response, Igs, delayed cutaneous hypersensitivity (DHS) to candida antigen and T-cell subsets by monoclonal antibodies. (OKT series 3-pan T marker; 4-helper/inducer subset; 8-suppressor/cytotoxic subset; 6-cortical thymocyte marker [8,9]).

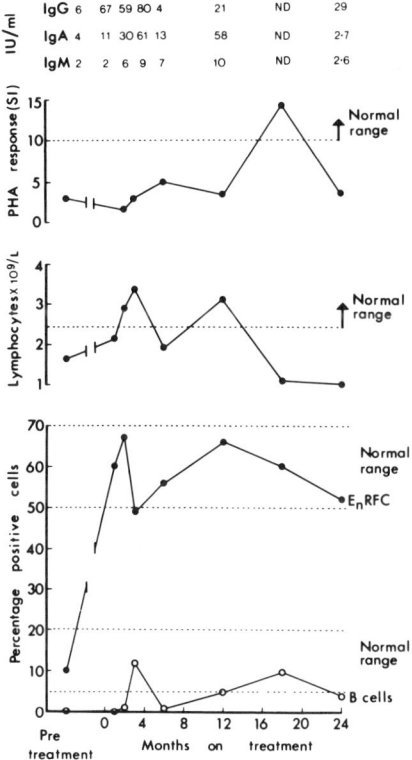

Fig. 1. Immunologic parameters in a child with SCID treated with calf thymic extract TP1.
SI = stimulation index
IU/ml = international units/ml
E_nRFC = E-rosette-forming cells (neuraminadase treated sheep red blood cells)

*Dr. Davies holds a training fellowship from Action Research–The National Fund for Research into Crippling Diseases.

TABLE 1. Lymphocyte Subpopulations in Immunodeficient Children After Therapy With TP5

Case	Time	L'cytes[a] × 10$^{9/L}$	E$_n$ RFC%[b]	B cells	OKT antisera 3[c]	4[c]	8[c]	6[c]	PHA response	Candida DHS[d]
1—Female	Before	0.8	12–32	4	32	11	6	<1	2	−
8 months old	1 month	0.7	32	11	30	16	20	19	15	+
T-cell deficiency	3 months	0.3	54	14	45	43	27	21	2.5	+
	1 month off TP5	0.9	40	10	30	15	18	5	6	+
	9 months on TP5	0.8	—	—	—	—	—	—	28	+
	1 year on TP5	0.3	47	—	30	13	25	0	—	−*
2—Male	Before	5.8	2	68	7	3	0	—	2	−
6 months old	1 month	8.4	12	54	3	3	4	3	1.5	−
SCID	3 months	7.0	3	58	3	19	13	<1	2	−
	1 month off TP5	10.5	5	60	8	22	16	<1	1.3	−
3—Female	Before	2.6	80	<1	65	10	30	0	21	−
5 years old	1 month	3.5	75	3	76	19	49	0	19	+
CVH	3 months	2.2	83	6	77	29	51	0	29	−
	1 month off TP5	3.7	88	2	76	25	85	0	16	−
	6 months on TP5	3.2	57	7	41	30	48	0	59	−
4—Female	Before	1.6	78	5	73	38	36	0	35	−
10 years old	1 month	1.6	74	4	83	38	53	0	29	−
CVH	3 months	2.0	64	3	61	35	27	0	105	−
	1 month off TP5	1.2	40	3	47	30	30	0	10	−

[a]L'cyte = Lymphocyte numbers × 10^{-9}/L.
[b]E$_n$RFC = E-rosette-forming cells (cells forming rosettes with neuraminidase treated red blood cells).
[c]3, 4, 8, 6, refer to % of cells reactive with the monoclonal antibodies OKT3, OKT4, etc.
[d]All % values are of mononuclear cells separated from venous blood.
Candida DHS = Delayed hypersensitivity intradermal test using candida antigen. Results expressed as positive or negative.
*At this occasion an Arthus reaction 6 hours after the test was observed.

CASE REPORTS

Case 1

A female with T-cell deficiency presented at 8 months of age with recurrent candidiasis, chest infections, and diarrhea. She suffered from recurrent generalized erythematous and bacterial rashes. She had scanty lymphoid tissue and no thymic shadow on chest x ray. She was lymphopenic, had low T-cell numbers, and very poor PHA response. DHS to candida antigen was negative. B-cell numbers and Ig levels were normal, but we could not demonstrate any functional antibody.

Case 2

A male with SCID (with B cells) presented at 5 months of age with diarrhea, failure to thrive, recurrent chest infections, and candidiasis. He had no palpable lymph nodes and no thymic shadow on chest x ray. He persistently excreted 5 viruses, including rotavirus and adenovirus. He had a normal lymphocyte count, but virtually no T cells and very high numbers of B cells. Igs were very low and PHA response and DHS to candida antigen were absent.

Case 3

A female with CVH presented at 3 years with chest and ear infections and failure to thrive. She was found to have Ig deficiency and was treated for this. At 4½ years, she developed generalized lymphadenopathy. Biopsy of a gland showed reactive hyperplasia, and adenovirus was cultured from the tissue. No rise in anti-adenovirus titers occurred. Tests showed low B-cell numbers and very low IgG and IgA. T cells and PHA response were normal, but the OKT4:8 ratio was reversed, and DHS to candida antigen was negative.

Case 4

From birth this female child with CVH suffered from chest and ear infections, multiple food allergies, and diarrhea. She had a profound yeast opsonization defect, which was treated with regular infusions of fresh frozen plasma. At age 5 years she developed Ig deficiency, initially affecting only IgA, but later (at 7 years), IgG. This was accompanied by an increased frequency of infections and the onset of recurrent arthritis. She had low B-cell numbers but normal T-cell numbers and PHA response. DHS to candida antigen was negative and the OKT4:8 ratio was very low. At 10 years of age she was given trial therapy with TP5.

RESULTS

None of the children showed any adverse effects of therapy clinically or on regular monitoring of blood count, and renal and hepatic function.

The main changes in immunologic parameters are shown in Table 1.

Case 1 showed marked clinical improvement, with cessation of diarrhea and clearing of candidiasis. She

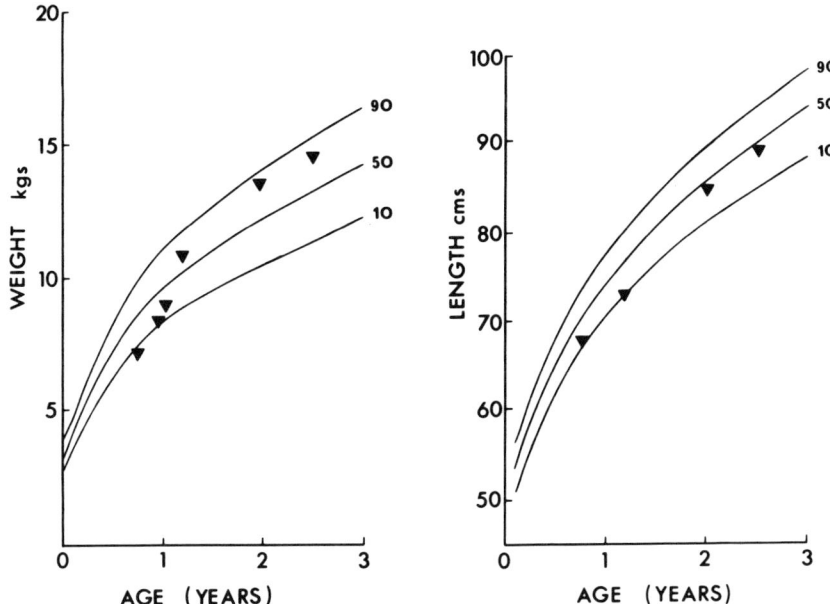

Fig. 2. Growth charts for *Case 1* after treatment with TP5 showing evidence of catch up growth. (Redrawn from the data of Tanner JM, Whitehouse RH, Tahaishi M: Arch Dis Child 1966, vol. 41, with permission.)

started to thrive and crossed percentiles for height and weight (Fig. 2). T-cell numbers rose to normal and PHA response improved. DHS to candida antigen became positive. However, analysis of T-cell subsets showed that many cells still had an immature phenotype with overlap between OKT4 and OKT8+ve cells and high circulating numbers of OKT6+ cells. She remains well on TP5 after a further 12 months and has suffered an adenovirus chest infection which she successfully cleared, producing specific antibody (titer 1:128) in the process.

Case 2 showed no benefit from therapy, which was not continued after the trial period. He has subsequently died. However, it can be seen that even in his case, there was some evidence of induction of T-cell markers during TP5 therapy.

Case 3 may have shown some benefit, since on therapy her lymphadenopathy regressed considerably, and her DHS test became transiently positive. B-cell numbers increased, but she failed to switch an IgG or IgA production and OKT4:8 ratio remained very abnormal. We have continued her on TP5 at a higher dose, but have so far found no further benefit.

Case 4 showed no benefit from therapy clinically or on any of the parameters tested.

DISCUSSION

In our trial of treating cell-mediated immunodeficiencies with a thymic extract (TP1) we have previously described that a small proportion of children respond very well [4]. These additional patients reported here illustrate that the same is true using TP5. As with TP1, we were unable to predict from in vitro tests with TP5 before treatment which children would respond (data not shown), and could only ascertain this by therapeutic trial. We have found no adverse effects of therapy, which makes this approach much more acceptable.

Monitoring of response to therapy is also difficult, as it was our impression in *Case 3* (as it had been our experience with TP1) that clinical benefit occurred out of proportion to the demonstrable changes in immunologic parameters.

It seems that the most dramatic effects of TP5 are seen on the T-cell markers defined by monoclonal antibodies. Even the child with SCID showed some induction of OKT4 and OKT8 markers. OKT8+ve cells appear to be more easily induced by TP5 than OKT4+ve cells (especially *Case 3*) but whether this correlates with helper and suppressor function remains unclear.

We are unsure of correct doses or routes of administration, or whether certain children will respond to one thymic hormone preparation rather than another. One way of solving this dilemma would be to treat initially with the synthetic pentapeptide, and subsequently follow with the crude extract to see if additional benefit occurs.

ACKNOWLEDGMENTS

We are grateful to Mrs. M. Butler for technical assistance.

REFERENCES

1. Gelfand EW, Dosch H-M, Shore A, Limatibul S, Lee WW: Role of the thymus in human T cell differentiation. In Gelfand EW, Dosch H-M (eds): "Biological Basis of Immunodeficiency." New York: Raven Press, 1980, p 39.
2. Schlesinger DH, Goldstein G: The amino acid sequence of thymopoietin II. Cell 5(4):361, 1975.
3. Goldstein G, Scheid P, Boyse EA, Schlesinger DH, Van Wauwe J: A synthetic pentapeptide with biological activity characteristic of the thymic hormone thymopoietin. Science 204:1309, 1979.
4. Davies EG, Levinsky RJ: Treatment of cell mediated immunodeficiency with calf thymic hormone (TP1). Pediatr Res 16:573, 1982.
5. Falchetti R, Caprino L: Immunological aspects of TP1 activity. In Aiuti F, Wigzell H (eds): "Proceedings of the Serono Symposia." London: Academic Press, 1980, vol 38, p 219.
6. Hayward AR: Immunodeficiency. In Turk J (ed): "Current Topics in Immunology Series 6." London: Arnold, 1977, p 75.

7. Trompeter RS, Layward L, Hayward AR: Primary and secondary abnormalities of T cell subpopulations. Clin Exp Immunol 34:388, 1978.
8. Reinherz EL, Moretta L, Roper L, Breard JM, Mingari MC, Cooper MD, Schlossman AF: Human T lymphocyte subpopulations defined by Fc receptors and monoclonal antibodies. J Exp Med 151:969, 1980.
9. Reinherz EL, Kung PC, Goldstein G, Levey RH, Schlossman SF: Discrete stages of intrathymic differentiation: Analysis of normal thymocytes and leukemic lymphoblasts of T lineage. Proc Natl Acad Sci USA 77:1588, 1980.

Delayed Marrow Aplasia Following Treatment for Thymic Hypoplasia: Correction by Marrow Transplant Without Immunosuppression*

Anthony R. Hayward, MD, PhD, John Githens, MD, Shirley Murphy, MD, Bennie McWilliams, MD, Peter Lane, MD, and Daniel R. Ambruso, MD

Department of Pediatrics, University of Colorado School of Medicine, Denver, CO (A.R.H., J.G., P.L., D.R.A.), and the Department of Pediatrics, University of New Mexico School of Medicine, Albuquerque, NM (S.M., B.McW.)

CASE HISTORY

This patient was the 3 kg product of a 36-week pregnancy, born by cesarean section for breech presentation to a 37-year-old gravida 7, para 7 mother. Neonatal examination revealed hypotonia and a cardiac murmur. When referred at 26 days of age he was hypocalcemic, and cardiac catheterization showed a patent ductus arteriosus (PDA) and ventriculoseptal defect. The PDA was ligated at 6 weeks of age, and he was started on vitamin D and calcium supplements because his serum Ca^{++} was low (2.8 mEq/L). In the week following surgery he developed a severe parainfluenza virus bronchiolitis, and lymphocyte studies showed reduced blood T-cell numbers and function (Fig. 1). He started to recover spontaneously, but 2 weeks later developed bronchiolitis due to respiratory syncytial virus. At 9 weeks of age, he was transfused with 45 ml of whole blood from an HLA-matched MLC-compatible male sib followed by a 10-day course of methotrexate. His T-cell number subsequently increased, and he gained weight. At 6-months follow-up he was hypogammaglobulinemic and was started on replacement IgG injections. The percentage of T cells in his blood fell and the percentage of B cells rose over the following year. He had a varicella infection with severe skin involvement. In vitro tests suggested decreased helper T-cell function. At age 16 months, he was given a second transfusion of 10 ml/kg of fresh blood from the same brother without subsequent methotrexate treatment. A skin rash (which was not biopsied) appeared about one month after this transfusion and resolved spontaneously. His blood T-cell number increased and 6 months later he demonstrated normal serum immunoglobulins; IgG replacement was discontinued. Additional findings at this age were vitiligo—affecting predominantly his trunk—and limping due to *Staphylococcus aureus* osteomyelitis of the distal femur. The osteomyelitis resolved following drainage and antibiotics, and no further symptoms occurred until age 3.5 years when he became increasingly pale and lethargic. Pancytopenia was found and aplastic anemia was diagnosed by marrow biopsy. Bone marrow transplantation from the HLA-compatible donor was planned. Typing data on which the marrow graft treatment was based is summarized in Table 1. It is not known with certainty whether the patient was still colonized with his brother's lymphocytes at this time, but the possibility exists as G-, Q-, and C-banding of PHA-stimulated blood lymphocyte metaphases failed to reveal any polymorphic differences between donor and recipient. Although the recipient's blood lymphocytes showed a normal PHA response, engraftment was attempted without immunosuppression.

CLINICAL COURSE

The patient was grafted with 5×10^8 marrow cells/kg and maintained with irradiated red cell and platelet transfusions for the following 9 days. The donor developed a fever to 40°C for 4 days following aspiration of his marrow but then recovered uneventfully. The first significant evidence of engraftment of the recipient (3.6% reticulocytes, 420 absolute neutrophils, and increase in platelets to 29,000) was obtained 15 days after grafting. Recovery (Fig. 2) was interrupted by a fever at 10 days and a Coombs-positive hemolytic anemia associated with a cold reactive IgM, anti-I antibody. An identical antibody was found in the donor's serum after his febrile illness. The recipient's lymphocytes did not then or subsequently proliferate in MLC with irradiated donor cells. The patient was started on 2 mg/kg of prednisone daily. Four weeks after grafting he developed a rash on his back and his serum bilirubin and transaminases were raised: a skin biopsy versus host disease (GVHD). The marrow graft remained functional

---

*Supported in part by NIH grants, Division of Research Resources RR-69 and HD 13733.

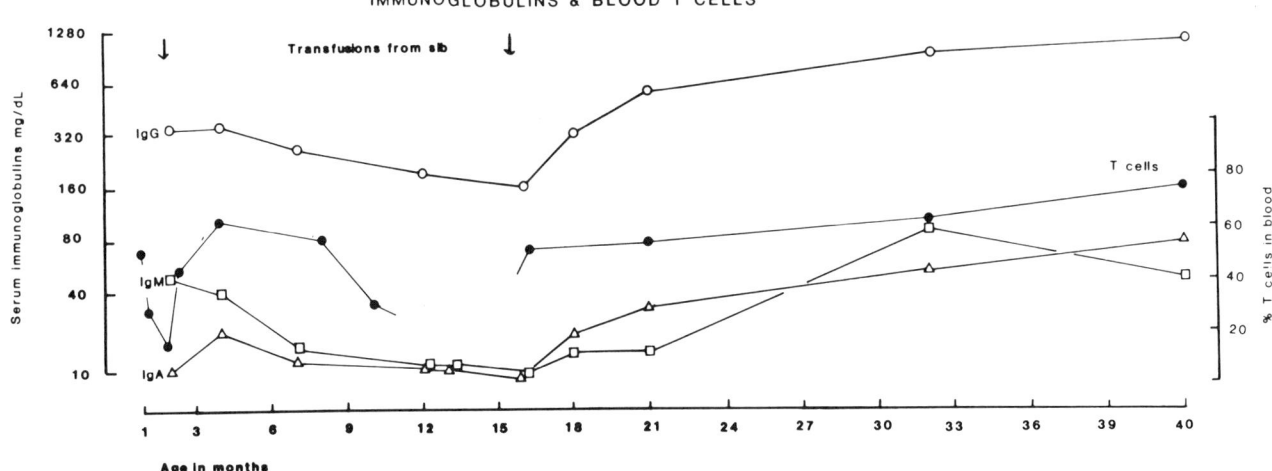

Fig. 1. Patient's pregraft course showing response to blood transfusions from his HLA-matched, MLC-compatible sib.

TABLE 1. Typing Results on Patient, Sib, and Parents

	ABO	HLA-A	HLA-B
Patient	0+	28, w30	5, 13
Sib donor	0+	28, w30	5, 13
Father	0+	1, w30	8, 13
Mother	0+	28, 2	5, w40

MLC results cpm × 10⁻²		
Responder	Stimulator	cpm
Patient	Patient	4.2
Patient	Sib donor	4.7
Patient	Control	47.6
Donor	Donor	4.2
Donor	Patient	2.6
Donor	Control	38.5

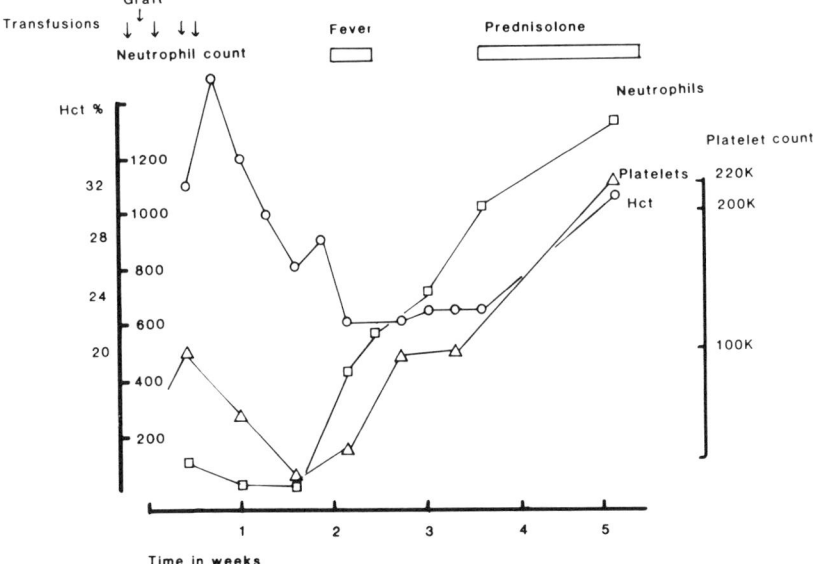

Fig. 2. Patient's postgraft course. Neutrophil count = —□—; platelet count = —△—; hematocrit = —○—.

and the hemolytic anemia reversed. Four months after grafting, the patient continues to manifest signs of mild chronic GVHD affecting only the skin, but has a completely normal Hgb, WBC, differential, and normal platelets. Reticulocytes remain slightly elevated at 3%.

DISCUSSION

The occurrence of aplastic anemia in a child with a thymic hypoplasia syndrome one year after a blood transfusion from a matched sib is unusual. The decision to treat thymic hypoplasia in our patient with 10 ml/kg of fresh matched blood at 9 weeks was prompted by the wish to reverse his susceptibility to severe virus infections rapidly, the lack of a fetal thymus, and the availability of an HLA-matched sib donor. Methotrexate was given to prevent or attenuate possible GVHD, and it is conceivable that this drug also limited subsequent antigen-driven expansion of donor cells accounting for the slow falloff in T cells. The second transfusion was followed by an increase in E-rosetting cells and serum Igs (Fig. 1) and may also have been followed by mild GVHD. Vitiligo has previously been associated with immunologic abnormalities [1], and GVHD [2], and may have been a consequence of our patient's primary immunodeficiency or of its treatment. Aplastic anemia is an occasional complication of GVHD [3], in which case it usually occurs within 3 months of grafting. If GVHD were responsible for the aplastic anemia in our patient the delay in onset could be attributed to the relatively small number of donor T cells given at each transfusion. We considered it likely that our patient's preexisting ID had indeed permitted engraftment by mature T cells from the two blood transfusions; therefore no preconditioning was used prior to the marrow graft. The occurrence of GVHD in the recipient after the marrow infusion is consistent with this view; in subsequent MLCs we never detected a response by recipient lymphocytes to those of the donor. The autoimmune hemolytic anemia was due to an IgM anti-I cold-reacting antibody and was most likely the result of infection in either the patient or the donor or both.

CONCLUSIONS

Our results suggest that HLA-matched sib T cells from peripheral blood can achieve at least partial reconstitution in patients with thymic hypoplasia, with an attendant risk of GVHD. Aplastic anemia arising under these circumstances can be reversed with marrow infusion. Procedures for T-cell depletion of the marrow graft might be advantageous under these circumstances to avoid further GVHD.

REFERENCES

1. Hertz KC, Gazze LA, Kirkpatrick CH, Katz SI: Autoimmune vitiligo. N Engl J Med 297:634, 1977.
2. Sullivan KM, Shulman HM, Storb R et al: Chronic graft versus host disease in 52 patients: Adverse natural course and successful treatment with combined immunosuppression. Blood 57:267, 1981.
3. Hathaway WE, Githens JH, Blackburn WR et al: Aplastic anemia hystocytosis and erythrodermia in immunologically deficient children. N Engl J Med 273:953, 1965.

Immunologic Reconstitution With Bone Marrow Transplantation and Thymic Hormones in Two Patients With Severe Pure T-Cell Defects*

Prof. Luisa Businco, P. Rossi, MD, R. Paganelli, MD, R. Seminara, MD, and F. Aiuti, MD

Department of Pediatrics (L.B.), and Department of Clinical Immunology (P.R., R.P., R.S., F.A.), University of Rome, 00185 Rome, Italy

INTRODUCTION

A number of patients with primary immunodeficiencies (ID) affecting primarily cell-mediated immunity (CMI)—previously classified as Nezelof syndrome—represent a large, heterogeneous group as yet not well defined [1]. Some of these patients have been successfully treated with thymic hormones (TH) [2, 3] or thymic and fetal liver transplants [4-6]. However, most of them, with the exception of classic DiGeorge syndrome, do not respond to such therapies and tend to develop features of severe combined immunodeficiency (SCID) after the age of one year. Moreover, these differ from the patients with classic SCID with B cell, due to the presence of plasmacells and near normal immunoglobulin production with some antibody activity against T-independent antigens.

The present paper reports 2 cases of pure T-cell defect who have been successfully treated with bone marrow transplantation (BMT) from HLA-identical sibs, which was associated with TH therapy. The engraftment occurred as early as 14 days after BMT without pretreatment of the recipients. Full immunologic reconstitution has been demonstrated by monoclonal antibodies analysis for T-cell subsets and precursors, in vitro functional test, in vivo delayed skin test reactivity and specific antibody production.

CASE REPORT

Case 1, a 9-month-old female suffered from the first month of life from severe diarrhea, chronic thrush, fever, interstitial pneumonia and failure to thrive. At the age of 9 months, she was admitted to the 1st Department of Pediatrics of the University of Rome. Body weight was 4 kg (< 5 SD); body temperature: 38°C. At physical examination the child appeared severely malnourished and pale. She had thrush, hyperpnea and diffuse lung rales; severe anorexia was also present. The immune system evaluation showed a severe defect of T-cell number and function, while B lymphocytes, Ig levels and hemagglutinins were normal, adenosine deaminase (ADA) as well as nucleoside phosphorylase (NP) enzymes were also normal (Table 1). On the basis of the case history and immunologic evaluation, the diagnosis of pure T-cell defect was made. A 1-month course of synthetic thymopoietin pentapeptide (TP5,Ortho) (0.5 mg/kg/im daily), and 1 month of calf thymic extract (TP1, Serono) (1 mg/kg/im daily) were given without any clinical and immunologic improvement. BMT was then performed and TP5 therapy was resumed. Seven days after the transplant the fever disappeared and diarrhea stopped. The infant became alert and began to enjoy her food, gradually gaining weight (4 kg over 4

TABLE 1. Immunologic Follow-Up of *Case 1* Before and After BMT

Days	-15	-7	+7	+14	+30	+60
WBC	8000	5000	13800	8000	10800	8900
T Lymph/mm^3	230	102	450	1540	2550	2100
B Lymph %	7	6	10	5	5	8
T3 %	0	0	23	62	50	59
T4 %	0	0	20	39	45	41
T8 %	0	0	20	19	20	29
T17	ND	26	35	73	ND	50
T6	0	0	10	2	6	7
T9	10	ND	23	10	5	15
T10	2	ND	3	18	7	11
HNK	ND	16	ND	25	19	12
PHA resp	3732	ND	3369	9919	19898	20480
IgG mg/dl	224	309	465	480	1980	2400
IgA	18	42	37	48	99	64
IgM	182	178	97	190	283	257
Skin test	neg	neg	neg	neg	neg	pos

resp = response in cpm

*This work has been supported by grants of C.N.R. and the Cenci-Bolognetti Foundation.

TABLE 2. Immunologic Follow-Up of *Case 2* Before and After BMT

Days	-15	-7	+7	+15	+30	+60
WBC	9600	11500	6000	5200	12400	6200
T Lymph/mm^3	474	600	432	1951	5208	2376
B Lymph %	5	6	5	15	12	ND
T3 %	37	30	16	54	60	66
T4 %	25	22	33	60	32	34
T8 %	18	29	17	22	63	43
T6 %	43	35	5	2	ND	5
T9 %	67	21	1	0	2	5
T10	66	27	18	2	21	ND
HNK	18	14	25	12	13	20
PHA resp	407	735	ND	ND	36995	38000
IgG mg/dl	377	384	ND	327	758	1832
IgA	63	65	ND	17	44	51
IgM	72	84	ND	60	194	27
Skin test	neg	neg	neg	pos	pos	pos

resp = response in cpm

months). All symptoms including interstitial pneumonia cleared without any treatment apart from TP5. The patient was discharged from the hospital in good health 45 days after the graft.

Case 2, a 13-month-old female, was the third living child of related parents; 2 brothers died in their first months of life of severe infections. From birth she experienced chronic diarrhea, failure to thrive, mucosal candidiasis and interstitial pneumonia. After several hospitalizations she was admitted to the 1st Department of Pediatrics. On admission, the infant appeared severely ill, malnourished and pale; body weight was 5.4 kg (< 5 SD), body temperature was 38.7°C. Physical examination showed thrush, dyspnea and diffuse lung rales. The diagnosis of pure T-cell defect with normal levels of ADA and NP enzymes was made on the basis of immunologic tests. A high percentage of lymphocytes reacting with monoclonal antibodies (OKT6, OKT10, OKT9) were found (Table 2).

Therefore, a 1-month course of TP1 followed by a course of TP5 were administered with the same schedule reported above for *Case 1*, without any change of clinical and immunologic conditions. BMT was performed and TP5 therapy was resumed. During the first week after BMT, the patient's condition worsened but beginning in the second week the infant gained weight (3 kg over 2 months), diarrhea stopped, and interstitial pneumonia cleared. The infant was dismissed in good condition 45 days after the graft.

MATERIALS AND METHODS

T- and B-lymphocyte markers, as well as in vitro response to polyclonal activators, were performed by methods previously described [7]. Analysis of T-cell subsets and T-cell precursors was carried out by the method of Reinherz et al with monoclonal antibodies [8]. Delayed skin test to *Candida* was performed using Dermatophytin "O" antigen (Hollister-Stier). Immunoglobulin levels, as well as specific antibodies, were detected by standard techniques.

BMT was performed from HLA-compatible donors (2-year-old brother for *Case 1*, a 9-year-old sister for *Case 2*) infusing 5×10^8 nucleated cells/kg/bw within 1 hour of collection. Simultaneously, TP5 was given daily for the first 2 weeks, followed by administration 3 times a week. The patients did not receive any pretreatment with immunosuppressive drugs and antibiotic cocktails to favor the engraftment and to avoid graft versus host disease (GVHD) nor were they placed in a sterile laminar flow system.

RESULTS

The immunologic results before and after the transplants are summarized in Tables 1 and 2, and in Figures 1, 2, 3, and 4. T-cell number increased in both patients as early as 2 weeks after the graft. Simultaneously T-cell subsets as defined by

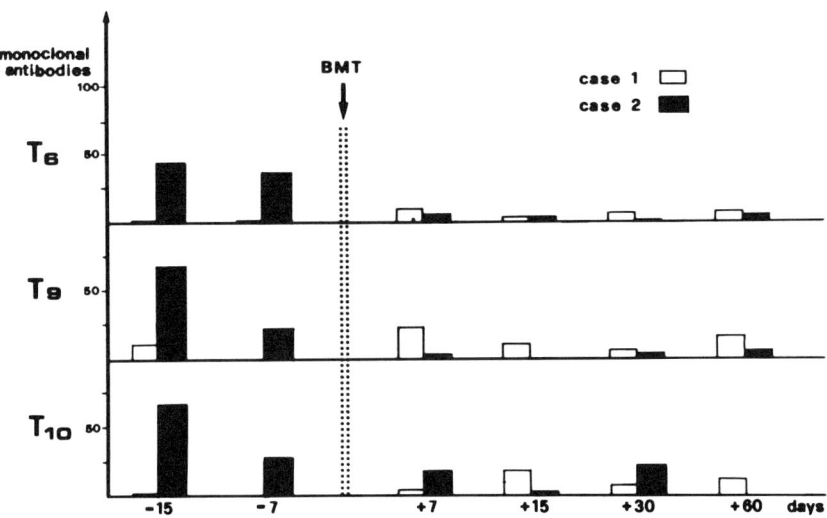

Fig. 1. Peripheral blood lymphocytes positive for OKT6, OKT9, OKT10 monoclonal antibodies in the 2 infants with pure T-cell defect, before and after BMT.

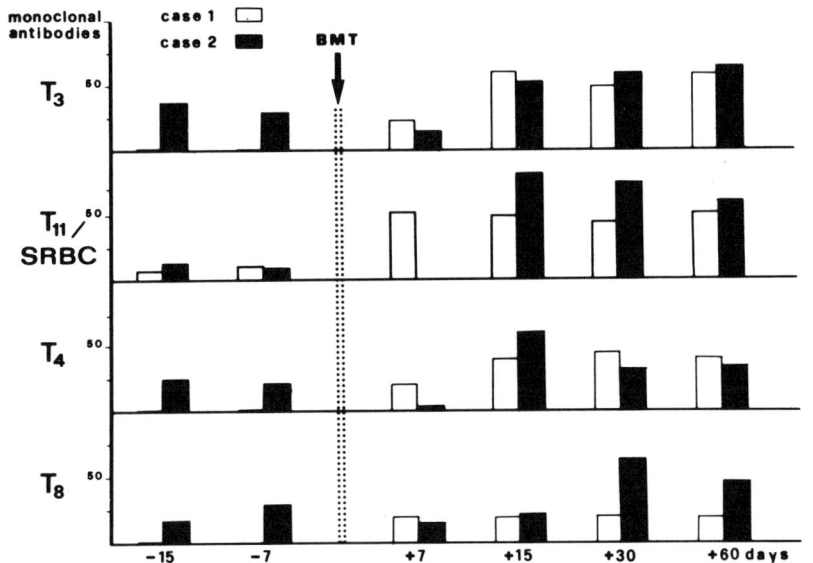

Fig. 2. Peripheral blood lymphocytes positive for OKT3, OKT4, OKT8, OKT11 and SRBC receptors in the 2 infants with pure T-cell defect, before and after BMT.

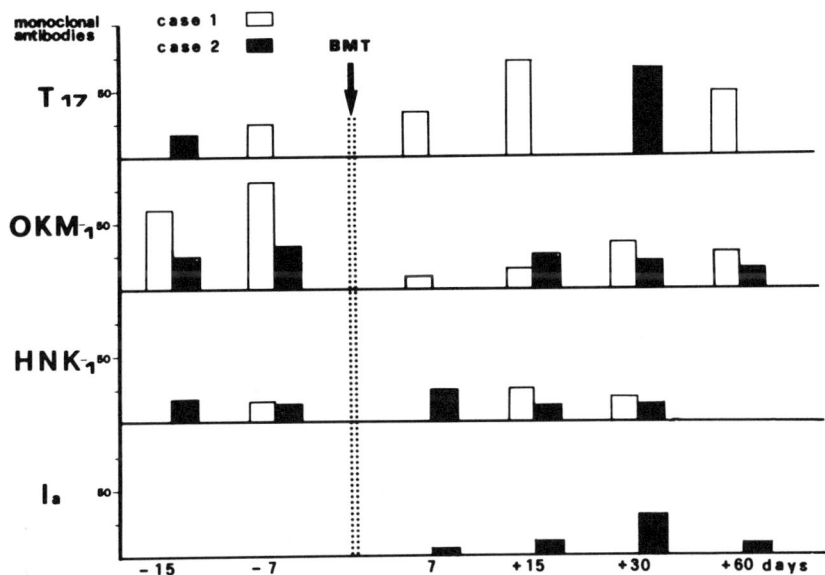

Fig. 3. Peripheral blood lymphocytes positive for OKT17, OKOM1, HNK1, Ia in the 2 infants with pure T-cell defect, before and after BMT.

OKT4, OKT8, OKT17 monoclonal antibodies normalized while T-cell precursors reacting with OKT6, OKT9, OKT10 decreased. The mitogen responsiveness to PHA, Con A and PWM appeared at the 4th week.

A marked increase of immunoglobulin levels was observed in both infants during the first 2 months after BMT. In *Case 1*, specific antibodies against CMV, Epstein-Barr virus (EBV), and influenza type A appeared 2 months after the graft without any sign or symptom of infection (Table 3). Delayed hypersensitivity reaction (DHR) to *Candida* was detected on day 18 and 65 in *Cases 1* and *2*, respectively. Y chromosome-bearing lymphocytes were detected in *Case 2*, 2 months after BMT. In *Case 1* a change in the red cell subgroups was observed 1 month after the graft.

DISCUSSION

In recent years, the analysis of T-subsets by specific monoclonal antibodies in patients with ID has provided new insights in the understanding and classification of such diseases [9]. From this point of view, pure T-cell defects can be recognized by very low T3, T11, T4, T8 bearing cells, various expression of precursor cells positive for T6, T9, T10, depressed CMI in vitro and in vivo, presence of bone marrow plasmacells and circulating B cells, normal or near normal serum immunoglobulin levels with specific antibody activity for T-independent antigens [10, 11]. Some of these patients can be treated successfully with thymic hormone TH [2, 3], but the majority are unresponsive to this therapy [1]. The recovery of the immune system observed after BMT in the 2 patients reported here, indicates that such treatment is highly effective in patients with pure T-cell defect. Indeed, the immunologic follow-up of these infants showed that T cells and their subsets, as defined by T3, T4, T8, T11, T17 monoclonal antibodies, reached normal values as early as 2 weeks after BMT. Several hypotheses may be offered to explain the early reconstitution of T-cell system observed in both infants. First, the TH therapy could have enhanced the proliferation and the differentiation of the infused stem cells thus inducing a more rapid amplification of T-cell system. Second, the different microenvironment of bone marrow and/or other lymphoid tissues of patients with pure T-cell defect in comparison with those with SCID might have played a role in the early engraftment. Third, the absence of an immunosuppressive conditioning regimen, usually performed in patients with aplastic anemia and leukemia, might have resulted in the

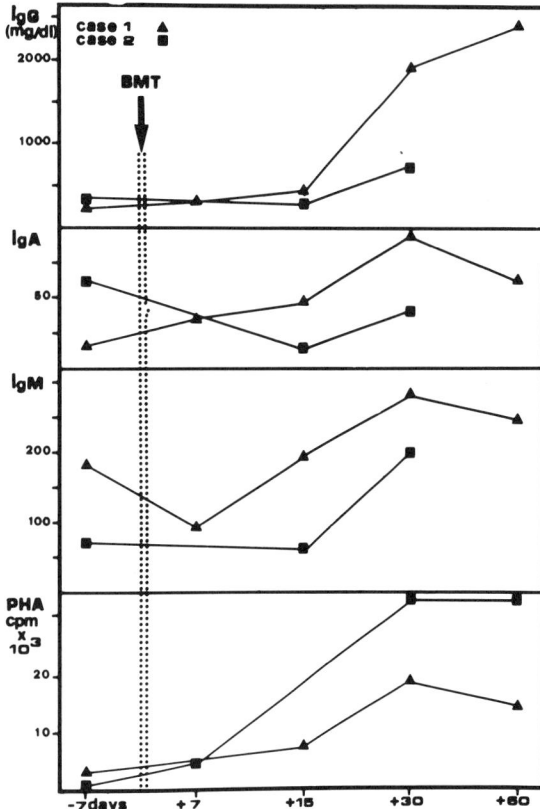

Fig. 4. Serum Ig levels and in vitro lymphocyte PHA response in the 2 infants with pure T-cell defect, before and after BMT.

TABLE 3. Specific Antibody Titers Against Viral Antigens in *Case 1* After BMT

Viral Antigen	Titer 60 days after BMT
Epstein-Barr viral antigens	
VCA	1:32
EA	< 1:5
EBNA	1:20
Adenovirus	< 1:8
Cytomegalovirus	< 1:32
Respiratory syncytial virus	< 1:8
Mycoplasma pneumoniae	< 1:8
Influenza Type A	1:16
Type B	< 1:8

No specific antibodies were present before BMT.

earlier immunologic and clinical recovery [12].

In contrast with the results of de Bruin et al [13], in patients suffering from aplastic anemia who underwent BMT, no immature T cells with T10 phenotype, no impairment of T4/T8 ratio was observed in the peripheral blood of *Case 1*. This pattern confirms that a very fast differentiative process occurred in these 2 patients who showed peripheral lymphocytes with postthymic T-cell antigens during the first weeks following BMT. This finding correlates with the early appearance of in vitro mitogen responsiveness and with the in vivo skin test reactivity to *Candida* antigens as early as 3 weeks in *Case 2*. The early engraftment of T-helper cells, as well as of B-cell lineage, demonstrated by the striking increase of immunoglobulin production with definite antibody activity against several viral antigens might also be related to TH treatment. Our data are relevant also since recovery from severe CID after allogeneic BMT does not usually occur until after one full year or more [14]. In addition, the period of susceptibility to fatal infections is over by about 4–5 months after BMT, therefore in accord with Santos [14], immunotherapy during the first 3–4 months after BMT with a T-cell system immunostimulant accelerate immune system recovery appears to be warranted. Furthermore, the absence of thymic hormones has been reported in such patients and normal TH values are reached only 4–6 months after BMT [14].

Finally, although TH have been noted to enhance and worsen GVHD in experimental studies, we did not observe any GVHD symptoms in our patients.

In conclusion, patients with pure T-cell defects who do not respond to TH therapy alone, may be successfully corrected by BMT without pretreatment with conditioning regimens. Immunotherapy with TH has been shown to induce an early reconstitution of the T- and B-cell systems and to protect against fatal posttransplant infections. Whether such treatment would also be useful in other ID and/or lymphoproliferative disorders has to be investigated further.

REFERENCES

1. WHO Bulletin: Immunodeficiency. Technical Report Series, 630, Geneva, 1978.
2. Goldstein AL, Cohen GH, Rossio J et al: Use of thymosin in the treatment of primary immunodeficiency diseases and cancer. Med Clin North Am 60:591–606, 1976.
3. Aiuti F, Ammirati P, Fiorilli M et al: Immunological and clinical investigations on a bovine thymic extract. Therapeutical applications in primary immunodeficiencies. Pediatr Res 13:797–802, 1979.
4. Cleveland WW, Fogel BJ, Brown WT et al: Foetal thymic transplant in a case of a DiGeorge syndrome. Lancet 2:1211–1215, 1969.
5. Businco L, Rezza E, Aiuti F et al: Thymus transplantation. Reconstitution of cellular immunity in a 4-year-old patient with T cell deficiency. Clin Exp Immunol 21:32–37, 1979.

6. Aiuti F, Businco L, Fiorilli M et al: Foetal liver transplantation in two infants with SCID. Transplant Proc 11:230–234, 1979.
7. Aiuti F, Cerottini JC, Coombs RA et al: Identification, enumeration and isolation of B and T lymphocytes from human peripheral blood. Scand J Immunol 3:521, 1974.
8. Reinherz EL, Kung PC, Goldstein G et al: Discrete stages of human intrathymic differentiation: Analysis of normal thymocytes and leukemia lymphoblasts of T cell lineage. Proc Natl Acad Sci USA 71:1588–1592, 1980.
9. Pandolfi F, Quinti I, Frielingsdorf A et al: Abnormalities of regulatory T-cell subpopulations in patients with primary immunoglobulin deficiencies. Clin Immunol Immunopathol 22:323–330, 1982.
10. Aiuti F, Businco L: Classification and therapy of T lymphocyte defects. In Doria G, Eshkal A (eds): "The Immune System Functions and Therapy of Dysfunctions." New York: Academic Press. 1980, pp 139–158.
11. Aiuti F, Pandolfi F, Fiorilli M et al: Monoclonal antibody analysis of T cell subsets in 40 patients with immunodeficiencies. J Clin Immunol (in press).
12. Mackowiak PA: The normal microbial flora. N Engl J Med 307:83–93, 1982.
13. de Bruin HG, Astaldi A, Leupers T et al: T lymphocyte characteristics in bone marrow-transplanted patients. II. Analysis with monoclonal antibodies. J Immunol 127:244–251, 1981.
14. Santos GW, Eltenbein GT, Sharkis S et al: Reconstitution of lymphohematopoietic function following allogenic, syngenic and autologous marrow transplantation. In Gelfand EW, Dosch HM (eds): "Biological Basis of Immunodeficiency." New York: Raven Press. 1980, pp 293–306.

SECTION 5
OTHER STATES ASSOCIATED WITH PRIMARY IMMUNODEFICIENCY

The Human Fetus and Newborn: Development of the Immune Response

Anthony R. Hayward, MD, PhD, MRCP

Department of Pediatrics, University of Colorado Medical School, Denver, CO 80262

This paper mainly describes experiments we have undertaken to clarify the pathogenesis of severe infections in infants due, for example, to herpes group viruses or to encapsulated bacteria such as *Haemophilus influenzae*. The discussion concentrates on T-cell responses and interactions as other contributors to this symposium deal with B-cell maturation. For convenience, the background to these studies is summarized first without detailed referencing; for reviews see Hayward [1].

LYMPHOCYTE DEVELOPMENT
B Cells

Commitment of a stem cell product to the B-cell series occurs with selection of one of each of the V, D, and J region genes which make up the variable region of the Ig heavy chain [2]. Rearrangement of these genes appears to involve the deletion of intervening DNA sequences, which provides a useful means for identifying the lineage of very immature cells such as acute lymphatic leukemia cells. The VDJ segment which codes for the complete variable region is next joined to a μ-region gene for transcription and translation. This stage has been reached by the time the cell is morphologically identifiable as a pre-B cell, since these cells have sufficient free heavy chain in the cytoplasm for it to be detectable by immunofluorescence. Maturation to the B-cell stage is signaled by the appearance of surface Ig and requires the selection of a kappa or lambda light-chain variable region by combining a light-chain V and J gene. It seems likely that kappa chain genes are normally rearranged first and, only if this fails to give a usable variable region, does the cell rearrange lambda genes. The appearance of surface IgD on fetal and adult B cells is made possible by the splicing of messenger RNA transcripts without DNA deletion; RNA splicing may also explain the ability of newborn B cells to express up to three different classes of surface Ig simultaneously. The most important conclusion of the molecular studies of Ig biosynthesis is that specificity of the B cell is determined early, and that antibody diversity can be explained largely as a result of the different possible combinations of the genomic library of V, D, and J regions.

T-Cell Development

Histologic studies show that the first lymphocytes appear in the thymus at about 8 weeks after conception and that separate cortical and medullary populations are seen by 12 weeks. T cells appear in the blood and spleen around 14 weeks. Nothing is known of the antigen-binding specificity repertoire which is available during fetal life: our initial experiments in this area are described below but their interpretation is limited by our current ignorance of the primary structure of the T-cell receptor. At least 3 different subsets of T cells can be distinguished by function. Helper-inducer cells respond to antigen which is presented in association with HLA-DR antigens on the surface of antigen-presenting cells. In man these include monocytes, macrophages, and vascular endothelial cells. In this linked recognition of antigen by T cells the HLA-DR antigens are referred to as the restricting elements of the response: comparable histocompatibility antigen restriction is well established for proliferative responses by mouse lymphocytes. Cytotoxic T cells lyse targets which have antigens such as virus-encoded proteins in association with an HLA antigen on their cell surface. This linked recognition resembles that of T helper (Th) cells, except that the restricting elements belong to the A, B, and C series of HLA antigens rather than to DR. Suppressor T cells may be able to respond to antigen in the absence of any restricting element, but this is not yet certain.

T- and B-Cell Subset Phenotypes

Table 1 summarizes the development of the T- and B- lymphocyte series in man regarding tissue distribution. The availability of monoclonal antibodies to define subsets has facilitated studies on blood; results from fetuses and full-term infants are given in Table 2.

Development of Immunoglobulins

Healthy human newborn serum contains about 1,000 mg/dL of IgG, <20 mg/dL IgM, and <10 mg/dL IgA. Almost all the IgG is maternal in origin and is transported across the placenta by a specific transport mechanism which starts at about 16 weeks' gestation and increases in rate so that the bulk of IgG is acquired by the fetus during the last 4 weeks of

TABLE 1. Lymphocyte Ontogeny in Man

T cells	Weeks after conception	B cells
Epithelial thymus	5	
	6	
	7	$c\mu^+$ pre-B cells in liver
Thymus becomes lymphoid	8	
	9	$s\mu^+$ B cells in liver
Corticomedullary differentiation in thymus	10	$s\gamma^+$ B cells in liver
	11	$s\alpha^+$ B cells in liver
Hassall corpuscles appear	12	Most μ^+ B cells have δ
	13	
T cells in spleen	14	B cells in blood and spleen

Key: $c\mu^+$ = positive for cytoplasmic μ-chains. $s\mu$, $s\gamma$, $s\alpha$ = positive for surface Ig.

gestation [4]. Consequently, premature infants are relatively poorly supplied with maternal antibodies. Infants normally start to make IgG antibodies in the first month of life, though at a rate slower than adults; therefore, their serum IgG levels do not reach adult values (about 1,000 mg/dL) until 3 years of age. IgM does not cross the placenta, so any which is found in the fetus or newborn is fetal in origin. Little is known about the specificities of the small amounts of IgM which healthy fetuses make, though it appears to include antibody to maternal T lymphocytes. The serum of newborn infants with congenital infection (rubella, CMV, toxoplasmosis) has increased levels of IgM, and the detection of antibody activity in this serum is used in diagnosis. Immunized infants make mainly IgM antibodies [5], probably because of relative immaturity of their B lymphocytes. Adult levels of IgM are usually reached by 9 months of age. IgA antibodies are made in the secretory system first (appearing between 2 and 4 weeks of age [6]), and adult serum levels are not attained until about 12 years of age. These physiologic delays in antibody production may be important in the pathogenesis of infantile allergy and present difficulty in immunizing infants with polysaccharides.

IMMUNITY AT BIRTH: FUNCTIONAL STUDIES ON B CELLS

Most of the plasma cells which appear in cultures of newborn lymphocytes following stimulation with polyclonal B-cell activators contain IgM and there is little if any IgG or IgA production [7]. This effect is clearly seen with PWM or with the T-cell independent stimuli: Cowan strain Staph A or Epstein-Barr virus (EBV). The IgM response is quantitatively less than that seen with adult lymphocytes. Furthermore, adult B cells make almost as much IgG or IgA as IgM in cultures stimulated with these polyclonal activators. Different kinetics of response might account for the differences between the adult and newborn responses. Miyagawa et al [8] found some late increase in IgG and IgA production in newborn PWM-stimulated cultures, but this was not confirmed by Andersson et al [9].

Predominance of IgM antibody production by congenitally infected fetuses [10] or by immunized newborns [6] had been recognized for many years, but it was unclear whether limitations of B- or T-lymphocyte or monocyte function were responsible. The restriction of the newborns' response to polyclonal B-cell activators suggests that B-cell immaturity limits the Ig isotype diversity of the newborns' antibody response. The biochemical basis of the immature responses of newborn B cells is of some practical interest because the B cells of some antibody-deficient patients show similarly restricted in vitro responses. The fact that newborn B cells can make surface γ- and α-immunoglobulin heavy chains makes defects in V-C region switching an unlikely explanation. Furthermore, newborn and adult B cells proliferate equally well in cultures stimulated with Cowan Staph A [11], so there do not appear to be differences in the cells' ability to be triggered and to make DNA. One possibility which has not yet been explored is that the newborn B-cell response may be biased toward the production of memory B cells rather than terminally differentiated plasma cells. Such a bias could have survival advantages through reducing the risk of B-cell tolerance induction. The significance of this limitation would probably depend on its duration after birth. In sequential studies of blood from infants of 2 months to 2 years of age, Andersson et al [9] found that IgG response to EBV stimulation approached adult levels by 2 years of age, while IgA production rose more slowly. The finding that responses in the IgG 2 subclass matured after 2 years of age is particularly interesting because antibodies to the capsular polysaccharides of H. influenzae occur mainly in this class. Both An-

TABLE 2. Phenotype of Fetal and Newborn Blood Lymphocytes as Percent Positive Cells*

Age in weeks	Pan-T	$T_{H/I}$	$T_{S/C}$	B
14	37	32	9	5
16	44	37	12	4
18–22	54	37	25	17
40	71	59	12	12

*Results from [14, 29, 30].

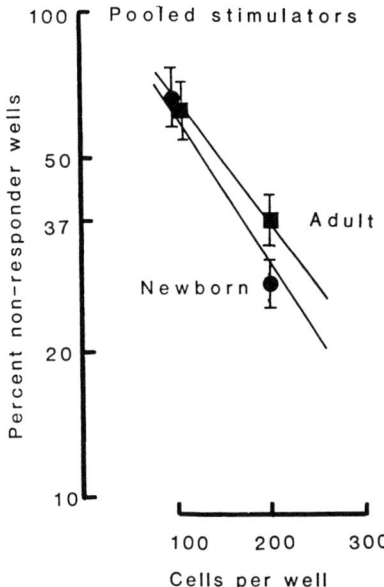

Fig. 1. Limiting dilution cultures of newborn and adult blood lymphocytes with irradiated T-cell-depleted pooled stimulator cells to determine responder-cell frequency in MLC. The results are plotted as percent non-responder wells of 24 replicates of 5 studies each of newborn and adult responders; they give a responder cell frequency of about 1:160 for newborns and 1:180 for adults.

TABLE 3. Thymidine Uptake by T-Cell Subsets Activated in MLC*

Responders	N	Counts in cells adhered through:		
		OKT4	OKT8	4:8 ratio
Newborn	5	1433 ± 160	384 ± 18	3.7
Adult	5	1073 ± 314	764 ± 203	1.6

*5×10^6 Newborn or adult cells were cultured for 6 days with 5×10^6 3,000 R irradiated single-donor stimulator cells. The cultures were pulsed for 2 hours with tritiated thymidine, then incubated with OKT4, or OKT8, or control. Antibody-coated cells were adhered to microwells which were then rinsed free of nonadherent cells before counting on a liquid scintillation counter. Results are expressed as cpm per 10^5 cells added to each well after subtraction of the nonantibody-treated control cpm. The mean cpm in the latter controls was 110 ± 20. The p value for the difference in OKT8$^+$ counts between newborn and adult responders is 0.05 for a two-tailed test.
Key: N = numbers of responders studied.

dersson et al [9] and Miyawaki et al [12] found that at 2 years of age the infants' B-cell response to PWM was still less than that of adults. These results suggest that intrinsic B-cell immaturity may be a major factor in restricting the antibody responsiveness of newborns [7]. Such restrictions, however, can only be partial because congenitally infected infants are known to make small amounts of IgG and sometimes IgA antibodies to the infecting agent. Probably the extended duration of a congenital infection affords time for some antigen-driven B-cell maturation to occur.

FUNCTIONAL STUDIES ON T CELLS

Fetal lymphocytes make rosettes with sheep erythrocytes and proliferate in mitogen or alloantigen-stimulated cultures almost as soon as they appear in the thymus [13]. The response to mitogens shows that the fetal and newborn T cells can make and use soluble factors, such as Interleukin 2, which are required for T-cell proliferation [14]. Initial reports indicated that newborn lymphocytes commonly respond to antigen to which their mothers are sensitive [15], while subsequent reports sometimes showed positive newborn responses with negative maternal responses [16]. Some of these studies made use of purified protein derivative (PPD) as the test antigen and so are open to the objection that the response might have been due to the mitogenicity of PPD [17]. In recent studies of newborn lymphocytes, the frequency of positive responses to antigen appears to be lower than that originally claimed. For example, Sirianni et al [18] found that none of 8 newborns responded to CMV or Candida, while Russell [19] found a frequency of response to HSV of 3 in 18; streptokinase, 1 in 17; vaccinia, 1 in 18; PPD, 3 in 14; and Candida, 0 in 15. In contrast to the minimal response to these microbial antigens, thymidine uptake by newborns' lymphocytes stimulated with alloantigens in MLC is similar to that of adults, as is the responder cell frequency (Fig. 1). The response to alloantigen may resemble the response to self-antigens associated with or modified by viruses. To pursue this analogy we have examined the phenotype of the newborn response to alloantigen in detail. Our results (Table 3) show that both helper and suppressor newborn T cells respond (as in adults); thus, there is no phenotypic evidence for immaturity or suppression. The simplest explanation for the low frequency of response to microbial antigens is that the relevant T-cell clones have not been expanded through antigen contact while the alloantigen response is presumably encoded in the germ line. Our own studies are consistent with this view in that we find that antigen-specific T cells can indeed be grown out of newborn blood by restimulation techniques (Table 4). An alternative hypothesis is that the response of newborn cells to microbial antigens is intrinsically suppressed.

Olding and Oldstone [20] and Lawler et al [21] showed that lymphocytes from human newborn blood tended to suppress the proliferative response of adult human lymphocytes stimulated with mitogen or antigen. These results were confirmed and expanded to show that human newborn cells suppressed in a variety of assays and that suppression persisted for months after birth [22]. The suppression requires the presence of newborn T cells and is abolished by

TABLE 4. Secondary Stimulation of Tetanus-Toxoid (TT) Prestimulated Newborn Lymphocytes*

Culture combination	Mean cpm tritiated thymidine uptake	
	No TT	1 Lf/ml TT
Responders + 10^5 irradiated cells	303	1202

*10^7 Newborn blood lymphocytes were cultured with 2 Lf/ml of TT in medium with human serum for 7 days. An aliquot of the same newborn's cells was frozen and stored at $-70°$. After 7 days the viable cells from the antigen-stimulated culture were recovered from a Ficoll-Hypaque gradient. The frozen cells were thawed, irradiated with 3,000 R, and used as antigen-presenting cells for the antigen-prestimulated cells. This result from a representative experiment shows increased thymidine uptake by the antigen-prestimulated newborn cells only in the presence of homologous antigen. Heterologous antigen or antigen-presenting cells gave no response.

TABLE 5. Origin of Dividing Cells in Newborn-Adult Mixed Lymphocyte Cultures as Judged by Karyotype

	Culture combination*					
	Unseparated		Separated		Irradiated separated	
Experiment	A	N	A	N	A	N
1	9	33	16	36	32	16
2	4	26	10	22	14	16
3	4	32	12	26	20	25
4	6	22	8	23	14	12
Mean % =	17	83	30	70	54	46

*In unseparated cultures the adult and newborn mononuclear cells were cultured without preliminary separation into T and non-T cells. The separated cultures comprised 4×10^6 each of newborn and adult T cells separated by E-rosetting, and 2×10^6 each of newborn and adult non-T cells. The irradiated separated cultures were identical except that the non-T cells were irradiated with 3,000 R before culture. All cultures were processed for metaphase spreads and the source of the dividing cell determined by the presence or absence of a fluorescent Y chromosome. The newborn was male in experiments 1–3 and female in experiment 4.
Key: A=adult; N=newborn mitoses.

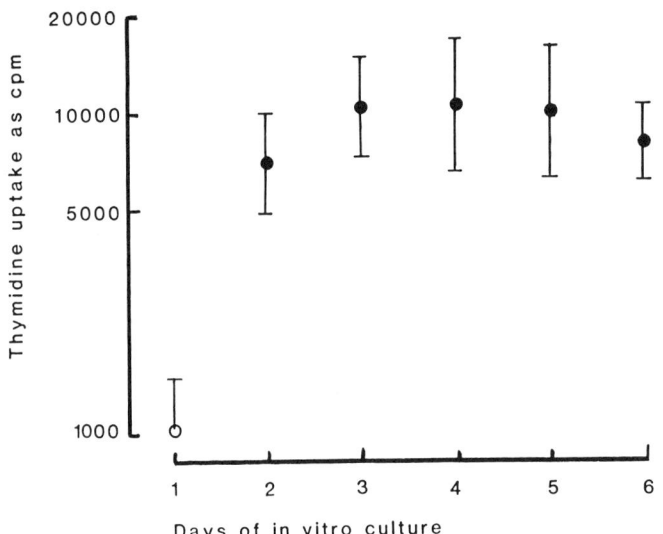

Fig. 2. Thymidine uptake by newborn blood mononuclear cells in culture with 10% human serum but no added mitogen or antigen. The newborn cells were cultured in 0.2 ml volumes at 10^6 cells/ml and triplicate aliquots were harvested on successive days.

irradiation or addition of cortisol to the cultures. Dialyzable factors may contribute to the suppression, and a recent report implicates prostaglandins as the suppression was prevented by indomethacin. The in vivo significance of suppression by newborn T cells can be questioned because it is generally detected only in the presence of mitogens [11] and it requires the activation of OKT8+ T cells [23]. Our recent studies suggest that even the MLC-induced suppression described by Lawler et al [21] may be open to other interpretations. In two-way MLCs between female adults and male newborns there is a striking predominance of mitoses of newborn origin as judged by the sex of the metaphases. No sex predominance is seen when both the male and female cells come from newborns. The predominance of newborn mitoses vanishes if the adult and newborn lymphocytes are first separated into T and non-T cells and the non-T cells are irradiated (Table 5). This result suggests that division by newborn non-T cells contributes to the excess of newborn mitoses in the two-way MLCs. Newborn non-T cells have long been recognized to include a subset with a high spontaneous uptake of tritiated thymidine (Fig. 2). These presumably dividing cells do not bear conventional T-cell antigen (OKT3,4,8) but they are Ia antigen positive. Their sustained proliferation during the 6-day incubation of an MLC is a likely explanation for the predominance of newborn mitoses in unseparated two-way cultures. This interpretation is consistent with the finding that there is no sex predominance when both donors are newborn.

Newborn T cells are clearly mature regarding phenotype and their proliferative response to mitogen. The susceptibility of newborns to severe HSV 2 infections suggests that more subtle defects exist. The delay in the appearance of CMV-responsive T cells in children with congenital CMV [24,25] might be due to a lack of natural killer cells or inducer T cells, to increased suppression, or to defective antigen handling by monocytes. There is some evidence to show that newborn natural killer cell activity is less than that of adults [26], but whether this is sufficient to account for the severity of newborn herpesvirus infections is uncertain. Excess suppressor activity seems an unlikely explanation both because newborns do not have an excess of suppressor cells by phenotype and because the absence of Ia antigens on those that are present suggests that they are not preactivated. Furthermore the T-cell response to foreign histocompatibility antigens (alloantigens) is not suppressed, nor does it differ in responder-cell frequency or phenotype from the adult response to alloantigens.

ANTIGEN PROCESSING BY NEWBORN MONOCYTES

Results in newborn mice and rats [27] suggest that monocyte immaturity may limit immune responses by newborns. We investigated this possibility in humans by testing the ability of newborn monocytes to process and present antigen to maternal antigen-specific T-cell blasts [28]. The result of one such experiment (Table 6) shows that newborn monocytes effectively present PPD: this confirms our previous results with tetanus toxoid antigen presentation. More recent studies suggest that newborn monocytes are also able to present CMV and VZV antigens.

CONCLUSIONS

Newborn antibody responses are likely to be restricted by a lack of memory B cells generated in the course of previous immune responses to cross-reacting antigens. T-cell clones with specificity for virus antigens are similarly unexpanded at birth and this is likely to limit significantly the response to rapidly growing viruses such as those of the Herpes group.

TABLE 6. Antigen Presentation by Newborn Monocytes*

Antigen-presenting cells	Thymidine uptake of maternal PPD-specific T-cell blasts cultured with:		
	No antigen	TT	PPD
None	602	775	865
Maternal	1,210	1,089	16,885
Newborn	996	947	17,940
Unrelated	967	856	1,068

*Maternal blood lymphocytes were cultured for 6 days with PPD to yield a population of T-cell blasts which could be used to test antigen presentation by the mother's own newborn's cells. Significant thymidine uptake by the blast is seen only in the presence of the appropriate antigen and with either autologous (maternal) or own-baby blood monocytes.

SUMMARY

Maturation of the immune system starts early in fetal life. Lymphocytes of the B series develop in the liver by 9 weeks' gestation and are present in the blood and spleen by 12 weeks. T lymphocytes start to leave the thymus from about 14 weeks' gestation and subsequently cells with helper and suppressor phenotypes are present in the spleen. The relative lack of development of secondary lymphoid tissues in healthy fetuses most probably reflects the lack of antigen stimulus. Newborn plasma contains adult levels of IgG which is acquired across the placenta from the mother. The small amounts of IgM (<20 mg/dL) which are normally present in healthy newborns have been reported to include antibody with specificity for maternal lymphocytes. IgA synthesis normally starts in the secretory immune system, about 2–3 weeks after birth. Poor antibody responses by newborns following immunization, especially with bacterial capsular polysaccharides, suggest that newborn immune responses are immature as compared with adults. The susceptibility of newborns to severe HSV and VZV supports this view. In vitro correlates of this immaturity include 1) deficiency of the response by newborn B cells to polyclonal activators, and 2) a lack of T cells which proliferate in HSV- or VZV-stimulated cultures. These characteristics more likely result from a lack of prior antigen stimulation and resulting clonal expansion than from intrinsic lymphocyte suppression. Antigen handling by newborn monocytes, in contrast, appears to be mature by the time of birth.

REFERENCES

1. Hayward AR: Development of lymphocyte responses and interactions in the human fetus and newborn. Immunol Rev 57:40–60, 1981.
2. Marcu KB, Cooper MD: New views of the immunoglobulin heavy chain switch. Nature 298:327–328, 1982.
3. Kung PC, Goldstein G: Functional and developmental compartments of human T lymphocytes. Vox Sang 39:121–127, 1980.
4. Gitlin D: Development and metabolism of the immune globulins. In Kagan BM, Stiehm ER (eds): "Immunologic Incompetence." Chicago: Year Book Medical Publishers, 1971.
5. Smith RT, Eitzman DV: The development of the immune response. Characterization of the immune response of the human infant and adult to immunization with salmonella vaccines. Pediatrics 33:163, 1964.

6. Selner JC, Merrill DA, Claman HN: Salivary immunoglobulin and albumin: Development during the newborn period. J Pediatr 72:685–689, 1968.
7. Hayward AR, Lawton AR: Induction of plasma cell differentiation of human fetal lymphocytes: Evidence for functional immaturity of T and B cells. J Immunol 119:1213, 1977.
8. Miyagawa Y, Sugita K, Komiyama A, Akabane T: Delayed in vitro immunoglobulin production by cord lymphocytes. Pediatrics 65:497–500, 1980.
9. Andersson U, Bird AG, Britton S, Palacios R: Humoral and cellular immunity in humans studied at the cell level from birth to two years of age. Immunol Rev 54:5–38, 1981.
10. Alford CA: Studies on antibody in congenital rubella infections. Arch Dis Child 110:455, 1965.
11. Tosato G, Magrath IT, Koski IR, Dooley NJ, Blaese RM: B cell differentiation and immunoregulatory T cell function in human cord blood lymphocytes. J Clin Invest 66:383, 1980.
12. Miyawaki Y, Moriya N, Nagaoki T, Taniguchi N: Maturation of B cell differentiation ability and T cell regulatory function in infancy and childhood. Immunol Rev 57:61–88, 1981.
13. Hayward AR, Soothill JF: Reaction to antigen by human fetal thymus lymphocytes. Ontogeny of acquired immunity. In "Ciba Foundation Symposium." Amsterdam: Elsevier, 1972.
14. Hayward AR, Kurnick JT: Newborn T cell suppression: Early appearance, maintenance in culture and lack of growth factor suppression. J Immunol 126:50, 1981.
15. Field EJ, Caspary EA: Is maternal lymphocyte sensitization passed to the child? Lancet 2:337, 1971.
16. Leikin S, Oppenheim JJ: Prenatal sensitization. Lancet 2:876, 1971.
17. Ringden O, Rynell-Dagöö R, Kunori T et al: Antibody production and DNA synthesis of human lymphocyte subpopulations induced by PPD tuberculin. Clin Exp Immunol 36:528, 1979.
18. Sirianni MC, Fiorilli M, Pana A, Pezzella M, Aiuti F: In vitro transfer of specific reactivity to cytomegalovirus and candida to cord blood leukocytes with dialyzable leukocyte extracts. Clin Immunol Immunopathol 14:300, 1979.
19. Russell AS: Cell mediated immunity to microbial antigens in mother and child. Clin Exp Immunol 22:457, 1975.
20. Olding LB, Oldstone MBA: Thymus derived peripheral lymphocytes from human newborns inhibit division of their mothers' lymphocytes. J Immunol 116:682–686, 1976.
21. Lawler SD, Ukaejiofo EO, Reeves BR: Interaction of maternal and neonatal cells in mixed lymphocyte culture. Lancet 2:1185, 1975.
22. Unander AM, Olding LB: Ontogeny and post natal persistence of a strong suppressor activity in man. J Immunol 127:1182–1186, 1981.
23. Hayward AR, Merrill D: Requirement for OKT 8+ suppressor cell proliferation by human newborn T cells. Clin Exp Immunol 45:468–474, 1981.
24. Gehrz RC, Marker SC, Knorr SO, Kalis JM, Balfour HH: Specific cell mediated immune defect in active cytomegalovirus infection of young children and their mothers. Lancet 2:844–847, 1977.
25. Starr SE, Tolpin MD, Friedman HM, Pauker K, Plotkin SA: Impaired cellular immunity to cytomegalovirus in congenitally infected children and their mothers. J Infect Dis 140:500–505, 1979.
26. Toivanen P, Uksila J, Leino A, Lassila O, Hirvonen T, Russkanen O: Development of mitogen responding T cells and natural killer cells in the human fetus. Immunol Rev 57:89–106, 1981.
27. Blaese RM, Lawrence EC: Development of macrophage function and the expression of immunocompetence. In Cooper MD, Dayton DH (eds): "Development of Host Defenses." New York: Raven Press, 1977.
28. Hoffman AA, Hayward AR, Kurnick JT, DeFreitas E, McGregor J, Harbeck RJ: Presentation of antigen by human newborn monocytes to maternal tetanus toxoid specific T cell blasts. J Clin Immunol 1:217, 1981.
29. Linch DC, Beverley PCL, Levinsky RL, Rodeck CH: Phenotypic analysis of fetal blood leucocytes: Potential for prenatal diagnosis of immunodeficiency disorders. Prenatal Diagnosis 2:211–218, 1982.
30. Durandy A, Oury C, Griscelli C, Dumez Y, Oury JF, Henrion R: Prenatal testing for inherited immune deficiencies by fetal blood sampling. Prenatal Diagnosis 2:109–113, 1982.

Deficient DR Antigen Expression on Human Neonatal Monocytes: Reversal With Lymphokines*

E. Richard Stiehm, MD, Dean Mann, MD, Carolyn Newland, PhD,
Marcelo B. Sztein, MD, Patricia S. Steeg, PhD, Joost J. Oppenheim, MD,
and R. Michael Blaese, MD

Department of Pediatrics and the Center for Interdisciplinary Research in Immunologic Diseases, UCLA School of Medicine, Los Angeles, CA 90024 (E.R.S.), National Cancer Institute and the Uniformed Services University for the Health Sciences, Bethesda, MD 20205 (D.M., C.N.), National Institutes of Dental Research, National Institutes of Health, Bethesda, MD 20205 (M.B.S., P.S.S., J.J.O.), Cellular Immunology Section, Metabolism Branch, National Cancer Institute, National Institutes of Health, Bethesda, MD 20205 (R.M.B.)

It has been demonstrated that macrophages expressing HLA-DR antigens play an important role in human macrophage-dependent T-cell activation to soluble antigens [1,2]. Two macrophage subpopulations, one bearing DR antigens (DR$^+$), and one DR-antigen deficient (DR$^-$), have been described. DR antigens on human cells appear to be analogous to Ia antigens in mouse cells [3]. Lu et al [4] reported diminished expression of Ia in newborn mice macrophages and this is correlated with a decrease in their antigen-presenting [4,5] and mixed leukocyte response-stimulating capabilities [6].

Since the human newborn has deficient antibody responses to certain antigens, we investigated the expression of DR antigens on human neonatal monocytes. We have also studied the role that soluble mediators play on the relative balance of DR$^+$ and DR$^-$ human cord blood monocytes in vitro.

We here report that DR expression by human cord blood monocytes is decreased, as compared to adult peripheral blood monocytes. In addition, we present evidence indicating that DR expression in cord blood monocytes can be increased after incubation with lymphokine-containing supernatants or recombinant interferon-α.

METHODS

Cord blood from 40 uncomplicated deliveries was collected into preservative-free heparined tubes. Isolation of monocytes was performed as follows: One-sixth part dextran (6% in saline) was added to 15–50 ml of cord blood, mixed and incubated at 37°C in 5% CO_2 for 30 minutes. The top plasma layer was removed and subjected to Ficoll-Hypaque separation. The washed cells were resuspended in RPMI with 10% human plasma. Aliquots (25–35 × 10^6) of the whole mononuclear cell suspensions were placed on Costar plastic dishes that had been preincubated at 37°C with 5 cc heat-inactivated fetal calf serum (FCS). The FCS was removed prior to adding the cells. The dishes were incubated in 5% CO_2 at 37°C for 1 hour and then the nonadherent cells removed by aspiration, followed by washing with three 10 cc aliquots of HBSS in 10% FCS, preheated to 37°C. Then 5 cc of EDTA was added and the dishes were reincubated at 37°C for 30 minutes. The adherent cells were removed with the aid of a stream of RPMI in 10% human plasma, generated by a #18 needle attached to a 20 ml plastic syringe. These cells were then concentrated by centrifugation and counted. The yield was approximately 5–10% of the whole mononuclear cell and > 98% viable by trypan blue exclusion.

These cells were kept overnight at 4°C or at 37°C in 5% CO_2. In some instances, they were allowed to incubate at 37°C for 48–72 hours prior to fluorescent-activated cell sorting (FACS) analysis. No statistically significant differences were noted following each treatment. Esterase staining, peroxidase staining, Channelizer analysis, and IL-1 assays were performed on these cells. FACS analysis, using a battery of DR monoclonal antibodies, was performed as described [7].

Other neonatal whole mononuclear cells (4-8 × 10^5 cells in 0.1 ml of RPMI 1640 containing 10% FCS per well) were added to 96 well, flat-bottom microtiter plates, incubated for 1 to 3 hours at 37°C, and the nonadherent cells removed by vigorously washing 4 to 6 times. The remaining adherent cells were cultured in 0.2 ml RPMI 1640 containing 10% FCS, 5 × 10^{-5} M 2-mercaptoethanol, and dilutions of either concanavalin A (Con A) stimulated peripheral blood mononuclear cell (PBMC) culture supernatant, a Con A-supplemented (unstimulated) PBMC culture supernatant or recombinant interferon-α (IFLrA, provided by Dr.

*Supported by USPHS grants AI-15332, HD-09800, and an NCI-USUHS Interagency Agreement.

TABLE 1. Comparison of Cell Surface Antigen Expression on Cord Blood and Adult Monocytes by Fluorescent-Activated Cell Sorting Analysis

Antisera	Cord Blood			Adult Blood		
	% Reacting	Mean Fluorescence	# Tested	% Reacting	Mean Fluorescence	# Tested
OKIA[a]	19.1 ± 8.05	516 ± 188.0	2	82.0 ± 3.06	1850 ± 373.1	4
DA-2[a]	25.6 ± 2.35	738 ± 119.8	4	71.7 ± 7.73	1364 ± 242.4	5
31.1[a]	24.0 ± 4.63	601 ± 143.5	4	79.5 ± 4.74	1122 ± 149.8	5
3.1[a]	33.2 ± 3.74	1196 ± 335.3	4	81.1 ± 2.95	2143 ± 479.3	5
4.4[a]	29.3 ± 4.38	1324 ± 313.8	4	78.4 ± 3.96	2954 ± 210.7	7
20.2[b]	32.5 ± 5.40	680 ± 215.6	4	73.3 ± 3.38	627 ± 246.5	7
7.2[b]	30.1 ± 3.51	638 ± 127.0	5	65.2 ± 7.19	797 ± 249.9	7
3F10[c]	45.6 ± 8.34	1370 ± 360.7	5	92.0 ± 2.17	3972 ± 460.1	7

[a]Monoclonal antibodies detecting HLA-DR monomorphic determinant.
[b]Monoclonal antibodies detecting monocyte antigen(s).
[c]Monomorphic anti-HLA-A, B, (C?) monoclonal antibody.

S. Peska, Hoffman LaRoche) for 2–3 days at 37° in a humidified atmosphere of 5% CO_2 in air.

Con A PBMC culture supernatants were obtained incubating 5×10^6 PBMC/ml, obtained by Ficoll-Hypaque separation from peripheral blood, with 1 µg/ml Con A for 48 hours at 37°C in a humidified atmosphere of 5% CO_2 in air. Con A-supplemented supernatants (control supernatants) were prepared under the same conditions, except that the Con A was added to the supernatants at the time of harvesting, instead of at the beginning of the culture.

To determine the percentage of DR antigen expressing cells the culture supernatants were removed, replaced with 50 µl of RPMI 1640 containing 1% FCS and a 1:60 final dilution of anti-DR (p 23,30) [3,8], and then incubated at 4°C for 1 hour. Subsequently a 1:5 final dilution of Low-Tox-H rabbit complement (Cedarlane Laboratories, Inc.) was added, and the cultures were reincubated for 30 to 60 minutes at 37°C. Viability was determined by trypan blue exclusion, and the percentage of DR^+ cells is reported as a mean Cytotoxicity Index (CI), with 95% confidence limits, based on arc sine square transformation.

RESULTS

The newborn cell fractions were subjected to cell sizing, using the Coulter Channelizer. This indicated that 10–25% of the mononuclear cells were large cells; following monocyte isolation, 90–95% of the cells were large cells. Nonspecific esterase staining of the neonatal monocyte preparations showed that only 45–55% of the cells were esterase-positive compared to adult monocyte preparations, which are 95% esterase-positive. Nearly all of the newborn (and adult) monocytes (> 95%) are peroxidase-positive. Analysis of the capacity of 12 newborn monocyte samples to produce IL-1 production following phytohemagglutinin, lipopolysaccharide or silica stimulation yielded levels of IL-1 activity that equaled that produced by adult peripheral monocytes.

The FACS analysis data are presented in Table 1. There was a consistent decrease in DR antigen expression on newborns as compared with adult monocytes, both in the degree of fluorescence mean 28% of adult cell fluorescence and the number of positive cells (19–33% in neonates versus 71–82% in adults). There also is decreased expression of other cell surface antigens. These data include all the samples studied, and neglect small fluctuations due to differences in temperature and incubation times after monocyte isolation.

Freshly obtained adherent human neonatal mononuclear cells were approximately 22% DR^+ as measured by anti-DR and complement-mediated

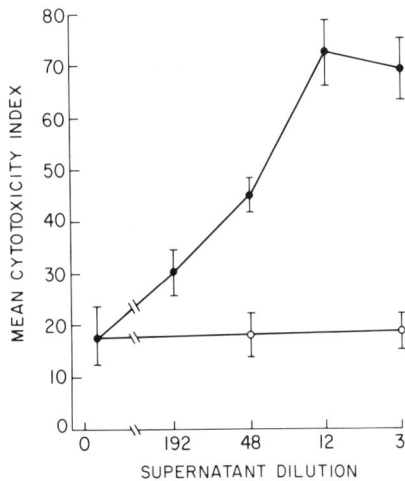

Fig. 1. Lymphokine enhancement of cord blood monocytes DR antigen expression. Cord blood monocytes obtained as described in **Methods** were incubated with dilutions of either a Con A-stimulated PBMC culture supernatant (●—●) or a control Con A-supplemented PBMC culture supernatant (○—○) for 2 days. The percent of DR^+ cells was determined by anti-DR and complement-mediated cytotoxicity, and is shown as mean cytotoxicity index ± 95% confidence interval.

cytotoxicity. Thus, the DR antigen expression of cord blood monocytes is significantly reduced as compared to human adult peripheral blood monocytes, which range from 70–85%.

We then studied the effects of lymphokines on neonatal monocytes. Figure 1 shows the effect that a Con A-stimulated PBMC culture supernatant has on cord blood monocyte DR expression in vitro. As can be

TABLE 2. In Vitro Induction of Cord Blood Monocyte DR Antigen Expression by Lymphokine After Anti-DR Plus Complement Pretreatment

Dilution	Mean Cytotoxicity Index (95% Confidence Interval)	
	Con A-Stimulated PBMC Culture Supernatant	Control PBMC Culture Supernatant
0		8.92 (5.6, 12.9)
1:192	32.86 (26.2, 39.9)	—
1:48	62.24 (56.5, 67.7)	—
1:12	58.35 (52.1, 64.4)	—
1:3	61.11 (56.5, 65.6)	8.85 (6.12, 12.02)

seen in this representative experiment, the percentage of DR+ cord blood monocytes was increased in a dose-dependent manner when dilutions of a lymphokine-containing supernatant were added to the cells. By contrast, no effect was observed with the Con A-supplemented PBMC culture supernatant. Thus, the percentage of DR+ cord blood monocytes can be increased by in vitro incubation with lymphokines. Additional observations suggest that the percentage of DR+ cord blood monocytes decreases with time of culture in medium alone (data not shown).

In order to determine if a lymphokine-containing supernatant induces DR− cord blood monocytes to become DR+, we pretreated freshly isolated cord blood monocytes with anti-DR plus complement in order to eliminate DR+ cells. These DR− pretreated cells were then washed and incubated for 2 days in the presence of dilutions of a Con A-stimulated or a Con A-supplemented (control) culture supernatant. As can be seen in Table 2, 62% of the pretreated cord blood monocytes became DR+, while cells incubated in the presence of control supernatant or medium alone remained about 10% DR+.

Kinetic experiments showed that maximum DR+ cord blood monocyte expression occurs in vitro by day 3–5 after the addition of lymphokine-containing supernatant to the cultures (data not shown). We then attempted to identify which lymphokine(s) in the Con A-stimulated PBMC culture supernatant mediate(s) the increased expression of DR+ cord blood monocytes in vitro.

TABLE 3. Enhancement of Cord Blood Monocyte DR Antigen Expression In Vitro by Recombinant Interferon

Units IFLrA	Mean Cytotoxicity Index (95% Confidence Limits)
0	19.11 (13.6, 25.4)
1.6	25.53 (21.3, 30.0)
6.25	42.46 (35.6, 49.4)
25	47.94 (41.3, 54.6)
100	41.38 (36.3, 46.6)

Since it had been reported [9] that an immune interferon-like lymphokine modulates Ia expression in mouse macrophages, we tested the effect of human recombinant interferon-α on cord blood monocyte DR antigen expression. Table 3 shows a typical experiment in which IFLrA induced an increase in the percent of DR+ cord blood monocytes after 2 days of incubation. In this experiment, maximal enhancement of DR antigen expression was observed at approximately 2–6 units/ml of IFLrA. In addition, we observed that the percentage of DR+ cells induced by IFLrA is typically lower than that obtained with lymphokine-containing supernatant.

DISCUSSION

The chief observation of lower HLA-DR expression on human neonatal monocytes is similar to the observation in neonatal mice macrophages made by Lu et al in 1979 [4]. More recent studies by this group [10] indicate that the failure of DR expression is due in part to the presence of a splenic suppressor cell that inhibits Ia expression in adult mouse peritoneal macrophages subjected to stimuli that normally cause increased Ia expression. This splenic cell was tentatively identified as an early phagocytic cell of the monocyte-macrophage series, present in adult bone marrow, that exerts its action through elevation of a prostaglandin-like substance.

A similar decrease in DR expression by human neonatal cord cells has been reported by Tweady et al [11]. They found that neonatal monocytes are less stimulatory than adult monocytes in MLC with adult responder cells.

These studies suggest that the DR deficiency of newborn monocytes is both relative and reversible. The reason for reduced DR antigen expression is unknown, although our experiments indicate neonatal monocytes can be stimulated to express DR antigens at levels comparable to normal peripheral blood monocytes. Possible explanations include a) alteration of monocyte-subsets in newborns favoring DR− expressing cells, b) reduced levels of DR antigen modulatory lymphokines in cord blood, and/or c) the presence of inhibitors of DR antigen modulatory lymphokines in cord blood. In this regard, prostaglandins have been demonstrated to inhibit lymphokine modulation of murine macrophage Ia antigen expression [12], and may therefore also exert modulatory effects in the human system.

Both crude lymphokine-containing culture supernatant and cloned IFLrA enhanced the percentage of DR+ cord blood monocytes in vitro. These results indicate that IFN can modulate human cord blood monocyte DR antigen expression; they do not indicate that IFN is the only mediator in crude culture supernatants with DR modulatory activity. Indeed, the observation that maximal enhancement of DR antigen expression by IFLrA is typically less than that by crude culture supernatants suggests that: a) a different IFN type (IFN-γ for instance) may be a more potent DR antigen modulatory agent, b) 2 types of IFN may act in concert to induce maximal DR expression, and/or c) a non-IFN lymphokine may act independently (additively) or synergistically with IFN to elevate DR antigen expression.

The duration of the diminished DR antigen expression in newborn monocytes is not yet known; nor do we know if there is a human equivalent of the murine suppressor of Ia expression. If DR expression remains diminished for several months after birth, this may contribute to the deficient antibody and cytotoxic responses of newborn cells [13,14] as a result of a diminished antigen presentation. Of note, Hoffman et al could find no in vitro deficiency of neonatal monocyte ability to process tetanus antigen for proliferation of toxoid-specific T-cell blasts [15]. These and other in vitro experiments of monocyte function must take into account the likelihood of lymphokine production in vitro that provides a stimulus for monocyte DR expression.

REFERENCES

1. Bergholtz BO, Thorsby E: HLA-D restriction of the macrophage-dependent response of immune human T lymphocytes to PPD in vitro: Inhibition of anti-HLA DR antisera. Scand J Immunol 8:63–73, 1978.
2. Rodey GE, Luehrman LK, Thomas DW: In vitro primary immunization of human peripheral blood lymphocytes to KLH: Evidence for HLA-D region restriction. J Immunol 123:2250–2254, 1979.
3. Lunney JK, Mann DL, Sachs DH: Sharing of Ia antigens between species. III. Ia shared between mice and human beings. Scand J Immunol 10:403–413, 1979.
4. Lu CY, Calamai EG, Unanue ER: A defect in the antigen-presenting function of macrophages from neonatal mice. Nature 282:327–329, 1979.
5. Beller DI, Ho K: Regulation of macrophage populations. V. Evaluation of the control of macrophage Ia expression in vitro. J Immunol 129:971, 1982.
6. Beller DI, Unanue ER: Regulation of macrophage populations. II. Synthesis and expression of Ia antigens by peritoneal exudate is a transient event. J Immunol 126:263–269, 1981.
7. Mann DL, Sharrow SO: HLA-DRw alloantigens can be detected on peripheral blood T lymphocytes. J Immunol 125:1889–1896, 1980.
8. Humphries RE, McCune JM, Chess AM, Herrman HM, Malenka AJ, Mann DL, Parham B, Schlossman SF, Strominger JL: Isolation and immunological characterization of a human B lymphocyte specific cell surface antigen. J Exp Med 144:99, 1976.
9. Steeg PS, Moore RN, Johnson HM, Oppenheim JJ: Regulation of murine macrophage Ia antigen expression by a lymphokine with immune interferon activity. J Exp Med 156:1780–1793, 1982.
10. Snyder DS, Lu CY, Unanue ER: Control of macrophage Ia expression in neonatal mice—role of a splenic suppressor cell. J Immunol 128:1458–1465, 1982.
11. Tweady DJ, Baley JE, Schacter BZ, Ellner JJ: Decreased surface expression of HLA-DR antigen on human neonatal cord blood monocytes. Clin Res 30:359a, 1982.
12. Steeg PS, Johnson HM, Oppenheim JJ: Regulation of murine macrophage Ia antigen expression by an immune interferon-like lymphokine. Inhibitory effect of endotoxin. J Immunol 129:2402–2406, 1982.
13. Blaese RM, Lawrence EC: Development of macrophage function and the expression of immunocompetence. In Cooper MD, Dayton DH (eds): "Development of Host Defenses." New York: Raven Press, 1977, pp 201–207.
14. Lubens RG, Gard SE, Soderberg-Warner M, Stiehm ER: Lectin-dependent and natural killer cytotoxic deficiencies in human newborns. Cell Immunol (In press).
15. Hoffman AE, Hayward AR, Kurnick JT, Defreitas EC, McGregor J, Harbeck RJ: Presentation of antigen by human newborn monocytes to maternal tetanus toxoid-specific T-cell blasts. J Clin Immunol 1:217–221, 1981.

T-Cell Cytotoxicity and Chemiluminescence Abnormalities in Newborns and Chronic Granulomatous Disease*

Allen G. Peerless, MD, and E. Richard Stiehm, MD

Department of Pediatrics and the Center for Interdisciplinary Research in Immunologic Diseases, UCLA School of Medicine, Los Angeles, CA 90024

INTRODUCTION

Newborns are unusually susceptible to infection by viruses and other organisms requiring an intact cellular (T cell) immune response. While some aspects of the newborns' T-cell system are intact (eg thymus size, T-lymphocyte numbers, T-lymphocyte proliferation), more differentiated T-cell functions (eg cutaneous delayed hypersensitivity reactions, lymphokine production, and certain cytotoxic reactions) are deficient when compared to adult T cells [1,2].

Accordingly, we sought to explore T-cell cytotoxicity further using lectin-dependent cellular cytotoxicity (LDCC) and T-cell chemiluminescence (CL). The latter was investigated because of the possibility that T cells lyse targets with the same enzymatic machinery that polymorphonuclears [3] have available for bacterial killing. Lymphocytes, lacking certain pieces of oxidative machinery found in granulocytes, generate less photon energy and require amplification using a luminescent compound, luminol.

During the course of these studies, 2 boys with proven chronic granulomatous disease (CGD) presented. Their T-cell CL was in the same low range as patients with CID. Further studies indicate that CL is a property of many cells and that a global membrane defect in CGD may result in defective CL in a variety of their cells.

*Supported in part by USPHS Research Grants AI-15332 and HD-09800.

METHODS

Peripheral blood samples were obtained from newborns (1 ml/kg), age 1-4 days, young children, and adults, with informed consent in accordance with the regulations of the UCLA Human Subjects Protection Committee. Cord bloods were obtained routinely at all deliveries and processed within 1 hour of collection.

Mononuclear cells were obtained using density centrifugation with Ficoll-Hypaque. The T-rosetted fraction (T-enriched > 90% rosette-forming cells (E-RFC), < 3% surface immunoglobulin (SIg), and < 3% lipase positive) pass through the gradient. The nonrosetting cells (T-depleted, < 5% E-RFC, 40-50% SIg positive and 30-50% esterase-positive) remain at the interface.

Alternatively, mononuclear cells, adjusted to a concentration of 0.5-0.75 × 10^8 cells/ml were loaded onto nylon-wool columns, presaturated with RPMI medium containing 10% fetal calf serum, 1 ml of 200 nm glutamine and 1 ml of a penicillin (10,000 μ/ml)-streptomycin (10,000 μg/ml) mixture. Filtration is initiated following a 30-minute incubation at 37°C. The cellular band is washed through the column with warmed medium so that the total volume of effluent does not exceed 15 ml [4,5]. T-cell purity utilizing this method approaches 90% by histochemical and serologic testing.

LDCC assay was performed as described by Bonavida et al [6]. Most assays utilized 8 × 10^5 mononuclear cells, 2 × 10^4 ^{51}chromium (Cr) labeled EL-4 (murine leukemia cells maintained in ascitic form in C57Bl male mice) target cells, and PHA (Burroughs-Wellcome) at final concentration of 1:250. The cells and PHA were pipetted into 10 × 75 mm disposable glass tubes, centrifuged briefly to enhance cell to cell contact, and incubated at 37°C in 5% CO_2 for 4 hours. The reaction was stopped with 1 ml cold Hanks' solution, centrifuged for 10 minutes at 300 g, and supernatants poured off for radioactive counting on a gamma scintillation counter. Target cells were labeled by incubating in the presence of 1 μc ^{51}Cr (New England Nuclear) for each 10^6 cells at 37°C for 1 hour. They were washed 3 times with cold Hanks before use.

CL generation by human T lymphocytes is established by the addition of Concanavalin A (Con A), 100 μg, to 2 × 10^6 purified T cells [7]. The standard reaction mix includes 800 μl of a 2.5 × 10^6 ml cell suspension, 100 μl of luminol solution, 100 μg of Con A or buffer control. Cell solutions are kept in a closed shaking water bath at 37°C and manually transferred to the counter. CL is measured in a liquid scintillation counter, set in the out of coincidence mode. To reduce background emission, scintillation vials are dark adapted. All manipulations are conducted in red light illumination.

Results are reported in terms of peak photon emission and as a chemiluminescence index (CI). This index reflects peak cellular photon emission minus nonspecific luminol drift divided by spontaneous emission of a cell-free dark-adapted vial and eliminates artifactual contributions to the measured emission.

RESULTS

LDCC was equivalent in cord, neonatal, and adult PBMC (Fig. 1). However, there was significant decrease in LDCC of newborn PBMC compared to adults (22% ± 3 vs 36% ± 2 SEM p < .001), but this corrected within 6 months. T-depleted cord cells (consisting of SIg positive B cells and esterase positive non-T cells) showed the highest cytotoxicity (48 ± 6%); this was significantly greater than T-depleted adult or newborn cells, although the latter had strong LDCC. There is a trend toward decreased LDCC with increasing age. LDCC of T-enriched cells from these groups is also shown in Figure 1. A marked LDCC deficiency is present in T-cord cells (22 ± 3) and newborn T cells (18 ± 5) compared to adult T cells (52 ± 2); this corrects gradually with increasing age. Combining these data, it is evident that the enhanced activity of LDCC in neonatal cells is due to increased LDCC in the non-T fraction, compensating for the deficient T-cell LDCC.

The CL response of adult T lymphocytes following the addition of Con A, as shown in Figure 2, is characterized by an early burst of CL, followed by a gradual taper and slow rise to the peak emission. Mean time to peak emission in 14 adult T-cell preparations was 18 minutes. CL of a luminol-free cell suspension does not vary from that of the dark-adapted blank, underscoring the absolute need for luminol in this reaction. Treatment of purified T-cell suspensions with opsonized zymosan does not change CL from spontaneous levels, affording a useful control against granulocyte contamination. Further proof of the T-cell origin of this CL is obtained by treatment of such preparations with pan-T monoclonal antibody and complement which abrogates 90% of the control response (Fig. 3).

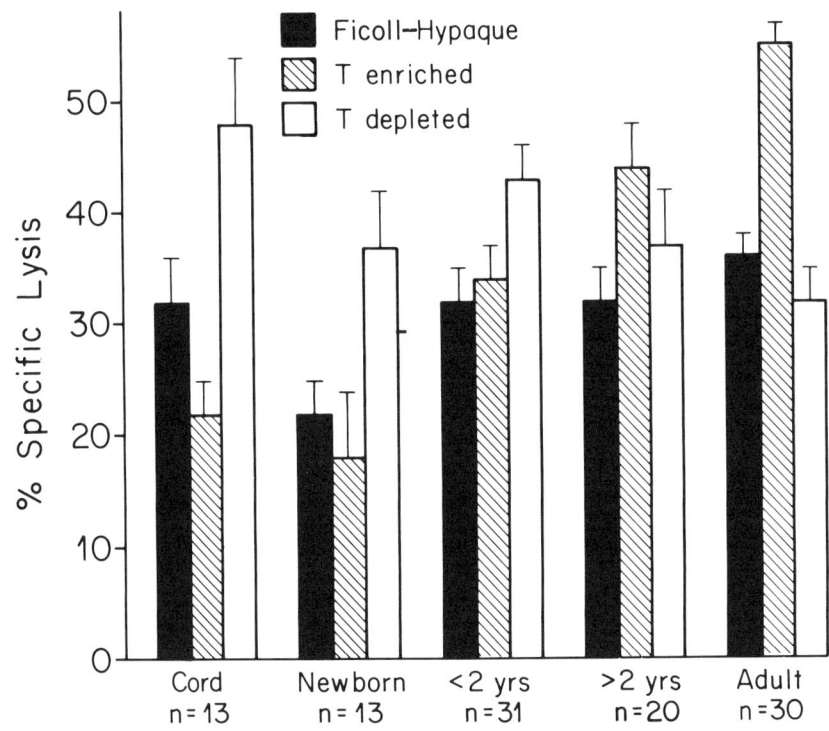

Fig. 1. Lectin-dependent cytotoxicity of Ficoll-Hypaque separated mononuclear cells T enriched (95%) from cord blood, newborns 1–3 days of age, children, and adults. The target was EL-4 chromated tumor cells. The assay utilized an effector:target ratio of 40:1, a PHA dilution of 1:50, and a 4-hour incubation time. Results are expressed as % specific lysis ± SEM. The significantly decreased T-cell cytotoxicity of newborn and cord cells is masked in the whole Ficoll-Hypaque preparations by the normal non-T-cell cytotoxicity. Some of the newborns have T-cell LDCC in the same low range as patients with primary T-cell immunodeficiencies such as SCID.

Fourteen adult and 8 cord T-cell preparations were tested for luminol-dependent CL. Mean spontaneous adult CI was 89 ± 23 compared to 19 ± 9 in cord T-cell preparations. The Con A stimulated adult mean CI was 112 ± 30 contrasted to 22 ± 10 in cord samples. The mean specific CI, a reflection of the incremental emission attributed to mitogen binding, was 24 ± 8.0 in adults and 3.6 ± 1.4 in cords (Fig. 4).

Participation of certain oxidants in the lymphocyte CL response was examined by the addition of antioxidant enzymes, superoxide dismutase (SOD), or catalase. Significant augmentation in total CPM over the 30-minute sampling period occurred in preparations treated with SOD. This effect was dose restricted, peaking at 7.5 μg. Catalase, by contrast, resulted in diminution of photon emission across the dosage range. Mean 50% inhibition of the control response resulted from treatment of the reaction mix with 100 μg of catalase. Combined treatment with 7.5 μg SOD + 100 μg catalase resulted in mild dissipation of the control CL response (Fig. 5).

CL generation by adult nylon-wool purified T lymphocytes following Con A (50 μg/ml final concentration) stimulation was significantly higher than spontaneous controls. Mean peak-stimulated CL in the 8 subjects studied was 95.9 ± 13.3 (CPM × 10^3 ± SEM) compared to 47.8 ± 4.8 in nontreated controls (p < .01). A dose-dependent response similar to

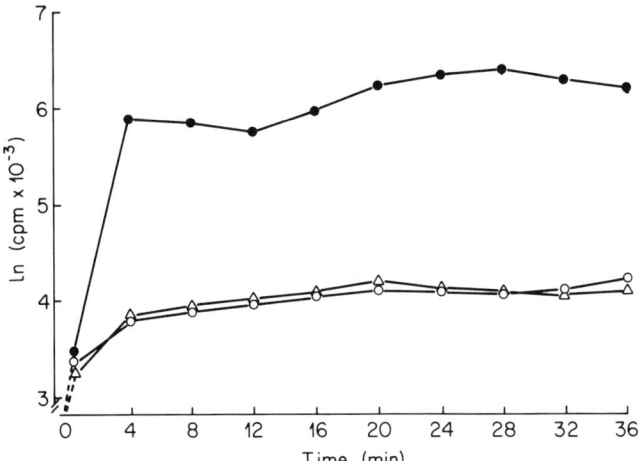

Fig. 2. REPRESENTATIVE CHEMILUMINESCENT RESPONSE OF A PURIFIED T-CELL PREPARATION TO MITOGEN STIMULATION, LUMINOL DEPENDENCY

Fig. 2. CL is generated by the addition of 2.0×10^6 nylon-wool or rosette-purified human T cells to a reaction mix containing 50–100 μg Con A, 100 μl luminol, and Hanks' balanced salt solution. Total volume of cellular reaction mix is 2.0 ml. Reaction proceeds in dark-adapted scintillation vials kept in a shaker bath at 37°C. CL is measured sequentially, in a liquid scintillation counter, set in the out of coincidence mode to facilitate optimum photon detection. Normal time-response profile (●) is compared to the luminol drift (no cells, 0) and a luminol-free cellular reaction (△). Stimulation with opsonized zymosan (not depicted) results in a CL response similar to that of the cell-free luminol drift. Failure in the normal CL response to opsonized zymosan stimulation and luminol-free lectin stimulation indicates the respective stimulant specificity and luminol dependency of this T-cell property.

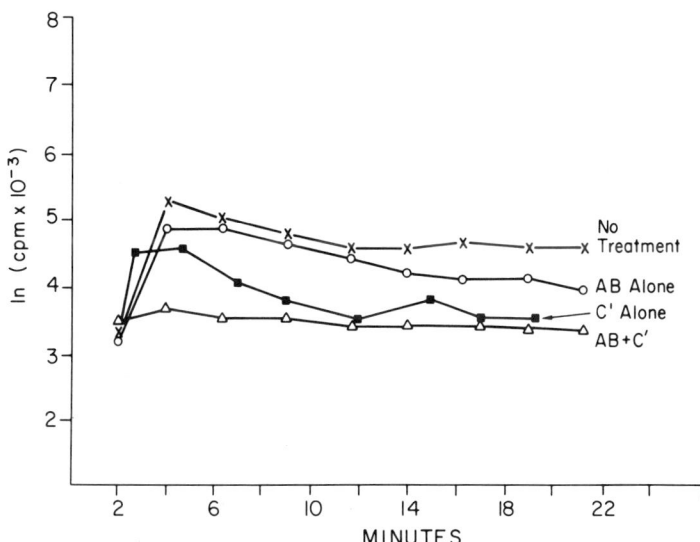

Fig. 3. EFFECT OF PAN-T MONOCLONAL ANTIBODY + COMPLEMENT TREATMENT ON MITOGEN STIMULATED CL RESPONSE

Fig. 3. Purity of T-cell chemiluminescence response to Con A (100 μg) stimulation is demonstrated by the significant abrogation of the control response (X) by pan-T monoclonal antibody treatment plus complement (△). Monoclonal antibody utilized was generated from a murine myeloma-Szeary cell hybridoma (B-7, Terasaki) and is specific for a ubiquitous T-cell membrane antigen. Complement source is Pelfreez rabbit complement. Complement is added in excess and may itself (■) be cytotoxic. Antibody, complement, and buffer controls are added in a stepwise fashion, followed by dark incubation at room temperature. Cells are then washed × 3 in RPMI medium, prior to lectin stimulation and CL measurement in the conventional fashion. Results depicted are the means of 2 separate experiments.

that noted in proliferation assays was demonstrated to increasing doses of Con A (50 to 200 μg). Wheat germ agglutinin (100 μg) was as effective as optimum stimulating doses of Con A in triggering T-cell CL. By contrast, pokeweed mitogen (PWM), at all doses tested, resulted in little change from spontaneous levels (data not shown). The inverse relationship between agglutinating potential and CL stimulating capacity was also found in rat thymocytes [7].

Luminol-dependent CL analysis was also performed in nylon-wool purified T-cell suspensions from patients with primary immune deficiency states. Two patients with SCID, but normal T-lymphocyte numbers, demonstrated profound deficiency in the Con A stimulated CL response. A similar defect was noted in the T cells of 3 patients with CGD. The utility of this probe in identify-

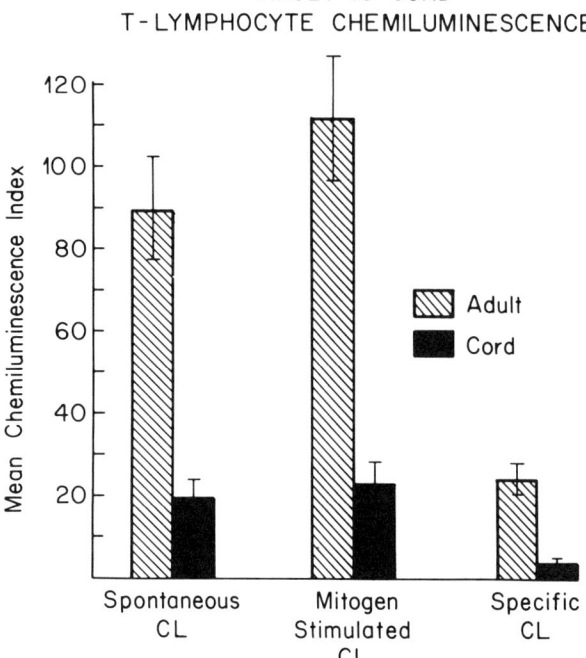

Fig. 4. Age-dependent rosette purified T-lymphocyte chemiluminescence, adult vs cord. Purified T-cell suspensions from 14 adult and 8 cord subjects were obtained by rosette purification of the mononuclear fraction. Stimulated CL is measured following the addition of 2.0×10^6 T cells to a reaction mix containing 100 µg Con A and 100 µl luminol. An appropriate volume of buffer is substituted for the lectin to determine spontaneous CL. Specific CL represents the difference between stimulated and spontaneous reactions. Results are expressed in terms of mean chemiluminescence index ± standard error (bars). The chemiluminescence index is calculated from the peak photon emission minus luminol drift divided by the spontaneous emission of a dark adapted blank. Stimulated CL, $p < 0.05$.

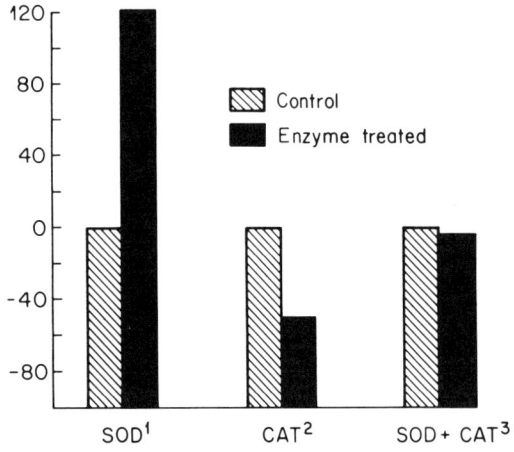

Reaction mix: cells (800 µl, 2.5×10^6/ml), luminol (100 µl), Con-A (50 µg), enzyme or HBSS control

[1] Superoxide dismutase, 7.5 µg
[2] Catalase, 100 µg
[3] Combined enzymatic conditioning; SOD 7.5 µg + CAT 100 µg

ing a global metabolic defect in CGD was then investigated in other CGD cells and membrane preparations.

Five CGD subjects, aged 8 months to 19 years, with X-linked CGD, 2 maternal carriers, and 5 controls were studied. Mean peak CL response of PMNs to opsonized zymosan stimulation was 30 ± 3 (CPM $\times 10^3$, mean ± SEM) in CGD compared to 197 ± 69 in adult controls. Mean stimulated CL of carrier PMNs was 56% of the control response. Luminol dependent, PMN membrane peak stimulated CL response was 66 ± 17 in CGD and 4041 ± 720 in controls.

Luminol dependent RBC CL to Con A stimulation revealed a mean peak stimulated response of 36 ± 5 in CGD compared to 84 ± 7 in controls (Fig. 6). Opsonized zymosan stimulation of RBCs resulted in mean peak responses of 40 ± 5 in CGD and 101 ± 8 in controls. Peak luminol dependent RBC membrane CL to Con A stimulation was 43 ± 5 in CGD compared to 89 ± 4 in adult controls. Peak luminol dependent RBC membrane CL to opsonized zymosan was 35 ± 5 in CGD and 49 ± 5 in normals (Table 1). Normal RBC and RBC membrane CL was demonstrated in 2 neutropenic subjects, eliminating the possible contribution of granulocytes in the control RBC response (Table 2).

Peak luminol dependent, Con A stimulated T lymphocyte CL was 33 ± 3 in CGD and 89 ± 1 in controls (Table 1).

Fig. 5. CL is generated by the addition of 2.0×10^6 rosette purified adult T cells to a reaction mix containing 50 µg Con A and 100 µl luminol solution. Superoxide dismutase (SOD) and catalase are reconstituted in Hanks' balanced salt solution (HBSS). SOD 7.5 µg, catalase 100 µg, or HBSS control are added to the luminol-lectin mix prior to the introduction of T cells. Percent change from the control responses in 2 separate experiments with SOD and catalase are depicted, as well as a single experiment with combined enzymatic conditioning.

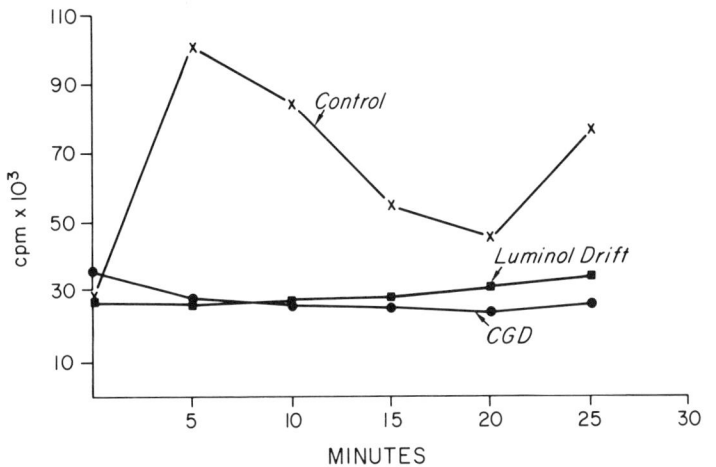

Fig. 6. Representative time-response curve of luminol dependent RBC chemiluminescence to 50 μg/ml Con A stimulation in CGD and control subjects. Low level photon emission requires amplification, using a luminescent compound, luminol. This pyridiazine compound (5-amino-2,3,-dihydro-1,4-phthalazinedione) is converted to an excited aminophthalate ion in the presence of minuscule amounts of oxidizing species, resulting in photon emission in the blue range (wavelength 425 nm).

RBCs are suspended to 2.5×10^6 ml; 800 μl of this suspension is added to a reaction mix containing 100 μl of luminol solution. Luminol drift over the sampling period is also depicted. Photon emission is expressed as CPM $\times 10^3$.

TABLE 1. Peak Cellular and Subcellular Chemiluminescence in CGD and Control Subjects: Mean Peak CPM $\times 10^3$

Cell Type or Fraction	Luminol	Stimulant	CGD Stimulated	CGD Index	Control Stimulated	Control Index	Difference CPM	Difference Index
PMN, intact		Ops Z	29.7 ± 3.2 (5)	1.0 ± 0.13	197.0 ± 69.0 (5)	5.5 ± 1.5	p < .02	p < .01
PMN, membr.	*	Ops Z	65.9 ± 16.9 (5)	2.3 ± 0.6	4041.2 ± 719.6 (5)	157.1 ± 26.8	p < .001	p < .001
RBC, intact	*	Con A	35.9 ± 5.1 (5)	1.1 ± 0.1	84.1 ± 7.1 (4)	3.3 ± 0.6	p < .001	p < .01
RBC, intact	*	Ops Z	40.3 ± 5.5 (5)	1.1 ± 0.2	101.4 ± 8.1 (4)	3.2 ± 0.3	p < .001	p < .001
RBC, membr.	*	Con A	42.9 ± 4.9 (3)	1.3 ± 0.2	89.2 ± 4.2 (3)	3.0 ± 0.3	p < .001	p < .02
RBC, membr.	*	Ops Z	35.0 ± 5.2 (3)	0.9 ± 0.2	49.3 ± 4.8 (3)	1.5 ± 0.3	p < .2	p < .20
T-Cell, intact	*	Con A	33.2 ± 3.4 (3)	1.4 ± 0.1	89.1 ± 1.5 (2)	4.2 ± 0.1	p < .001	p < .001

Mean peak stimulated CL responses in CPM $\times 10^3$ ± standard error of the mean for various cellular and subcellular purified suspensions from CGD and control subjects. Number in parentheses refers to the number of subjects studied. Luminol dependent reactions are expressed as a *chemiluminescence index*; peak emission minus luminol drift divided by the spontaneous emission of a dark adapted blank. Statistical comparisons utilize the *t test*.
Tabular display, responses of PMN, PMN membranes, RBC, RBC membranes and T lymphocytes to soluble and nonsoluble stimuli. Luminol dependent reactions are indicated. Soluble stimulus is Con A, final concentration 50 μg/ml. Particulate stimulus is zymosan (1 mg) opsonized with 100 μl serum.

TABLE 2. RBC Luminol Dependent Chemiluminescence in Neutropenic Subjects and Controls: Peak CPM $\times 10^3$

A)

Subject	ANC[a]	AMC[b]	Neutropenia Spontaneous	Stimulated	Index[c]	Control	Spontaneous	Stimulated	Index
1	522	288	91.3 (2.1)[d]	107.5	2.6	1	48.6 (1.0)[d]	108.8	2.6
2	174	1015	45.9 (1.3)[d]	53.3	1.6	2	42.8 (1.2)[d]	55.3	1.7
Mean				80.4	2.1			82.0	2.1

RBC Membrane Luminol Dependent Chemiluminescence in Neutropenic Subjects and Controls: Peak CPM $\times 10^3$

B)

Subject	ANC[a]	AMC[b]	Neutropenia Spontaneous	Stimulated	Index[c]	Control	Spontaneous	Stimulated	Index
1	522	288	69.5 (1.6)[d]	124.0	3.4	1	50.5 (1.0)[d]	75.2	1.7
2	174	1015	66.2 (2.0)[d]	94.5	3.0	2	73.6 (2.3)[d]	68.4	2.1
Mean				109.2	3.2			71.8	1.9

Luminol dependent CL of 2.0×10^6 A) intact RBC, and B) purified membrane preparations, derived from 5×10^8 whole RBC, to Con A (50 μg/ml final concentration) stimulation. 100 μl of luminol is added to the total 2.0 ml reaction mix. All luminol dependent reactions are expressed as a *chemiluminescence index (ci)*, peak response minus luminol drift divided by the emission of a dark-adapted blank. *Subject 1* is an 8-year-old female with aplastic anemia, status post-BMT, on azathioprine therapy. *Subject 2* is an 8-year-old male with Wiskott-Aldrich syndrome, complicated by severe leukopenia and thrombocytopenia. Control 2 is the 4-year-old normal male sib of *Subject 2*. Note to superscripts: [a] = absolute neutrophil count; [b] = absolute monocyte count; [c] = CI; [d] = CI of spontaneous reaction.

Statistical comparison of CGDs to normals demonstrated highly significant differences in the CL responses of PMNs, PMN membranes, RBCs, T lymphocytes, and Con A stimulated RBC membranes. The CL responses of CGD subjects and controls are summarized in Figure 7.

DISCUSSION

The main observations in this study include deficient T-cell lectin dependent cytotoxic responses in newborn cells, deficient mitogen-stimulated luminol dependent chemiluminescence in neonatal T cells, and deficient mitogen-stimulated luminol dependent CL in T cells, red cells, red cell membranes, and PMN membranes of patients with CGD. The poor CL response of control RBC membranes to opsonized zymosan stimulation suggests absence of a cell surface receptor or alteration of this receptor during membrane derivation.

The occurrence of deficient T-cell activity in newborns in an assay which utilizes lectin to bridge the effectors and targets, thus circumventing the necessity for presensitization and MHC identity between target and effector, suggests a defect in a late stage of lysis, rather than in the recognition or binding stages. This is compatible with the finding of deficient cell-mediated lympholysis (CML) in the face of a normal mixed leukocyte culture (MLC) response and enhanced cytotoxicity to the sensitizing cell rather than to 3rd party cells [8]. The normal neonatal CML, when lymphoblastoid lines are used as sensitizers and targets as reported by Rayfield et al [9], may result in a more susceptible target or a different mechanism for killing in the presence of Epstein-Barr virus in the target cell genome.

This T-effector defect might be paralleled by deficiency of activated T rosettes in the newborn [10], which Felsburg and Edelman have shown to be effector T cells [11]. It is of

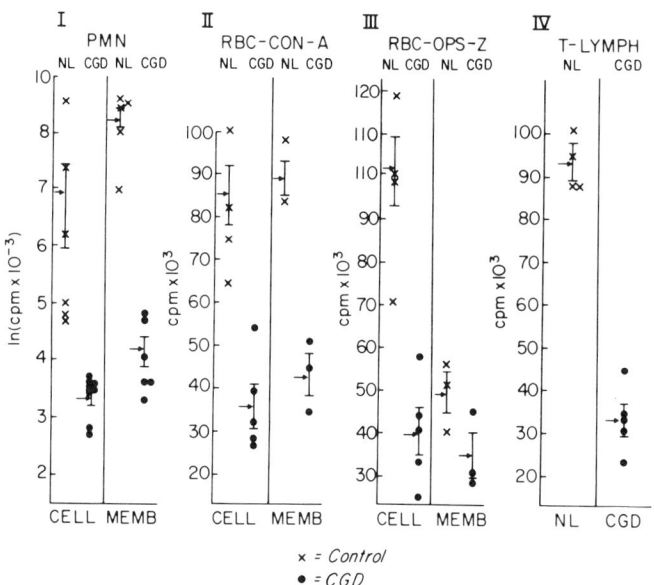

Fig. 7. Peak stimulated CL of whole cell and membrane preparations. Panel I = peak CL response, expressed as natural log CPM × 10^3, of $2.0 × 10^6$ plasma gel separated PMN and PMN membranes to opsonized zymosan stimulation. PMN membrane CL is luminol dependent. Panel II = peak CL response, expressed as CPM × 10^3, of $2.0 × 10^6$ RBC and RBC ghosts to Con A stimulation. RBC and RBC membrane CL are luminol dependent. Panel III = peak CL response, expressed as CPM × 10^3, of $2.0 × 10^6$ RBC and RBC ghosts to opsonized zymosan stimulation. RBC and RBC membrane CL are luminol dependent. Panel IV = peak CL response, expressed as CPM × 10^3, of $2.0 × 10^6$ nylon-wool purified T lymphocytes to Con A stimulation. T-cell CL is luminol dependent. Experiments are conducted on control (X) and CGD (●) cell and membrane suspensions, according to methods described in the text. Means and standard error of the mean are depicted by arrows and bars, respectively.

interest that suppressor activity is enhanced in newborn T cells, and that cytotoxic and suppressor activity in the adult may be derived from the same lymphocyte subset as that defined by the OKT8 monoclonal mouse antibody [12]. However, no consistent T-cell subclass abnormalities in newborn cord blood have been identified [13], suggesting that the diminished cytotoxicity and the enhanced suppression are functional defects rather than unusual subclass distribution.

The LDCC activity is not totally absent but, in many instances, is as deficient as in children with SCID. Most of these latter children have virtually no T-cell function as manifested by flat PHA responses and low numbers of T lymphocytes. Since newborns have near normal T-cell numbers, this defect is a late-maturing event, not dependent on T-cell proliferation.

Lymphocyte CL has heretofore been characterized only in rat thymocytes [7,14–16]. The studies reported here support CL as a property of human T lymphocytes following specific lectin stimulation. The artifactual contribution of contaminating granulocytes to this response is unlikely, based on the differential responsiveness of these cell types to opsonized yeast and successful abrogation of the detected CL by serologic removal of T cells. Antioxidant treatment suggests a prominent role for H_2O_2 in this CL. SOD may enhance photon emission by accelerated conversion of superoxide to H_2O_2 or its peroxidation of H_2O_2 to the hydroxyl radical [7,17]. The effect of SOD in human T-lymphocytes is opposite to the dramatic dissipation observed in granulocyte chemiluminescence. T lymphocytes possess high levels of intrinsic SOD activity, more than 3 times the activity noted in granulocytes [18]. The intracellular level of SOD among various hemic cell lines parallels the circulatory half-life of those cells, although a causal role in this longevity or other functional significance remains unproven.

Catalase participates in the conversion of H_2O_2 to water and oxygen. As in rodent thymocytes [15], dissipation of the chemiluminescence response by catalase implicates H_2O_2 as critical to this response. This is of particular interest since hydrogen peroxide has been detected during the interaction of effector cells with tumor targets [19]. Hydrogen peroxide treatment of tumor cells is directly cytolytic; catalase treatment abrogates this cytotoxic activity.

Correlation of the lymphocyte respiratory burst to conventional in vitro proliferation and cytotoxicity assays, though tantalizing in SCID, is not supported by the demonstration of a profound deficiency in CGD, where T-cell function is normal. The significance of defective T-lymphocyte CL in cord blood, SCID, and CGD, therefore, remains undefined.

Demonstration of deficient CL in nonphagocytic CGD cells may imply a global metabolic defect, functionally manifest only in those cells responsible for ingestion and elimination of foreign material. CL may, in fact, be a property of all respiring cells, requiring amplification for detection. Ongoing studies with cultured amniotic epithelial cells and skin fibroblasts in a similar luminol dependent system tend to support this hypothesis.

The availability of large numbers of RBCs for sampling and utility of this CL probe for localization of the abnormality should facilitate chromatographic delineation of the enzymatic defect in CGD. Furthermore, RBC CL may serve as a valuable screening test for CGD prenatally (using RBCs obtained by fetoscopy), as well as in infants and young children.

REFERENCES

1. Miller ME: The immunodeficiencies of immaturity. In Stiehm ER, Fulginiti VA (eds): "Immunologic Diseases in Infants and Children," 2nd Ed. Philadelphia: WB Saunders, 1980, pp 219–238.
2. Lubens RG, Gard SE, Soderberg-Warner M, Stiehm ER: Lectin-dependent and natural killer cytotoxic deficiencies in human newborns. Cell Immunol (In press).
3. Allen RC, Stjernholm RL, Steele RH: Evidence for the generation of an electronic excitation state in human polymorphonuclear leukocytes and its participation in bactericidal activity. Biochem Biophys Res Commun 47:679–684, 1972.
4. Trizio D, Cudkowicz G: Separation of T and B lymphocytes by nylon wool columns: Evaluation of efficacy by functional assays in vivo. J Immunol 113:1093–1097, 1974.
5. Julius MH, Simpson E, Herzenberg LA: A rapid method for separation of thymus-derived murine lymphocytes. Eur J Immunol 3:645–649, 1973.
6. Bonavida B, Robins A, Saxon A: Lectin-dependent cellular cytotoxicity in man. Transplantation 23:261–270, 1977.
7. Mockerjee BK, Ferber E, Ernst M, Sharon N, Fischer H: Chemiluminescence and immune cell activation: General features of the thymocyte chemiluminescent response to plant lectins. Immunol Commun 9:653–676, 1980.
8. Granberg C, Hirvonen T, Toivanen P: Cell-mediated lympholysis by human maternal and neonatal lymphocytes: Mother's reactivity against neonatal cells and vice versa. J Immunol 123:2563–2567, 1979.
9. Rayfield LS, Brent L, Rodeck CH: Development of cell-mediated lympholysis in human foetal blood lymphocytes. Clin Exp Immunol 42:561–570, 1980.
10. Davis RH, Galant SP: Non-immune rosette formation: A measure of the newborn infant's cellular immune response. J Pediatr 87:449–452, 1975.
11. Felsburg PJ, Edelman R: The active E-rosette test: A sensitive in vitro correlate for human delayed-type hypersensitivity. J Immunol 118:62–66, 1977.
12. Reinherz EL, Schlossman SF: Regulation of the immune response-inducer and suppressor T-lymphocyte subsets in human beings. N Engl J Med 303:370–373, 1980.
13. Hayward AR, Kurnick J: Newborn T cell suppression, early appearance, maintenance in culture and lack of growth factor suppression. J Immunol 126:50–53, 1981.
14. Hume DA, Wrogemann K, Ferber K, Kolbuch-Braddon ME, Taylor RM, Fischer H, Weidemann MJ: Concanavalin A induced chemiluminescence in rat thymus lymphocytes: Its origin and role in mitogenesis. Biochem J 198:661–667, 1981.
15. Wrogemann K, Weidemann MJ, Peskar BA, Staudinger H: Chemiluminescence and immune cell activation. I. Early activation of rat thymocytes can be monitored by chemiluminescence measurements. Eur J Immunol 8:745–752, 1978.
16. Wrogemann K, Weidemann MJ, Ketelson UP, Weherle H, Fischer H: Chemiluminescence and immune cell activation. II. Enhancement of Concanavalin A-induced chemiluminescence following in vitro pre-incubation of rat thymocyte: Dependency on macrophage-lymphocyte interaction. Eur J Immunol 10:36–40, 1980.
17. Trush MA: The generation of chemiluminescence by phagocytic cells. Methods Enzymol 57:462–494, 1978.
18. Kobayashi J, Okahata S, Sakano T, Tanaka K, Usui T: Superoxide dismutase activity of thymocytes. FEBS Lett 98:391–393, 1979.
19. Thorne KI, Svvennsen RJ, Franks D: Role of hydrogen peroxide in the cytotoxic reaction of T-lymphocytes. Clin Exp Immunol 39:486–495, 1980.

Protean Appearances of Immunodeficiencies: Syndromes and Inborn Errors Involving Other Systems Which Express Associated Primary Immunodeficiency

Walter H. Hitzig, MD

Department of Pediatrics, University of Zurich, 8032 Zurich, Switzerland

Proteus in Greek mythology was an old man of the sea who knew past, present, and future, but was unwilling to utter prophecies. He assumed different shapes to avoid being questioned . . . [1]. I was reminded of this figure when I tried to review the many more or less well-defined conditions and syndromes with immunodeficiency (ID) as one aspect. They either present a striking similarity but not identity with well-defined syndromes, or they can hardly be accommodated within our present classification without pressing and squeezing them.

I will review odd descriptions of diseases with ID, and then try to propose a possible classification.

SEVERE COMBINED IMMUNODEFICIENCY

Severe combined immunodeficiency (SCID) is close to my interest, and at the same time, also one of the most frequent IDs. The clinical features: severe polytopic infections involving all contact surfaces of the body and leading to septic invasions, and the broad spectrum of microorganisms—bacteria, viruses, protozoa and fungi—are quickly summarized. I want to stress the fact that this straightforward clinical approach is still correct and of considerable importance in daily practice. As specialists, however, we must look at heterogeneities and distinguishing features.

Deficiency of Adenosine Deaminase (ADA)

The first new finding to break up this uniform picture was ADA deficiency, discovered just 10 years ago [2]. Up to that time an early block in the normal development of immunocytes was assumed as the cause of SCID [3]—inactivity of an enzyme did not fit into this concept. In the meantime this apparent contradiction has been elucidated by biochemical studies of purine metabolism and of the consequences of ADA inactivity. We have learned that a normally developed immune system at birth is gradually destroyed by metabolic intoxication: ADA catalyzes the one-way reaction of adenosine to inosine, which can hardly be circumvented. Some of the metabolites accumulating behind the enzymatic block are toxic to the lymphoid system, in particular deoxyadenosine, adenosine-monophosphate, and others [4]. Therefore, the peripheral lymphatic system is unable to expand, but, on the contrary, is progressively damaged, particularly T cells, and later also the B-cell system. Early reports on heterogeneity of the SCID syndrome before ADA inactivity was discovered are now better understood [5].

Prenatal Infection

Certain viruses, in particular the rubella virus, can destroy the developing embryonic immune system, which will not recover. If the fetus survives, the newborn child presents combined immunodeficiency (CID) [6]. In this case, the thymus is dysplastic, however this is not due to an isolated developmental block but to the general interruption of organ formation.

Membrane Transport Disturbance

In a few patients with SCID the deficient in vitro response of lymphocytes to mitogens could be corrected by adding a calcium ionophore (A 23187) [7]. They seem to have a local membrane defect which, as a side effect, also manifests itself as failing immune response.

These examples demonstrate that the final result of both cellular and humoral immune deficiency can be due to numerous causes; in other words, hereditary SCID has a number of phenocopies (Fig. 1).

IMMUNODEFICIENCY AND SKELETAL CHANGES

A characteristic metaphyseal dysostosis (short-limbed dwarfism) has been found to be connected with CID [8]. When ADA deficiency was discovered, it showed that these patients were dysostotic. Apparently chondrocytes need ADA to proliferate just as immunocytes do. However, the story that ADA deficiency and dysostosis are closely linked is not so simple. As a result of careful

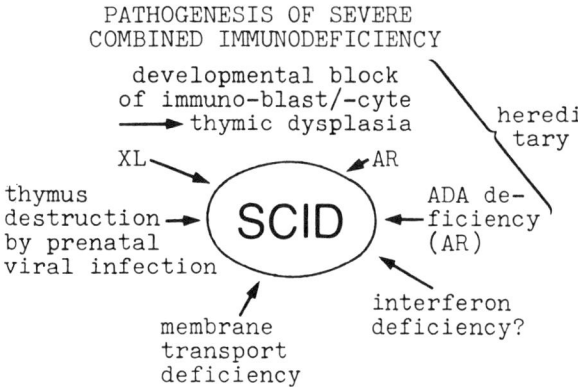

Fig. 1. SCID results from many different causes, partly hereditary, partly acquired (eg prenatal infection). Disturbed development of thymic precursor cells leads to thymic dysplasia, enzyme inactivity to metabolic intoxication and destruction.

TABLE 1. Immunodeficiency and Bone Disease

Metaphyseal dysostosis (short-limbed dwarfism) may or may not be linked with ID:
 dysostosis c̄ normal immune reactions
 dysostosis c̄ isolated humoral ID
 dysostosis c̄ isolated cellular ID
 dysostosis c̄ CID
  with normal ADA activity
  with deficient ADA activity
associated features: hair, skin, gut disease

investigations 5 combinations can be distinguished (Table 1).

Close association between dysostosis or chondropathy and growth of hair has also been described (Table 2). In cartilage hair hypoplasia (CHH) [9], sparse, very fine, brittle hair is an additional feature. Finally, malformation of the gut, in particular megacolon congenitum, is often seen. These patients again present different degrees of ID. Some of the originally described Amish patients [9] had severe infections and died early. Systematic investigation of similar patients in Finland has shown varying degrees of immunodeficiencies, but clinically they were not subjected to repeated infections [10]. Some of these patients were in the 3rd and 4th decade of their lives despite laboratory findings typical of CID. Variable expression of immunologic functions has also been described within the same family [11].

To understand this obvious contradiction, we must look for additional factors which are not measured by the tests used today.

Two probably unrelated conditions of ID and skin disease should be mentioned here: Griscelli et al [12] described a congenital hereditary partial albinism and immunodeficiency. The hair of these children was silver-grey from birth, and on microscopic examination it contained clusters of pigment. The children had recurrent infections of skin and mucosa with severe attacks of diarrhea which were usually accompanied by neutropenia and thrombocytopenia. The obvious clinical suspicion of Chédiak-Higashi syndrome could be excluded, since the granulocytes showed normal morphology (no giant inclusion bodies which are typical in Chédiak-Higashi syndrome) and also normal functions.

A second probably acquired association has been described by Ipp and Gelfand [13]: 3 of their patients with congenital or common variable agammaglobulinemia suddenly developed alopecia closely resembling alopecia areata, and in all 3 cases it rapidly proceeded to complete loss of all hair, including brows and eyelashes. A number of single cases with ID combined with dysmorphic signs like absent thumbs, flat facies, and anosmia [14] or Hallermann-Streiff syndrome and hypothyroidism [15], or Schwartz-Jampel syndrome [16] may be mentioned here, but cannot be classified at present.

To these ill-defined syndromes I have added (in brackets) enteropathic acrodermatitis (Table 2). Although its etiology is rather clear, it will be treated elsewhere in this volume.

DEFICIENT VITAMIN B_{12} TRANSPORT

Our patient with congenital lack of transcobalamin II (a vitamin B_{12} transporting protein) presented with agammaglobulinemia in addition to the typical signs of pernicious anemia [18]. With a daily supplement of pharmacologic doses of oral vitamin B_{12} (2 mg daily) his hematologic and immunologic parameters remain normal. However, a deficiency of phagocytosis could only be normalized by adding tetrahydrofolic acid (Leukovorin 10–30 mg once every 10–20 days) [19]. We have evidence that the lack of intracellular vitamin B_{12} and of tetrahydrofolic acid is the cause of all these disturbances, and that supplementation reverses all of them. The boy is now almost 10 years old, normal in weight, height,

TABLE 2. Immunodeficiency and Diseases of Bone, Skin, Hair, Gut

	Immunodeficiencies					
	Humoral	Cellular	Skin	Hair	Bone	Gut
CHH (Amish)	+	+	−	+	+	+/−
CHH (Finnish)	+/−	+/−	−	+	+	−
ID+albinism	+	+	+	+	−	−
ID+alopecia	+	−	+/−	+	−	−
(enteropathic acrodermatitis)	+	+	+	+	−	+

physical and mental development, and in every immunologic and hematologic parameter (antitetanus antibodies 16 IU/ml). As a matter of fact, he is very good in mathematics and speaks 3 languages! I am stressing this point, since lack of vitamin B_{12} is deleterious to the nervous system, and in all probability is particularly dangerous to the developing brain.

In addition, the study of this patient generated the elaboration of excellent and rapid methods to measure vitamin B_{12} and transcobalamin, and the detection of a transcobalamin II isoprotein system [20]. The heterozygote carriers can be identified, and present interesting disturbances: eg one man developed macrocytic anemia while modestly drinking alcohol, which disappeared without vitamin B_{12} or folic acid supplements in periods of alcohol abstinence.

CHRONIC MUCOCUTANEOUS CANDIDIASIS

Candida colonization is the rule in neonates. Growth on the surface of the oral mucosa at an early age is very frequent, but at a later age is a sign of bad health. Invasive and extensive *Candida* growth is always a sign of impaired resistance.

Different causes can lead to chronic mucocutaneous candidiasis (CMC) (Table 3). Overwhelming infection in the maternal vagina during birth may lead to an isolated immune tolerance against *Candida*. In CID and pancytopenia, *Candida* infections are frequent, but not specific. The syndrome of polyendocrinopathy involving thyroid, parathyroids, and adrenals may be complicated or preceded by CMC [21]. Deficiency of mannosidase in macrophages explains the pathogenesis in some patients, since these cells are unable to degrade mannosides, the cell wall constituents of *Candida* [22].

Finally, a favorable reaction to large doses of biotin has been found in a few patients with hereditary disease. It is associated with predominant T-cell and occasional B-cell deficiency [23]. Administration of biotin is followed by marked improvement of immune functions and clinical features of candidiasis. Another case report [24] relates similar clinical findings, but this patient responded only to pharmacologic doses of biotin, and therefore specific biotin malabsorption was assumed. The skin changes were similar to those in acrodermatitis enteropathica. At least 4 carboxylases require biotin as a coenzyme (Table 4). Patients with deficiencies of these enzymes also present with organic acidemia; they excrete excessive amounts of leucine, isoleucine, and valine.

INTRACTABLE DIARRHEA

Diarrhea is frequent and generally trivial in children. If large areas of the mucosa are destroyed, it may become intractable and be followed by malabsorption, as is usually the case in advanced stages of SCID. Intractable diarrhea with acrodermatitis as a clinical entity was described in 1936 [25]. It is a rare, often familial disease with chronic diarrhea leading to malabsorption, dermatitis, lesions of the mucocutaneous areas, and hair loss resulting in alopecia. It usually starts in the first year of life—the onset often coincides with weaning, and remission can be achieved by reintroducing human milk in the diet. By a chance observation the favorable action of diodoquin was discovered [26]. Subsequently, deficiency in serum zinc was found as a constant feature [27]. Peroral or parenteral application of large doses of zinc salts leads to prompt improvement. Recently ID was also recognized, with predominant involvement of T cells. Since it is normalized equally by zinc supplements, this diagnosis must not be missed.

TABLE 3. Chronic Mucocutaneous Candidiasis (CMC)

Etiology multiple and variegated:
  overwhelming infection of neonate → immune tolerance?
CID
pancytopenia, + cachexia
polyendocrinopathy c̄ CMC
mannosidase deficiency in macrophages (MØ)
biotin dependency

TABLE 4. Enzymes Requiring Biotin as Co-Enzyme

carboxylases and transcarboxylases
1) pyruvate carboxylase (PC)
2) propionyl-CoA-carboxylase (PCC)
3) β-methyl-crotonyl-CoA-carboxylase (MCC)
4) acetyl-CoA-carboxylase (ACC)
key functions in gluconeogenesis (1), amino acid catabolism (2,3), and lipogenesis (4). Biotin deficiency leads to multiple enzyme inactivities.

TABLE 5. Zinc-Requiring Enzymes

alcohol dehydrogenase
RNA polymerase
DNA polymerase
alkaline phosphatase
carboxypeptidase A
carboxypeptidase B
dipeptidase
aldolase
carbonic anhydrase
superoxide dismutase

Biochemically a great number of zinc-containing enzymes and metallo-proteins are known (Table 5), among others, polymerases for DNA and RNA which are indispensable for cell replication. In experimental zinc deprivation of animals, T-cell functions are impaired, in particular T-helper cells, but in more advanced stages B cells can also be depressed. These findings may explain the variety of clinical descriptions in man, including normal immune function, isolated T-cell deficiency, and CIDs. Thus, depending on the degree and duration of the zinc deprivation, immunocytes may function normally, or only T cells, or both T and B cells may be depressed [27].

HYPER IgE SYNDROME

The clinical features of this syndrome are quite characteristic [28]. One laboratory finding may be the key for the understanding of the entire pathogenesis [29]. Infectious episodes in these patients are generally due to *Staphylococcus aureus*, and these patients may not be able to make anti-staphylococcal antibodies of the IgG-class. Apparently IgE comes in as a substitute. The consequences are deleterious, particularly for areas of the body with many mast cells (Fig. 2). These are covered by the abundant IgE antibodies which, in the presence of staphylococcal antigens, trigger an allergic reaction. Histamine and similar bioactive substances paralyze the PMNs which therefore become unable to cope with the invading Staphylococci. This explains the overshooting inflammatory reactions predominantly in the face and the rapid formation of abscesses. Repeated episodes of this kind lead to hypertrophy of connective tissues producing a very characteristic coarse aspect of the face, particularly around

TABLE 6. Etiology of Immunodeficiency Syndromes

Basic Cause	Clinical Correlate
1. Malformation	DiGeorge syndrome
2. Chromosomal defects	Down syndrome + CID
	ataxia telangiectasia
3. Prenatal destruction of fetal immune system	
by infection	SCID
by graft-vs-host	SCID
4. Differentiation defects hemopoietic cells	
stem cell	reticular dysgenesis
myeloblast	cong. neutropenia
immunoblast	SCID: bare lymphocyte syndrome thymic dysplasia
lymphoblast	isol. T- or B-cell deficiency
lymphocyte	IgA deficiency
	IgG subgroup deficiency
	hyper IgM syndrome
	hyper IgE syndrome
5. Metabolic defects	
Enzyme deficiency	
e. purine m.:ADA	SCID, dysostosis
PNP	aplastic anemia, CID
e. requiring Zn	enteropath. acroderm.
e. requiring biotin	chron. candidiasis
mannosidase in MØ	chron. candidiasis
e. ion transport	SCID
e. glycosylation	a-γ-glob., AR
Plasma protein deficiency	
all immunoglobs.	a-γ-glob., XL
complement Clq	a-γ-glob., AR
transcobalamin 2	a-γ-glob., AR
single Ig class	IgA deficiency
Intracellular protein deficiency	
actomyosin in PMN	phagocyte failure
mallein in cilia	ciliary dyskinesia s.

Key: cong. = congenital; s. = syndrome; isol. = isolated; e. = enzyme; chron. = chronic; XL = X-linked; AR = autosomal recessive; m. = metabolism; MØ = macrophage; a-γ-glob. = agammaglobulinemia.

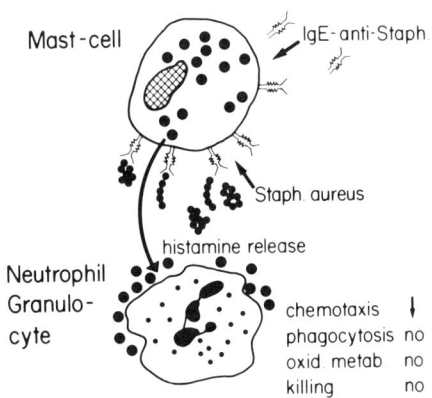

Fig. 2. Hyper IgE syndrome: lack of anti-staphylococcal IgG-antibodies leads to excessive synthesis of IgE with specificity anti-staph. They are mostly fixed on mast cells. Staphylococcal antigens trigger release of histamine, which in turn paralyzes granulocytes: Impaired chemotaxis renders their normal accumulation impossible and enables Staphylococci to proliferate rapidly.

eyes, nose, and mouth. For a systematic classification the disturbed antibody production against Staphylococci, namely failure of IgG and overshooting IgE response, might be the leading criteria.

CHROMOSOME FAILURES

Ataxia telangiectasia presents a complex clinical picture. A common denominator for all these signs is not yet clear. Chromosome fragility [30] which was found in all cases examined, might provide such a general base. It is due to impaired DNA-repair, and the consequences are chromosome breaks, losses, translocations, unusual sensitivity to ionizing radiation, and greatly increased frequency of malignancies. This deficiency is already present in the fetus, thus enabling the prenatal diagnosis of a sick child [31].

NEW CLASSIFICATION

An attempt is now being made to logically classify such odd diseases. It is meant to serve as a base for further discussion (Table 6). Two things should be stressed:

1) Purely developmental considerations cannot explain all the phenomena in the large host of clinical observations collected to date. Other pathogenetic principles must be equally considered.

2) Similar clinical syndromes can emerge as the result of different etiologic factors. Therefore, a clinical system must include different etiologies for one disease; on the other hand, in an etiologic classification the same clinical syndrome must reappear under different headings.

Finally we must admit that several distinct clinical diseases such as the Wiskott-Aldrich syndrome, or familial erythrocytophagic lymphohistiocytosis [32] are not yet satisfactorily classified, and many associations are poorly understood.

SUMMARY

Developmental defects interrupting the normal evolution of immunocytes can explain many of the congenital immunodeficiency syndromes. Observations accumulated during the last decade have, however, shown that this is not the only cause, and that many diseases have signs of immunodeficiency as an accompanying feature. Severe combined immunodeficiency (SCID) is a good example of the multiple etiology of similar clinical features—they are phenocopies of a well-delineated hereditary disease.

A number of recently described syndromes are reviewed, albeit an incomplete list. Metabolic disorders due to inactivity of enzymes may present characteristic ID. Some of them are explained by lack or increased need of co-enzymes (like biotin or zinc). In other syndromes, better understanding of the pathogenesis might pin down the primary failure to one single point, as shown in the hyper IgE syndrome. Other fundamental disturbances are located in the chromosome itself, eg decreased repair capacity, deletion, translocation.

An attempt is made to propose a general classification accommodating all etiologic factors known to date which lead to immunodeficiency. It is obvious that within this framework the same clinical syndrome may be repeated.

REFERENCES

1. Homer: Odyssey. Chapter 4, 364+.
2. Giblett ER, Anderson JE, Cohen F, Pollara B, Meuwissen HJ: Adenosine deaminase deficiency in two patients with severely impaired cellular immunity. Lancet 2:1067–1069, 1972.
3. Cooper MD, Faulk WP, Fudenberg HH, Good RA, Hitzig W, Kunkel HG, Roitt IM, Rosen FS, Seligmann M, Soothill JF, Wedgwood RJ: Primary immunodeficiency diseases in man. Clin Immunol Immunopathol 2:416–445, 1974.
4. Carson DA, Kaye J: Deoxyribonucleoside toxicity in adenosine deaminase and purine nucleoside phosphorylase deficiency: Implications for the development of new immunosuppressive agents. In "Enzyme Defects and Immune Dysfunction." Ciba Found Symposium 68. Amsterdam: Excerpta Medica, 1979, pp 115–144.
5. Hitzig WH, Landolt R, Müller G, Bodmer P: Heterogeneity of phenotypic expression in a family with Swiss-type agammaglobulinemia: Observations on the acquisition of agammaglobulinemia. J Pediatr 78:968, 1971.
6. Garcia AGP, Olinto F, Fortes TGO: Thymic hypoplasia due to congenital rubella. Arch Dis Child 49:181–185, 1974.
7. Kersey JH, Fish LA, Cox ST, August CS: Severe combined immunodeficiency with response to calcium ionophore: A possible membrane defect. Clin Immunol Immunopathol 7:62, 1977.
8. Gatti RA, Pomerance HH, Langer LO, Good RA: Hereditary lymphopenic agammaglobulinemia associated with a distinctive form of short-limbed dwarfism and ectodermal dysplasia. J Pediatr 75:675, 1969.
9. McKusick VA, Eldridge R, Hostetler JA, Ruangwit U, Egeland JA: Dwarfism in the Amish. II. Cartilage hair hypoplasia. Bull Johns Hopkins Hosp 116:285–326, 1965.
10. Ranki A, Perheentupa J, Andersson LC, Hayri P: In vitro T- and B-cell reactivity in cartilage hair hypoplasia. Clin Exp Immunol 32:352–360, 1978.
11. Wilson WG, Aylsworth AS, Folds JD, Whisnant JK: Cartilage hair hypoplasia (metaphyseal chondrodysplasia, type McKusick) with combined immune deficiency: Variable expression and development of immunologic functions in sibs. In Summitt RL, Bergsma D (eds): "Cell Surface Factors, Immune Deficiencies, Twin Studies." New York: Alan R Liss for The National Foundation-March of Dimes, BD:OAS XIV(6A):117–129, 1978.
12. Griscelli C, Durandy A, Guy-Grand D, Daguillard F, Herzog C, Prunieras M: A syndrome associating partial albinism and immunodeficiency. Am J Med 65:691–702, 1978.
13. Ipp MM, Gelfand EW: Antibody deficiency and alopecia. J Pediatr 89:728–731, 1976.
14. Shokeir MHK: Short stature, absent thumbs, flat facies, anosmia and combined immune deficiency (CID). Supra #11, pp 103–116.
15. Chandra RK, Joglekar S, Antonio Z: Deficiency of humoral immunity and hypoparathyroidism associated with the Hallermann–Streiff syndrome. J Pediatr 93:892–893, 1978.
16. Mollica F, Messina A, Stivala F, Pavone L: Immuno-deficiency in Schwartz-Jampel syndrome. Acta Paediatr Scand 68:133–135, 1979.
17. Dawson J, Hodgson HJF, Pepys MB, Peters TJ, Chadwick VS: Immunodeficiency, malabsorption and secretory diarrhea. A new syndrome. Am J Med 67:540–546, 1979.
18. Hitzig WH, Kenny AB: The role of vitamin B12 and its transport globulins in the production of antibodies. Clin Exp Immunol 20:105–111, 1975.
19. Seger R, Galle J, Wildfeuer A, Fràter M, Linnell J, Hitzig WH: Impaired functions of lymphocytes and granulocytes in transcobalamin II deficiency and their response to treatment. INSERM Symp 16:353–362, 1980.
20. Fràter-Schröder M, Hitzig WH, Bütler R: Studies on transcobalamin. Detection of TC II isoproteins in human serum. Blood 53:193–203, 1979.
21. Blizzard RM, Gibbs JH: Candidiasis: Studies pertaining to its association with endocrinopathies and pernicious anemia. Pediatrics 42:231–237, 1968.
22. Desnick RJ, Sharp HL, Grabowski GA, Brunning RD, Quie PG, Sung JH, Gorlin RJ, Ikonne JU: Mannosidosis: Clinical, morphologic, immunologic, and biochemical studies. Pediatr Res 10:985–996, 1976.
23. Cowan MJ, Wara DW, Packman S, Ammann AJ: Multiple biotin-dependent carboxylase deficiencies associated with defects in T-cell and B-cell immunity. Lancet 2:115–118, 1979.
24. Charles BM, Hosking G, Green A, Pollitt R, Bartlett K, Taitz LS: Biotin-responsive alopecia and developmental regression. Lancet 2:118–120, 1979.
25. Brandt T: Dermatitis in children with disturbances of the general condition and the absorption of food elements. Acta Derm Venereol (Stockh) 18:513–546, 1936.
26. Dillaha CJ, Lorincz AL, Asvik OR: Acrodermatitis enteropathica. Review of the literature and report of a case successfully treated with Diodoquin. JAMA 152:509–572, 1953.

27. Moynahan EJ: Acrodermatitis enteropathica: A lethal inherited human zinc-deficient disorder. Lancet 2:399–440, 1974.
28. Buckley RH: Immunoreconstitution. Pediatr Clin North Am 24:313, 1977.
29. Schopfer K, Baerlocher K, Price P, Krech U, Quie PG, Douglas SD: Staphylococcal IgE antibodies, hyperimmunoglobulinemia E and staphylococcus aureus infections. N Engl J Med 300:835–838, 1979.
30. Schmid W, Jerusalem F: Cytogenetic findings in two brothers with ataxia-telangiectasia (Louis Bar's syndrome). Acta Genet Med Gemellol (Roma) 45:49–52, 1952.
31. Ahmed FE, Setlow RB: Excision repair in ataxia telangiectasia, Fanconi's anemia, Cockayne syndrome, and Bloom's syndrome after treatment with ultraviolet radiation and N-acetoxy-2-acetylaminofluorene. Biochim Biophys Acta 521:805–817, 1978.
32. Ladisch S, Holiman B, Poplack DG, Blaese RM: Immunodeficiency in familial erythrophagocytic lymphohistiocytosis. Lancet 1:581–583, 1978.

Hereditary Orotic Aciduria: A Defect of Pyrimidine Metabolism With Cellular Immunodeficiency

Robert Girot, MD, Anne Durandy, MD, Jean-Louis Perignon, MD, and Claude Griscelli, MD

Laboratoire Central d'Hématologie et d'Immunologie Necker, Paris (R.G.); Unité d'Immunologie et d'Hématologie Pédiatriques, Département de Pédiatrie, INSERM U 132, Hôpital des Enfants Malades, 75730 Paris Cedex 15 (A.D., C.G.); Laboratoire de Biochimie, Faculté de Médecine Necker, Paris (J.-L.P.), France

Hereditary orotic aciduria is a rare inborn error of pyrimidine metabolism associated with autosomal recessive inheritance [1]. The disease is characterized usually by retarded growth and development, anemia, and megaloblastic bone marrow. To date, only 9 patients with this disease have been reported. The enzymatic defect involves 2 sequential enzymes of de novo pyrimidine biosynthesis—orotate phosphoribosyltransferase (OPRT, EC 2.4.2.10) and orotidine 5′phosphate decarboxylase (ODC, EC 4.1.1.23) (type I) or, as described by Fox et al [2], only ODC (type II). Because severe infections were observed in some patients with the disease (2 of them died from varicella [3] and meningitis [4]), an immunodeficiency has been suspected but has never been demonstrated [1]. We report on 2 sibs with hereditary orotic aciduria associated with an immunodeficiency syndrome characterized by impaired cellular immunity but with normal humoral immunity. This observation widens the spectrum of inborn errors of metabolism associated with immunodeficiency disease.

MATERIALS AND METHODS

Biochemical Studies

Urinary orotic acid was determined by the method described [5], and orotidine was identified by anion exchange chromatography. The radioisotopic assays of enzymatic activities have been previously described [2, 6]; PRPP synthetase was assayed by the method of Snyder et al [7].

Immunologic Evaluation

Peripheral blood lymphocytes were isolated on Ficoll-Hypaque gradient. T lymphocytes were evaluated by sheep erythrocyte rosetting (E-RFC) and/or by monoclonal antibodies OKT3 (T lymphocytes), OKT4 (T helper) and OKT8 (T-suppressor cytotoxic) (Ortho Pharm., Raritan NJ) in an indirect immunofluorescence assay [8]. B lymphocytes were evaluated by membrane immunofluorescence studies (SIg) using a rhodamine-labeled F(ab)'2 fragment of IgG against human F(ab)IgG (Nordic Lab., Tilburg, Nederland). In vitro T/B cooperation studies were performed according to Wu et al [9]: briefly, immunoglobulin-containing cells revealed by immunofluorescence using anti-μ, α, and γ-chain antisera (Meloy Lab., Springfield Va) were counted at the end of a 7-day PWM-stimulated leukocyte culture. In some experiments, helper effect of T lymphocytes (isolated by E-rosetting) was tested on control B lymphocytes (E$^-$ populations).

CASE REPORTS

Patient Y.S. was a Senegalese male born in 1971. His parents were first cousins. During the first years of life, he suffered from recurrent diarrhea, stomatitis, and anemia not cured by iron, folic acid, or vitamin B_{12}. At age 7, hematologic data showed an anemia: hemoglobin 7.9 gm/dl; erythrocytes 3.46 M/mm^3, mean corpuscular volume 76 fl, reticulocytes 1%, white blood cells 9,300/mm^3, differential count: 75% PMN, 22% lymphocytes, 3% monocytes, platelets 325,000/mm^3. Bone marrow smears contained megaloblastic red cells, myeloid precursors, and large megakaryocytes. Plasma iron, serum vitamin B_{12}, serum folic acid, and serum and urinary amino acids were normal. Urinary orotic acid excretion was 836 mg/day (normal value < 5), and no orotidine was detected. Microscopic examination of the urine sediment revealed typical crystals. OPRT and ODC activities in red blood cells were both very low as in type I orotic aciduria (Table 1). Enzyme activity was below 1% in separated leukocytes (Ficoll-Hypaque).

Uridine (75 mg then 150 mg/kg/day) was first given orally for 9 weeks with a poor clinical and biologic response. Uridine therapy was started again orally and intramuscularly for 7 months using the dosage of 75 mg then 150 mg/kg/day. This therapy was marked by a stable level of hemoglobin (10 gm/dl) without blood transfusion. During therapy, mean urinary orotic acid excretion was 500 mg/day (380–600 mg/day). However, diarrhea became severe with malabsorption. *Candida albicans* was isolated in duodenal aspirate (5.2 × 10^4 organisms/ml). In

TABLE 1. Hereditary Orotic Aciduria: Enzyme Studies

Enzyme	Patient Y.S.	Patient R.S.	Normal Values* (nmol/min/ml RBC)
OPRT + ODC**	< 0.03	< 0.03	1.35 ± 0.43
OPRT	< 0.02	< 0.02	1.7 ± 0.99
ODC	0.005	0.004	4.2 ± 2.2
ADA	895.0	790.0	494.0 ± 60
PNP	42,820.0	51,700.0	47,500.0 ± 6,200
Adenosine kinase	116.9	86.2	104.5 ± 18.8
P-ribosyl PP synthetase	42.0	54.8	48.9 ± 8.4
Adenine phosphoribosyltransferase	150.1	151.1	147.9 ± 26.9
Hypoxanthine phosphoribosyltransferase	825.0	811.0	555.0 ± 110
Guanine phosphoribosyltransferase	1,045.0	1,145.0	910.0 ± 220
5' Pyrimidine nucleotidase	66.9	37.7	56.3 ± 11.8

Enzymatic activities in the red blood cells of the patients.
*Mean ± SD [See references 4, 6].
**OPRT + ODC activity: synthesis of uridine monophosphate from orotate (phosphoribosyltransferase followed by decarboxylation).

July 1979, the patient died from meningitis.

Patient R.S., born in 1979, is the sister of Y.S. She was referred at the age of 3 months because of pallor and transient diarrhea. Diagnosis of type I orotic aciduria was made on the following data: anemia and megaloblastic bone marrow precursors; urinary orotic acid excretion 150 mg/day (bw 4 kg), no urinary orotidine, and very low OPRT and ODC activities in red blood cells (Table 1). Oral uridine therapy was started in March 1980 at a dose of 20 mg/kg/day for one year, then 50 mg/kg/day until the time of reporting. We observed a reticulocyte peak, stable hemoglobin level (10 gm/dl) for 2 years without any blood transfusion and the disappearance of megaloblastic changes on bone marrow. Urinary orotic acid excretion performed in January 1981 and January 1982 was 220 (bw 9 kg) and 260 mg/day (bw 11.5 kg). Since beginning uridine therapy, the patient's general health improved with weight gain and increased strength. No peculiar susceptibility to infections was noted.

The parents were found heterozygous for hereditary orotic aciduria (OPRT-ODC activities 0.28 and 0.63 nmol/min/ml RBC in father and mother, respectively, as compared with normal values: 1.35 ± 0.43). The 2 patients' sisters were normal (1.37 and 3.76). Urinary orotic acid excretion was slightly increased in the parents (father: 8.64 mg/day; mother: 11.55 mg/day).

IMMUNOLOGIC STUDIES (Table 2)

Immunologic investigations of *Patient Y.S.* were performed before uridine therapy. Serum Ig levels were increased for the 3 main classes, and antibody formation to blood substances and vaccinal antigens were normal. Delayed skin reactivity to antigens was negative. A severe lymphopenia was observed with 10% E-RFC and an increased percentage of B cells (32 and 17%). Proliferative responses to mitogens were lower than control range. Patient's leukocytes normally proliferated in the presence of allogeneic cells (MLR) but cell-mediated lymphocytolysis (CML) was depressed. Generation of plasma cells in the PWM system was severely impaired and was not reversed by in vitro addition of uridine (10^{-3} and 10^{-5} M). Immunologic study was also performed while the patient received uridine therapy. No modifications were observed except for the MLR which was not normal.

Patient R.S. was tested before uridine therapy. Serum Ig levels were normal for age, and antibody formation to blood substances and vaccinal antigens were within normal values. Blood lymphocyte count was normal and E-RFC were mildly decreased (40%). Skin tests for PPD were negative although she was inoculated with the BCG at birth. Skin test for PHA (2 µg) was positive, and in vitro mitogenic responses were normal for mitogens. MLR was normal, but CML was repeatedly impaired. Generation of plasma cells in the PWM system was negative even after in vitro addition of uridine (10^{-3} to 10^{-5} M). Three months after starting uridine at 50 mg/kg/day immunologic studies showed even more pronounced abnormalities. E-RFC were very low (15%) as well as the number of T cells detected by monoclonal antibodies. T-cell subsets were both very decreased: 1% OKT4-positive cells and 5% OKT8-positive cells. PHA-induced proliferation and MLR were impaired, and generation of plasma cells in PWM-stimulated culture was still absent. Seven months later (10 months after uridine therapy), E-RFC were 35% and OKT3-positive cells 32%, with 12% OKT4 and 14% OKT8-positive cells. PHA-induced proliferation was normal, but generation of plasma cells in PWM-stimulated cultures was still severely impaired.

DISCUSSION

We report 2 sibs with clinical, hematologic and biochemical findings consistent with the diagnosis of type I hereditary orotic aciduria. In both patients, humoral immunity was normal and serum Ig levels were even increased in the older one. Immunologic abnormalities observed involved only CMI and were characterized in vivo by an absence of

TABLE 2. Hereditary Orotic Aciduria: Immunologic Studies

	Patient Y.S.	Patient R.S. Mar. '80 Before Therapy	Patient R.S. Jan. '82 Under Uridine Therapy	Normal Values
Total lymphocytes/mm^3	300–2,100	3,000	4,000	2,000
Serum immunoglobulin				
IgG gm/liter	20.0	8.1	11.2	9.2–14.8
IgA gm/liter	3.8	0.74	1.1	1.4–2.6
IgM gm/liter	5.6	0.69	0.85	0.9–1.9
B-cell lymphocytes SIg%	17–32	13.0	29.0	5–15
E-RFC%	10–20	15.0	40.0	65–76
T-cell subset				
OKT3%	NT	13.0	32.0	68–86
OKT4%	NT	1.0	12.0	46–51
OKT8%	NT	5.0	14.0	27–36
Skin reactivity	0*	PPD−PHA+		
Proliferation response to				
PHA cpm × 10^{-3}	3 ± 05–45 ± 3.0	97 ± 9.0	78 ± 6	60–150
PWM cpm × 10^{-3}	1 ± 0.2–22 ± 4.0	9 ± 0.5	NT	10–45
Con A cpm × 10^{-3}	2 ± 04–46 ± 6.0	18 ± 2.1	NT	25–110
Unstimulated cultures cpm × 10^{-3}	0.8 ± 0.3–1 ± 0.2	2.6 ± 0.4	3 ± 1.2	0.5 ± 2.0
MLR**				
Unstimulated P leukocytes cmp × 10^{-3}	1.1 ± 0.4–14 ± 0.3	3 ± 1	NT	0.5–3
P + Rx C$_1$ leukocytes cpm × 10^{-3}	15 ± 5.0–18 ± 5.0	33 ± 6	NT	10–45
C$_2$ + Rx C$_1$ leukocytes cpm × 10^{-3}	34 ± 4.0–38 ± 4.0	35 ± 5	NT	10–40
CML†	NT		NT	
PWM-induced plasma cells %	0	0	0	50–500

*PPD, candidin and streptococcal antigens.
**One way MLR study compared responses of patients (P) and control (C$_2$) leukocytes stimulated with the same irradiated (Rx 3,000 rads) unrelated control (C$_1$) leukocytes.
†CML generated in MLR.
NT = Not tested.

delayed type skin reactivity to antigens and in vitro by a decreased number of blood T cells and subsets. T-cell functions, including mitogen- or antigen-induced proliferations and CML were impaired while MLR was normal or slightly decreased. An absence of generation of plasma cells in the PWM system was repeatedly found.

As previously described in hereditary orotic aciduria, uridine therapy in our patients provoked an improvement of hematologic status, but immunologic abnormalities were only partially improved in the younger patient.

Immunodeficiency has previously been suspected in hereditary orotic aciduria [1]. Suggestions of an immunodeficiency in the disease are the death of 2 patients secondary to varicella in the report by Huguley et al [3] and, similar to Y.S., meningitis in the patient reported by Fox et al [2]. Although a lymphopenia was described in almost all reported patients [3, 4, 10, 11], specific T- and B-cell functions have not been studied, to our knowledge. Our observation strongly suggests a direct relationship between enzymatic defect and the documented T-cell immunodeficiency. Accumulation of pyrimidine nucleotide precursors may be specifically toxic to T rather than B lymphocytes. This observation represents a situation similar to other immunodeficiencies associated with inborn errors of purine metabolism, ADA, or PNP deficiency. There are similarities between the immunologic abnormalities documented in our patients and those described in patients with PNP deficiency, ie the delayed onset of the susceptibility to infections and the selective impairment of T-cell function with apparently intact humoral immunity.

REFERENCES

1. Kelley WN, Smith LH: Hereditary orotic aciduria. In Stanbury JB, Wyngaarden JB, Fredrickson DS (eds): "The Metabolic Basis of Inherited Disease." New York: McGraw-Hill, 1978, pp 1045–1071.
2. Fox RM, Wood MH, Royse-Smith D, O'Sullivan WJ: Hereditary orotic aciduria: Types I and II. Am J Med 55:791–798, 1973.
3. Huguley CM, Bain JA, Rivers SL, Scoggins RB: Refractory megaloblastic anemia associated with excretion of orotic acid. Blood 14:615–634, 1959.
4. Fox RM, O'Sullivan WJ, Firkin BG: Orotic aciduria. Differing enzyme patterns. Am J Med 47:332–336, 1969.
5. Rosenbloom FM, Seegmiller JE: An enzymatic spectrophotometric method for determination of orotic acid. J Lab Clin Med 63:492–500, 1964.
6. Hamet M, Bonissol C, Cartier P, Houllier AM, Kona P: Enzymatic activities of purine and pyrimidine metabolism in nine mycoplasma species contaminating cell cultures. Clin Chim Acta 103:15–22, 1980.
7. Synder FF, Mendelsohn J, Seegmiller JE: Adenosine metabolism in phytohemagglutinin-stimulated human lymphocytes. J Clin Invest 58:654–666, 1976.
8. Reinhertz EL, Kung PC, Golstein G, Schlossman SF: Further characterization of the human inducer T cell subset defined by monoclonal antibody. J Immu-

nol 123:2894–2896, 1979.
9. Wu LY, Lawton AR, Cooper MD: Differentiation capacity of cultured B lymphocyte from immunodeficient patient. J Clin Invest 52:3180–3189, 1973.
10. Tubergen DG, Krooth RS, Heyn RM: Hereditary orotic aciduria with normal growth and development. Am J Dis Child 118:864–870, 1969.
11. Wada Y, Nishimura Y, Tanabu M, Yoshimura Y, Iinuma K, Yoshida T, Arakawa T: Hypouricemic, mentally retarded infant with a defect of 5-phosphoribosyl-1-pyrophosphate synthetase of erythrocytes. Tohoku J Exp Med 113:149–157, 1974.

Heterogeneity of Immunologic and Enzymatic Deficiencies in the Familial Reticuloendotheliosis Syndrome

Alain Fischer, MD, Françoise Ledeist, MD, Anne Durandy, MD, Michèle Hamet, PhD, Frank Arnaud-Battandier, MD, and Claude Griscelli, MD

Unité d'Immunologie et d'Hématologie Pédiatriques, Département de Pédiatrie (A.F., F.L., A.D., M.H., C.G.), and Unité de Gastro-Enterologie et Nutrition Pédiatriques (F.A.-B.), Département de Pédiatrie, INSERM U 132, Hôpital Necker-Enfants Malades, 75730 Paris Cedex 15, France

In 1965, Omen described an entity called familial reticuloendotheliosis [1]. A CID has been described by Ochs et al [2] in this syndrome and was recently shown to be associated with a defect of ecto 5'nucleotidase activity in lymphocytes [3]. The syndrome is characterized by a diffuse skin exudative erythroderma, hepatosplenomegaly, lymph nodes enlargement, severe repeated infections, diarrhea, and failure to thrive. Blood eosinophil counts are increased, skin biopsy shows an infiltration of histiocytic cells, lymphocytes and eosinophil. Lymph node and spleen histology is marked by T- and B-cell depletion replaced by a diffuse histiocyte-like cell infiltration. A profound thymic hypoplasia without any cell infiltration is also described [1–5]. This syndrome is accompanied by a severe functional deficiency in T- as well as in B-cell functions, although the blood T-cell number is usually subnormal. The lymphocytic ecto 5'nucleotidase deficiency is suggestive of a T-cell immaturity since the enzyme activity was found normal in T-cell blasts [3].

All patients reported in the literature died within the first year of life because of malnutrition and infections despite intensive care with antibiotics and various cytotoxic drugs [1–4, 6].

Several questions remain in this rare and peculiar syndrome: 1) The nature of the cell(s) infiltrating skin, lymph nodes, spleen, and other organs. 2) The causal relationship between the diffuse cell infiltration and the CID. 3) The heterogeneity of the syndrome, and 4) the therapeutic approach of this disorder.

We report 4 observations (Table 1) meeting the previously enumerated criteria for diagnosis to emphasize some aspects illustrating the discussion on the pathogenesis of this syndrome.

In *Patient 1*, born in germ-free condition and maintained in a sterile environment in a Trexler's isolator, we observed the onset of skin involvement at day 2 of life (hair loss, erythroderma). In this patient, all clinical manifestations developed successively while she remained germ-free except for diarrhea that only appeared following bacterial contamination. This unique observation indicates that most symptoms of the disease may occur independently of exogenous antigen challenge. In a second patient (#4), the efficiency of a treatment associating parenteral renutrition, cutaneous and general steroid administration, and VP 16-213 (150 mg/m^2/day IV for 3 days, then one injection every 3 weeks) was observed. While in previous patients mentioned in the literature, elementary enteral nutrition, steroids, associated with cyclophosphamide, vinblastine, vincristine or methotrexate constantly failed, a progressive improvement occurred in our patient. Organomegaly and bronchopulmonary symptoms rapidly disappeared and, progressively, also the diarrhea. Growth rate was restored with a high caloric input. Enteral nutrition was progressively substituted successfully to parenteral nutrition. After 8 months of treatment, the patient exhibits only occasional skin manifestations, and a mild eosinophilia ($\simeq 1000/m^2$). However, some degree of ID persisted. In vitro T-cell proliferation and PHA skin tests were significantly improved, but an antibody production deficiency and a relative decrease in T-lymphocyte proportion (30–40% of blood lymphocytes) are observed. One should stress that this patient, who displayed all the clinical and histologic criteria of the disease, was different by having a partially distinct CID (Table 1) since there was no hyper IgE, no deficiency of IgM, IgG, and IgA and decrease in the T-cell number. Finally, no lymphocyte ecto 5'nucleotidase deficiency was found.

This observation deserves the following comments:

Immunologic and Enzymatic Heterogeneity

For similar clinical and histologic pictures, distinct immunologic and enzymatic features could be seen. For instance, in a case reported by Cohen et al [3], the presence of blood B lymphocytes is mentioned. In patients described by Cederbaum et al [5] serum Ig levels were either increased or low. Similar variations were observed in our patients. We also observed variation of T-cell number. However, the functional deficiency appears relatively constant in all cases (mitogen and antigen-induced cell proliferation, as well as T-cell helper function and antibody production which are defective).

In our series, the ecto 5'nucleotidase deficiency could not be considered as a constant feature of the syndrome. It was found only in 3 of our 4 patients, and it is striking to note that no enzyme deficiency was found in the patient with normal number of blood B lymphocytes (*Patient 4*). Since it is well known that the enzyme activity is much higher in B- than in T-lymphocytes, it is plausible that the ecto 5'nucleotidase deficiency parallels the B-cell deficiency. However, in Cohen's patient, purified T cells appeared to be deficient in the enzyme. On the contrary, *Patient 4*'s T cell did exhibit a normal ecto 5'nucleotidase activity. These data raise the question of the heterogeneity of the expression of the ecto 5'nucleotidase activity in this syndrome.

NATURE OF INFILTRATING CELLS AND THERAPEUTIC APPROACH

The fact that a cytotoxic therapy associated with renutrition can largely improve the disease could suggest the important role of the visceral cell infiltration. The clue to distinguish a primary from a secondary immune deficiency would be the observation of the complete correction of the immune functions in this unique patient. The follow-up is, however, too short as yet for a definitive conclusion.

Since VP 16-213 has been shown to have a preferential, although not specific, cytotoxic effect for the macrophage lineage [8], the satisfying results add a fragile argument for the histiocytic nature of the invading cell. For Omen [1], Barth et al [2], Cederbaum et al [5], there was no doubt of the histiocytic nature but, recently, Wyss et al [7] have suggested that cells infiltrating lymph nodes in their patient could be immature T cells since they had the following characteristics: E+, phosphatase acid +,

TABLE 1. Familial Reticuloendotheliosis

Patients	1	2	3	4
Age of onset	Day 2	6 weeks	3 weeks	2 weeks
Skin involvement (clinical + histology)	+	+	+	+
Hepatosplenomegaly	+	+	+	+
Lymph node enlargement	+	+	+	+
Chronic diarrhea	+	+	+	+
Failure to thrive	+	+	+	+
Infections	+	+	+	+
Eosinophilia	+	+	+	+
T cell	N	N	↗	↘
B cell	↘	↘	↘	↗
T-cell proliferation	↘	↘	↘	↘
Serum IgG, M, A	↘	↘	↘	↗
Serum IgE	↗	↗	↗	↘
Antibody production	↘	↘	↘	↘
Ecto 5' nucleotidase activity	↘	↘	↘	N
Treatment	steroids	steroids Vincristine	steroids Vincristine Cyclophosphamide	steroids VP 16-213 parenteral nutrition
Outcome	death (9 months)	death (12 months)	death (15 months)	alive (11 months old)

absence of lysosomes. However, in 3 of our patients (*1,2,* and *4*), lymph nodes were carefully studied by C. Nezelof, who found that infiltrating cells were phosphatase acid +, non-specific acidic esterases +, and contained granulations suggesting a rather histiocytic nature. However, the debate remains open in absence of the use of well-defined monoclonal antibodies.

EXCESSIVE IMMUNE SUPPRESSION

We found in 3 out of 3 patients studied (including the patient described by Wyss et al [7]) a spontaneous T-cell mediated suppression of in vitro polyclonal Ig production (in the pokeweed system) and mitogen-induced cell proliferation. Furthermore, an excessive monocyte suppression was shown in 2 patients, together with an excess of prostaglandin E2 production by blood adherent cells [9] as compared to age-matched controls. The significance

and the in vivo relevance of these data remain unknown but are compatible, at least in some cases, with a possible macrophage proliferation and activation inducing a secondary T and B immunodeficiency. This working hypothesis should be added to that of a primary CID mentioned above.

REFERENCES

1. Omen GS: Familial reticuloendotheliosis, a new syndrome. N Engl J Med 273:427, 1965.
2. Ochs HD, Davis SD, Mickelson E, Lerner KG, Wedgwood RJ: Combined immunodeficiency and reticuloendotheliosis with eosinophilia. J Pediatr 85:463, 1974.
3. Cohen A, Mansour H, Dosch M, Gelfand EW: Association of a lymphocyte purine enzyme deficiency (5'nucleotidase) with combined immunodeficiency. Clin Immunol Immunopathol 15:245, 1980.
4. Barth RF, Vergara GC, Khurana SK, Lowman JT: Rapidly fatal familial histiocytosis associated with eosinophilia and primary immunological deficiency. Lancet 2:503, 1972.
5. Cederbaum SD, Niwayama G, Stiehm ER, Neerhout RC, Ammann AJ, Berman W:

Combined immunodeficiency presenting as the Letterer-Siwe syndrome. J Pediatr 85:466, 1974.
6. Edwards NL, Gelfand EW, Burk L, Dasch HM, Fox IH: Distribution of 5'-nucleotidase in human lymphoid tissues. Proc Natl Acad Sci USA 76:3474, 1979.
7. Wyss M, Fliedner V, Jacot-Descombes E, Jeannet M, Despont JP, Kapanci Y, Cox JN: A lymphoproliferative syndrome, "cutaneous dystrophy," and combined immune deficiency with lack of helper T-cell factor. Clin Immunol Immunopathol 23:34, 1982.
8. Ambruso DR, Hays T, Zwartjes WJ, Tubergen DG, Favara BE: Successful treatment of lymphohistiocytic reticulosis with phagocytosis with Epipodophyllotoxin VP 16-213. Cancer 45:2516, 1980.
9. Fischer A, Durandy A, Mamas S, McCall E, Dray F, Griscelli C: Lack of prostaglandin E2-mediated monocyte suppressive activity in newborn and mothers. Clin Exp Immunol 49:377, 1982.

X-Linked Lymphoproliferative Syndrome: Abnormal Antibody Responses to Bacteriophage ΦX 174*

Hans D. Ochs, MD, John L. Sullivan, MD, Ralph J. Wedgwood, MD, Janet K. Seeley, PhD, Kiyoshi Sakamoto, MD, and David T. Purtilo, MD

Department of Pediatrics, University of Washington, Seattle, WA 98195 (H.D.O., R.J.W.), University of Massachusetts Medical Center, Worcester, MA 01605 (J.L.S.), Department of Pediatrics, Health Center, The University of Connecticut, Farmington, CT 06032 (J.K.S.), and Department of Pathology and Laboratory Medicine, University of Nebraska Medical Center, Omaha, NE 68105 (K.S., D.T.P.)

Epstein-Barr virus (EBV) has been shown to infect B cells [1], cause polyclonal B-cell activation [2], and induce T-lymphocyte suppressor cells that inhibit polyclonal B-cell activation [3–5]. This ubiquitous virus may induce "silent" seroconversion in children [6], cause infectious mononucleosis in young adults, and has been associated with Burkitt lymphoma and nasopharyngeal carcinoma [7,8].

In the normal host, multiple immune responses are activated by a primary EBV infection. If these immune mechanisms fail to develop, uncontrolled B-cell proliferation or B-cell destruction will occur. In the X-linked lymphoproliferative syndrome (XLP), following EBV infection, affected male patients will develop fatal or chronic infectious mononucleosis, progressive hypogammaglobulinemia, aplastic anemia, or malignant B-cell lymphoma [9].

Studies of 100 patients with XLP have identified a number of immunologic defects: 1) hypogammaglobulinemia occurred in 19 of 100 XLP patients [9]; 2) abnormal in vitro Ig synthesis by PBL was observed in most XLP patients; however, lymphoblastoid cell lines established from XLP patients produced normal quantities of all major Igs, suggesting a regulatory rather than a primary B-cell defect [10]; 3) a vigorous anti-EBNA response failed to develop in all XLP patients [11]; 4) antibody-dependent cellular cytotoxicity (ADCC) against EBV infected cells has been found low in 6 of 11 patients studied [12]; 5) lymphocyte subsets were abnormal (low OKT4:OKT8 ratio) [13]; 6) failure to effect regression to autologous EBV-infected lymphoblastoid cell lines was observed in many XLP patients, indicating a deficiency in long-lived T-cell mediated immunity to EBV [12]; 7) defective natural killer cell (NK) activity [14]; 8) destruction of thymic epithelium and depletion of T-dependent regions [15]; 9) malignant lymphomas were observed in 35 of 100 XLP patients (6 of the 35 also had hypogammaglobulinemia) [9].

It has been hypothesized that the XLP gene, located on the X chromosome, is responsible for a defective immune response to EBV and possibly other microorganisms. The cause for this deficiency may be defective T-cell regulation. As a consequence, following EBV infection, a proliferative B-cell disorder (lymphoma) may develop or antibody-producing B cells may be eliminated.

To test this hypothesis we measured antibody responses to bacteriophage ΦX 174 in 5 patients with XLP and 3 boys at risk for XLP (mother or maternal grandmother known to be a carrier). Phage was prepared as previously described [16] and given intravenously at a dose of 2×10^9 plaque-forming units (PFU) per kg body weight. Antibody activity to ΦX 174 was determined by a phage neutralization assay and was expressed as the rate of phage inactivation or K value, as derived by a standard formula [16]. Susceptibility of neutralizing activity to 2-mercaptoethanol (2-ME) was estimated using the method of Grubb and Swahn [17]. Antibody titers to various EBV-related antigens were determined by immunofluorescent methods as described previously [11].

RESULTS

Table 1 lists the patients studied, the diagnosis, the presenting clinical abnormality ("phenotype"), serum Ig levels, and the anti-EBV antibody titers. All 5 patients with XLP have serologic evidence of EBV infection. Two of these individuals have chronic infectious mononucleosis, and 3 have hypogammaglobulinemia. The 3 individuals at risk for XLP have developed anti-VCA antibody; one of the 3 boys, *DA*, shows a progressive decline of his serum Ig levels although the most recent values are still within the normal range. None of the individuals studied have developed significant anti-EBNA antibody.

Antibody responses to bacteriophage ΦX 174 are shown in Figure 1. All 8 individuals studied cleared phage normally and produced measurable antibody. Four of the 5 XLP

---

*Supported in part by NIH grants (AI-07073 and CA-30196), and from the March of Dimes Birth Defects Foundation (6-273).

TABLE 1. Characteristics of Patients Studied: Serum Ig Levels and Antibody Titers to EBV Antigen

Patient	Dx	Presenting Abnormality "phenotype"	Serum Ig (mg/dl)			Anti-EBV Titers					
							VCA		EA		
			IgG	IgA	IgM	IgM	IgA	IgG	DR	D	EBNA
KM (□)	XLP	CIM*	1285	3	496	<2	<2	<10	10	<10	<1:2
RM (●)	XLP	CIM	630	13	125	<2	<2	718	<10	<10	<1:2
DM (△)	XLP	Hypogamma-globulinemia	195	27	52	<2	14	285	<10	<10	1:5
LM (▲)	XLP	Hypogamma-globulinemia	36	16	36	<2	<2	<61	<10	<10	<1:2
KW (○)	XLP	Hypogamma-globulinemia	80	41	27	<2	<2	101	<10	<10	1:3
CMK (■)	At risk for XLP**	—	1050	90	122	<2	<2	1:80	<10	<10	1:10
DA (◇)		— 1980	680	43	96	<2	<2	1:160	1:20	<10	<1:2
		1981	495	19	56	<2	<2	1:40	<10	<10	<1:2
RA (◆)		1981	875	44	127	<2	<2	<10	<10	<10	<1:2 (3/82)
		1982	980	21	127	<2	<2	1:80	<10	<10	<1:2 (7/82)

*CIM = chronic infectious mononucleosis
**Mother or maternal grandmother are known carriers

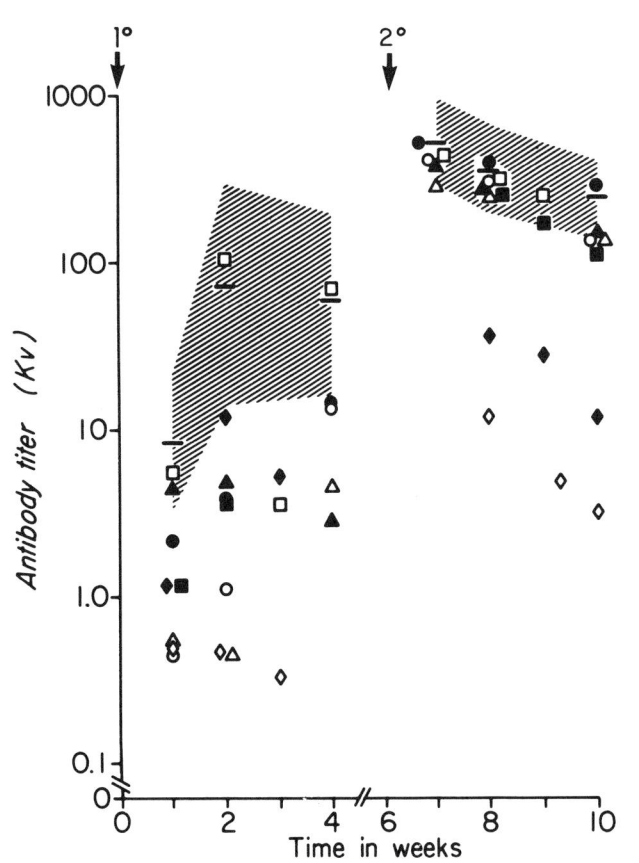

Fig. 1. Primary (1°) and secondary (2°) antibody responses to bacteriophage φX 174. The Kv of each individual patient is indicated by a symbol. Two XLP patients have chronic infectious mononucleosis (□, ●); 3 have hypogammaglobulinemia (△,▲,○); and 3 are at risk for XLP (■,◇,◆). The ranges of Kvs from 10 normal male controls are indicated by the hatched area, the geometric mean by the horizontal bar. The 3 patients at risk for XLP received their 2° dose of φX 174 three weeks following the primary immunization.

patients and all 3 patients at risk for XLP showed a very low 1° antibody response. The antibody titers following a 2nd phage injection were within the normal range, except for 2 brothers at risk for XLP. However, analysis of the antiphage antibody with 2-ME demonstrated that all XLP patients and those at risk for XLP failed to switch from IgM to IgG during the 2° response to phage (Fig. 2). In 10 normal male controls (young adults) approximately one-half (geometric mean percent = 44%, range 25–78%) of the antibody present at 2 weeks following 2° immunization were of the IgG class.

DISCUSSION

The clinical findings and laboratory abnormalities characteristic for male patients with XLP [9] suggest a defective immune system. This hypothesis is further supported by the abnormal antibody responses to the T-cell dependent antigen, bacteriophage φX 174. Failure to switch from IgM to IgG suggests defective T-inducer or T-suppressor functions. This X-linked regulatory defect may be responsible in part for the development of the XLP syndrome following EBV infection. Normal individuals,

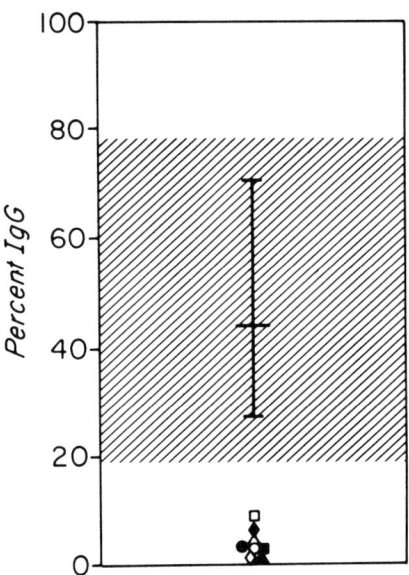

Fig. 2. Percent IgG of the antibody to bacteriophage φX 174 at 2 weeks post-2° immunization. The geometric mean of 10 normal male controls is indicated by the horizontal bar, the 66% confidence limit by the vertical bar, and the range by the hatched area. Symbols indicating individual XLP patients and individuals at risk for XLP are described in Table 1 and Figure 1.

during the early phase of acute infectious mononucleosis, will respond with proliferation of immunoregulatory T cells causing temporary in vitro and in vivo suppressor activity [3–5], including abnormal antibody responses to bacteriophage φX 174 [18]. These suppressor/cytotoxic cells may be necessary to contain B-cell proliferation [3–5]. The generation of functionally abnormal suppressor/cytotoxic T cells may result in the development of chronic progressive mononucleosis, or hypogammaglobulinemia, or B-cell lymphoma.

REFERENCES

1. Pattengale PK, Smith RW, Gerber P: B-cell characteristics of human peripheral and cord blood lymphocytes transformed by Epstein-Barr virus. J Natl Cancer Inst 52:1081–1086, 1974.
2. Kirchner H, Tosato G, Blaese RM, Broder S, Magrath IT: Polyclonal immunoglobulin secretion by human B lymphocytes exposed to Epstein-Barr virus in vitro. J Immunol 122:1310–1313, 1979.
3. Tosato G, Magrath I, Koski I, Dooley N, Blaese M: Activation of suppressor T cells during Epstein-Barr virus-induced infectious mononucleosis. N Engl J Med 301:1133–1137, 1979.
4. Haynes BF, Schooley RT, Payling-Wright CR, Grouse JE, Dolin R, Fauci AS: Emergence of suppressor cells of immunoglobulin synthesis during acute Epstein-Barr virus-induced infectious mononucleosis. J Immunol 123:2095–2101, 1979.
5. De Waele M, Thielemans C, Van Camp BKG: Characterization of immunoregulatory T cells in EBV-induced infectious mononucleosis by monoclonal antibodies. N Engl J Med 304:460–462, 1981.
6. Andiman WA: The Epstein-Barr virus and EB virus infections in childhood. J Pediatr 95:171–182, 1979.
7. Henle G, Henle W, Diehl V: Relation of Burkitt's tumor-associated herpes-type virus to infectious mononucleosis. Proc Natl Acad Sci USA 59:94–101, 1968.
8. Klein G: The Epstein-Barr virus and neoplasms. N Engl J Med 293:1353–1354, 1975.
9. Purtilo DT, Sakamoto K, Barnabei V, Seeley J, Bechtold T, Rogers G, Yetz J, Harada S: Epstein-Barr virus-induced diseases in boys with the X-linked lymphoproliferative syndrome (XLP). Am J Med 73:49–56, 1982.
10. Lindsten T, Seeley JK, Ballow M, Sakamoto K, Saint Onge S, Yetz J, Aman P, Purtilo DT: Immune deficiency in the X-linked lymphoproliferative syndrome: II. Immunoregulatory T cell defects. J Immunol (In press)
11. Sakamoto K, Freed HJ, Purtilo DT: Antibody responses to Epstein-Barr virus in families with the X-linked lymphoproliferative syndrome. J Immunol 125:921–925, 1980.
12. Harada S, Sakamoto K, Seeley JK, Lindsten T, Bechtold T, Yetz J, Rogers G, Pearson G, Purtilo DT: Immune deficiency in the X-linked lymphoproliferative syndrome. I. Epstein-Barr virus-specific defects. J Immunol. (In press).
13. Seeley J, Sakamoto K, Ip SH, Hansen PW, Purtilo DT: Abnormal lymphocyte subsets in X-linked lymphoproliferative syndrome. J Immunol 127:2618–2620, 1981.
14. Sullivan JL, Byron K, Brewster F, Purtilo DT: Deficient natural killer cell activity in the X-linked lymphoproliferative syndrome. Science 210:543–545, 1980.
15. Purtilo DT: Immune deficiency predisposing to Epstein-Barr virus-induced lymphoproliferative disease: The X-linked lymphoproliferative syndrome as a model. Adv Cancer Res 34:279–312, 1981.
16. Wedgwood RJ, Ochs HD, Davis SD: The recognition and classification of immunodeficiency diseases with bacteriophage φX 174. In Bergsma D (ed): "Immunodeficiency in Man and Animals." Sunderland MA: Sinauer Associates for the National Foundation—March of Dimes, BD:OAS 11(1):331–338, 1975.
17. Grubb R, Swahn B: Destruction of some agglutinins but not of others by two sulfhydryl compounds. Acta Pathol Microbiol Scand 43:305–309, 1958.
18. Bowen TJ, Wedgwood RJ, Ochs HD, Henle W: Transient immunodeficiency during asymptomatic Epstein-Barr virus infection. Pediatrics (In press)

Down Syndrome: A Model of Immunodeficiency

G. Roberto Burgio, MD, Alberto Ugazio, MD, Luigi Nespoli, MD, and Rita Maccario, PhD

Department of Pediatrics, University of Pavia, 27100 Pavia, Italy

For a long time, clinical and laboratory findings have suggested that deficiency of the immune system contributes to the clinical picture of Down syndrome (DS):

a) the high susceptibility to polytopic infections, the high mortality from infectious diseases [1], and the extremely high frequency of HBs Ag carriers [2,3] (Fig. 1);
b) the high frequency of malignancies, especially leukemia, which is 20 times more frequent in DS than in the general population [4,5];
c) the high frequency of autoantibodies, particularly those directed against thyroid antigens [3,6] often associated with clinical and laboratory evidence of thyroid disorders [7].

It is also well recognized that, in children with primary immunodeficiencies, high susceptibility to infections is often associated with an increased susceptibility to malignancies and autoimmune disorders [8].

Growing clinical and laboratory evidence has accumulated over the last decade indicating that a combined deficiency of antibody- and cell-mediated immunity (CMI) is an integral feature of DS.

DERANGEMENTS OF HUMORAL IMMUNITY

Serum Ig levels are normal for age during the first 5 years of life but IgG and IgA increase thereafter reaching very high levels, while IgM decreases slightly in DS subjects after adolescence [9].

Titers of "natural" antibodies such as those directed against sheep erythrocytes (SE), *Salmonella adelaide* flagellar antigens, *E. coli* and rabbit erythrocytes [10,11], as well as antibodies against several viral antigens [12], have been reported as severely depressed. Furthermore, defective antibody responses to influenza vaccine [13] and bacteriophage ϕX 174 [14] have been documented; however, studies of the antibody response to tetanus toxoid (TT) and other bacterial antigens have resulted in conflicting data [15,16].

The frequency of autoantibodies directed against human thyroglobulin is much higher in DS than in age-matched controls living under the same environmental conditions [3]. The percentage and absolute number of circulating B lymphocytes are normal [9].

DERANGEMENTS OF T-CELL IMMUNITY

The finding that lymphocytes from DS proliferate poorly in vitro in response to polyclonal T-cell activators such as PHA [17] provided the first laboratory evidence of a T-cell deficiency in DS. Lymphocyte response to PHA, normal for age during the first 10 years of life, has been shown to decline rapidly and irreversibly thereafter [9,18]. Furthermore, DS lymphocytes proliferate poorly in response to soluble antigens [19] and show depressed lymphokine production in vitro [20]. Delayed hypersensitivity skin test responses are also impaired in DS [10].

Data concerning the number of circulating T lymphocytes have been more controversial: some studies using the E-rosette test, as well as anti-T-cell sera, have shown that DS subjects of all ages, including newborns, have fewer peripheral T lymphocytes than normal children [9,21,22]; others, however, have found normal numbers of circulating T lymphocytes [10,23]. This discrepancy is more apparent than real, since it probably results from the presence of a large subset of circulating lymphocytes with very low avidity for SE in DS [24]. This is in keeping with recent data with monoclonal antibodies suggesting that in DS, in contrast with normal controls, a relatively large proportion of lymphocytes expressing the OKT3 antigen forms rosettes only with 2-aminoethylisothiouronium (AET) bromide-treated SE (Table 1). The strikingly high percentage of large granular lymphocytes (LGL) expressing the HNK1 as well as the OKT8 and Leu 2a antigens [25,26] found in the peripheral blood of DS (Table 1) may pertain to the above subset of lymphocytes with low avidity for SE and represent NK cells.

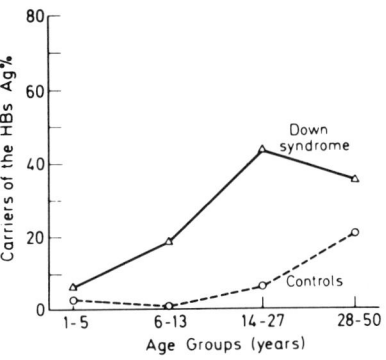

Fig. 1. Frequency of carriers of the HBs Ag in subjects with DS ($\triangle$) and controls ($\bigcirc$). Controls were carefully matched for age, sex and socioenvironmental conditions (adapted from reference 3).

TABLE 1. Membrane Markers of Peripheral Blood Lymphocytes in Children With DS and Age-Matched Controls Living Under the Same Environmental Conditions

Membrane receptor or antigen	Positive cells (%)		P
	DS	Controls	
E	[a]56 ± 12 (42)	72 ± 4 (36)	<0.001
E$_{AET}$	71 ± 3 (38)	71 ± 4 (30)	NS
OKT3	71 ± 12 (40)	74 ± 6 (29)	NS
OKT4	38 ± 9 (24)	43 ± 11 (33)	NS
OKT8	44 ± 12 (51)	23 ± 7 (36)	<0.001
Leu 2a	52 ± 9 (22)	23 ± 6 (36)	<0.001
OKT6	4 ± 4 (26)	2 ± 2 (18)	NS
HNK1[b]	40 ± 12 (18)	16 ± 6 (15)	<0.001

[a]Mean ± 1 SD; number of subjects in parentheses.
[b]Courtesy of Dr. Max Cooper.

Whatever the nature of this cellular subset, the functional involvement of the T lymphocytes, as well as the evidence for a reduced number of fully differentiated T lymphocytes in peripheral blood, point to a central role of the thymus in the pathogenesis of the immunodeficiency in DS. In fact, morphologic evidence of thymic derangement in DS was first provided by Benda and Strassmann [27]: a small thymus with poor corticomedullary differentiation and anomalous Hassall corpuscles. Degeneration of Hassall corpuscles—a morphologic index of the function of thymic epithelial cells—is already present in newborns with DS [28]. In fact, there is now direct and indirect evidence that thymus-dependent humoral factors are deficient in DS from the first few months of life [29,30].

MOLECULAR BASIS: FACTS AND SPECULATIONS

The gene responsible for the species-specific response to interferon (IFN) has been mapped to chromosome 21 [31] and is thought to code for a cell-surface receptor for IFN [32]. As a direct or indirect result of gene-dosage, trisomic cells are several times more sensitive than normal cells to the effect of IFN [19]. Since IFN is known to affect several immunologic functions [33], it has been suggested that the immune defects of DS may result from "hypersensitivity" of trisomic cells to IFN. So far, pertinent experiments have failed either to substantiate or to rule out conclusively this hypothesis. Inferferon has also been shown to enhance NK activity [34]: whether the high *number* of lymphocytes with an NK phenotype reported in the present study has anything to do with the increased susceptibility to IFN of trisomic cells remains to be established. There is indirect evidence that DS lymphocytes—but not fibroblasts—have faulty DNA repair, possibly leading to accumulation of somatic mutations [35]; however, the eventual role of abnormal DNA repair in the pathogenesis of immune derangements or malignancy, although theoretically attractive, remains purely speculative at the moment.

Low levels of serum zinc have been found in DS, and treatment with zinc sulphate has been reported to improve some immunologic parameters [36]. This finding is particularly appealing in view of the evidence that zinc deficiency results in a severe reversible T-cell deficiency in acrodermatitis enteropathica [37] as well as in nutritional zinc deficiencies [38].

THYMUS DEFECT AND STRESS DEFICIENCY: A TENTATIVE CONCLUSION

There is now very little, if any, doubt that immunodeficiency is an integral feature of DS. Many controversies in the literature concerning the degree of this immunodeficiency appear to have resulted from two often overlooked factors: age and institutionalization. Retrospectively, most studies pointing to a marked immunodeficiency were carried out in institutionalized and/or postpubertal subjects with DS [10,17]. On the other hand, studies limited to noninstitutionalized trisomic infants and children often led to the opposite conclusion, that the immunodeficiency of DS is marginal [23]. As shown in Figure 1, institutionalization per se results in a striking increase of the HBs Ag carrier rate among karyotypically normal subjects, but subjects with DS are far less able to eradicate HB virus than age-matched inmates. Thus, institutionalization cannot be considered a major factor in the pathogenesis of the immunodeficiency in DS.

Whatever the underlying molecular defect, the earliest site of immune derangement in DS appears to lie in thymic epithelial cells which fail to synthesize or secrete adequate amounts of one or more hormone(s), thus resulting in failure of T-cell differentiation, which probably underlies the early appearance of autoantibodies and also contributes to the emergence of lymphoid malignancies in the trisomic newborn and infant. Recurrent infections certainly contribute to progressive "exhaustion" (or "stress deficiency") of the immune system and eventually lead to the extensive deficiency of T- and B-cell functions usually seen in trisomic adults. Institutionalization, with its high rate of infection, would therefore be expected to accelerate the exhaustion of the immune system, resulting in an earlier and more severe immunodeficiency. It is conceivable that the striking increase in lymphocytes with phenotypic characteristics of NK cells may be a result of the recurrent viral infections, the high susceptibility of trisomic cells to IFN, or both.

REFERENCES

1. Oster J, Mikkelsen M, Nielsen A: Mortality and life-table in Down's syndrome. Acta Paediatr Scand 64:322–326, 1975.
2. Sutnick AI, London WT, Gerstley BJS, Cronlund MN, Blumberg BS: Anicteric hepatitis associated with Australia antigen. JAMA 205:670–674, 1968.
3. Ugazio AG, Jayakar S, Marcioni AF, Duse M, Monafo V, Pasquali F, Burgio GR: Immunodeficiency in Down's syndrome: Relationship between presence of human thyroglobulin antibodies and HBs Ag carrier status. Eur J Pediatr 126:139–146, 1977.
4. Miller RW: Neoplasia and Down's syndrome. Ann NY Acad Sci 171:637–644, 1970.
5. Krivit W, Good RA: Simultaneous occurrence of mongolism and leukemia. Am J Dis Child 94:289–293, 1957.
6. Burgio GR, Severi F, Rossoni R, Vaccaro R: Mongolism and thyroid autoimmunity. Lancet 1:166–167, 1965.
7. Baxter RG, Larkins RG, Martin FIR, Heyma P, Mylex K, Ryan L: Down syndrome and thyroid function in adults. Lancet 2:794–796, 1975.
8. Good RA: Crucial experiments of nature that have widened analysis of the immunologic apparatus. In Stiehm ER, Fulginiti VA (eds): "Immunologic Disorders in Infants and Children." Philadelphia: WB Saunders, 1980, pp 3–19.
9. Burgio GR, Ugazio AG, Nespoli L, Marcioni AF, Bottelli AM, Pasquali F: Derangements of immunoglobulin levels, phytohemagglutinin responsiveness and T and B cell markers in Down's syndrome at different ages. Eur J Immunol 5:600–603, 1975.
10. Whittingham S, Pitt DB, Sharma DLB, MacKay IR: Stress deficiency of the T lymphocyte system exemplified by Down's syndrome. Lancet 1:163–166, 1977.
11. Ugazio AG, Lanzavecchia A, Jayakar S, Plebani A, Duse M, Burgio GR: Immunodeficiency in Down's syndrome: Titers of "natural" antibodies to E. coli and rabbit erythrocytes at different ages. Acta Paediatr Scand 67:705–708, 1978.
12. Fekete G, Kulcsar G, Daun P, Nasz I, Schuler D, Dobos M: Immunological and virological investigations in Down's syndrome. Eur J Pediatr 138:59–62, 1982.
13. Gordon MC, Sinha SK, Carlson SD: Antibody responses to influenza vaccine in patients with Down's syndrome. Am J Ment Defic 75:391–399, 1971.
14. Lopez V, Ochs HD, Thuline HC, Davis SD, Wedgwood RJ: Defective antibody response to bacteriophage ϕX 174 in Down syndrome. J Pediatr 86:207–211, 1975.
15. Siegel M: Susceptibility of mongoloids to infection. II. Antibody response to tetanus toxoid and typhoid vaccine. Am J Hyg 48:63–73, 1948.
16. Griffith AW, Silvester PE: Mongols and non-mongols compared in their response to active tetanus immunization. J Ment Defic Res 11:263–266, 1967.
17. Agarwal SS, Blumberg BS, Gerstley BJS, London WT, Sutnick AI, Loeb LA: DNA polymerase activity as an index of lymphocyte stimulation: Studies in Down's syndrome. J Clin Invest 49:161–169, 1970.
18. Seger R, Buchinger G, Ströder J: On the influence of age on immunity in Down's syndrome. Eur J Pediatr 124:77–87, 1977.
19. Epstein LB, Epstein CJ: T lymphocyte function and sensitivity to interferon in trisomy 21. Cell Immunol 51:303–318, 1980.
20. Hahn T, Levin S, Handzel ZT: Leukocyte migration inhibition factor (LIF) production by lymphocytes of normal children, newborns, and children with immune deficiency. Clin Exp Immunol 24:448–454, 1976.
21. Levin S, Nir E, Mogilner BM: T system immune deficiency in Down's syndrome. Pediatrics 56:123–126, 1975.
22. Franceschi C, Licastro F, Paolucci P, Masi M, Cavicchi S, Zannotti M: T and B lymphocyte subpopulations in Down's syndrome. A study on non-institutionalized subjects. J Ment Defic Res 22:179–191, 1978.
23. Reiser K, Whitcomb C, Robinson K, MacKenzie MR: T and B lymphocytes in patients with Down's syndrome. Am J Ment Defic 80:613–619, 1976.
24. Burgio GR, Lanzavecchia A, Maccario R, Vitiello A, Plebani A, Ugazio AG: Immunodeficiency in Down's syndrome: T lymphocyte subset imbalance in trisomic children. Clin Exp Immunol 33:298–301, 1978.
25. Ortaldo JR, Sharrow SO, Timonen T, Herberman RB: Determination of surface antigens on highly purified human NK cells by flow cytometry with monoclonal antibodies. J Immunol 127:2401–2409, 1981.
26. Grossi CE, Cadoni A, Zicca A, Leprini A, Ferrarini M: Large granular lymphocytes in human peripheral blood. Ultrastructural and cytochemical characterization of the granules. Blood 59:277–283, 1982.
27. Benda CE, Strassmann GS: The thymus in mongolism. J Ment Defic Res 9:109–117, 1965.
28. Levin S, Schlesinger M, Handzel Z, Hahn T, Altman Y, Czernobilsky B, Boss J: Thymic deficiency in Down's syndrome. Pediatrics 63:80–86, 1979.
29. Duse M, Brugo MA, Martini A, Tassi C, Ferrario C, Ugazio AG: Immune deficiency in Down's syndrome: Low levels of serum thymic factor in trisomic children. Thymus 2:127–131, 1980.
30. Handzel ZT, Dolfin Z, Levin S, Altman Y, Hahn T, Trainin N, Gadot N: Effect of thymic humoral factor on cellular immune functions of normal children and of pediatric patients with ataxia-telangiectasia and Down's syndrome. Pediatr Res 13:803–806, 1979.
31. Tan YH: Chromosome-21-dosage effect on inducibility of anti-viral gene(s). Nature 253:280–282, 1975.
32. Revel M, Bash D, Ruddle FH: Antibodies to cell surface components coded by human chromosome 21 inhibit action of interferon. Nature 260:139–141, 1976.
33. Friedman RM: Interferons. In Oppenheim JJ, Rosensstreich DL, Potter M (eds): "Cellular Functions in Immunity and Inflammation." London: Edward Arnold, 1981, pp 283–300.
34. Sonnenfeld G: Modulation of immunity by interferon. Lynfokine Rep 1:113–131, 1980.
35. Yotti LP, Glover TW, Trosko JE, Segal DJ: Comparative study of X-ray and UV induced cytotoxicity, DNA repair, and mutagenesis in Down's syndrome and normal fibroblasts. Pediatr Res 14:88–92, 1980.
36. Björkstén B, Back O, Gustavson KH, Hallmans G, Hägglöf B, Täruvik A: Zinc and immune function in Down's syndrome. Acta Paediatr Scand 69:183–187, 1980.
37. Barnes PM, Moynahan AJ: Zinc deficiency in acrodermatitis enteropathica: Multiple dietary intolerance treated with synthetic diet. Proc R Soc Med 66:325–333, 1973.
38. Golden MH, Harland PS, Golden BE, Jackson AA: Zinc and immune competence in protein-energy malnutrition. Lancet 1:1226–1227, 1978.

Hypogammaglobulinemia and Malakoplakia—Effect of Bethanechol

John F. Soothill, FRCP, B.A.M. Harvey, FIMLT, M. Webb, MB,
W.C. Marshall, MD, L. Spitz, FRCS, and J.R. Pincott, MRCPath

Department of Immunology, Institute of Child Health, London WC1N 1EH (J.F.S., B.A.M.H.), Department of Surgery, Institute of Child Health, London WC1N 1EH (L.S.), Department of Histopathology, Hospital for Sick Children, London WC1 (J.R.P.), and Hospital for Sick Children, London WC1 (M.W., W.C.M.), England

Abdou et al [1] described a patient with recurrent infections, intestinal fistulae, hypogammaglobulinemia, malakoplakia, and a monocyte lysosomal abnormality, who improved on treatment with Bethanechol. Here is a brief report of a similar patient, also treated successfully, who will be described in detail elsewhere.

CASE HISTORY

S.E., born in 1972 in Teheran, Iran, was well until 1976 when he developed recurrent fever, bloody diarrhea, abdominal pain, and weight loss. His parents (first cousins) and 3 sibs are well. He was treated for *Giardia lamblia*, and *Salmonella* infection. Stricture of transverse colon was diagnosed in 1979 and he was referred to London. The stricture was confirmed. Igs and B lymphocytes were deficient, and one sample showed neutropenia (Table 1). Other immunologic tests and bone marrow were normal. Transverse colon and appendix were resected; histology showed ulceration and an inflammatory exudate; localized malakoplakia was noted on later reexamination of this tissue. No pathogenic organisms were isolated. Ig injections (25 mg/kg/week) were started, and he was followed by Dr. A. Farhoudi in Iran. He was well, apart from occasional abdominal pain and blood in the feces, until March 1981 when he was admitted to hospital in Teheran for an abdominal emergency. An inflamed ascending colon and a retrocecal abscess was found; a right hemicolectomy was performed. The histology showed extensive ulceration, granulation tissue, and diffuse malakoplakia throughout the thickness of the bowel wall. He developed 2 chronic abdominal sinuses and lost weight, and was transferred to London. *Salmonella typhimurium*, *Klebsiella aerogenes*, *Acinetobacter*, *Enterobacter*, and *Proteus* were grown from the discharge. Many antibacterial agents and fresh frozen plasma were given, and the sinuses, which communicated, were drained.

Colonoscopy showed strictures of the transverse descending and sigmoid colon. A 3rd sinus developed in the old hemicolectomy scar. The sinuses then leaked jejunal fluid, and a jejunal fistula was resected and a colostomy was performed. The resected colon showed similar malakoplakia. He then developed a vesicocolic fistula. Despite IV feeding, and full supportive treatment, he deteriorated; he was emaciated and had lost his brave and happy spirit, and was thought to be moribund. An increased proportion of adherent mononuclear cells contained large granules which stained with acridine orange as described by Abdou et al [1]; these became fewer on culture with carbachol (Table 2). His father showed similar granules but normal Igs. S.E.'s blood film showed marked vacuolation of the monocytes. One sample from S.E. and each of his parents had low mononu-

TABLE 1.

	1979	1981	1982
Height (UK %)	25	3	10
Weight "	10	<3	>3
Hg (G/L)	10.3	10.3	14.3
Neutrophils (× 10⁹/L)	1.8	2.7	2.5
Lymphocytes	3.7	2.2	1.7
Monocytes	1.1	0.5	0.2
Serum albumin (g/L)	35	33	—
IgG (IU/ml)	30	32	46
IgA "	6	6	2.2
IgM "	24	47	4.4
PHA response	normal	normal	—
E rosettes %	57	70	—
Lymphocyte surface Ig (polyvalent) %	0.5	0	<1

Other tests giving normal values include hemolytic complement, C3, yeast opsonization, monoclonal antibody tests for T-cell subsets (OKT3,4, and 8), NBT, neutrophil staph. phagocytosis and killing, and neutrophil mobility.

TABLE 2.

	Bethanechol Treatment	% With Large Granules		
		Medium Alone	With Colchicine	With Carbachol
S.E.	before	68	80	42
	9 days	38	84	36
	18 days	43	90	39
	9 months	28	49	15
Father		47	64	
Mother		18	60	
5 Healthy Controls	mean:	15	54	
	observed range:	6–20	44–78	

Percentage of adherent mononuclear cells (Ficoll-Triosil preparation from heparinized blood) showing large (>1M) granules stained with acridine orange, after culture for 30 minutes in vitro in medium alone, or with Colchicine 10^{-5}M, or Carbachol 10^{-4}M.

clear cyclic GMP (radioimmunoassay), but one sample from S.E. was normal; all values were higher than those reported by Abdou et al [1].

He was given Bethanechol 10 mg/tid and a remarkable improvement occurred. The discharge from the sinuses stopped in 3 days, and they healed in 2 weeks. He became cheerful, energetic, and his appetite returned; he was discharged after 2 weeks.

He was readmitted in July 1982. He was well and the colostomy was closed. Resected colon showed hypertrophic muscularis and a mild inflammatory exudate only; a lymph node showed sinus histiocytosis; there was no malakoplakia. A possible excess of blood monocytes with large granules was still noted, though these were fewer than before treatment started (Table 2). Ig levels were unchanged (apart from the increase of IgG from injections).

COMMENT

S.E. confirms many aspects of the report of Abdou et al [1]. The younger age, and consanguineous parents, who showed partial abnormality, strengthen the case for a primary defect and that the monocyte abnormality is not an effect of the hypogammaglobulinemia. The extreme illness when the diagnosis was made prevented delay of treatment for more extensive investigation.

The very rapid improvement when Bethanechol treatment was started strongly suggests that it was effective, though the inconsistency of the abnormality of cyclic GMP metabolism raises some doubt on the theory which led Abdou et al [1] to use it. Like them, we noted no effect on Ig production. The excellent course of both patients while on the treatment, and the death from septicemia of their patient some weeks after stopping the treatment against advice (Abdou 1982, personal communication), suggests that this line of treatment is lifesaving, and can lead to good health. S.E. remains on treatment.

REFERENCES

1. Abdou NI, NaPombejara C, Sagawa A, Ragland C et al: Malakoplakia: Evidence for monocyte lysosomal abnormality correctable by cholinergic agents in vitro and in vivo. N Engl J Med 297:1413, 1977.

Basophil and Eosinophil Deficiency in a Patient With Hypogammaglobulinemia Associated With Thymoma

E. Bruce Mitchell, MD, FRCP(C), Thomas A.E. Platts-Mills, FRCP*, R. Scott Pereira, MRCPath, Vera Malkovska, and A. David Webster, FRCP

Clinical Research Centre, Harrow HA1 3UJ, England

Patients who have late-onset hypogammaglobulinemia in association with thymoma have been reported to be deficient in eosinophils [1–3]. These patients also have abnormal suppressor T-cell activity and very few circulating B cells and are thus distinct from the majority of patients with late-onset hypogammaglobulinemia [4,5]. We report here a patient (J.C.) who had thymoma, hypogammaglobulinemia, and absence of eosinophils, who was found to be severely deficient in basophils.

The patient is a 55-year-old man who presented at age 47 with a history of recurrent bacterial and viral infection and was found to have a mediastinal mass and low serum globulins (IgG 0.9 gm/liter; IgM < 0.1 gm/liter; IgA < 0.1; and IgE 2.0 IU/ml), although his salivary IgA was normal [5]. Thymectomy revealed a benign spindle cell thymoma. Initially, he had eosinophils in his peripheral blood, but these were no longer present after 2 years. At present, he has no eosinophils in peripheral blood or bone marrow. In addition, he was found to have very low peripheral blood histamine ($\leqslant$ 60 nmole/liter; normal range 871 ± 422 nmole/liter), and on review no basophils were present in repeated blood films or in spears from 2 bone marrow aspirations. Following passive sensitization with IgE antibodies (P-K test) he showed immediate skin tests, and skin biopsy confirmed the presence of normal numbers of skin mast cells. By contrast, using an allergen patch technique after passive sensitization which is known to recruit eosinophils to the skin, he showed no eosinophils in skin biopsy [6]. His peripheral blood mononuclear cells contained a normal percentage of T cells (71%), but 54% of these cells were OKT5+ve, while only 39% were OKT4+ve. Furthermore, his T cells showed grossly abnormal suppressor activity for PWM-induced Ig production in vitro [5]. Only 0.8% of his mononuclear cells were SmIg+ve and in keeping with this his non-T cells made no Ig in response to PWM even with normal T cells. However, when stimulated with Epstein-Barr virus (EBV) these cells produced normal quantities of IgG and IgM [7]. J.C. has had normal hemoglobin throughout this period, but his total white cell count has been falling and is now 3.0–4.0 × $10^3/\mu l$.

This patient lacks basophils and eosinophils and has a reduced number of B cells. The possibility that these 3 cell types have a common precursor seems unlikely. Alternatively, it may be that the abnormal T cells seen in J.C. act on "helper" T cells required for the maturation of each of these 3 cell types. Basophils and eosinophils are known to participate in a form of delayed hypersensitivity, cutaneous basophil hypersensitivity (CBH). CBH is thought to be involved in allograft rejection, tumor rejection, and parasite rejection, as well as in allergic diseases. The absence of these cells may well contribute to the progressive deterioration of immunity often seen in these patients, or to the immune defect apparent in other patients with deficiency of both cell types [8].

REFERENCES

1. Good RA, Varco RL: A clinical and experimental study of agammaglobulinaemia. Lancet 75:245–271, 1955.
2. Waldmann TA, Strober WS, Blaese RM, Strauss AJL: Thymoma, hypogammaglobulinaemia and absence of eosinophils. J Clin Invest 46:1127, 1967.
3. Asherson GL, Webster ADB: Thymoma and immunodeficiency. In "Diagnosis and Treatment of Immunodeficiency Diseases." Oxford: Blackwell, 1980, pp 78–98.
4. Waldmann TA, Broder S, Durm M, Blackman M, Krackauer R, Meade B: Suppressor T cells in the pathogenesis of hypogammaglobulinaemia associated with thymoma. Trans Assoc Am Physicians 88:120, 1975.
5. Platts-Mills TAE, de Gast GC, Webster ADB, Asherson GL, Wilkins SR: Two immunologically distinct forms of late onset hypogammaglobulinaemia. Clin Exp Immunol 44:383–388, 1981.
6. Mitchell EB, Chapman MD, Pope FM, Crow J, Jouhal SS, Platts-Mills TAE: Basophils in allergen-induced patch test sites in atopic dermatitis. Lancet 1:127–130, 1982.
7. Pereira RS, Webster ADB, Platts-Mills TAE: Immature B cells in fetal development and immunodeficiency. Studies of IgM, IgG, IgA and IgD production *in vitro* using Epstein-Barr virus activation. Eur J Immunol 12:540–546, 1982.
8. Juhlin L, Michaëlson G: A new syndrome characterised by absence of eosinophils and basophils. Lancet 1:1233–1235, 1977.

---

*Present address: Department of Medicine, University of Virginia, Charlottesville, VA 22908.

Bone Marrow Transplantation in a Patient With Chédiak-Higashi Syndrome

Claude Griscelli, MD, and Jean-Louis Virelizier, MD

Unité d'Immunologie et d'Hématologie Pédiatriques, Département de Pédiatrie, INSERM U 132, Hôpital des Enfants Malades, 75730 Paris Cedex 15, France

Chédiak-Higashi disease (CHD) is a rare familial disorder characterized by an incomplete oculocutaneous albinism, photophobia, and severe recurrent infections [1]. Neutrophils from these patients are deficient in chemotactic [2] and bactericidal activities [3]; and there is delayed fusion of the abnormal granules with phagocytic vacuoles [4]. It was recently shown that microtubular abnormalities may be responsible for these defects and that ascorbic acid therapy may correct certain functions of these cells [5,6]. We have also observed that ascorbic acid in vitro (and in vivo) induces a partial correction of the abnormal polar distribution of membrane Con A receptor of the PMNs [7]. However, this therapy given for several weeks or months to 3 patients was unable to prevent the severe "accelerated phase" characteristic of the disease. A major immunologic defect in patients with Chédiak-Higashi syndrome (CHS) is a profound decrease in the natural killer activity of peripheral leukocytes, as described simultaneously by Roder et al [8] and by us [9]. Although it has been claimed that in vitro natural killer activity of leukocytes in CHS can be partially restored by interferon (IFN) [10], we have been unable to modify the natural killer cytotoxic indexes of 4 patients with CHS by in vitro addition of IFN, even after a 24-hour incubation in medium containing up to 10,000 U/IFN/ml. Furthermore, we have shown that in vivo administration of 200,000 U/kg/bw daily for 5 days in a patient with CHS did not modify the very low natural killer activity of his peripheral leukocytes [9].

CASE REPORT

A patient born of consanguineous parents of Laotian origin was shown to have CHS on the association of partial albinism and typical giant leukocyte granules. One of his brothers, who also had albinism, died of infection in 1967. The patient presented several infections from the 1st year of life but no symptoms of "accelerated phase." A first bone marrow transplantation (BMT) was performed in September 1979 (3 years of age) with 3.5×10^8 cells/kg from his HLA-A, B, and D compatible, MLR-negative sister after the following regimen: cyclophosphamide, 50 mg/kg × 4 (day 5, 4, 3, and 2 before BM cells transfusion). Prevention of GVH reaction was performed with methotrexate. This BMT was unsuccessful. The patient presented a severe, diffuse varicella 12 days after BMT and he was reconstituted with autologous cells with the CH morphology. Varicella was treated with specific gamma globulins and IFN (2,000,000 U/day × 5). In October (45 days posttransplantation), signs of accelerated phase were present with hepatosplenomegaly, decrease in serum fibrinogen levels, hypertriglyceridemia, leukopenia, and thrombocytopenia. This episode was treated with steroids and VP 16 (epipodophyllotoxin). A second BMT was performed in January 1981 with 3×10^8 cells/kg from the HLA-identical sister, after cyclophosphamide (50 mg/kg × 2, day 5 and 4 before BMT) and total body irradiation (700 rads with lung protection = 350 rads). At day 30 after grafting, hematologic and immunologic reconstitution was complete, with 100% of the leukocytes showing female markers and absence of abnormal granules. Twenty months after transplantation, the patient is clinically and immunologically normal and free from infections. As expected, the partial albinism was not modified. We tested natural killer activity by calculating the specific chromium-51 release from K562 target cells incubated with peripheral leukocytes. Leukocytes had previously been incubated with either control medium or 10^4 units of IFN alpha (Institut Pasteur, Paris) for 24 hours at 37° C and were washed before the test. Reversal of the profound natural killer defect observed before grafting was complete as soon as day 46 after transplantation [11]. We observed the reversal of both the spontaneous levels of natural activity and its activation in vitro with IFN.

This successful BMT in CHS shows that replacement of hematopoietic and lymphoid precursor cells may result in a correction of the functional anomalies of this severe disease. It also shows that natural killer effector cells are of BM origin in humans and that an intrinsic, IFN-resistant defect of natural killer activity can be reversed by BMT.

REFERENCES

1. Blume RS, Wolff SM: The Chédiak-Higashi syndrome: Studies in four patients and a review of the literature. Medicine (Baltimore) 51:247–280, 1972.
2. Clark RA, Kimball HR: Defective granulocyte chemotaxis in the Chédiak-Higashi syndrome. J Clin Invest 50:2645–2652, 1971.
3. Root RK, Rosenthal AS, Balestra DJ: Abnormal bactericidal, metabolic, and lysosomal functions of Chédiak-Higashi syndrome leukocytes. J Clin Invest 51:649–665, 1972.
4. Stossel TP, Root RK, Vaughan M: Phagocytosis in chronic granulomatous disease and the Chédiak-Higashi syndrome. N Engl J Med 286:120–123, 1972.
5. Olivier JM, Zurier RB: Correction of characteristic abnormalities of microtubule function and granule morphology in Chédiak-Higashi syndrome with cholinergic agonists: Studies in vitro in man and in vivo in the beige mouse. J Clin Invest 57:1239–1247, 1976.
6. Boxer LA, Watanabe AM, Rister M et al: Correction of leukocyte function in Chédiak-Higashi syndrome by ascorbate. N Engl J Med 295:1041–1045, 1976.
7. Griscelli C, Durandy A, Guy-Grand D, Daguillard F, Herzog C, Prunieras M: A syndrome associating partial albinism and immunodeficiency. Am J Med 65:691–702, 1978.
8. Roder JC, Haliotis T, Klein M et al: A new immunodeficiency disorder in humans involving NK cells. Nature 284:553–555, 1980.
9. Virelizier JL, Griscelli C: Interferon administration as an immunoregulatory and antimicrobial treatment in children with defective interferon secretion. In Seligmann M, Hitzig WH (eds): "Primary Immunodeficiencies." Amsterdam: Elsevier/North Holland, Biomedical Press, 1980, pp 473–484.
10. Haliotis T, Roder JC, Klein N, Ortaldo J, Fauci AS, Herberman RB: Chédiak-Higashi gene in humans. Impairment of natural killer function. J Exp Med 151:1039–1048, 1980.
11. Virelizier JL, Lagrue A, Durandy A, Arenzana F, Oury C, Griscelli C, Reinert P: Reversal of natural killer defect in a patient with Chédiak-Higashi syndrome after bone marrow transplantation. N Engl J Med 306:1055–1056, 1982.

Humoral Immune Deficiency and Recurrent Otitis Media

C.S. Hosking, MD, FRACP, FRCPA, M.J. Shelton, MSc, J. Ward, MD, and D.M. Roberton, MD, FRACP

Department of Immunology, Royal Children's Hospital, Parkville, Victoria 3052, Australia

The purpose of this study was to assess the clinical and laboratory data related to otitis media of a group of children referred for investigation of recurrent infections. The results from these patients form part of a data base of results from children referred because of a variety of different types of infections who had investigations of their clinical and immunologic status.

Basically the data were examined in two different ways. First, the whole group, consisting of 328 patients and 30 controls, was assessed to determine whether or not there was a difference in incidence of otitis media between different groups of patients, and patients and controls. In the second part of the study, a subgroup of patients whose major complaint was recurrent otitis media was selected and the incidence of a number of factors compared. As well, these latter patients were grouped using a clustering algorithm.

MATERIALS AND METHODS

Parents of outpatients referred to the Department of Immunology for investigation of immune function filled in a questionnaire relating to the numbers and types of infections the patient had had in the previous 12 months, the family history of allergy, and the family history of infections. The questionnaire was completed in the presence of one of the authors (C.S.H. or D.M.R.), or a trained nursing sister. All of the infection episodes were categorized using strict clinical criteria [1] and entered into files on a Hewlett Packard 1000 computer. The identical clinical data were sought from a group of 131 randomly chosen control children and similarly entered into files. All of the patients and 30 of the controls had a wide range of immune function tests performed [2]; these results were also stored in files linked to the clinical data.

From this data base a major subgroup was analyzed. These were those patients who had had >95th%

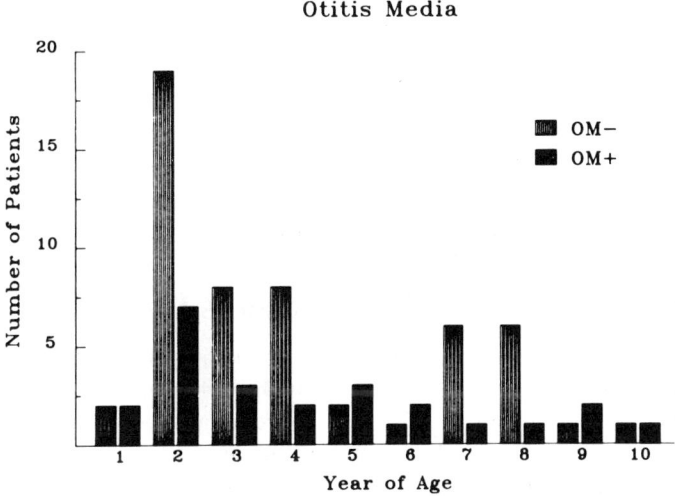

Fig. 1. Age of patients when questionnaire was completed and tests were performed.

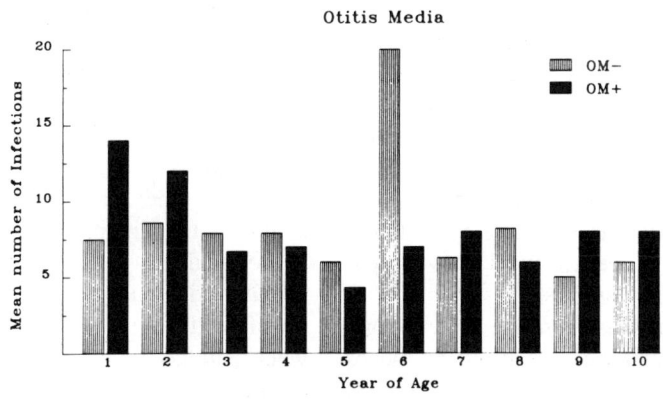

Fig. 2. Mean number of attacks of otitis media at each age.

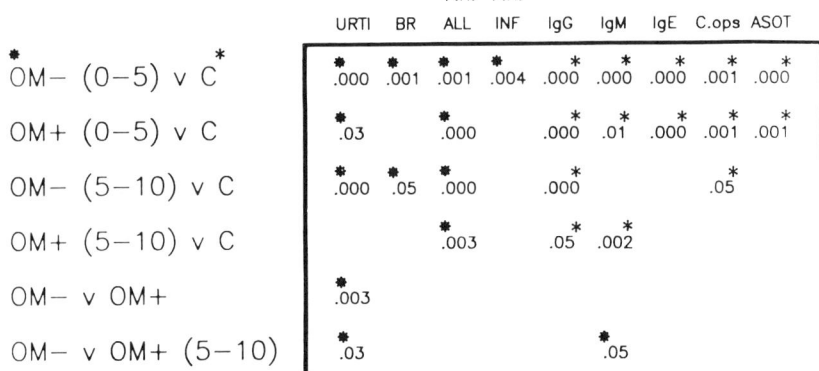

Fig. 3. Differences between groups of patients and between patients and controls for 9 clinical or laboratory features. Nonsignificant (>0.05) differences are left blank. An asterisk at the left upper corner of a significance figure indicates that the first named group was significantly higher than the second named group. An asterisk at the right upper corner indicates that the second group was higher than the first. A significance figure of .000 indicates that the level is <.001.

of the number of infections of the control group in the previous 12 months using the infection scoring system of Hosking and Roberton, 1981 [3]. Three hundred twenty-eight patients fulfilled the above criteria. Their clinical data were compared with that of the group of 131 children randomly chosen as part of a community survey of the incidence of infections in childhood.

A subgroup of patients whose major problem was otitis media was chosen from the above 328 patients using the following criteria: They were younger than 11 years of age, they had had 4 or more attacks of otitis media in the previous 12 months, and otitis media represented >40% of the infection score. This latter group consisted of 78 patients.

Statistical analysis using nonparametric methods was used to assess the differences between different groups of patients and between patients and controls.

The results from the larger group of patients were analyzed by means of a K-means clustering algorithm [4] using clinical and laboratory variables chosen on the basis of the initial analyses. The relationships between clusters were analyzed using a single linkage method utilizing Euclidean distances [4].

RESULTS AND DISCUSSION

In the initial analysis of data, a number of comparisons were made concerning the incidence of otitis media in various groups. Not surprisingly, the 328 patients had more attacks of otitis media than the controls $p < .001$. Patients who had had one or more attacks of bronchitis in the previous 12 months had more otitis media than controls ($p < .001$) as did patients who had had at least one attack of pneumonia ($p < .001$). Patients who had had more than 3 severe colds in the previous 12 months also had more attacks of otitis media than controls ($p < .001$).

On the other hand, a difference could not be demonstrated ($p > .05$) in the incidence of otitis media when patients with pneumonia were compared with those with bronchitis, when patients with a family history of allergy were compared with those without a family history of allergy, when patients with greater than 4 severe colds and a family history of allergy were compared with patients with greater than 4 severe colds but without a family history of allergy. There was also no difference in the incidence of otitis media in controls with a family history of allergy and controls without a family history of allergy.

The ages of the subgroups of patients with otitis media as a major problem and whether or not the otitis media was perforating are shown in Figure 1. There appears to be a bivariate distribution divided at about 5 years of age, so a division at 5 years was made in some of the analyses. The mean number of attacks at each age is shown in Figure 2.

Figure 3 shows the differences between groups for 9 features of clinical or laboratory data.

In general, patients with otitis media have more severe colds (URTI) than controls. This is most marked in the groups of patients whose major problem is otitis media without perforation (OM−). It is also this group of patients who have more bronchitis than controls.

All groups of patients with otitis media have a higher incidence and degree of family history of allergy

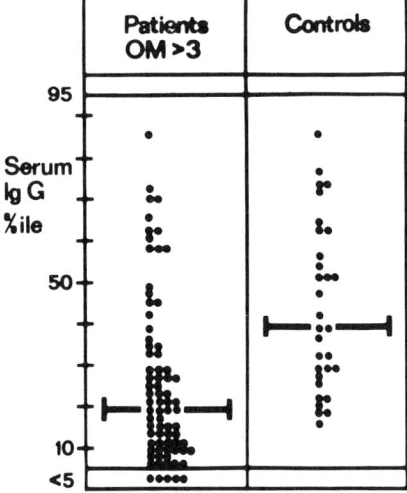

Fig. 4. Comparison between serum IgG percentiles of patients with otitis media and controls.

compared with controls but only the younger patients with OM− have a significantly increased family history of infections. All groups of patients have lower IgG percentiles than controls, and all but the older children with OM− have lower IgM percentiles than controls. The younger patients have lower IgE levels than controls. Opsonins to *Candida albicans* and antistreptolysin O titers (ASOT) were lower in the younger patients. In the older patients there was a difference in IgM levels in that patients with OM+ had lower levels than those with OM−. The serum IgG percentiles are compared between all the patients and the controls in Figure 4.

The group of patients with otitis media described above were then analyzed by a K-means clustering algorithm. The variables used were those shown at the left-hand side of Figures 5–7. These variables were chosen as they appeared from earlier analysis to be those most likely to produce discrimination.

Twenty-four clusters were described by the algorithm but those containing fewer than three members were excluded from the figures. The diagrams give an indication of the importance of the factors used to distinguish each cluster. Thus by examining clusters 1 and 2 one can see that the mean numbers of OM− in both clusters were high, though higher in cluster 2. Both clusters had low IgG, IgA, and IgM percentiles, though cluster 2 was lower for IgG and IgM. The major difference between the clusters is that cluster 1 has a higher family history of allergy than cluster 2, whose members have more severe colds (URTI) than cluster 1. All but two of the controls were allocated into clusters 13, 14, 15, or 16. The difference in these clusters is based on the different patterns of serum Igs.

As further exploration of this type of data handling, we examined the relationship between each of the clusters of patients using a single linkage algorithm. The results are shown in Figure 8 as a taxonomic tree.

While none of the clusters is very close to any other cluster (the diameter of even the most alike clusters is large), which is to be expected following the previous manipulation of the data, there are some relationships of interest. Thus, clusters 13–15

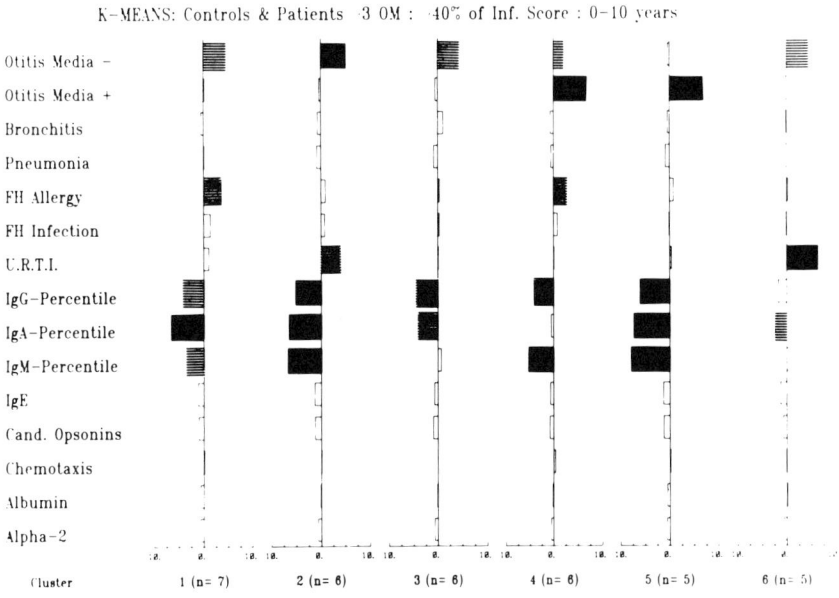

Fig. 5. Results of K-means clustering on patients and controls. The distance that the mean weighted Z scores for the cluster differ from the control means are indicated by the length and direction of the blocks.

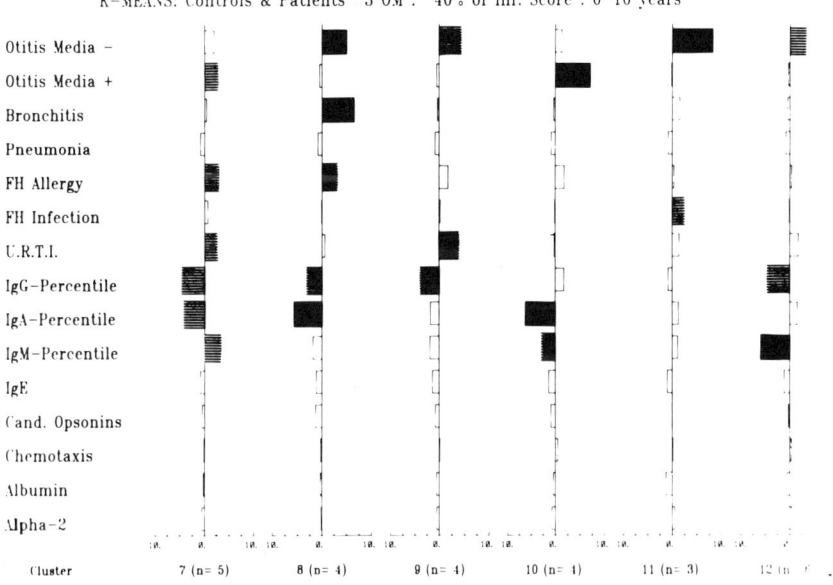

Fig. 6. Results of K-means clustering on patients and controls. The distance that the mean weighted Z scores for the cluster differ from the control means are indicated by the length and direction of the blocks.

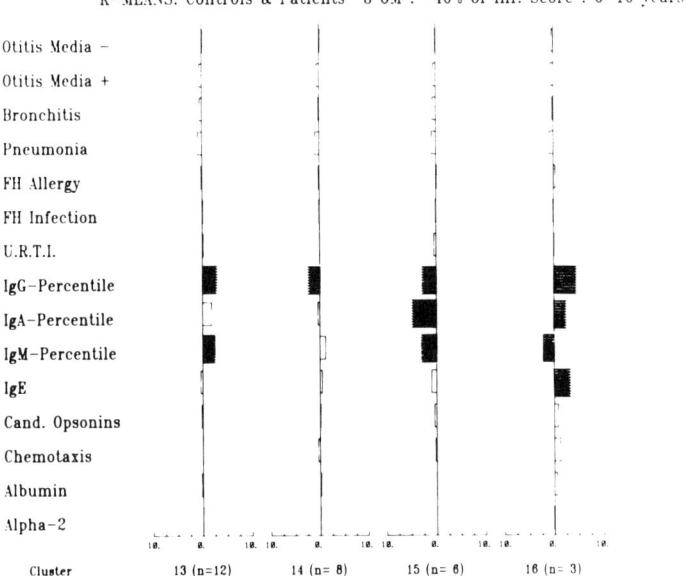

Fig. 7. Results of K-means clustering on patients and controls. The distance that the mean weighted Z scores for the cluster differ from the control means are indicated by the length and direction of the blocks.

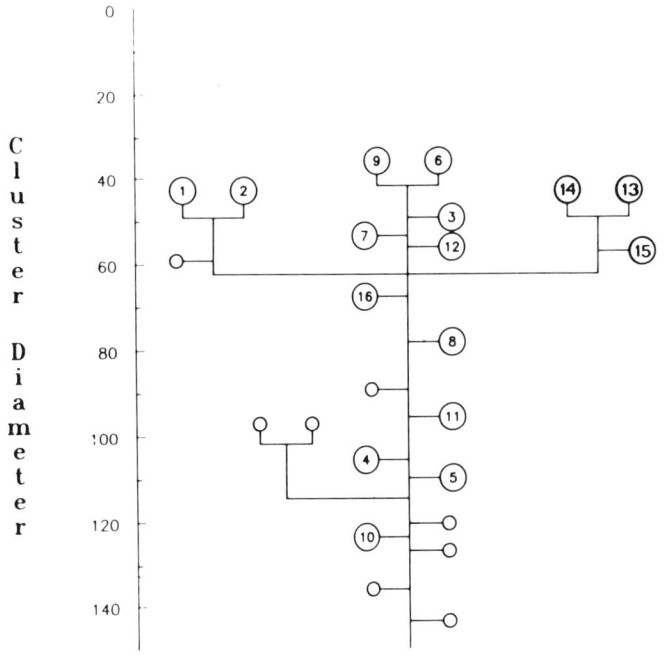

Fig. 8. Single linkage cluster analysis applied to the clusters defined by K-means.

which contain the majority of the controls form a small subcluster. Clusters 1 and 2 which differ mainly in the family history of allergy and the number of severe colds fall close to one another. Clusters 6 and 9 whose members have only moderate differences in the number of severe colds and IgG, IgA, and IgM percentiles are the most alike clusters.

CONCLUSIONS

These techniques have permitted a much closer look at both otitis media as it occurs as part of the syndrome of children with recurrent infections and also as it occurs in children in a Western society who have recurrent otitis media as a major problem.

The most important element that is lacking in this analysis is an assessment of outcome and/or of the effects of treatment on these groups. Long-term follow-up will demonstrate whether there is clinical usefulness in this approach. If it can be shown that patients in one cluster improve while those in another cluster deteriorate, then more rational and perhaps radical decisions can be made about treatment in some patients.

REFERENCES

1. Hope-Simpson RE, Miller DL: The definition of acute respiratory illness in general practice. Postgrad Med J 49:763–770, 1973.
2. Hosking CS, Fitzgerald MG, Shelton MJ: The immunological investigation of children with recurrent infections. Aust Paediatr J 13(Suppl):56–60, 1977.
3. Hosking CS, Roberton DM: The diagnostic approach to recurrent infections in childhood. In "The Assessment of Immunocompetence." Vol 1, no. 3 of Clinics in Immunology & Allergy. London: Webster ADB Saunders Company Ltd, 1981.
4. Hartigan JA: "Clustering Algorithms." New York: J Wiley & Sons, 1975.

Immunization Reactions and Immunodeficiency

John F. Soothill, FRCP, and J.A. Dudgeon, MD

Department of Immunology, Institute of Child Health, London WC1N 1EH (J.F.S.), and Department of Microbiology, Hospital for Sick Children, London WC1 (J.A.D), England

Immunization may be followed by a number of illnesses, local or general; of the latter, some may rarely be severe, involving permanent brain damage. Recent studies show that though rare, these are significantly associated with the immunization, particularly diphtheria, tetanus, and pertussis vaccine [1]. Such reactions have received much publicity in Britain in the last 10 years, leading to parental and medical refusal to accept immunization, especially pertussis. This has been followed by a pertussis epidemic with several deaths, and our first recent diphtheria death.

Patients with SCID, given certain live vaccines (smallpox vaccine and BCG), may get disseminated infections which may be fatal [2,3] and may also develop hemolytic uremia syndrome following killed vaccines, perhaps because of failure to clear endotoxin [4]. Patients with Ig deficiency may continue to excrete the live polio vaccine virus in their feces for many months; it regains its neurotoxicity [5] and possibly may cause paralysis in them and others [6].

Though most of these adverse effects result from the failure to eliminate attenuated organisms, some of these reactions may be immunopathologic. Immunodeficiency (ID) is one predisposing factor for immunopathology induced by killed antigen in experimental animals, since common polygenically inherited low-affinity antibody response and defective antigen clearance predisposes to nephritis [7-9]; but we know of only one study of ID in patients presenting with abnormal responses to immunization and this concerns dissemination of a live vaccine. Chandra et al [10] reported that patients who developed disseminated nonprogressive vaccinia, following the use of an unusual, perhaps rather virulent, strain of smallpox vaccine, had relative Ig deficiency, especially of IgM. However, a remarkable patient pointed the way. A perfectly healthy 16-year-old man (*Patient 1*, Table 1) wanted to join the Royal Air Force Officer training scheme, as a pilot, but his parents declined to consent to smallpox vaccination because an aunt and an uncle had died following it, and he had had some vague general symptoms during a cautious incomplete immunization program. Very low Igs G and A, with IgM at the lower limit of normal, were found, so we saw him in 1976. His blood count, PHA response, E rosettes, and number of lymphocytes with surface Ig were normal, and he makes antibodies. Despite a further fall in Ig levels, he remains perfectly well, apart from a possible slight excess of upper respiratory infections (URI), herpes zoster (having had varicella), and measles (diagnosed twice).

After that, we measured Ig in all of the 8 patients who had since consulted us for advice on immunization because of a history of adverse reaction in relatives or in themselves. All but 2 had more than one relative affected (Table 1). All but one had abnormal Ig concentrations (Table 2). The exception (*Patient 2*) was the older of 2 brothers, the younger of whom (*Patient 3*) had relative IgA deficiency, which was transient. All were symptomless when they first saw us, but 4 subsequently developed an excess of URI and otitis; one was given prophylactic Septrin (Table 3). Though the ID of 4 of the patients was transient, 4 remained clearly deficient throughout the follow-up (Table 3). Apart from high IgE in *Patients 2* and *8*, and unusually high antitetanus antibody response after a low dose of vaccine (*Patient 3*), other immunologic tests were normal; these included, blood count (in 8), allergy skin tests (5), PHA (3), hemolytic complement (3), C3 (3), and yeast opsonization (5).

Patient 1 received all routine vaccines apart from smallpox, *Patient 3* received all except pertussis, and *Patient 2* received oral polio vaccine only. Only vague general symptoms (*Patient 1*) and local symptoms (*Patients 2* and *3*) occurred.

The detection of abnormality in all but one of the 9 patients, presenting when well largely because of their relatives' illness, must partly be influenced by chance, but the association of familial immunization reactions with ID, often transient, seems clear. If most are transient, the phenomenon may well be undetectable retrospectively in those who have been severely damaged. The avoidance of damage in the patients studied could have been due to the modified immunization regimens, or to the development of new vaccines, but, since the mechanism of the reaction is unknown, we cannot say whether the changes would have reduced the reactions.

Clearly this preliminary study needs extensive confirmation, but these findings can already influence our policy for immunization. Severe reactions leading to chronic brain damage are very rare in previously

TABLE 1. Family History of Reactions to Immunizations of Relatives of 9 Infants and Children

Patient	Age	Who Reacted	To What*	How
1	16	aunt, uncle,	V	died
		self	T (5)	vague, general
2 } brothers	3¾	self, brother,	DT (2)	local
		mother,	P	fit
		aunt	T	local swelling
3 }	1¼	self, brother	T (1)	local
4	2	father,	T (4)	swelling
		mother	DT (1)	rash & swelling
5	1	self	DT (1)	local
6	¾	2 uncles	? DPT (1)	fever, delirium, mental defect, facial palsy (1)
7	¾	half brother	DPT (1)	fit
		half brother	DPT (1)	fit, developmental delay
		great-uncle	D (early)	died
8	¾	father	DPT (2)	fever & swelling
		great-uncle, great-aunt, 2nd cousin	?	?
9	½	aunt	DPT (1)	fits, dementia

*Vaccines: V=smallpox; T=tetanus; D=diphtheria; P=pertussis. Number of dose of vaccine is indicated in parentheses; ?=unknown or uncertain.

TABLE 2. IgG, IgA, and IgM Concentrations When First Seen in 9 Infants and Children With a Family History of Reaction to Immunization

Patient	Age	IgG IU/ml (mg%)	IgA IU/ml (mg%)	IgM IU/ml (mg%)
1	16	19 (152)	<u>≤3 (<4)</u>	66 (56)
2 } brothers	3¾	152 (1220)	66 (92)	134 (114)
3 }	1¼	81 (650)	<u>10 (14)</u>	**51 (43)**
4	2	80 (640)	<u>19 (27)</u>	36 (31)
5	1	53 (420)	<u>8 (11)</u>	**56 (48)**
6	¾	<u>17 (140)</u>	<u>8 (11)</u>	<u>38 (32)</u>
7	¾	<u>25 (200)</u>	<u>3 (4)</u>	73 (62)
8	¾	<u>33 (260)</u>	36 (50)	<u>42 (36)</u>
9	½	<u>38 (300)</u>	<u>8 (11)</u>	<u>44 (37)</u>

Underlined values are below age-matched control values (log mean-2SD) and bold values are at the lower limit.

TABLE 3. Follow-Up Ig Results (maximum period 5 years) in Children With a Family History of Reaction to Immunization

Patient	IgG	IgA	IgM	Excess infection
1	→	→	↘	? minor URI
2	(→)	(→)	(→)	—
3	(→)	(↑)	(→)	—
4	(→)	(↑)	(↑)	—
5	(→)	↗	↗	—
6	↗	→	(↑)	URI, otitis
7	↗	↗	↘	? URI, otitis
8	(↑)	(↑)	(↑)	URI, otitis, deaf, Septrin
9	(↑)	(↘↑)	(↑)	Otitis

Key: →=unchanged; ↑=rise to normal for age; ↗=rise, not normal for age; ↘=fall; ( )=normal for age.

healthy children (about 1 in 110,000 injections of triple vaccine [1]). This alone suggests that the fault lies in the child rather than the vaccine, but our data provide positive support for this view. Similar, and other chronic disabilities, and death, are associated with pertussis, and with the other infections against which we immunize. In an ideal world we would identify the vulnerable child, and not immunize him, because he could depend on the herd immunity achieved in his peers. However, with immunization rates so low that epidemics still occur, it is likely that the natural disease would be a much greater risk than the immunization in the vulnerable child, so even he is probably safer with the vaccine than without, and there is probably no risk to the vast majority. Ig measurements might be used to identify the vulnerable, but clearly only a few of those who are deficient have trouble with modern vaccines (an interaction with a coincidental infection, and the role of artificial feeding should be considered). Our data provided no evidence that the commonest minor ID, the yeast opsonization defect, contributed to this problem, but it is likely that other defects may play a part. The observation on the individual is therefore probably not important, but as with the interaction of immunodeficiency, infant feeding, and atopic allergy [11], the demonstration of the immunologic heterogeneity of man, especially relevant in infancy, leads to more rational infant care.

REFERENCES

1. Miller DL, Ross EM, Alderslade R, Bellman MH, Rawson NSB: Pertussis immunisation and serious acute neurological illness in children. Br Med J 282:1595, 1981.
2. Fulginiti VA, Kempe CH, Hathaway WE, Pearlman DS, Sieber OF Jr, Eller JJ, Joyner JJ Sr, Robinson A: Progressive vaccinia in immunologically deficient individuals. In Bergsma D (ed): "Immunologic Deficiency Diseases in Man." New York: The National Foundation, BD:OAS IV(1):129–145, 1968.

3. Bouton MJ, Mainwaring D, Smithells RW: BCG dissemination in congenital hypogammaglobulinaemia. Br Med J 11:1512, 1963.
4. M.R.C. Report on Hypogammaglobulinaemia in the United Kingdom (1971). MRC Special Report Series 310, H.M.S.O., London.
5. Hitzig WH, Biro Z, Bosch H, Huser HJ: Agammaglobulinaemie und Alymphozytose mit Schwund des lymphatischen Gewebes. Helv Paediatr Acta 13:551, 1958.
6. Wyatt HV: Poliomyelitis in hypogammaglobulinaemia. J Infect Dis 128:802, 1973.
7. Soothill JF, Steward MW: The immunopathological significance of the heterogeneity of antibody affinity. Clin Exp Immunol 9:193, 1971.
8. Alpers JH, Steward MW, Soothill JF: Differences in immune elimination in inbred mice. The role of low affinity antibody. Clin Exp Immunol 12:121, 1972.
9. Devey M, Steward MW: The induction of chronic antigen-antibody complex disease in selectively bred mice producing either high or low affinity antibody to protein antigens. Immunology 41:303, 1980.
10. Chandra RK, Kaveramma B, Soothill JF: Generalized non-progressive vaccinia associated with IgM deficiency. Lancet 1:687, 1969.
11. Soothill JF: The atopic child. In Soothill JF, Hayward AR, Wood CBS (eds): "Paediatric Immunology." London: Blackwell Scientific Publications, 1983.

SECTION 6
SUMMARY

PRIMARY IMMUNODEFICIENCY DISEASES*

INTRODUCTION

Immunity results from many complex interacting mechanisms. The skin and mucous membranes are nonspecific barriers to infection. There are numerous other nonspecific factors such as complement or interferon. Many of these nonspecific factors act in conjunction with specific immunity mechanisms. Deficiency of an immunity mechanism may involve specific factors such as antibody or lymphocytes, or nonspecific factors such as a complement component. In any case, the deficiency results in some failure of the inflammatory response and more or less severe, but repeated, bacterial, fungal and viral infections ensue as a consequence.

Both primary and secondary deficits in immunity may lead to the same clinical spectrum of disease. Malignancy, malnutrition, cytotoxic drugs, and a variety of pathologic conditions and metabolic diseases may all lead to secondary immunodeficiency. Furthermore, the relationship between immunity and infection is a complex one: infection may cause, as well as result from, immunodeficiency (ID). A variety of infectious agents can cause both specific and nonspecific ID.

During the past decade, knowledge of the immune response has expanded rapidly as a result of experimental work in animals and the study of human patients with both primary and nonspecific IDs. Because of this progress, the primary IDs can now be further classified in part on the basis of the ontogeny of cells that interact to create the immune response and various genetic and biochemical factors that influence these cells.

CELLULAR BASIS OF THE IMMUNE RESPONSE

The progenitors of T cells and B cells are derived from multipotent hematopoietic stem cells (HSC). Cells of the monocyte-macrophage series and other antigen presenting cells, important collaborators in the immune responses of T and B cells, are also derived from the HSC (see Fig. 1).

Within the thymus, bone marrow-precursor cells are induced by epithelial cell interaction to begin dividing and to express T-cell characteristics which include surface glycoproteins that can serve as differentiation markers. Following migration to peripheral tissues, T-cell differentiation continues to be influenced by thymic hormones. The best known subpopulations of peripheral T cells are helpers (Th) and suppressors or cytotoxic cells (Ts); other functionally distinct subclasses or sublines of T cells also exist. The developmental level at which T-cell subclass diversification occurs has not been precisely defined.

The development of B cells begins within fetal liver and thereafter in bone marrow. Precursor cells give rise to a rapidly dividing population of pre-B cells that produce cytoplasmic μ-heavy chains, but lack immunoglobulin receptors on their surface. Many of the major decisions on the selection of immunoglobulin genes to be expressed by sublines of B cells are made at this level of differentiation. Immature surface immunoglobulin bearing (SIg) B lymphocytes, already committed with regard to the specificity of the antibodies that they and their plasma cell progeny will subsequently synthesize and secrete, represent the next stage of differentiation and express $SIgM^+$. The immature $SIgM^+$ lymphocytes, easily rendered immunologically tolerant, are critical to the ontogenic expression of Ig class (isotype) diversity. Most B cells acquire SIgD with further maturation. One of the subclasses of IgG or IgA is expressed in sequence on separate subpopulations of $SIgM^+ IgD^+$ cells. The SIgM and SIgD are lost at a later stage in differentiation of these B-cell sublines. During this process of isotype diversification, B lymphocytes acquire other cell surface receptors (eg for C3, IgG and T-cell factors) that allow them to respond to antigens and T-cell help by division and terminal plasma cell differentiation.

The initiation and completion of specific immune responses involve a complex series of genetically restricted interactions between antigen presenting cells and T-cell subpopulations for cell-mediated immunity (CMI), and between these cells and B cells for antibody response. The Th and Ts cells exert positive and negative regulatory effects, respectively, on B-cell responses. In turn, IgM and IgG antibodies may affect the activities of functionally distinct subpopulations of T cells through specific Fc receptors.

---

*This Summary was prepared by a scientific group on Immunodeficiency sponsored by the WHO, which met subsequent to the Workshop. In preparing the report for the WHO, extensive use was made of the WHO Technical Report Series 630, "Immunodeficiency" (WHO Geneva 1978), which in turn was derived from the "Meeting Report on Primary Immunodeficiency Diseases in Man," *Clinical Immunology and Immunopathology*, 2:415–445, 1974. This report will appear in the *Journal of Clinical Immunology and Immunopathology* 28(3), 1983, and is reprinted here with permission of Academic Press, Inc.

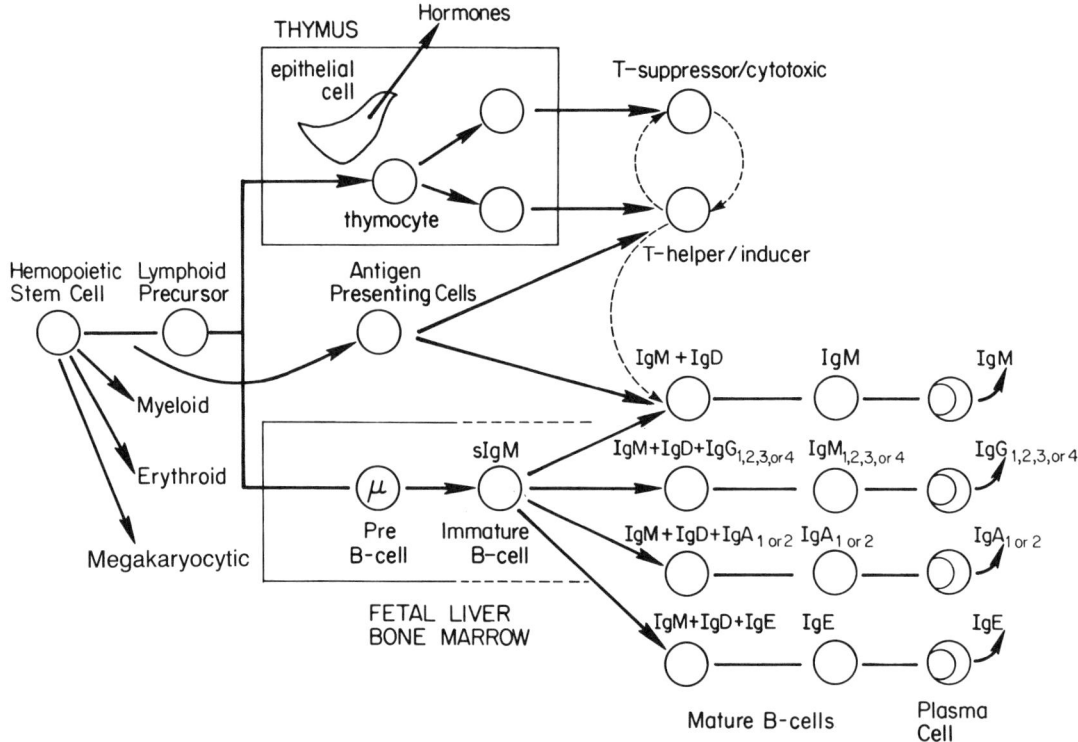

Figure 1.

TESTS FOR ASSESSING IMMUNITY

Immunoglobulins and Antibodies

Measurement of immunoglobulin concentration.

Serum immunoglobulins may be measured by single radial diffusion, double diffusion in agar gel, immunoelectrodiffusion, radioimmunoassay, enzyme-linked immunoassay (ELISA), and automated laser nephelometry. Electrophoresis is not a satisfactory technique for the measurement of immunoglobulins: gross immunoglobulin deficiencies may be obscured by this technique. Immunoglobulin can also be measured in body secretions, eg saliva, tears, and milk. Discrepancies in results have arisen from the use of different standards by different laboratories. WHO now makes available reference preparations for the 5 classes of human serum immunoglobulins,* and it is recommended that these be used. The source of antisera is also an important factor. Goat or sheep antisera may give spuriously high estimates for serum IgA in patients with selective IgA deficiency who have circulating antibodies to ruminant proteins. IgA levels in such patients should be assayed with antisera produced in nonruminant species such as the rabbit or horse.

Concentrations of immunoglobulins cannot be used as the sole criteria for the diagnosis of primary ID. Serum immunoglobulin concentrations vary with age and environment; thus, appropriate local age-related norms must be used. Since the concentration of immunoglobulin is the net result of synthesis, breakdown, and loss, interpretation of immunoglobulin levels must also take these factors into account. An indication of loss may be obtained by measuring serum albumin. Limited heterogeneity of immunoglobulins and abnormal kappa-lambda light-chain ratios may be indicative of ID syndromes. Normal immunoglobulin concentrations do not exclude antibody deficiency, and responses to antigenic stimulation should be tested if ID is strongly suspected. Failure to respond to one or more antigens has been observed in patients with normal or high levels of all immunoglobulins, and in patients with isolated immunoglobulin deficiencies.

Assessment of antibody formation following immunization.

Humoral immunity may be assessed by antibody responses to antigens to which the population is com-

---

*Obtainable through: Dr. David Rowe, WHO, Geneva.

monly exposed, or following active immunization. Protein or polysaccharide antigen may be used. Live vaccines (BCG, and vaccines for smallpox, poliomyelitis, measles, rubella, mumps) should never be given when primary or severe secondary ID is suspected.

The following tests are recommended:

1. "Natural" antibodies: A and B isohemagglutinins, heteroagglutinins and heterolysins (eg against sheep or rabbit red cells), antistreptolysin and bactericidal antibodies against *Escherichia coli*.

2. Antibody response to usual immunization.

a) In unimmunized children, commercial diphtheria/tetanus (DT) vaccine may be given in recommended doses. Blood is taken 2 weeks after each injection and tetanus antibodies determined. A Schick test is performed. Three doses of killed poliomyelitis vaccine (1.0 ml intramuscularly, at intervals of 2 weeks) can also be used; blood is taken 2 weeks after the last injection and antibody determined, usually by virus neutralization.

b) In patients who have been immunized with DT or diphtheria/pertussis/tetanus (DPT) vaccine, one booster injection is given, followed by determination of antibodies and performance of a Schick test.

3. Additional active immunizations that may be recommended:

a) Bacteriophage ϕX 174 has been shown to be a potent, safe, and useful antigen; it allows measurement of antigen clearance and primary and secondary immune responses.[a]

b) Polyribose phosphate *Hemophilus influenza* polysaccharide is also a potent and harmless antigen. A single dose (0.05 mg subcutaneously) is sufficient to immunize a healthy person. Blood is drawn after 2 weeks, and antibody is determined.[b] This and other polysaccharide antigens should not be used in infants under one year of age, particularly when ID is suspected.

Other useful antigens include:
(i) Monomeric flagellin[c]
(ii) Pneumococcal polysaccharide (Pneumovax)[d]
(iii) Vi antigen
(iv) Keyhole limpet hemocyanin (KLH).[e]

B lymphocytes.

Lymphocytes are usually isolated for assay from peripheral blood using density gradients such as Ficoll-Hypaque. Tests for B lymphocytes include detection of membrane-bound immunoglobulin, a receptor for Epstein-Barr virus (EBV), and B-cell antigens identified by antibodies. C3 and Fc receptors are not found exclusively on B cells, but also occur on monocytes and certain T cells. Latex particles and peroxidase may distinguish monocytes, an important control because they also bind autologous and heterologous IgG and complement.

B cells may be counted by the use of fluorescein-labeled antibody. The isolated lymphocytes are incubated at 37°C for 45 min and then are incubated with labeled rabbit Fab$_2$ antibody fragments or with intact goat antibodies to the heavy or light chain determinants to be studied. Fluores-

---

[b]This requires special facilities: the antigen and antibody determinations may be arranged by writing to Dr. F.S. Rosen, Department of Pediatrics, Children's Hospital Medical Center, Boston, MA 02115, USA.

[c]Obtainable from Dr. I.R. Mackay, Walter and Eliza Hall Institute of Medical Research, Melbourne, Victoria 3050, Australia.

[d]Obtainable from Dr. G. Schiffman, Downstate Medical Center, 450 Clarkson Avenue, Brooklyn, NY 11203, USA.

[e]Obtainable from Sigma Chemical Co., P.O. Box 14508, St. Louis, MO 63178, USA; or Calbiochem-Behring, P.O. Box 12087, San Diego, CA 92112, USA.

cein and rhodamine labels are commonly used. After thorough washing of the lymphocytes in protein solution, the cells are examined under a fluorescence microscope, preferably equipped with epi-illumination. Fluorescent spots or crescents on lymphocytes indicate the presence of surface immunoglobulins in high density. If initial incubation at warm temperature is not performed or if intact rabbit antibodies are fluorescein-labeled, spuriously high estimates for the B-cell percentage may be obtained from IgG binding by the receptors of other cell types.

Pre-B cells may be identified among bone marrow cells with purified fluorochrome-labeled antibodies to μ-heavy chains. Pre-B cells are large-to-small lymphocytes without demonstrable surface immunoglobulins but with small quantities of cytoplasmic μ-heavy chain.

EBV receptors on B cells may be detected with fluorescein-labeled human antisera directed toward EBV after incubation of B cells with this virus.

Cell-Mediated Immunity

A number of tests are commonly employed for assessing CMI, including: a) delayed-type skin reactions; b) enumeration of T cells and T-cell subsets; c) in vitro stimulation of lymphocytes to proliferate and form blast cells; d) other in vitro tests of T-cell function.

Skin-testing.

Delayed cutaneous hypersensitivity (DCH) is a localized immunologic skin response: the prototype is the tuberculin skin test. Because DCH is dependent on functional thymus-derived lymphocytes (T lymphocytes), it is used in screening for immunodeficiency. Antigens generally used are: mumps, trichophyton, purified protein derivative (PPD), Candida or Monilia, streptokinase-streptodornase (SK-SD), tetanus toxoid, and diphtheria. To ascertain defective CMI several antigens must be

---

[a]These determinations require special facilities and can be arranged by writing to Dr. R.J. Wedgwood or Dr. H.D. Ochs, Department of Pediatrics RD-20, University of Washington, Seattle, WA 98195, USA.

used. All skin tests are by intradermal injection of 0.1 ml of antigen into the volar aspect of the forearm with the needle introduced in a transverse axis, and should be read in 48–72 hours for the maximal diameter of induration.

1. Tuberculin: 0.1 ml containing 10 IU of Tween-stabilized soluble PPD. If negative, the test should be repeated using 50 IU.
2. Candida or Monilia:[a] Initially test at 1:100 dilution.[*] If no reaction, test at 1:10 dilution.[*]
3. Trichophyton:[b] Use at 1:30 dilution.[*]
4. Streptokinase-streptodornase (SK-SD):[c] In patients under 10 years of age, SK-SD test initially with 40 units of streptokinase. If negative, repeat, using 100 units. In patients 10 years or older, use 4 units; if negative, 40 units. If still negative, 100 units of streptokinase.[*]
5. Mumps:[d] Use undiluted; read at 6–8 hours for early Arthus reaction (antibody-mediated) and then at 48 hours for DCH.
6. Tetanus and diphtheria toxoid:[e] Use at 1:100 dilution.[*]

A positive skin test is defined by induration greater than or equal to 5 mm of induration, and indicates intact CMI. Erythema is *not* an indication of DCH.

---

[*]DILUTIONS - Make all dilutions in Hollister-Stier buffered saline; make up fresh every two months; store at 4°C.

[a]Undiluted glycerin-free Dermatophytin O, Hollister-Stier Labs, Box 3145 Terminal Annex, Spokane, WA, USA.

[b]Dermatophytin (Trichophyton), Hollister-Stier Labs.

[c]Streptokinase-streptodornase (Varidase), Lederle Labs, Pearl River, NY 10965, USA.

[d]Mumps skin test, Eli Lilly and Company, Indianapolis, IN 46206, USA.

[e]Pediatric diphtheria and tetanus toxoid, Wyeth Laboratories, P.O. Box 8299, Philadelphia, PA 19101, USA.

T lymphocytes.

T cells may be counted by the sheep-red cell rosette method or by the use of monoclonal antibody immunofluorescence. Monoclonal antibodies may be used to estimate the ratio of T helper (Th) to T suppressor (Ts) cells.

In vitro stimulation of lymphocytes.

Lymphocytes transform in the presence of a) nonspecific mitogens such as phytohemagglutinin (PHA), pokeweed mitogen (PWM), or concanavalin A (Con A); b) antigens such as PPD, candidin, SK-SD, tetanus and diphtheria, if the patient has had prior encounter with the antigen; c) allogeneic cells.

The cell response is assayed by ^{3}H- or ^{14}C-labeled thymidine incorporation for 16–24 hours, followed by DNA extraction techniques or cell precipitation on filter paper and subsequent liquid scintillation counting. Control values of unstimulated cultures vary from person to person and from day to day. Data on unstimulated and stimulated cultures should always be given and control cells from at least 2 healthy people should be tested simultaneously. All cultures should be performed in triplicate. Interpretation of mitogenic responses to various stimuli must be made with caution as to the type of responding cells. Soluble PHA and Con A require the presence of T cells; under certain conditions, however, such as when bound to particulate matter, they may also stimulate B cells. PWM stimulates a response in both T and B cells, although T cells must be present for the B cells to be stimulated. The mixed lymphocyte reaction (MLR) results from T-cell reactivity to antigen displayed on B cells and monocytes. It should be noted that, when normal irradiated or mitomycin C-treated lymphocytes are the stimulators of an MLR, the normal T cells in the culture may secrete factors inducing blastogenesis in the patient's lymphocytes. Therefore, it is preferable to use B-cell lines or T-cell depleted normal cells as the stimulators.

Assays for helper and suppressor T-cell activity.

Several research laboratories have developed antigen-specific and nonspecific assays for Th and Ts activity. A description of the details of any specific approach is beyond the scope of this report.

MORPHOLOGY AND HEMATOLOGY

Histologic and cytologic examination of lymphoid tissue and blood lymphocyte counts are useful for the diagnosis of ID. In addition, postmortem examination of thymus and lymphoid tissue may permit diagnosis of a potentially familial defect, important for genetic counseling and for understanding the pathogenesis of ID.

Peripheral Blood

A total lymphocyte count is a useful screening test for primary ID. The majority of patients with severe combined ID (SCID) and thymic hypoplasia have a persistently low total lymphocyte count (less than 1×10^9/L or 1000/mm^3). However, lymphopenia can also be secondary to viral infections, malnutrition, gastrointestinal loss, and autoimmune diseases. Normal lymphocyte counts do not exclude the diagnosis of SCID. Variable lymphocyte counts have been observed in other forms of ID. Blood monocytes should also be enumerated, employing several histochemical tests for metabolic function and inclusions. Thrombocytopenia and small platelets in a male infant should arouse the suspicion of the presence of the Wiskott-Aldrich syndrome. Anemia is present in some patients with ID. Coombs-positive hemolytic anemia is associated with many forms of ID. Hypoplastic anemia has been described in 2 patients with polynucleotide phosphorylase defect. Transcobalamin 2 (TC 2) deficiencies are invariably associated with megaloblastic anemia.

Bone Marrow

Bone marrow aspiration (for assessment of the presence of plasma cells and pre-B cells) may be important in the evaluation of ID.

Rectal and Intestinal Biopsy

Examination of rectal tissue for plasma cells and lymphoid cells by histologic and immunohistologic methods is useful in patients with common varied ID and selective IgA deficiency. Lymphoid cells are present in rectal and intestinal biopsies in normal infants only at 15-20 days of age. The immunofluorescent study of secretory component is helpful for the diagnosis of secretory component deficiency. Sometimes *Giardia lamblia* can be found only by intestinal biopsy.

Skin Biopsy

Biopsy of this tissue is useful to establish a diagnosis of graft-vs-host (GVH) reaction in patients with SCID after blood transfusion, bone marrow and fetal tissue transplantation, or from transfer of lymphocytes into the immunodeficient fetus in utero.

Lymph Nodes

Lymph node biopsy is not necessary to establish a diagnosis of ID, but can be important in classification. Rapid enlargement of lymph nodes in patients with ID is an indication for a biopsy. If lymph node biopsies are performed, the biopsy should be done 5-7 days after local antigenic stimulation by diphtheria and tetanus toxoids. A biopsy of a lymph node draining the location can then be performed. The criteria for morphologic assessment of the lymphoid tissue published by WHO* should always

---
*Bulletin of the World Health Organization 47:257, 1972.

be used in describing the tissues. Lymph nodes of patients with SCID involving both T and B cells are characterized by a completely disorganized architecture, without any distinction between cortical and paracortical areas; the medullary cords are absent. Germinal centers are absent and follicles are only rudimentary. There are very few lymphoid cells and no plasma cells. Only stromal cells, monocytes, and histiocytes are present. Lymph nodes of patients with SCID with B cells and thymic hypoplasia show a similar pattern, but there are more lymphoid cells in cortical areas. Follicles are present in some patients, but there are very few lymphocytes in the so-called T-dependent areas. Lymph node biopsies are potentially hazardous in SCID, heal poorly, and may produce a portal of entry for infection. When tonsillar tissue is available, its histologic examination can assist definition of ID.

Thymus

Thymic biopsy may be difficult and should be performed in children with ID only by skilled surgeons in special situations. The morphology of the thymus is important for the diagnosis of certain forms of SCID. The embryonal pattern of lymphoid disorganization and developmental failure has been described extensively; some of the pathologic features may not reflect thymic abnormality per se, but rather the lack of normal T cells which may be necessary for normal thymic development. Thymic biopsy tissue may be very useful in studying the capacity of thymic epithelium to sustain lymphoid development, and for planning therapeutic strategies. Serial sections of neck tissue at postmortem may be necessary to find small residua of normal thymus in otherwise athymic persons.

Chimerism

Chimerism (the occurrence in an individual of 2 genetically different cell lines) has been observed in different forms of SCID. The chimerism can be congenital or acquired. The former is due to intrauterine fetal implantation of maternal cells, while acquired chimerism can occur in SCID after blood transfusion, bone marrow transplantation, and fetal tissue implants. The presence and origin of lymphoid chimeric cells can be ascertained by karyotype, human leukocyte (HLA) or other antigenic typing, and MLC reaction.

Special Studies

Adenosine deaminase (ADA) and purine nucleoside phosphorylase (PNP) levels should be determined in all patients with possible SCID and T-cell deficiency, respectively. An assay of serum α-fetoprotein levels measured by sensitive radio immunoassay (RIA) may be of value in separating patients with ataxia telangiectasia (AT) from those with other neurologic disorders; it is raised (46-2,200 mg/L) in at least 95% of persons with AT. TC 2 deficiency must be suspected when there is megaloblastic anemia, with normal vitamin B_{12} concentrations and a lack of unsaturated vitamin B_{12}-binding capacity; TC 2 should be determined.

PRIMARY SPECIFIC IMMUNODEFICIENCY

Genetics

Inheritance is known for many of the primary specific IDs (Table 1). In addition, many of the so-called "late/adult onset" variable IDs are also genetically determined, although the exact mode of inheritance is unknown.

At least six distinct IDs are inherited in an X-linked pattern (Table 1 under 1, 2, 4, 17, 18). Autosomal recessive transmission is recognized in some groups of ID and in certain conditions with specific protein or enzyme deficiencies, such as deficiency of ADA, PNP, or TC 2. Autosomal dominant inheritance is seen in rare

TABLE 1. Primary Specific Immunodeficiencies
a) Predominantly Antibody Defects

Designation	Usual Phenotypic Expression					Presumed Pathogenesis/ Differentiation Defect	Inheritance
	Serum Ig	Serum Antibodies	Circulating B Cells	Circulating T Cells	CMI		
1. X-linked agammaglobulinemia	all isotypes decreased	decreased	usually absent	normal	normal	intrinsic defect pre-B to B-cell differentiation	X-linked
2. X-linked hypogammaglobulinemia with growth hormone deficiency*	all isotypes decreased	decreased	absent or very low	normal	normal	unknown: probably defect pre-B to B-cell differentiation	X-linked
3. Autosomal recessive agammaglobulinemia	all isotypes decreased	decreased	decreased	normal	normal	? intrinsic defect pre-B to B-cell differentiation	Autosomal recessive (AR)
4. Ig deficiency with increased IgM (and IgD)	A) IgM and IgD increased	IgM increased, other isotypes decreased	normal IgM and IgD bearing cells	normal	normal	intrinsic isotype switch defect; failure of IgM^+, IgD^+, B-cell maturation to IgG^+, IgA^+, IgE^+ B cells	X-linked or AR or autosomal dominant (AD) or unknown
	B) IgG and IgA decreased	IgG & IgA decreased	no IgG or IgA bearing cells	normal	normal		
5. IgA deficiency*	A) IgA_1, IgA_2 decreased	IgA decreased	immature SIgA B cells	usually normal	usually normal	defective IgA ($\pm$ IgG subclass) B-cell maturation. Intrinsic? Extrinsic (T cell)?	unknown: some AR, some AD (frequent in families with CVID)
	B) IgA_1, IgA_2, IgG_2 decreased with or without IgG_4 decrease	IgA & IgG decreased	immature SIgA B cells	normal	normal		
	C) IgA_1 or IgA_2 decreased	IgA_1 or IgA_2 decreased	immature SIgA B cells	normal	normal		
6. Selective deficiency of other Ig isotypes	decrease in IgM or $IgG_{1,2,3, or 4}$	decrease of the deficient isotype	?normal	normal	normal	differentiation defect of IgM B cell to isotype-specific plasma cell	unknown
7. κ-chain deficiency	Ig (κ) decreased	decreased	normal or decreased κ^+ B cells	normal	normal	unknown	unknown
8. Antibody deficiency with normal- or hyper-gammaglobulinemia	normal	decreased	near normal	normal	variable	B-cell differentiation defect: defective T-cell help	unknown
9. ID with thymoma*	all isotypes decreased	decreased	absent or very low	variable	variably decreased	unknown defect HSC to pre-B-cell maturation; (? excessive T-suppressor activity)	none
10. Transient hypogammaglobulinemia of infancy	IgG and IgA decreased	decreased	normal	decreased T-help	variable	IgG/IgA B cell to IgG/IgA plasma cell differentiation defect: delayed maturation of T-help, ? other	unknown (frequent in heterozygous individuals in families with SCID)

*Characteristic Associated Features:
  2. X-linked hypogammaglobulinemia with growth hormone deficiency: short stature.
  5. IgA deficiency: chromosomal defects in some patients.
  9. ID with thymoma: eosinopenia, erythroblastopenia, aplastic anemia (some).

b) Common Variable Immunodeficiency (CVID)

Designation	Usual Phenotypic Expression					Presumed Nature of Basic Defect	Inheritance
	Serum Ig	Serum Antibodies	Circulating B Cells	Circulating T Cells	CMI		
11. CVID with predominant B-cell defect:							
A) Near normal B-cell number with primarily $\mu^+ \delta^+$ without $\mu^+ \delta^-$, γ^+ or α^+ cells	decreased	decreased	near normal numbers but abnormal proportion of subtypes	variable	variable	intrinsic defect in cell differentiation of immature to mature B cells	unknown, AR, AD
B) Very low B-cell number	decreased	decreased	decreased	variable	variable	intrinsic defect in pre-B to B- cell maturation	unknown, AR, AD
C) $\mu^+ \gamma^+$ or γ^+ "nonsecretory" B cells with plasma cells	decreased	decreased	normal number but abnormal proportion of subtypes	normal	normal	intrinsic defect in B-cell maturation at plasma cell level; H-chain deletion	unknown
D) Normal or increased B-cell number with $\mu^+ \delta^+ \gamma^+$, $\mu^+ \delta^+ \alpha^+$, γ^+ and α^+ B cells	decreased	decreased	normal or increased	variable	variable	intrinsic defect in B-cell to plasma cell maturation	unknown
12. CVID with predominant immunoregulatory T-cell disorder:							
A) Deficiency of Th cells	decreased	decreased	normal	variable	variable	immunoregulatory T-cell disorder: defect in thymocyte to Th cell differentiation	unknown
B) Presence of activated Ts cells	decreased	decreased	normal	variable	variable	immunoregulatory T-cell disorder—cause unknown	unknown
13. CVID with autoantibodies to B cells or T cells*	decreased	decreased	decreased	decreased	variable	variable no differentiation defect known	unknown

*Characteristic Associated Features:
  13. Common variable immunodeficiency with autoantibodies to B cells or T cells; other autoimmune disorders.

cases of IgA deficiency. Many cases of ID not known to be heritable are clinically indistinguishable from inherited forms of the disease.

Early Diagnosis of Primary Specific Immunodeficiency

Diagnosis soon after birth is important because, where treatment is possible, it should be instituted before chronic damage has occurred. Early symptoms may include repeated or persistent infection (especially treatment-resistant thrush), failure to thrive, diarrhea, and eczema. The associated features of diagnostic value given in Table 1 may help in early diagnosis. A family history of immunodeficiency or infant death from infection, allergy, etc, should increase suspicion. Recognition of heterozygote carriers is of utmost importance for early diagnosis, as well as for sound genetic counseling. It is now possible for ADA, PNP, and TC 2. It is of interest that prolonged transient hypogammaglobulinemia of infancy has been observed in a number of ADA heterozygotes. Antenatal diagnosis, where possible, can assist family counseling, both in regard to abortion and to

c) Predominantly Cell-Mediated Immunity (CMI) Defects

Designation	Usual Phenotypic Expression					Presumed Nature of Basic Defect	Inheritance
	Serum Ig	Serum Antibodies	Circulating B Cells	Circulating T Cells	CMI		
14. Combined immunodeficiency (CID) with predominant T-cell defect	near normal or progressive decrease	decreased	normal	decreased	decreased	unknown: defect involves T-cell differentiation	unknown, AR
15. Purine nucleoside phosphorylase deficiency (PNP)*	normal	normal	normal	progressive decrease	progressive decrease	T-cell defect from toxic metabolites due to enzyme deficiency	AR
16. SCID with adenosine deaminase (ADA) deficiency*	decreased	decreased	decreased	decreased	decreased	T-cell (and B-cell) defects from toxic metabolites due to enzyme deficiency	AR
17. SCID*							
A) Reticular dysgenesis	decreased	decreased	decreased	decreased	decreased	defective differentiation of T and B cells; lymphomyeloid maturation defect	AR
B) Low T-B-cell numbers	decreased	decreased	decreased	decreased	decreased	lymphoid maturation defect of both T and B cells	AR or X-linked
C) Low T, normal B cell (Swiss)	decreased	decreased	normal	decreased	decreased	lymphoid maturation defect of both T and B cells	AR or X-linked
D) "Bare lymphocyte syndrome"	decreased	decreased	decreased	decreased	decreased	differentiation defect with lack of HLA determinants on T & B cells	AR
18. ID with unusual response to EBV*	decreased after EBV infection in some	decreased after EBV infection in some	decreased after EBV infection in most	normal	normal	unknown	X-linked or AR

*Characteristic Associated Features:
- 15. PNP: hypoplastic anemia; mental retardation (in some).
- 16. SCID with ADA deficiency: dysostosis (some).
- 17. SCID
  - A) Reticular dysgenesis: aplastic anemia (some); neutropenia; granulocytopenia.
  - B) Low T-B-cell numbers: dysostosis (some).
  - C) Low T, normal B cell (Swiss): dysostosis (some).
- 18. ID with unusual response to EBV: fatal EBV infection (some); aplastic anemia (some); lymphoproliferative disease (some).

early therapy. Reliable prenatal diagnosis of ADA and TC 2 deficiency can be made using amnion fibroblast cultures. SCID, ADA deficiency, AT, and various forms of chronic granulomatous disease (CGD) may be identified using fetal blood samples taken prior to 20 weeks of gestation. Sexing of fetuses may identify X-linked inherited diseases. Cord blood lymphocyte PHA responses and E-rosette tests may be abnormal in SCID. B cells bearing surface Ig may be absent in X-linked agammaglobulinemia.

Classification of Primary Specific Immunodeficiency States

Primary specific immunodeficiency results in failure to manifest an efficient antibody and/or cell-mediated response. The functional interaction of B and T cells and monocytes in the full expression of the immune response makes division of the primary immunodeficiency diseases solely on the basis of B- or T-cell abnormalities artificial. Nevertheless, the spectrum of these diseases may be usefully separated (see Tables 1a, 1b, 1c, 1d) into 4 general categories:

1a) Predominantly Antibody Defects;

d) ID Associated With Other Major Defects

Designation	Usual Phenotypic Expression					Presumed Nature of Basic Defect	Inheritance
	Serum Ig	Serum Antibodies	Circulating B Cells	Circulating T Cells	CMI		
19. Transcobalamin 2 deficiency*	all isotypes decreased	decreased	normal	normal	normal	defect in B12 transport resulting in defective cell proliferation; B-cell to plasma cell differentiation	AR
20. WAS*	increased IgA, IgE; decreased IgM	decreased	normal	progressive decrease	progressive decrease	cell membrane defect affecting all hematopoietic stem cell derivatives	X-linked
21. AT*	often decreased IgA, IgE, and IgG; increased IgM (monomers)	variably decreased	normal	decreased	decreased	unknown: defective T-cell maturation	AR
22. 3rd and 4th pouch/arch syndrome (DiGeorge)*	normal (?)	decreased	normal	decreased	decreased	embryopathy: abnormal thymus with resultant T-cell defects	none

*Characteristic Associated Features:
  19. TC 2 deficiency: pancytopenia with megaloblastic anemia; intestinal villous atrophy; defect in granulocytes, bactericidal activity.
  20. Wiskott-Aldrich syndrome: thrombocytopenia; eczema.
  21. Ataxia telangiectasia: cerebellar ataxia; telangiectasia; ovarian dysgenesis; chromosomal instability; decreased α-fetoprotein.
  22. 3rd and 4th pouch/arch syndrome (DiGeorge): hypoparathyroidism; cardiac outflow tract malformation; abnormal facies; mental retardation (some); GI tract malformation (some).

1b) Common Variable Immunodeficiency (CVID);
1c) Predominantly Cell-Mediated Immunity (CMI) Defects;
1d) ID Associated With Other Major Defects.

Although recent advances in immunobiology may permit a precise etiologic classification in the near future, at present the identification of diseases within these 3 general categories is best based upon the expression of 5 generally assessed immunologic attributes: type and amount of serum immunoglobulins, serum antibody levels, the nature and number of circulating B cells, the nature and number of circulating T cells, and T-cell function as expressed in cell-mediated immune responses. These attributes are identified in the classification schema presented in Table 1. Also presented is current opinion on the nature of the presumed level of faulty cell differentiation, utilizing the schematic model of cell development given in Figure 1. In many instances we have attempted to indicate the possible pathogenetic mechanism(s) involved. Where known, the nature of the basic defect, and the inheritance of the disorder is given. Since many immunodeficiencies have characteristic nonimmunologic associated features which may assist in diagnosis, these also have been indicated.

The fact that many defects of humoral immunity reflect regulatory T/B cell interactions emphasizes the combined nature of immunodeficiencies. The term "severe combined immunodeficiency" (SCID), however, should be restricted to those patients, usually infants, who have severe defects of both CMI and antibody deficiency. For those patients with defects predominantly of CMI with some antibody deficiency, we use the term "combined immunodeficiency" (CID).

SCID includes a broad spectrum of syndromes, most of which include thymic dysplasia. The heterogeneity, as now defined, depends on various factors such as defined enzymatic defects (eg ADA deficiency), mode of inheritance, and level of faulty cellular differentiation. Patients lacking both T and B cells are likely to have a genetic defect precluding normal stem cell differentiation. SCID with normal numbers of B cells (not infrequent) may reflect an early flaw in T-cell differentiation (eg due to an intrinsic abnormality or faulty induction by thymic epithelium), though the possibility of a defective lymphoid stem cell should not be discarded if the B lymphocytes fail to display normal Ig diversity.

The presence in infants of CMI deficiency and an embryonic thymus, but with normal circulating immunoglobulins, has been called the "Nezelof syndrome." There has been no consistency in the literature on the use of this term. It does not appear to be a distinct entity, and such patients are classified as a variant of SCID.

A limited supply of normal lymphoid stem cells may also result in SCID, reflected by a reduced number of T- and B-cell clones, restricted allograft rejection and antibody responses, and homogeneous Ig. SCID can occasionally be seen in the presence of normal numbers of B and T cells which are functionally defective. In some cases, surface products of the major histocompatibility gene complex are lacking ("bare lymphocyte syndrome"). Apart from genetic defects, congenital viral infections (eg congenital cytomegalovirus) can play an important pathogenetic role in SCID. Other exogenous causes of ID syndromes include congenital rubella, which can result in Ig deficiencies with increased IgM or in selective IgA deficiency.

Among the selective Ig deficiencies, that of the IgA class is the most common and best characterized. Several pathogenetic mechanisms appear to be responsible for the failure of IgA-bearing cells to mature into plasma cells. Associated selective deficiencies of one other class, such as IgM, or of IgG subclasses, could also be due to abnormalities of structural genes or regulatory mechanisms such as selective Ts cells or deficiencies in Th cells.

Many patients with ID cannot yet be unequivocally classified, and are therefore grouped under the heading of "varied immunodeficiencies." This group presumably encompasses several syndromes about which there is a paucity of information on definite patterns and causes. Included in the subgroup of predominant Ig deficiencies are cases previously classified as "congenital" and non-X-linked (or sporadic) hypogammaglobulinemia, primary "dysgammaglobulinemia" of both childhood and adult life, and "acquired" primary hypogammaglobulinemia. Enumeration of Ig-bearing lymphocytes in such patients has led to the delineation of several patterns presumably reflecting different underlying mechanisms. Some patients with nodular lymphoid hyperplasia belong to the subgroup defined by normal or increased numbers of B cells. Other patients in this group may have reduced numbers of B lymphocytes. In some of them, correspondingly low frequencies of pre-B cells are found in bone marrow. When examined on multiple occasions, fluctuations in both pre-B and circulating B-lymphocyte levels can be observed, suggesting abnormalities in regulatory mechanisms yet to be defined.

Patients with varied ID and hypogammaglobulinemia present with a variety of clinical defects and potential pathogenetic mechanisms. A minority is deficient in B cells. A second group has B lymphocytes that fail to respond with normal plasma cell differentiation to any polyclonal activators but have no demonstrable regulatory T-cell defect; they appear to have an intrinsic B-cell defect. A third group has B cells that can be activated to synthesize Ig, which is not secreted. These B cells lack a receptor for EBV and also fail to glycosylate newly synthesized Ig intracellularly. A fourth group has B cells that synthesize and secrete Ig in vitro after polyclonal activation. Because they fail to do so in vivo an extrinsic defect has been suggested, and in some of these cases a circulating inhibitory factor has been described. Yet a fifth group has B cells with a marked increase in Ts activity. For this group, separation of T from B cells in vitro leads to normal Ig synthesis. Other mechanisms of failure of T and B cooperation may also prove to be pathogenetic in common variable ID.

A number of immunodeficient patients with variable ID appear to have predominant T-cell deficiency reflecting a primary abnormality of T-cell development. When treated with thymic extracts or factors, or by thymic grafts, some of these patients have shown rapid improvement in T-cell maturation and function.

Finally, ID can result from the activity of autoantibodies to B or T cells in patients whose normal production and potential differentiation of these cells is not impaired.

ID Associated With Other Major Defects

Chromosomal abnormalities.

a) Bloom syndrome: Affected children have chromosomal instability, retarded growth, facial telangiectasias with erythema and light sensitivity, frequent ear and respiratory infections, and a predisposition to malignancies. Hypogammaglobulinemia including one, two, or three of the major Ig classes and poor antibody production is seen, as well as decreased in vitro T-cell responsiveness.

b) Fanconi anemia: These patients with chromosomal aberrations have bone marrow failure with anemia and neutropenia and may have associated skeletal abnormalities. They may also have increased infections, decreased IgA, and signs of diminished T-cell function.

c) Down syndrome: The increased frequency of respiratory tract infections, hepatitis, and leukemia is unexplained. Slight depression of antibody responses, T-cell functions, and phagocytic dysfunction have been reported.

Metal transport defects.

a) Acrodermatitis enteropathica is an autosomal recessive disease characterized by eczema, diarrhea, malabsorption, and recurrent sinopulmonary infections. Hypogammaglobulinemia and abnormalities of CMI occur but are not constant features. The symptoms and immunologic abnormalities respond to zinc therapy.

b) A possible calcium transport defect has been described in 2 patients with the clinical picture of SCID, with normal numbers of unresponsive T and B cells, and a blastic transformation to calcium ionophore. They had progressive declining immunoglobulin levels and circulating lymphocyte numbers. Their lymphocytes failed to respond to mitogens and antigen but transformed normally in the presence of calcium ionophore, suggesting a calcium transport membrane defect.

Metabolic disease.

Several hereditary metabolic disorders have an associated immunodeficiency state and an increased incidence of infection.

Patients with Type I *hereditary orotic aciduria* have retarded growth, recurrent diarrhea, megaloblastic anemia, and an increased incidence of infections, including fatal meningitis and varicella. There is associated lymphocytopenia, a decrease in the number of T lymphocytes, and impaired CMI. A few infants with *biotin-dependent carboxylase deficiency* and a rapid urinary excretion of β-hydroxy-propionic acid have been reported to have had convulsions, ataxia, alopecia, candida dermatitis and keratoconjunctivitis, isolated IgA deficiency, and a reduced number of circulating T cells. Biotin administration led to biochemical and clinical improvement.

Hypercatabolism of immunoglobulin.

Patients with *myotonic dystrophy* have reduced levels of IgG due to selective hypercatabolism. Hypercatabolism affecting many serum proteins has also been described in a kindred with an increased incidence of infections, bone abnormalities, abnormal glucose metabolism, and low albumin and immunoglobulin levels. The nephrotic syndrome is associated with a profound hypercatabolism of IgG.

Excessive loss of immunoglobulins into the gastrointestinal tract is common to many gastrointestinal diseases, including intestinal lymphangiectasia and inflammatory bowel disease. Lymphocytes as well as immunoglobulins may be lost; the lymphopenia may lead to defects in CMI.

Other syndromes.

Short-limbed dwarfism has been associated with immunodeficiency. A subgroup of these patients have cartilage hair hypoplasia with or without megacolon. Some of these patients may have severe cell-mediated, humoral, or combined immunodeficiency.

Severe pyogenic infections, usually with staphylococcal abscesses (often cold), very high levels of IgE, eosinophilia, and aberrant Ts for IgE synthesis are found in the *Job* or *hyper-IgE syndrome*. The interrelationship between the T-cell regulatory defect and infection is not understood. Familial cases have been encountered.

Patients with persistent severe candidal infections of skin and mucosa (*chronic mucocutaneous candidiasis*) have markedly impaired CMI. The relationship of the infection to the defect of immunity is not understood. Mannase deficiency of monocytes has been noted in some of these patients. Mannans inhibit cytotoxic T cells.

Immunodeficiency and viral infections.

Transient immunodeficiency may occur with many viral infections. As noted in Table 1, certain viral infections may also be associated with persistent immunodeficiency. Of special note are cytomegalovirus (CMV) infections which may result in persistent inversion of circulating Th/Ts ratios.

Patients with antibody ID may be susceptible to a variety of types of meningitis and encephalitis with particular susceptibility to chronic ECHO virus infection. Such patients have been shown to shed ECHO virus for prolonged periods (more than 2 years). They have all developed a chronic meningoencephalitis, and in some a dermatomyositis-like syndrome has been observed. Rare ECHO types have been isolated from cerebrospinal fluid and postmortem from all viscera. Untreated, the infection is nearly always fatal.

An acquired combined immunodeficiency syndrome (AIDS) has recently been reported in homosexual males, drug abusers, frequently transfused persons such as hemophiliacs, immunosuppressed patients, and male Haitians. These individuals have lymphopenia, markedly reduced T-cell numbers and profoundly diminished CMI with an inversion of the Th/Ts ratio. The patients frequently develop opportunistic infections and an aggressive Kaposi sarcoma at a relatively young age. The cause of AIDS has not been defined.

Associated Disorders

Malignancies and immunodeficiency.

Age-specific mortality rates for cancer in primary ID groups exceed by 10–200 times the expected rates for the general population. The majority of cancers are observed in patients with ataxia telangiectasia and Wiskott-Aldrich syndrome. In patients with ataxia telangiectasia the cancers may be attributable, at least in part, to chromosomal instability, as is also the case in Fanconi and Bloom syndromes. Patients with CVID, and patients with selective absence of IgA also have a somewhat increased frequency of epithelial and lymphoreticular malignancy. Malignant lymphomas and rare cases of epithelial tumors and leukemias have also been reported in ID patients.

The types of tumors in ID patients of all groups are completely different from those observed in nonselected populations: lymphoreticular malignancies in patients with primary immunodeficiency disease show an unusually high proportion of B-cell lymphomas. Some of these malignancies have shown clear evidence of clonal proliferation. Some have been associated with EBV infection. The data on lymphoproliferative disorders in ID are thus sufficient to suggest an association between at least some forms of ID and oncogenesis. Possible mechanisms for the association include: defective immunologic surveillance; defective immune response to oncogenic viruses; chronic overstimulation or proliferation of responsive cells to antigen; independent effects of the same common cause (ie defective DNA repair in ataxia telangiectasia).

Autoimmunity and immunodeficiencies.

A significant number of autoimmune syndromes have been described in association with ID. These include autoimmune hemolytic anemia, systemic lupus erythematosus (SLE), rheumatoid arthritis (RA), thyroiditis, pernicious anemia, Sjögren syndrome, idiopathic thrombocytopenic purpura, chronic active hepatitis, and myasthenia gravis. In addition, autoantibodies against blood cells, immunoglobulins, and various tissue antigens have been observed.

Atopic allergy and immunodeficiency.

ID plays an important role in atopic allergy. A small proportion of atopic subjects have low levels of serum IgA at the time of their symptoms; a prospective study of the newborn offspring of atopic parents showed that those who later developed atopic allergy had transiently lower levels of IgA before their illness. In patients with selective IgA deficiency or with CVID, antigenemia following ingestion of food antigens can often be demonstrated. This defect may permit unusual antigenic stimulation, and result in the development of atopic responses to these antigens. The prevention of eczema by exclusive breast-feeding of babies with potential atopy has been reported.

Treatment of Specific Immunodeficiency

Individual infections should be treated early with full doses of antimicrobial agents. Where possible, narrow spectrum drugs selected on the basis of microbial sensitivity testing should be used. Prophylactic antibiotics are not generally recommended; they increase the hazard of infection with fungi or other resistant organisms. Long-term treatment with combination sulfa drugs (co-trimoxazole, sulfamethoxazole-trimethoprim) is believed to be of some benefit, but this has not been critically evaluated.

Intestinal infestation with *Giardia lamblia* is common in ID patients and may lead to intestinal protein loss and malabsorption, and thus to superimposed secondary ID. Treatment with metronidazole or mepacrine is usually effective. Intestinal disease is frequent in ID patients and, in addition to treatment of infection or infestation, disaccharide- or gluten-free diets may be of benefit. In some instances, intravenous hyperalimentation of limited duration may be justified.

Blood transfusions should be avoided and never given to patients with CMI deficiency, unless fully oxygen-saturated blood has been irradiated with 7.7×10^{-4} C/kg (3 κ R) to eliminate viable white blood cells which may inappropriately engraft the patient. Blood transfusion is also safe when processed by freezing and centrifugation. However, lymphocytes are still viable in old blood, washed red blood cells, unprocessed plasma, and platelet preparations. Plasma infusions may be used for the correction of immunoglobulin or some complement defects. White cell transfusions can be lifesaving in patients with leukocyte defects.

Replacement of immunoglobulins.

Immunoglobulin replacement has demonstrated efficacy in all patients with demonstrable ID affecting humoral immunity. Both intramuscular and intravenous preparations are available. The optimal dose of neither has yet been determined. Generally, for intramuscular preparations a minimum dose of 0.1 gm/kg/month is recommended. More frequent injections permit reducing the volume of individual injections and may be more effective. The gamma globulin injections are painful for some patients but can be better tolerated if procaine 1% is mixed at 1 part in 10 with the gamma globulin, and if the rather large volume is injected into 4–6 intragluteal sites.

There are now a variety of immunoglobulin preparations available for intravenous use which meet acceptable standards for antibody content, preservation of immunoglobulin structure, stability on storage, safety, efficacy (including reasonable in vivo half-life), and patient acceptability.* Certainly in adults where large doses of Ig are required, the intravenous route has advantages over the intramuscular and should be considered for treatment. Indeed, since intravenous administration of immunoglobulin is less painful than intramuscular and is at least as efficacious, it should perhaps be considered in the treatment of all ID patients requiring Ig replacement.

Untoward reactions (dyspnea, flank pain, hypotension, collapse, fever, rashes, and even death) which

---

*Appropriate uses of human immunoglobulin in clinical practice: Memorandum from an IUIS/WHO meeting. Bulletin of the World Health Organization 60 (1):43–47, 1982.

may occur with both IM and IV replacement are usually due to immunoglobulin aggregates. They tend to occur more frequently in severely hypoimmunoglobulinemic patients.

Enzyme replacement.
Frozen irradiated red blood cells may provide partial replacement of enzymes in infants with ADA or PNP deficiency. Apparently, the great amounts of purine degradation enzymes within the red cells permit some degradation of toxic metabolites within lymphocytes; however, the results of this therapy have been variable and do not compare favorably with bone marrow transplantation.

Thymic factors.
Different extracts of thymus have been prepared in recent years, including thymic factors, thymosin, and THF. In spite of encouraging results reported in the treatment of primary ID, these preparations have not yet been critically evaluated.

Vitamin B_{12} in TC 2 deficiency.
With pharmacologic doses of vitamin B_{12} (1–2 mg daily by enteral or parenteral route), all disturbances of hematopoietic, gastrointestinal, and immunologic functions can be overcome.

Transplantation

Bone marrow.
Transplantation of bone marrow cells from HLA genotypically identical donors (ie matched sib donors or genotypically identical or other phenotypically appropriate member of a family) has led to complete immunologic reconstitution of nearly 100 patients with SCID. Ideally, donor and recipient should be identical at A, B, C, D, and DR loci of the major histocompatibility complex. Unfortunately, the majority of patients with SCID do not have a donor compatible at the major histocompatibility locus. The results of bone marrow transplantations from HLA-D incompatible donors in SCID patients invariably have been bad; with engraftment all patients developed fatal GVH reactions. Successful bone marrow transplantation from a matched unrelated donor has been performed; such donors may be found in one of the registries of HLA testing, special attention being paid to the HLA-D match. It also appears possible to overcome the major histocompatibility barrier by the elimination of cells responsible for GVHD with a lectin column or monoclonal antibodies. These procedures are still in an experimental phase.

Graft-versus-host disease (GVHD), when it occurs, generally appears 8–20 days after a transplant and is usually manifested by fever, Coombs test-positive hemolytic anemia, erythematous maculopapular skin rash, bloody diarrhea, hepatosplenomegaly, aregenerative pancytopenia, and death. The prophylactic treatment often recommended with small doses of methotrexate has never been proven effective. Persistent low-grade GVH reactions, characterized by hepatomegaly, jaundice or skin rashes, can continue for many months and become chronic and severely debilitating.

The establishment of immune competence ("take" of the graft) may be indicated by: improvement of clinical status (eg rapid resolution of moniliasis); the appearance of T and B cells in the circulating blood; genetic markers on cells including enzyme activity in previously deficient patients; increase of immunoglobulin levels (including Ig of donor origin); the appearance of humoral antibodies (including those following antigenic stimulation); return of C1q level to normal; and the appearance of CMI reactions. Of these, the establishment of chimerism is the most reliable evidence of engraftment. Appropriate tests for mosaicism in all available systems (sex and other chromosomal studies, HLA and red cell antigens, plasma protein or enzyme markers) should be performed.

Tests of immunologic competence should be repeated periodically in successful cases, since subsequent gradual decline has been observed in some instances. Children dramatically restored immunologically have also occasionally died of preexisting pulmonary infections with *Pneumocystis carinii* or other organisms when immunologic capacity has been established. Prophylactic treatment with pentamidine or sulfamethoxazole-trimethaprim has proven useful in the treatment of the complications. Several deaths from varicella have occurred in successfully transplanted ID patients; such patients should be passively protected with VZIG following exposure if no circulating antibody can be demonstrated.

Fetal liver.
Hematopoiesis in the liver starts at a gestational age of about 4 weeks, but immunocompetent lymphocytes appear only at week 12 (surface immunoglobulin-bearing cells) and week 18 (PHA-responsive cells). Successful fetal liver transplantation, sometimes in combination with the thymus of the same fetus, has been reported in several patients with SCID. There was generally a slow immunologic reconstitution, mainly of T-cell function, with only a mild-to-moderate degree of GVH reaction. Unfortunately, several of these infants died after a prolonged survival period, either of complications (nephrotic syndrome) or of apparent loss of the graft.

Fetal thymus.
Transplantation of thymus from fetuses of 10–16 weeks' gestation has appeared to reconstitute thymus-dependent immune functions, particularly in children with the third and fourth arch syndrome. However, evaluation of the influence of corrective therapy is difficult because the thymic maldevelopment is variable, and some patients have developed immune capacity spontaneously in spite of deficiencies in early life.

Cultured thymus epithelial fragments have been reported to partially correct immunologic function in some patients with SCID. A few long-term survivors have been achieved. The reasons for the successes and failures are not clear. Further study of this approach seems justified.

COMPLEMENT DEFICIENCY

The classic complement system consists of 9 numbered components and 4 regulatory proteins. The first component comprises 3 subcomponents, C1q, C1r, and C1s. It is the molecular interaction between C1q and aggregated IgG or IgM (as in an antigen-antibody complex) that initiates activation of the classic complement sequence.

An alternative pathway to C3 activation was discovered some 20 years ago and named the properdin system. The known proteins in the system are factor B, factor D, and properdin. Activation of factor D proceeds in the presence of a cleavage fragment of C3 which is similar to or identical with C3b. In the presence of factor D, C3b and the major cleavage fragment of factor B, Bb, form the alternative pathway C3 convertase C3bBb, which appears to cleave and activate C3 in a fashion similar to C4b2a. Properdin appears to stabilize this alternative pathway C3 convertase.

A large number of biologic activities important in the inflammatory response and in host resistance to infection take place at various points in the complement sequence. The lytic property for bacterial or animal cells requires the activation of C3 to C9 by the classic or alternative pathway. The complement enhancement of phagocytosis is probably of great biologic significance and requires the deposition of C3 on the particle to be ingested. Certain viruses are neutralized after interaction with antibody and only the first 2 complement components (C1 and C4); other viruses require C2 and C3 in addition. Immune adherence, a property whereby certain blood cells, including B lymphocytes, adhere to antigen-antibody complexes, occurs with complement activation through the C4 and C3 steps. Histamine release from mast cells, smooth muscle contraction, and increased vascular permeability arising from anaphylatoxin activity are properties of each of the 2 small fragments, C3a and C5a. These fragments are also chemotactic for polymorphonuclear leukocytes, particularly C5a, which also causes exocytosis of neutrophils. The classic complement pathway also appears to be important in the dissolution of immune complexes.

Genetic Defects in Human Complement

Genetic defects have been described for almost all the complement components in man, including C1q, C1r, C4, C2, C3, C5, C6, C7, C8, and C9. In all instances, defects are transmitted as autosomal-recessive traits, and the heterozygotes are readily detected because their sera contain approximately half the normal level of the deficient component as determined by functional and/or immunochemical tests (Table 2). Hemolytic and other functional activity are completely restored by adding back to the deficient serum the isolated complement component. Ge-

TABLE 2. Complement Deficiencies

Deficiency	Inheritance	HLA linkage	Symptom
C1q	AR	−	SLE-like syndrome
C1r	AR	−	SLE-like syndrome
C4	AR	+	SLE-like syndrome
C2	AR	+	SLE-like syndrome, vasculitis, polymyositis
C3	AR	−	Recurrent pyogenic infections
C5	AR	−	SLE, Neisserial infection
C6	AR	−	SLE, Neisserial infection
C7	AR	−	SLE, Neisserial infection, vasculitis
C8	AR	−	SLE, Neisserial infection
C9	AR	−	None
C1 inhibitor	AD	−	Hereditary angioedema
C3b inactivator	AR	−	Recurrent pyogenic infection

netic defects have also been recognized for 2 inhibitors of the complement system: the C1 inhibitor and the C3b inactivator. Although the latter defect has been found in only 6 kindred, where it is inherited as an autosomal recessive, deficiency of the C1 inhibitor is inherited as an autosomal dominant and is the most common of the hereditary complement defects. This deficiency is associated with hereditary angioedema, or Quincke disease. Several hundred cases of this disease have been reported in the literature. In 15% of kindred affected with hereditary angioedema, the sera contain normal or elevated amounts of an immunologically cross-reacting (CRM$^+$), nonfunctional protein. C9 deficiency has a very high incidence among the Japanese; it appears to be without clinical consequence.

Nonfunctional variants of C1q also have been described in 4 kindred. C8 deficiency is unusual in that the gene for the β-chain is not linked to the gene for the α- and γ-chains. Thus, all affected C8 deficients are either deficient in the β-chain or in the α-, γ-chains, and thus have nonfunctional immunoreactive incomplete C8 molecules in their serum.

The genes for factor B, C2 and C4, are located on the short arm of chromosome 6 in linkage disequilibrium

TABLE 3.

Disease	Affected Cells	Inheritance	Associated Feature
a) Defects of Mobility and Adherence			
Actin dysfunction	N	AR	None
Chédiak-Higashi	N + M	AR	Hair pigment change, granules in phagocytes
Shwachman disease	N	AR	Pancreas malfunction, bone abnormalities, defective NK cells
GP110 deficiency	N	AR	Delayed separation of umbilical cord, defective NK cells
b) Defective Endocytosis and Killing			
GP150 deficiency	N	AR	None
X-linked CGD	N + M	XL	?Mothers with discoid LE
Autosomal-recessive CGD	N	AR	None
Neutrophil G6-PD deficiency	N	AR	None
Myeloperoxidase deficiency	N	AR	None

with the HLA loci. The C4 gene is duplicated and the 2 genes are designated C4A and C4B, C4A being identical to the Rogers blood group substance, and C4B to the Chido blood group substance. C4 deficiency results only when all 4 alleles (the 2 of C4A and the 2 of C4B) are not expressed. The genes for factor B, C2, C4A, and C4B, are so tightly linked that no crossover has yet been observed between them, although unequal crossover may rarely result in the expression of three C4A alleles and one C4B allele, or vice versa.

Genetic polymorphisms are now known for C4A, C4B, C2, Factor B, C3, C6, C7, C8α,γ and C8β. It is thus possible to demonstrate the inheritance of nonexpressed alleles in the kindred of deficient propositi.

Impeded androgens have proven extremely effective in the treatment of hereditary angioedema. Purified C1 inhibitor preparations are available for intravenous administration and should be used in the treatment of acute attacks of angioedema. There is no satisfactory replacement therapy for the other complement deficiencies, largely because the catabolic rate of these proteins is very high. Sometimes patients with late component deficiencies require antibiotic prophylaxis because of recurrent *Neisseria* infections.

A group of infants with recurrent infections, diarrhea, and atopic disease, particularly eczema, cannot successfully opsonize yeast particles with C3 deposition. They clinically benefit from fresh plasma infusions. The nature of their complement defect is not known.

DEFECTS OF PHAGOCYTIC FUNCTION

Apart from neutropenia, which has many causes and is not considered here, there may be genetically determined defects of phagocyte function, polymorphonuclear and mononuclear. Neutrophil function depends on movement in response to chemotactic stimulus, adherence, endocytosis, and killing or destruction of the ingested particles. Mobility and endocytosis both depend on adherence and the integrity of the cytoskeleton and the contractile system.

Defects of intracellular killing usually result from failure of the "respiratory burst" following ingestion of organisms, which is critical to production of superoxide radicals, oxygen singlets, hydroxyl radicals, and hydrogen peroxide. The organisms cultured from the lesions are generally catalase-producing and include staphylococcus, *E. coli*, molds, and other opportunistic organisms. Patients with defects in mobility and adherence (see Table 3a) usually present with infections of skin, periodontitis, and intestinal and perianal fistulae. On the other hand, patients with defective endocytosis and killing (see Table 3b) tend to have chronic infected granulomas in addition. The measurement of nitroblue tetrazolium dye reduction by actively phagocytosing leukocytes has been accepted as a standard measure for the adequacy of the respiratory burst. A number of assays for chemotaxis and associated phenomena such as adherence and contractility as well as tests of bacterial killing, superoxide production, and chemiluminescence have been developed but are not satisfactorily standardized at this time for routine clinical use. GP 110 and GP 150 are glycoproteins of cell walls; the GP 110 deficiency is associated with defective adherence and mobility, and defective natural killer cells.

Phagocyte function may also be defective in a number of generalized diseases, such as diabetes, liver failure, glycogen storage disease type b, etc. The phagocytic dysfunction does not constitute a characteristic or diagnostic feature of these diseases. Certain syndromes (such as the hyper-IgE or Job syndrome) may be associated with a secondary phagocytic defect.

Infections should be treated with appropriate antibiotics, surgery, and perhaps neutrophil transfusion. Sulfamethoxazole-trimethoprim prophylaxis is valuable, especially for CGD. There are reports of improvement of some defects with ascorbic acid (Chédiak-Higashi and GP 110 deficiency). In severe cases, tissue-matched sib bone marrow transplantation should be considered.

F.S. Rosen
United States Of America

R.J. Wedgwood
United States Of America

Co-Chairmen

F. Aiuti	**L.Å. Hanson**	**M. Seligmann**
Italy	Sweden	France
M.D. Cooper	**W.H. Hitzig**	**J.F. Soothill**
United States Of America	Switzerland	England
R.A. Good	**S. Matsumoto**	**T.A. Waldmann**
United States Of America	Japan	United States Of America

Index

Abelson virus, 177
N-Acetylglucosamine, 183–185
Aciduria. See Orotic aciduria, hereditary
Acquired immunodeficiency syndrome (AIDS), 355
Acrodermatitis enteropathica, 354–355
Adenosine deaminase, 315
   isozymes, 77–78
Adenosine deaminase deficiency and SCID, 67, 69, 70, 73–78, 97, 98, 108, 258, 260, 263, 268, 307
   abnormal metabolites and pathophysiologic mechanisms, 75–76
   BMT, 117, 199
      soybean lectin treatment of BMT, 148–149
   bony abnormalities, 74
   case report, 117
   dipyridamole and IV deoxycytidine therapy, 117–120
   fetal liver transplants, 139
   genetic heterogeneity, 73, 77–78
   metabolism, schema, 74
   neurologic abnormalities, 74–75
   partial, 77–78
   prenatal diagnosis, 73–74, 121–123, 125
   testing, 349, 351–352
   therapy, 76–77
   THU inhibitor, 118, 120
   transfusion (enzyme replacement), 117
S-Adenosyl homocysteine, 75–76
Agammaglobulinemia, 185
   poliovirus in, 229–234
   in purine nucleoside phosphorylase deficiency, 73
   treatment with IgA, secretory, oral administration, 229–236
   see also Hypogammaglobulinemia
Agammaglobulinemia, X-linked (SLA)
   bronchiectasis, 223, 224
   Bruton-type, 239–240
   dietary protein antigenemia, 239–241
   incidence, 224
   incomplete μ H-chains, 177–181
   otitis media, chronic, 223, 224
   pre-B cells, 177–181
      mRNA, 179–180
   prevalence, 223
   primed cDNA, 179, 180
   with SCID, 125–127
   T cells and T-cell subsets, 187–191
   treatment, gammaglobulin, 224
      IV pH 4.0, 201–203
      subcutaneous infusion, 213–215
   V_H region, 177–181
      fluorescence, 177–179
   see also Hypogammaglobulinemia, Severe combined immunodeficiency (SCID)
Agglutinin, peanut, 147
Albinism, 308, 333

Algorithm
   K-means clustering, 336–338
   single linkage clustering, 336, 338
Allergies, 335–336
   atopic, 356
Alopecia, 308
Alymphocytosis, 125, 127
AMP, cyclic. See Cyclic AMP
Anaphylaxis, IM gammaglobulin, 218
Anemia
   aplastic, 129, 131, 277–279
   Fanconi, 354
   hemolytic, 150, 356
   and fetal liver transplant, 144
Antibodies
   anti-IFN, 110–111
   anti-SIII, 44
   formation after immunization, 346–347
   in vitro anti-mannan production by peripheral blood lymphocytes, 41–44
   juvenile rheumatoid arthritis, 17, 19
   -mediated elimination of B cells in defective humoral immunity, 158
   monoclonal. See Monoclonal antibodies
   -producing cells in peripheral blood in response to immunization, 47–50
      isotype switch, 48–49
      T-cell dependence, 49
   production in combined immunodeficiency with defective HLA expression, 90, 91
Antibody deficiency syndromes, 226
   with normal Igs
      T cells and T-cell subsets, 187–191
      treatment with IV pH 4.0 gammaglobulin, 201–203
   treatment
      infections, 217
      replacement therapy by plasma transfusions, 218
      subcutaneous gammaglobulin, 217–220
Antigen(s)
   pokeweed, 32, 33
   recognition, Th cells, 11
   response, neonatal monocytes, 51–55, 293
   thymus, abnormal epithelial surface expression, 255–258
   Thy1, 255–256
   see also HLA
Antigenemia, dietary protein, 239–241
Antithymocyte globulin and fetal liver transplants, 131, 134, 135
α_1-Antitrypsin deficiency, and SCID, 68
Aplastic anemia, 129, 131, 277–279
Arthritis, rheumatoid, 356
   juvenile, 15–16, 220
      antibodies, 17, 19
Assay(s)
   CMI, 347–348
   functional, for humoral immune response

assessment, 31–35
   thymus, abnormal development, 248–249
Ataxia telangiectasia, 33, 154
   chromosome fragility, 310
   and GPL-115 deficiency, 97
   and IgA deficiency, 262
   and neoplasia, 163
   thymus, abnormal development, 248–249
   TP-5 therapy, 267–271
ATP/deoxy ATP ratios in ADA deficiency, 75, 76, 77, 79, 117–120
   in prenatal diagnosis of SCID with ADA deficiency, 121–123, 125
Autoimmunity, 356; see also specific diseases

Bacteriophage ϕX 174, 47–50, 158, 321–323
Bare lymphocyte syndrome, 67, 90
   clinical features, 83–84
   combined immunodeficiency, 83
   immunogenetic effect, 84
   lack of HLA antigen expression, 83–85
   β_2-microglobulin, 84, 85
   registry, 83
   T-lymphocyte function and differentiation, 84–85
   lymphocyte homing, 85
Basophil deficiency, thymoma, 331
B cells
   antibody-mediated elimination in defective humoral immunity, 158
   deficiency. See Humoral immunity defects
   development, 289, 290
      failure of isotype progression, 165–166
      faulty, in defective humoral immunity, 154–155
      subset phenotypes, 289
   differentiation, 25–28
   growth factor, 38
   helper-macrophage interaction in combined immunodeficiency, 94–95
   IgG gene rearrangements in lymphocytic leukemia, 31–32
   mature, schematic model, 26
   pokeweed responsive, 26–28
      three major subpopulations, 27
   polyclonal, activation factor, 37–38
   pre-, in X-linked agammaglobulinemia, 177–181
      mRNA, 179–180
   in SCID, 68
   SM14 cell line, 180
   cooperation, 12
   and T cells, 26–28
      controlling isotype switching, 33
      cooperation, 12
   tests for assessing immunity, 347
   see also Lymphocytes, T cells
Bethanechol, 329–330
Biopsies, various, in SCID, 349

Biotin, 309, 311
  -dependent carboxylase deficiency, 355
Bloom syndrome, 354
Bone marrow aspiration, 349
Bone marrow transplants (BMT), 357
  and ADA deficiency, 76
  busulfan and cyclophosphamide, 129, 130
  correction of marrow aplasia without immunosuppression, 277–279
  HLA-identical sib donors, 129, 141
  for lethal congenital immunodeficiencies, 129–135
  in SCID, 65
    mismatched, 147–150
    with NK-cell predominance, 101
    unmodified, from HLA-nonidentical but compatible donors, 129–130
  Wiskott-Aldrich syndrome, 129
  see also Hematopoietic cell transplantation
Bony abnormalities, SCID with ADA deficiency, 74
Bovine gammaglobulin, 239–240; see also Gammaglobulin
Brain damage in immunodeficiency, 339–340
Breast milk and IgA, secretory, oral administration, 229, 235
Bronchiectasis, 223, 224
Burkitt lymphoma, 184

Candida albicans, 41–44, 57, 131, 133
  mannan, 90
Candidiasis
  chronic mucocutaneous, 162, 309
    and buccal carcinoma, 263
    delayed hypersensitivity reaction, 274–275, 283, 284
Carboxylase deficiency, biotin-dependent, 355
Carcinoma, buccal, and chronic candidiasis, 263
Cartilage hair hypoplasia, 261, 308
Catalase, 300, 302
Cell(s)
  B. See B cells
  cord blood mononuclear (CBMC), 51–55
  Kupffer, 4
  LSM myeloma, 179–180
  murine leukemia, 299
  natural killer. See Natural killer (NK) cells
  plaque-forming, regulatory role of neonatal monocytes in in vitro antigen specific response, 51–55
  stem, hematopoietic, 245, 345
  T. See T cells
  θ-positive, 147
  WISH system, 109
  fetal liver transplant, 143–144
Cell sorting, fluorescent-activated (FACS), 121–123, 295–298
Cellular immunodeficiency
  impaired production of interleukins, 115
  OKT4$^+$:OKT8$^+$ lymphocyte ratios, 115
  with pyrimidine metabolism defect, 313–315
  see also specific syndromes
CFU-S, 245

Chédiak-Higashi syndrome, 103, 308, 359
  BMT in, 333
Chemotactic factor, lymphocyte-derived, 183
Chromosome(s)
  abnormalities, primary specific immunodeficiency, 354
  fragility in ataxia telangiectasia, 33, 154
Chronic granulomatous disease (CGD), 125, 130, 352, 359
  vs SCID, 301
  T-cell cytotoxicity and chemiluminescence abnormalities, 299–305
Colds, 336
Colostrum and IgA, secretory, oral administration, 229, 235
Combined immunodeficiency
  in bare lymphocyte syndrome, 83; see also Bare lymphocyte syndrome
  selective deficiency of OKT4$^+$ lymphocytes, 105–106
Combined immunodeficiency with defective HLA expression, 87–91, 93–95
  case reports, 87, 89, 93
  in Dutch, 93–95
  "experiment of nature," 83, 95
  hypogammaglobulinemia, 87
  immunoglobulin and antibody production, 90, 91
  interferon treatment, 87, 90, 91
  lack of delayed skin reactivity, 87
  macrophage-B cell interaction, 94–95
  macrophage-T helper interaction, 94
  β_2-microglobulin, 87–88, 91, 93
  OA-induced T-helper factor (ThF120), 93–95
  see also Severe combined immunodeficiency (SCID)
Common variable immunodeficiency (hypogammaglobulinemia), 162
  synthetic TP-5 in, 267–271, 273–275
  T cells and T-cell subsets, 187–191
  treatment with IV pH 4.0 gammaglobulin, 201–203
  see also Humoral immunity, Hypogammaglobulinemia
Complement
  activation, humoral immunity defects, 195–196
  C5a, 5
  deficiency, 358–359
    pathways, and gammaglobulin infusion, 213–215
    response to IV pH 4.0-treated gammaglobulin in humoral immunodeficiency disease, 202
    treatment of transplant material, 134–135
Concanavalin A, 183
Cord blood mononuclear cells, 51–55
Coxsackie virus, 87
Cyclic AMP, 69, 75
  and thymic humoral factor, 246
Cyclic GMP, 330
Cyclophosphamide, 131, 134, 135, 333
  and busulfan, 129, 130

Cyclosporin A, 149
Cytomegalovirus, 198, 218, 355
Cytotoxicity
  lectin-dependent cellular, 299–305
  T-cell, in newborns, 299–305

Deoxycytidine and dipyridamole therapy in ADA deficiency, 117–120
Diagnosis
  prenatal. See Prenatal diagnosis
  primary specific immunodeficiency, 351–352
  tests for assessing immunity, 346–348
Diarrhea, 309–310
  and IgA, secretory, oral administration, 229–235
DiGeorge syndrome, 97, 103, 162
  T cells and T-cell subsets, 187–191
  thymus, abnormal development, 248, 249, 251
  TP-5 therapy, 267–271
Dipyridamole and IV deoxycytidine therapy, ADA deficiency, 117–120
DNA, complementary, primed, and X-linked agammaglobulinemia, 179, 180
Down syndrome, 325–326, 354
Dutch, combined immunodeficiency with defective HLA expression, 93–95
Dwarfism, short-limbed, 67, 355
Dysmorphic signs, 308

ECHO virus, 193, 217, 220, 355
  -5, 236
  -8, viral encephalitis, 223, 226
ELISA, 41–42, 213, 215, 225, 346
Encephalitis, ECHO-8 virus, 223, 226
Enteric viruses and SCID, 65
Enzyme replacement in ADA deficiency, 117
Eosinophil deficiency, thymoma, 331
Epidemiology, hypogammaglobulinemia, 223–227
Epstein-Barr virus, 32–33, 51, 165, 177, 184, 198, 290, 354
  B cells, 12
  newborns, 302–305
  in severe pure T-cell defects, 283, 284
  X-linked lymphoproliferative syndrome, 321–322
Escherichia coli, 195

Fab fragments, defective humoral immunity, 194–195
Factor(s)
  growth. See Growth factors
  IgA-PFC-helper, in T-T hybridomas, 38
  -increasing monocytopoiesis, 4–5
  lymphocyte-derived chemotactic, 183
  OA-induced T-helper (ThF120), 51–53, 93–95
  polyclonal B-cell activation, 37–38
  serum thymic (FTS), 246, 247, 249, 251, 267, 271
  thymic, 357
  thymic humoral, 246, 267

Familial reticuloendotheliosis syndrome, 317–318
Fanconi anemia, 354
Fc
    fragments, defective humoral immunity, 194–195
    receptors, T-cell, 15, 18
Fetal liver transplantation, 130–135, 357
    ADA deficiency, 139
    causes of death, 140
    cell cooperation despite HLA mismatch, 143–145
    chimeras, 132, 140, 143–145
    and CMI, 131, 143–144
    with FTT, 139–140
    GVHD, 140–141
    hemolytic anemia, 144
    immune reconstitution, 143–144
    in SCID, European experience, 139–141
Fetal thymus transplantation, 259–260, 357–358
    cortical vs medullary, 262
    cultured thymus fragments, 260–264
    with FLT, 139–140
    GVHD, 139
    in SCID, 139, 259–264
Fetal tissue transplantation, in SCID, European experience, 139–141
Fluorescence-activated cell sorting (FACS), 121–123, 295–298

Gammaglobulin, bovine, 239–240
Gammaglobulin treatment
    in antibody deficiency syndromes with normal Igs, 217–220
    effect on IgG metabolism, 210–211
    IM, 217–218, 226
        anaphylaxis, 218
    IV, 218–219, 224–226
        pH 4.0, treated, 201–203
    maltose-treated vs non-treated, 225
    vs S-IgA in IgA deficiencies, 234–235
    various routes, advantages and disadvantages, 217
    U.K. MRC trial, 224
Gene(s)
    IgG, 25, 31–32
    MHC, 84, 93
Genetics
    complement deficiency, 358–359
    primary specific immunodeficiency, 349, 351
GPL-115 deficiency, 97–98
Graft resistance, SCID, 135
Grafts, thymus, 250
Graft-vs-host disease, 125, 277–279, 357
    abrogation, 130–131
    fetal liver transplants, 140–141
    fetal thymus transplantation, 139
    after lectin treatment of transplant material, 132–134
    mismatched BMT, 149
    OKT3 monoclonal antibody and complement pretreatment, 134–135
    and SCID, 66, 68, 129–130
    and thymic hormones, 284
    thymic humoral factor, 246
    and thymus, 250, 251
    transplantation, 259
Granulomatous disease, chronic. See Chronic granulomatous disease (CGD)
Growth factors
    B-cell, 38
    T-cell, 32, 34–35, 247–248
    see also Factors
GTP, deoxy, 79

Heavy chains
    isotype switching in B-cell differentiation, 25, 27–28
    μ, incomplete, in X-linked agammaglobulinemia, 177–181
Hematology of immunodeficiency, 348–349
Hematopoietic cell transplantation
    antithymocyte globulin, 131, 134, 135
    cell-mediated immune function, 131
    cyclophosphamide, 131, 134, 135
    fetal liver transplants, 130–135
        chimeras, 132
    marrow-derived, from HLA-nonidentical donors, 130–135
    see also Bone marrow transplants, Fetal liver transplantation
Hematopoietic stem cells, 245, 345
Hemocyanin, keyhole limpet (KLH), 41, 44, 47, 49, 117, 119, 347
Hemolytic anemia, 150, 356
    and fetal liver transplant, 144
Hepatitis B, 217, 218
Herpes simplex type I, 101, 102
HLA, 284
    donor matching, See Bone marrow transplants, Fetal liver transplantation, Hematopoietic cell transplantation
    -DR, 9–12, 26
        antigen deficiency on neonatal monocytes, 295–298
        and neonatal monocytes in antigen-specific PFC response, 51–55
    lack of antigen expression in bare lymphocyte syndrome, 83–85
    phenotypes in T-T hybridomas, 37
    and prenatal diagnosis of SCID, 125–127
    see also Combined immunodeficiency with defective HLA expression
Hormones, thymic. See Thymic hormones
Human T-cell leukemia/lymphoma virus, 34
Humoral immune response
    assays, 31–35
    regulation, 31–35
Humoral immunity defects (B-cell deficiency, severe hypogammaglobulinemia)
    in Down syndrome, 325
    fetal liver transplant, 143–144
    otitis media, recurrent, 335–338
Humoral immunity defects, primary
    antibody-mediated elimination of B lymphocytes, 158
    B-cell differentiation, faulty, 154–155
    clinical abnormalities, 154
    common variable (CVID), 153, 155, 158
    diagnostic criteria and classification, 153–158
    κ/λ ratio, 155
    T cells
        control of B-cell differentiation, defective, 155, 158
        helper, defective, 158
        suppressor activity, excessive, 158
    see also specific syndromes
Humoral immunity defects, treatment, 193–198
    chemically modified products, 196
    complement activation, 195–196
    ECHO virus infections, 193
    enzyme-treated products, 195–196
    Fab and Fc fragments, 194–195
    gammaglobulin infusions
        adverse reactions to IV, 197
        effect on IgG metabolism, 210–211
        individualization, 209–212
        pH 4.0, treated, 201–203
        safety, IV, 196–198
        three types, IV, 194–195
    serum immune globulin, human, 193
        enriched, 194
Hybridomas, T-T
    generation, 37
    HLA phenotypes, 37
    induction of Ig secretion by supernatants, 38
    IgA-PFC-helper factor, 38
    secreting factors for B-cell differentiation and proliferation, 37–39
Hydrogen peroxide, 304–305
Hypercatabolism of Ig, 355
Hyper-IgE (Job) syndrome, 13, 309, 310, 355
    clinical features, 57, 58
    immune regulation, 57–60
    inheritance, 57
    in vitro assessment, 58–60
    lung abscesses, 57, 58
    OKT monoclonal antibodies, 57–59
    possible allogeneic suppressor defect, 57–60
    PWM, 58–60
    T cells and T-cell subsets, 187–191
    TP-5 therapy, 267–271
Hyper-IgM, X-linked, T cells and T-cell subsets, 187–191
Hypogammaglobulinemia, 153, 185
    dietary protein antigenemia, 239–241
    epidemiology, 223–227
    failure of isotype progression, 165–166
    incidence, 223–224
    and lung function, 205–206
    and malakoplakia, effect of bethanecol, 329–330
    prevalence, 223
    and SCID, 66
    secondary to lymphoma and leukemia, treatment with IV pH 4.0-treated gammaglobulin therapy, 201–203
    therapy, 205–206
        subcutaneous gammaglobulin, 217–220
        U.K. MRC trial, 224

364 / Index

Hypogammaglobulinemia *(continued)*
   thymoma, basophil and eosinophil deficiency, 331
   transient, of infancy, 155
      T cells and T-cell subsets, 187–191
   see also Agammaglobulinemia, Combined immunodeficiency, Common variable hypogammaglobulinemia, Humoral immunity defects, Immunodeficiency, Severe combined immunodeficiency (SCID)

Idiopathic thrombocytopenic purpura, 196
Immune response
   assessing, 346–348
   cellular basis, 345, 346, 347–348
   in fetal liver transplant, 131, 143–144
   development in fetus and newborn, 289–294
   HLA, 284
   immunity at birth, 290–291
   newborn monocytes, 293
   phases, 3
   see also Humoral immune response
Immune suppressor supernatant, soluble, 183–184
Immunization reactions in immunodeficiency, 339–340; *see also* Poliomyelitis
Immunodeficiency
   hematology, 348–349
   immunization reactions, 339–340
   morphology, 348–349
   skeletal changes, 307–308
   syndromes, classification and etiology, 310–311
   see also specific types and syndromes
Immunodeficiency, primary
   associated neoplastic and autoimmune disorders, 161–163
   cytofluorographic analysis of blood lymphocytes, 187–191
   Italian National Registry, 161–163
   NK activity, 189–191
   viral infections, 355
   see also specific syndromes
Immunodeficiency, primary specific
   associated disorders, 355–356
   chromosome abnormalities, 354
   classification, 352–354
   diagnosis, 351–352
   genetics, 349, 351
   Ig replacement, 356–357
   metal transport defects, 354–355
   table listing, 350–353
   T cells and T-cell subsets in a large population, 187–191
      T4:T8 ratios, 189–190
   TP-5 therapy, 267–271
   treatment, 356
   see also specific syndromes
Immunoglobulin(s)
   concentration test, 346
   development, 289–290
   hypercatabolism, 355
   production in combined immunodeficiency with defective HLA expression, 90, 91
   profile in recurrent otitis media, 337, 338
   replacement in primary specific immunodeficiency, 356–357
   and SCID, 67
Immunoglobulin A (IgA)
   deficiency, and ataxia telangiectasia, 170, 174, 262
   deficiency, selective
      associated diseases, 169
      with IgG subclass deficiencies, 169–170, 173–175
      Ig therapy, 170, 173
      recurrent infections in children, 169–170
      in U.S. vs Sweden, 174
   secretory (S-IgA), oral administration
      antibodies, function, 229, 233, 235
      anti-diarrheal, 229–235
      in breast milk and colostrum, 229, 235
      case reports, 229–232
      vs gammaglobulin, 234–235
      in hypogammaglobulinemia, 240
      with IV hyperalimentation, 235
      oral administration in SCID with B cells, 229–234
      -PFC-helper factor in T-T hybridomas, 38
      preparation, 230
Immunoglobulin E (IgE). *See* Hyper-IgE (Job) syndrome
Immunoglobulin G (IgG)
   genes, 31–32
   in B-cell differentiation, 25
   metabolism, effect of gammaglobulin infusions, 210–211
   regulation of synthesis, 31
   secretion in T-T hybridomas, 38
   subclass deficiencies, with selective IgA deficiency, 169–170, 173–175
   in X-linked lymphoproliferative syndrome, 322
Immunoglobulin M (IgM) deficiency, treatment with IV pH 4.0 gammaglobulin, 201–203
Indomethacin, 54
Infections
   and antibody-deficiency syndromes, 217
   congenital, 290, 307
   in selective IgA deficiency, 169–170
   see also Virus(es), specific agents
Infectious mononucleosis, 184–185
Inflammation, humoral regulation of monocyte production, 4–5
Influenza virus A/X31, 42–44, 90
Interferon, 270
   α, 295–298
   and Down syndrome, 326
   γ, 297
   treatment of combined immunodeficiency, 87, 90, 91
Interferonopathy, possible, in SCID, 109–113
Interleukin(s)
   impaired production in cellular immunodeficiency, 115
   -2, 32, 34–35, 133, 134, 247, 248
Intestinal biopsy, 349
Isotype
   progression, failure in B-cell ontogeny, 165–166
   switching in antibody production in peripheral blood in response to immunization, 48–49
   see also under B cells, T cells
Isozymes, ADA, 77–78; *see also* Adenosine deaminase

Job syndrome. *See* Hyper-IgE (Job) syndrome

Keyhole limpet hemocyanin, 41, 44, 47, 49, 117, 119, 347
K-means clustering algorithm, 336–338
!Kung tribe, 77
Kupffer cells, 4

Lectin
   -dependent cellular cytotoxicity, 299–305
   -like receptor molecules, mononuclear phagocytes, 183–186
   soybean, treatment of BMT material, 132–134, 147–150
      vs monoclonal antibodies, 149
Letterer-Siwe syndrome, 65, 67
Leukemia
   acute lymphoblastic, 246
   chronic lymphocytic, thymus transplantation, 264
   HTLV, 34
   murine, cells, 299
   and secondary hypogammaglobulinemia, treatment, 201–203
   T-cell, Japanese, associated with new type C retrovirus, 34
Listeria monocytogenes, 5
Liver. *See* Fetal liver transplants
Luminol, 301–303
Lung
   abscesses in hyper-IgE syndrome, 57, 58
   function in hypogammaglobulinemia, 205–206
Lupus erythematosus, systemic, 19, 356
Lymph node biopsy in SCID, 349
Lymphoblastogenesis in SCID, 110–111
Lymphocyte(s)
   $ANAE^+$, 105–106
   assessment of in vitro responsiveness to PHA, 21–23
   -derived chemotactic factor, 183
   glycoprotein. *See* GPL-115 deficiency
   large granular, 101–104
   membrane
      abnormalities, and SCID, 67–68
      markers in SCID, 190–191
   $OKT4^+:OKT8^+$ ratios in cellular imunodeficiency, 115, 126
   peripheral blood (PBL), in vitro anti-mannan antibody production, 41–44
   phenotyping, in SCID with NK-cell predominance, 102
   Stimulation Index, 21
   subpopulations, and TP-5 therapy, 274–275
   see also Bare lymphocyte syndrome, B cells, T cells

Lymphokine(s)
  MIF, 183
  reversal of HLA-DR antigen deficiency on neonatal monocytes, 295-298
Lymphoma
  Burkitt, EBV, 184
  HTLV, 34
  secondary hypogammaglobulinemia, treatment, 201-203
Lymphoproliferative disease, X-linked, 103, 321-323

Macrophages
  origin and kinetics, 3-4
  role in immune process, 3-6
  T-helper and B-cell interaction in combined immunodeficiency with defective HLA expression, 94-95
Major histocompatibility complex
  genes, 84, 93
  and thymus, 245, 247
Malakoplakia and hypogammaglobulinemia, effect of bethanecol, 329-330
Maltose-treated gammaglobulin, 225
Marrow aplasia, delayed, and treatment for thymic hyperplasia, 277-279
Marrow transplantation. See bone marrow transplantation
Membrane markers
  Down syndrome, 326
  in SCID, 190-191
Membrane transport, SCID, 307
Metal transport in primary specific immunodeficiency, 354-355
Methotrexate, 134
α-Methyl-mannoside, 183-184
β_2-Microglobulin
  in bare lymphocyte syndrome, 84, 85
  in combined immunodeficiency, 87-88, 91, 93
  in prenatal diagnosis of SCID, 125-127
Miscarriage risk, amniocentesis, 123
Mitogen, pokeweed (PWM)
  and hyper-IgE syndrome, 58-60
  and Nocardia water-soluble mitogen, 51
  -responsive B cells, 26-28
Moniliasis, chronic mucocutaneous, T cells and T-cell subsets, 187-191
Monoclonal antibodies
  vs abnormal epithelial thymus surface antigen, 255-258
  anti-Tac, 34
  HNK-1, 107-108, 283
  in hyper-IgE (Job) syndrome, 57-59
  Leu7, 107-108
  OKM-1, 107-108
  OKOM1, 283
  OKT, 15-17, 282-283
    hyper-IgE (Job) syndrome, 57-59
    in SCID with NK predominance, 102
    treatment of transplant material, 134-135
  in prenatal diagnosis of SCID, 121-123, 125
  vs soybean lectin treatment in BMT, 149
  vs thymus hormones, 246-248
  VEP, in SCID with NK predominance, 102

Monocytes
  humoral regulation of production during inflammation, 4-5
  neonatal
    antigen processing, 293
    HLA-DR antigen deficiency, 295-298
    regulatory role in in vitro antigen-specific PFC response, 51-55
  origins and kinetics, 3-4
  production inhibitor, 5
Monocytopoiesis, factor increasing, 4-5
Mononuclear cells, cord blood (CBMC), 51-55
Mononuclear phagocytes, lectin-like receptor molecules, 183-186
Mononucleosis, infectious, 184-185
Mucocutaneous moniliasis, T cells and T-cell subsets, 187-191; see also Candidiasis
Murine leukemia cells, 299
Mycobacterium avium, 132
Myeloma, LSM cells, 179-180
Myotonic dystrophy, 355

Natural killer (NK) cells, 135, 268, 270
  in DiGeorge syndrome, 107-108
  primary immunodeficiency, 189-191
  in SCID, 101-104, 107-108, 113
  in X-linked lymphoproliferative syndrome, 321-323
Navajo children, SCID, 109, 110, 112
Neurologic abnormalities, ADA deficiency and SCID, 74-75
Newborns
  EBV, 304
  monocytes. See Monocytes, neonatal
  RBCs, 302-305
  T-cell cytotoxicity and chemiluminescence abnormalities, 299-305
  transient hypogammaglobulinemia of infancy, 155, 187-191
Nezelof syndrome (immunodeficiency with normal serum Igs), 354
  T cells and T-cell subsets, 187-191
  thymus, 255, 257, 258
  TP-5 therapy, 267-271
  treatment with IV pH 4.0 gammaglobulin, 201-203
  see also Severe pure T-cell defects
Nocardia opaca, 154
  water-soluble mitogen, 51
Nucleoside phosphorylase. See Purine nucleoside phosphorylase deficiency

Omenn syndrome, 65, 67
Orotic aciduria, hereditary, 313-315, 355
Otitis media, 223, 224, 335-338

Parallel tubular arrays (PTA), 112-113
Paraproteinemia and SCID, 67
Patent ductus arteriosus, 277
Peanut agglutinin, 147
Peptides, thymus, 246
Pertussis vaccine, reaction in immunodeficiency, 339
Phagocytes
  function defects, 359-360
  mononuclear, lectin-like receptor molecules, 183-186

Phagocytosis, 5-6
Phytolacca americana, 26
Plaque-forming cells, 15, 18, 51-55
Pneumocystis carinii, 65
Pokeweed
  mitogen, 32, 33, 51
    and hyper-IgE syndrome, 58-60
    -responsive B cells, 26-28
    three major subpopulations, 27
Poliomyelitis virus, 217, 229-236
  in agammaglobulinemia, 229-234
  fecal shedding, 235-236
Prekallikrein activator, 197
Prenatal diagnosis in SCID with ADA deficiency, 70, 73-74, 121-123, 125-127
Primary defects of humoral immunity. See Humoral immunity, primary defects of
Primary immunodeficiency syndromes. See Immunodeficiency syndromes, primary
Proliferative abnormality, RES, and SCID, 67
β-Propiolactone, 194, 196, 209-212
Prostaglandin E_2, 54, 55
Proteus, 307
Purine nucleoside phosphorylase deficiency, 78-79, 125, 315, 349, 351-352
  metabolism, schema, 74
  transcobalamin II absence and agammaglobulinemia, 73
  T-suppressor function abnormalities, 78-79
Pyrimidine metabolism defect with cellular immunodeficiency, 313-315

Rectal biopsy, 349
Red cells, newborn, 302-305
Registry
  bare lymphocyte syndrome, 83
  Italian National, primary immunodeficiency syndromes, 161-163
  Swedish, primary immunodeficiency diseases, 162
Reticuloendothelial system, proliferative abnormality, and SCID, 67
Reticuloendotheliosis, familial, 317-318
Retrovirus, new type C, and T-cell leukemia, 34
Rheumatoid arthritis, 356
  juvenile, 15-16, 220
  antibodies, 17, 19
RNA, messenger, pre-B cell, and X-linked agammaglobulinemia, 179-180
Rotavirus infection, 234

S-Adenosyl homocysteine, 75-76
Sandoglobulin, 196
Self-recognition, T cells, 11-13
Septrin prophylaxis of immunization reactions, 339
Serratia marcescens, 195
Serum immune globulin, human, 193
  enriched, 194
Serum thymic factors (FTS), 246, 247, 249, 251, 267, 271
Severe combined immunodeficiency (SCID), 9
  ADA deficiency. See Adenosine deaminase deficiency in SCID
  α_1-antitrypsin deficiency, 68

Severe combined immunodeficiency *(cont.)*
   and bare lymphocyte syndrome, 67; *see also* Bare lymphocyte syndrome
   B-cell differentiation and function, 68
   BMT, 21–23, 65, 101
   calcium transport defects, 355
   vs CGD, 301
   chimerism, 349
   classification, 353–354
   clinical features, 65–66, 256
   as consequence of lymphocyte membrane abnormalities, 67–68
   diagnosis and classification, 65–71
   enteric viruses, 65
   enzyme replacement, 357
   etiology, multiple, 311
   fetal thymus and liver transplants, 139–141
   graft resistance, 135
   GVHD, 66, 68
   with Igs, 67
   immunologic characteristics, 256
   interferonopathy, 109–113
      anti-IFN antibody and lymphoblastogenesis, 110–111
   laboratory features, 66–67
   lymph node biopsy, 349
   lymphocytes
      large granular, 101–104
      membrane markers, 190–191
      phenotyping, 102
   membrane transport disturbance, 307
   monoclonal antibodies OKT and VEP, 102
   in Navajo children, 109, 110, 112
   and neoplasia, 163
   NK cells, 107–108, 113
      case reports, 101
      predominance, 101–104
      parallel tubular arrays, 112–113
   with paraproteinemia, 67
   pathogenesis, 308
   peripheral blood, 348
   Pneumocystis carinii, 65
   PNP and ADA testing, 349, 351–352
   prenatal diagnosis, 70, 121–123, 125–127
   prenatal infection, 307
   with proliferative abnormality of the RES, 67
   vs severe pure T-cell defects, 281, 282
   T cells
      differentiation and abnormalities, 68–70
      subsets, 107–108
   thymus, abnormal
      development, 248–250
      epithelial surface antigen expression, 255, 257, 258
   treatment
      IgA, secretory, oral administration, 229–234
      TP-5, 267–271, 273–275
      with IV pH 4.0 gammaglobulin, 201–203
   see also Agammaglobulinemia, Hypogammaglobulinemia
Severe pure T-cell defects
   immunologic reconstitution with BMT and thymic hormones, 281–284
   vs. SCID, 281, 282
   TP-5 therapy, 281, 282
   see also Nezelof syndrome (immunodeficiency with normal serum Igs)
Short-limbed dwarfism, 67, 355
Single linkage clustering algorithm, 336, 338
Skeletal changes in immunodeficiency, 307–308
   bony abnormalities in SCID with ADA deficiency, 74
   cartilage hair hypoplasia, 261, 308
Skin biopsy, 349
Smallpox vaccine, reaction in immunodeficiency, 339
Soluble immune suppressor supernatant (SISS), 183–184
Soybean lectin. *See* Lectin(s)
Splenomegaly, 241
Staphylococcus aureus, 195, 196, 310
Stem cells, hematopoietic, 245, 345
Superoxide dismutase (SOD), 300, 302, 304–305
Sweden
   IgA deficiency, selective, 174
   primary immunodeficiency syndrome registry, 162
Syndrome(s)
   acquired immunodeficiency (AIDS), 355
   bare lymphocyte. *See* Bare lymphocyte syndrome
   Bloom, 354
   Chédiak-Higashi, 103, 308, 359
      BMT in, 333
   DiGeorge. *See* DiGeorge syndrome
   Down, 325–326, 354
   familial reticuloendotheliosis, 317–318
   hyper-IgE. *See* Hyper-IgE (Job) syndrome
   Letterer-Siwe, 65, 67
   Nezelof. *See* Nezelof syndrome
   Omenn, 65, 67
   Wiskott-Aldrich. *See* Wiskott-Aldrich syndrome
Systemic lupus erythematosus, 19, 356

T cell(s)
   in antibody production in peripheral blood in response to immunization, 49
   antigenic moieties recognized by, 9–11
   in bare lymphocyte syndrome, 84–85; *see also* Bare lymphocyte syndrome
   and B cells, 12, 26–28
      defective control of differentiation in defective humoral immunity, 155, 158
   controlling isotype switching, 33
   development and differentiation, 9, 289, 290
      functional studies, 291–293
      model, 70
      subset phenotypes, 289
      self-recognition, 11–13
      self + X cf. allo + X recognition structure, 145
   in Down syndrome, 325–326
   Fc receptors, 15, 18
   growth factor, 13, 32, 34–35, 133, 134, 247, 248
   helper
      allelic exclusion at receptor level, 11–12
      factor (ThF120), OA-induced, and combined immunodeficiency, 51–53, 93–95
      –macrophage interaction in combined immunodeficiency, 94
      mechanisms of antigen recognition, 11
   leukemia. *See* Leukemia, T-cell
   newborns, 299–305
   OKT4:T8 ratio, 189–190
      and TP-5 therapy, 270
   in primary immunodeficiency, 187–191
   production of anti-mannan antibodies by peripheral blood lymphocytes, 43
   subsets, 9, 10, 289
      and activation markers, 12–13
      in DiGeorge syndrome, 107–108
      in SCID, 68–70, 107–108
   suppressor
      abnormalities in PNP deficiency, 78–79
      circuit in man, 15–20
      defect in hyper-IgE (Job) syndrome, 57–60
      excessive activity in defective humoral immunity, 158
      precursor (Ts_p), 15, 17–18
      $T\mu\gamma^-$, 15–16, 18
      TSE factor preparation, 16, 18
      TSI cells, 16–19
   tests for assessing immunity, 348
   see also B cells, Lymphocyte(s)
Tests for assessing immunity, 346–348
Tetanus toxoid, 10–11, 41, 47
Theophylline, 16, 17, 68, 69
Thrombocytopenic purpura, idiopathic, 196
Thymic factors, 357
   humoral, 267
      and cAMP, 246
      GVH, 246
   serum (FTS), 246, 247, 249, 251, 267, 271
Thymic hormones, 246–247, 251–252
   and GVHD, 284
   monoclonal antibodies vs , 248
   therapeutic considerations, 250–251
   see also specific hormones
Thymoma, 165
   basophil and eosinophil deficiency, 331
   treatment with IV pH 4.0 gammaglobulin, 201–203
Thymopoietin, 246, 255, 256, 257
Thymopoietin pentapeptide (TP-5)
   in severe pure T-cell defects, 281–282
   synthetic, 267–271
   in T-cell immune deficiency, 273–275
   vs Tpl, 273, 275
Thymosin(s), 68, 69, 246, 247, 249, 250, 256–258
   fraction 5, 267, 271
   therapy of CID, 105–106
Thymostimulin, 267, 271
Thymulin, 246–247, 251
Thymus
   abnormal development, 248–250
   epithelial surface antigen expression, 255–258

Thymus *(continued)*
  biopsy, 349
  chemically defined thymus peptides, 246
  differentiation functions of epithelium, 245–248
  Down syndrome, 326
  grafts, 250
  hormones. *See* Thymic hormones
  maturation signals, 247
  and MHC, 245, 247
  Nezelof syndrome, 255, 257, 258
  T-cell growth factors, 247–248
  T-cell precursor migration to, 245–246
  therapeutic considerations, 250–251
  Thy1 antigen, 255–256
  transferrin receptors, 257
  transplantation. *See* Fetal thymus transplantation
Transcobalamin II deficiency, 73, 157, 158, 308–309
Transferrin receptors, thymus, 257

Transfusion
  enzyme replacement, in ADA deficiency, 117
  plasma, antibody deficiency syndromes, 218

United States
  IgA deficiency, selective, 174
  primary immunodeficiency syndrome registry, 162

Vaccination, 347
  reaction in immunodeficiency, 339–340
Ventriculoseptal defect, 277
Virus(es), 355
  Abelson, 177
  A/X31 influenza, 42–44, 90
  CMV, 198, 218, 355
  Coxsackie, 87
  ECHO, 193, 217, 220, 355
    -5, 236
    -8, encephalitis, 223, 226
  enteric, and SCID, 65
  Epstein-Barr. *See* Epstein-Barr virus
  HTLV, 34
  polio-, 217, 229–236
  retro-, new type C, and T-cell leukemia, 34
  rota-, infection, 234
  vesicular stomatitis, 109, 355
Vitamin B_{12}, 308–309, 357
Vitiligo, 277, 278
VP 16-213, 317, 318, 333

WISH cell system, 109
Wiskott-Aldrich syndrome, 97–98, 129, 154
  and neoplasia, 163
  peripheral blood, 348
  T cells and T-cell subsets, 187–191
  TP-5 therapy, 267–271

Zinc, 251, 309, 311

BOOKS PUBLISHED BY ALAN R. LISS, INC.
FOR THE MARCH OF DIMES BIRTH DEFECTS FOUNDATION

BIRTH DEFECTS: ORIGINAL ARTICLE SERIES

1975 — Volume XI

No. 7 **Morphogenesis and Malformation of Face and Brain,** Daniel Bergsma and Jan Langman, *Editors*

1976 — Volume XII

No. 1 **Cancer and Genetics,** Daniel Bergsma, R. Neil Schimke, Robert L. Summitt, and David J. Harris, *Editors*

No. 3 **The Eye and Inborn Errors of Metabolism,** Daniel Bergsma, Anthony J. Bron, and Edward Cotlier, *Editors*

No. 4 **Developmental Disabilities: Psychologic and Social Implications,** Daniel Bergsma and Ann E. Pulver, *Editors*

No. 5 **Cytogenetics, Environment and Malformation Syndromes,** Daniel Bergsma and R. Neil Schimke, *Editors*

No. 6 **Growth Problems and Clinical Advances,** Daniel Bergsma and R. Neil Schimke, *Editors*

No. 8 **Iron Metabolism and Thalassemia,** Daniel Bergsma, Anthony Cerami, Charles M. Peterson, and Joseph H. Graziano, *Editors*

1977 — Volume XIII

No. 1 **Morphogenesis and Malformation of the Limb,** Daniel Bergsma and Widukind Lenz, *Editors*

No. 2 **Morphogenesis and Malformation of the Genital System,** Richard J. Blandau and Daniel Bergsma, *Editors*

No. 3 **Annual Review of Birth Defects, 1976,** Daniel Bergsma and R. Brian Lowry, *Editors* Proceedings of the 1976 Vancouver Birth Defects Conference. Published in 4 volumes:
  3A **Numerical Taxonomy of Birth Defects** *and* **Polygenic Disorders**
  3B **New Syndromes**
  3C **Natural History of Specific Birth Defects**
  3D **Embyology and Pathogenesis** *and* **Prenatal Diagnosis**

No. 5 **Urinary System Malformations in Children,** Daniel Bergsma and John W. Duckett, *Editors*

No. 6 **Trends and Teaching in Clinical Genetics,** Daniel Bergsma, Frederick Hecht, Gerald H. Prescott, and Joan H. Marks, *Editors*

1978 — Volume XIV

No. 1 **Genetic Effects on Aging,** Daniel Bergsma and David E. Harrison, *Editors*

No. 2 **The Molecular Basis of Cell-Cell Interactions,** Richard A. Lerner and Daniel Bergsma, *Editors*

No. 3 **The Genetics of Hand Malformations,** *by* Samia A. Temtamy and Victor A. McKusick

No. 5 **Neurochemical and Immunologic Components in Schizophrenia,** Daniel Bergsma and Allan L. Goldstein, *Editors*

No. 6 **Annual Review of Birth Defects, 1977,** Robert L. Summitt and Daniel Bergsma, *Editors*. Proceedings of the 1977 Memphis Birth Defects Conference. Published in 3 volumes:
  6A **Cell Surface Factors, Immune Deficiencies. Twin Studies**
  6B **Recent Advances** *and* **New Syndromes**
  6C **Sex Differentiation** *and* **Chromosomal Abnormalities**

No. 7 **Morphogenesis and Malformation of the Cardiovascular System,** Glenn C. Rosenquist and Daniel Bergsma, *Editors*

1979 — Volume XV

No. 1 **Sex Chromosome Aneuploidy: Prospective Studies on Children,** Arthur Robinson, Herbert A. Lubs, and Daniel Bergsma, *Editors*

No. 2 **Genetic Counseling: Facts, Values, and Norms,** Alexander M. Capron, Marc Lappe, Robert F. Murray, Jr., Tabitha M. Powledge, Sumner B. Twiss, and Daniel Bergsma, *Editors*

No. 3 **Recent Advances in the Developmental Biology of Central Nervous System Malformations,** Ntinos C. Myrianthopoulos and Daniel Bergsma, *Editors*

No. 4 **Continuous Transcutaneous Blood Gas Monitoring,** A. Huch, R. Huch, and J. Lucey, *Editors*

No. 5 **Annual Review of Birth Defects, 1978,** Proceedings of the 1978 San Francisco Birth Defects Conference. Published in 3 volumes:

    5A **Diagnostic Approaches to the Malformed Fetus, Abortus, Stillborn, and Deceased Newborn,** Mitchell S. Golbus and Bryan D. Hall, *Editors*

    5B **Penetrance and Variability in Malformation Syndromes,** James J. O'Donnell and Bryan D. Hall, *Editors*

    5C **Risk, Communication, and Decision Making in Genetic Counseling,** Charles J. Epstein, Cynthia J.R. Curry, Seymour Packman, Sanford Sherman, and Bryan D. Hall, *Editors*

No. 6 **Dermatoglyphics—Fifty Years Later,** Wladimir Wertelecki and Chris C. Plato, *Editors*

No. 7 **Newborn Behavioral Organization: Nursing Research and Implications,** Gene Cranston Anderson and Beverly Raff, *Editors*

No. 8 **Developmental Aspects of Craniofacial Dysmorphology,** Michael Melnick and Ronald Jorgenson, *Editors*

No. 9 **External Ear Malformations: Epidemiology, Genetics, and Natural History,** *by* Michael Melnick and Ntinos C. Myrianthopoulos

1980 — Volume XVI

No. 1 **Enzyme Therapy in Genetic Diseases: 2,** Robert J. Desnick, *Editor*

No. 2 **In Vitro Epithelia and Birth Defects,** B. Shannon Danes, *Editor*

No. 3 **Diet in Pregnancy: A Randomized Controlled Trial of Nutritional Supplements,** *by* David Rush, Zena Stein, and Mervyn Susser

No. 4 **Morphogenesis and Malformation of the Ear,** Robert J. Gorlin, *Editor*

No. 5 **Dentistry in the Interdisciplinary Treatment of Genetic Diseases,** Carlos F. Salinas and Ronald J. Jorgenson, *Editors*

No. 7 **Genetic and Environmental Hearing Loss: Syndromic and Nonsyndromic,** L. Stefan Levin and Connie H. Knight, *Editors*

1981 — Volume XVII

No. 1 **Annual Review of Birth Defects, 1980, The Fetus and the Newborn,** Arthur D. Bloom and L. Stanley James, *Editors*

No. 2 **Morphogenesis and Malformation of the Skin,** Richard J. Blandau, *Editor*

No. 3 **Pregnancy and Childbearing During Adolescence: Research Priorities for the 1980s,** Elizabeth R. McAnarney and Gabriel Stickle, *Editors*

No. 4 **Reproductive Pasts, Reproductive Futures: Genetic Counseling and Its Effectiveness,** James R. Sorenson, Judith P. Swazey, and Norman A. Scotch

No. 6 **Perinatal Parental Behavior: Nursing Research and Implications for Newborn Health,** Regina Placzek Lederman, *Conference Coordinator–Consulting Editor,* and Beverly S. Raff, *Editor*